Joseph Babinski

Joseph Babinski

A Biography

JACQUES PHILIPPON, MD
JACQUES POIRIER, MD, PHD

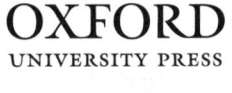
UNIVERSITY PRESS

2009

OXFORD
UNIVERSITY PRESS

Oxford University Press, Inc., publishes works that further
Oxford University's objective of excellence
in research, scholarship, and education.

Oxford New York
Auckland Cape Town Dar es Salaam Hong Kong Karachi
Kuala Lumpur Madrid Melbourne Mexico City Nairobi
New Delhi Shanghai Taipei Toronto

With offices in
Argentina Austria Brazil Chile Czech Republic France Greece
Guatemala Hungary Italy Japan Poland Portugal Singapore
South Korea Switzerland Thailand Turkey Ukraine Vietnam

Copyright © 2009 by Oxford University Press, Inc.

Published by Oxford University Press, Inc.
198 Madison Avenue, New York, New York 10016
www.oup.com

Oxford is a registered trademark of Oxford University Press

All rights reserved. No part of this publication may be reproduced,
stored in a retrieval system, or transmitted, in any form or by any means,
electronic, mechanical, photocopying, recording, or otherwise,
without the prior permission of Oxford University Press.

Library of Congress Cataloging-in-Publication Data
Philippon, Jacques.
Joseph Babinski : a biography / Jacques Philippon, Jacques Poirier.
p. ; cm.
Includes bibliographical references and index.
ISBN: 978-0-19-536975-5
1. Babinski, J. (Joseph), 1857–1932. 2. Neurologists—France—Biography
I. Poirier, Jacques, 1937- II. Title. [DNLM: 1. Babinski, J. (Joseph),
1857–1932. 2. Neurology—France—Biography.
3. Neurology—history—France. WZ 100 P552j 2008]
RC339.52.B32P45 2008
616.80092—dc22 [B]   2008003646

1 3 5 7 9 8 6 4 2
Printed in the United States of America
on acid-free paper

Acknowledgments

This volume could not have been completed without the friendly help of numerous individuals, whom we thank warmly: Professor Jean-François Bernaudin at Paris-6 University; Professor Michel Bonduelle Honorary Professor of Neurology at the Saint Joseph Hospital; General Jean Briolle, director of the Archives of the French Army Health Service, Paris; Dr. Hubert Déchy former chief-resident at the Salpêtrière Hospital; Mr. Albert Gargar, curator of the Archives of the French Army Health Service, Paris; Agnès Gomez, archivist of the Pontoise bishopric; Dr. Pierre Konopka, president of the Association of French physicians of Polish origin; Stéphane Kraxner, curator of the Archives of the Pasteur Institute, Paris; Lucyna Haaso-Basta and Malgorzata Paluch, for the French translations of Polish sources; Véronique Leroux-Hugon, chief librarian, Charcot Library, Salpêtrière Hospital, Paris; Marie-Noëlle Maisonneuve, chief librarian, École des mines de Paris; Evelyne Maury, curator of the archives of the Collège de France, Paris; Jean-François Minot, curator at the Musée de l'Assistance publique, Paris; Kazimierz Molenda, president of the Alumni Association of the Polish School in Paris; Annick Perrot, curator of the Pasteur Museum, Paris; Professor Jean-Paul Poirier, member of the Academy of Sciences, for the French translation of German, Portuguese, Swedish, and Lithuanian sources; Dr. Diana Rivas and Mariella Aleman, for the photographs of the Habich Monument in Lima, Peru; the staff and employees of the Bibliothèque nationale de France, the Archives nationales, the archives of the Academy of Sciences, the library of the Academy of Medicine, the archives of the Assistance publique–Hôpitaux de Paris, and the Paris Opera; and all the colleagues who have discussed Babinski's work with us.

We gratefully acknowledge in particular Natalie Philippon-Tulloch for her kind supervision of our English-language writing and for her numerous and fruitful suggestions.

Preface

Sir Percival Bailey once wrote: "There is no complete biography of Babinski in any language and there is no complete compendium of his work in English.... The literature on the life and works of Babinski in the United States is sparse and scattered."[1] Our ambition is to fill this gap.

We first heard of Joseph Babinski as young medical students, initially through learning about the Babinski sign and later when we encountered the particular diagnostic method that he held so dear. We soon realised that, while he was perhaps most known for the 'sign', it was indeed his strict diagnostic method and adherence to facts which we would come to appreciate the most. Even if the tools for neurological diagnosis have dramatically changed since Babinski's time, especially with the fantastic breakthroughs in neuroimagery, neurobiology, and neurogenetics, the need to ensure a rational thought process in diagnosis and therapeutics remains as crucial as ever.

Taking up the challenge of revisiting Joseph Babinski and his work by no means implies a desire to question his undisputed achievements, diminish other giants of medicine, or rewrite the history of neurology. Rather, this is an adventure in which Babinski's own methodology will be applied to a new look at his work, avoiding the temptation to join the ranks of his unconditional admirers and panegyrists. We explore sources in forgotten archives and library collections, leading us to territory above and beyond the traditional

---

[1] P. J. Bailey, "Joseph Babinski (1857–1932): The Man and His Works," *World Neurology* 2, 2 (1961): 134–140.

view of the man. Above all, we intend to accept nothing as true that cannot be demonstrated. As Babinski himself often said, *observatio summa lex*.

There is undoubtedly an aura around Babinski's name, amplified by his family's fame. His father, Aleksander, was a Polish revolutionary committed to the Paris Commune, and his brother, Henri, was a famous gastronome, better known under the pseudonym Ali-Bab. Myth and reality merge, contributing to a cult following. While Babinski is often associated with Jean-Martin Charcot, the two men were in reality quite different. Whereas Charcot tended to abuse his professional power and gradually involved himself and others in pseudoscientific investigations (notably in regard to hysteria), Babinski was unflinching in his quest for documented and demonstrable conclusions.

Morally unassailable, without the slightest hint of personal ambition or vanity, Babinski embodied the best qualities of Charcot while avoiding his negative characteristics, notably as a result of his having been obliged to renounce any aspirations to a university career after his undeserved failure in the competitive examination (*agrégation*) of 1892. Many of his biographers agree that because he was not overburdened with teaching and administrative duties, he had more time for his research (though this overlooks those who were able to produce remarkable bodies of work despite their professorial responsibilities, such as Jules Dejerine and Pierre Marie). Babinski was a pure clinician in every sense of the term, and even if he was not the father of a true neurological school, he had many students and associates, all enthusiastic admirers, who helped to keep his work alive.

To be fully appreciated, Babinski's achievements must be placed within the context of his time and place. In many aspects he was the scientific heir of Charcot, a fact that he never denied. At the same time he felt the need to make a break with the Salpêtrière school's paradigm: a nonobjective neurology concentrated mainly on hysteria. His desire to create a new approach to neurology based upon objective signs is certainly the unifying thread of his scientific work. By refining neurological semiology, Babinski established his place in the scientific community of his era, and his work has stood the test of time: it would be hard to find many members of the contemporary health community who would not recognize the Babinski sign. No doubt the most important progress in medicine has been made through basic research, but this fact in no way lessens the central role of the clinician in patient treatment, which remains the fundamental purpose of medicine. Babinski's contribution to the development of this role is reflected in the fact that, a hundred years after his discovery of the reflex that now bears his name, that name now graces an important new building at the Salpêtrière that houses all the specialities he dealt with during his professional life.

If Joseph Babinski was neither a genius nor a god, he demonstrated throughout his professional career the talents of an exceptional clinician, retaining at the same time an rigorous intellectual honesty. He was, finally, a man: "Just a man, as every man, equal to all and better than none."[2]

To complement our spheres of competence, we have called in for three chapters a pair of colleagues more specialized than ourselves. 15, on hysteria versus pithiatism, has been written by Christian Derouesné, professor emeritus at the University of Paris VI and honorary head of the 3rd neurological department at the Salpêtrière Hospital, while chapter 11, on reflexes and the Babinski sign, and chapter 12, on cerebellar and vestibular semiology, was a collaborative effort with Philippe Ricou, former chief resident at the Chair for the study of diseases of the nervous system and *médecin des hôpitaux*.

We wish also to acknowledge the extensive background material found in Christopher Goetz, Michel Bonduelle, and Toby Gelfand, *Charcot: Constructing Neurology* (Oxford University Press, 1995), which is a basic reference for all those interested in this period of French medical history.

Jacques Philippon
Jacques Poirier

---

[2] Jean-Paul Sartre, *Les mots* (Paris: Gallimard, Collection Folio, 1964), 214.

Foreword

Among neurologists, the *Babinski sign* is the most widely appreciated and globally entrenched eponym in our field. In 1896, Joseph Babinski described this primitive reflex in a modest, 28-line communication. This young physician was a student of the recently deceased and highly celebrated French neurologist, Jean-Martin Charcot. Having lived in the halo of his mentor while Charcot was alive, Babinski struggled to emerge from the shadow of his powerful teacher throughout his career. The delicate balance of deference to his teacher's heritage and a clear understanding of the need for growth and independence likewise marked the careers of a full generation of French neurologists. Babinski's humble communication remained only modestly recognized for many years, but, even before international acknowledgment, the contribution was an important symbolic step for Babinski and his generation of post-Charcot French neurologists.

Babinski painstakingly examined patients with neurological diseases, and the Babinski sign, among other examination techniques and phenomena, helped to codify the method of the neurological examination that persists today as the anchor of neurological practice worldwide. While Charcot was pivotal in categorizing neurological diagnoses and teaching how to interview patients, Babinski and the neurologists of his generation built the neurological examination as it is today. In this way, acknowledging the heritage of Charcot, but entering a field untouched by his mentor, Babinski and his generation of younger neurologists carried the Charcot heritage into the twentieth century. In their successes and failures, this generation collaborated and competed for recognition that would never be as focused or monolithic as they had witnessed during their own training with the all-powerful Charcot.

Joseph Babinski: A Biography traces the period and life of this Frenchman of Polish descent whose neurological career and private life have been sparsely studied in spite of the immediate recognition of his name in medicine. The authors, Jacques Philippon and Jacques Poirier, are highly successful French neuroscientists, widely published in the scientific arenas of neurology and neurosurgery. Both are familiar with the modern Salpêtrière-La Pitié complex that historically bridges Babinski's career. Having spent many long sojourns studying the archives of the Bibliothèque Charcot, I am personally familiar with the dedicated and thorough research style of both authors. The fruit of their study is a highly readable and comprehensive evaluation of an important neurologist's career. The authors anchor their biography in extensive historical documentation based on primary source materials and, at the same time, provide interpretive reflections on the impact of Babinski on modern neurological thinking.

Both the man and period are fairly and subtly treated. Prior biographical studies were composed by authors who knew Babinski as a friend or colleague, but the close proximity in relationship and time make many of these sources sugary and myopic. Enough time has passed and sufficient primary documents remain in archival sources to allow a modern and carefully objective evaluation of the Babinski legacy. The authors have enriched their text with many pictures, and as a researcher who has spent long hours in search of iconography, I laud the quality and number of the photographs and diagrams collected.

Neurologists, neurosurgeons, neuroscientists, and the larger medical field will find this book of immediate relevance to their appreciation of a man whose name is remarkably familiar but whose life and career have never been extensively studied. The themes of power struggles and a mentor's double-edged gift of support will resonate to all physicians who owe their first career chances to a caring mentor and then were forced to extricate themselves to define their own path. Beyond a strictly medical audience, students of the late nineteenth and early twentieth centuries will appreciate the well-developed themes of French society's emergence from the comfort of the *fin-de-siècle* to the modern era. This evolution is especially pertinent in light of the duality of the French culture and its capacity to integrate immigrants into the social fabric.

In arrangement and organization, this biography is not strictly chronological, but, instead, deals with pivotal themes. The introductory and final two chapters are extremely useful for placing Babinski in the context of his time and for introducing the reader to the cast of characters who were his allies and foes. Neuroscientists will be naturally most interested in the scientific sections that populate the middle chapters of the book. These essays cover Babinski's publications, the celebrated Babinski sign, his work on the cerebellum, and his participation in the evolution of neurosurgery as a specialty. Readers with more interest in social and medical-political movements will find the chapters on the history of competitive examinations for faculty posts in the French medical hierarchy, Babinski's struggle to develop a neurological service outside the Salpêtrière, and his relationship with the powerful Anatomical Society particularly important to an understanding of academic career development. Throughout the book and throughout Babinski's life, the undercurrent influence of Charcot is unceasingly present, and whereas Babinski spent most of his career in safer territories of neurology untouched by his mentor, the chapter late in the book on pithiatism brings all readers to a vivid consciousness of the consequences of confronting one's teacher directly. With this thematic organization, each chapter is largely an independent essay that covers one aspect of a multidimensional personality. The synthesized whole provides the reader with a breadth and context to understand Babinski in a way that has not been provided before.

Christopher G. Goetz, MD
Chicago, IL, USA

Contents

1	Babinski's Life and Times	3
2	A Complex and Captivating Personality	23
3	The Babinskis and Their Polish Roots	53
4	The Babinski Circle	85
5	The Competitive Examinations	97
6	His Revered Teachers	115
7	Babinski and the Anatomical Society	133
8	Babinski, Head of a Department at La Pitié	151
9	The Affectionate Admiration of His Students	167
10	The Babinski Papers	187
11	The Reflexes and the Sign *Written in collaboration with Philippe Ricou*	217
12	Cerebellar and Vestibular Symptomatology *Written in collaboration with Philippe Ricou*	249
13	Babinski and the Birth of French Neurosurgery	265
14	Babinski as Therapist	283
15	Pithiatism Versus Hysteria *by Christian Derouesné*	297
16	Neurology in the Time of Babinski	321
17	Babinski's Public Image	345
	Bibliography	365
	Index	429

Joseph Babinski

··· *one* ···

Babinski's Life and Times

Babinski's life spanned a period of great change in France, both in science and in society. Although he left few personal observations, a rapid glance at what was going on in the world around him at various stages in his career may shed some light on why he became so committed to proven facts as opposed to suppositions.

Babinski's Youth (1857–1875)

Personal Landmarks

Joseph Babinski's parents, Aleksander Babinski (1823–1899) and Henryeta Weren (1819–1897), were born and married in Poland, coming to France shortly after the Polish revolution of 1848 (see chapter 3). The couple gave birth to two children, Henri in 1855 and Joseph in 1857, both born in Paris in their parents' apartment at 142 boulevard du Montparnasse.[1]

---

[1] A legend nourished by some authors set his birth in Peru—for example, in J. J. Lhermitte's eulogy of Babinski, published in *Bull Acad Nat Méd* 1957 (32–33): 727–740, and J. M. Cuba, "Influencia de la medicina francesa en la medecina peruana" [Influence of French medicine on Peruvian medicine], *Revista peruana de Neurologia*, 2002 (8): 31–40. This supposition is totally refuted by civil status documents and the testimony of his friends (A. Tournay, "Babinski dans la vie" [Babinski in everyday life], *La Presse Médicale* 1958 (66): 1485–1489). The building on Montparnasse in which they were born was demolished; the one presently at that address was constructed in 1892. The Babinski family moved in 1871 to 153 boulevard Montparnasse and later to 70 bis then 54, rue

Though Aleksander found work as a municipal employee of the city of Paris, their financial situation at the beginning was rather difficult, though it improved when he obtained a position as surveyor-engineer. A new rebellion in Poland called him back to Warsaw in 1863 and he left behind his wife and two young children. The boys were both enrolled in the Polish School, where they would stay till 1870, when they entered the Lycée Descartes (previously called the Lycée Impérial Louis-le-Grand), from which Joseph received his baccalaureate in 1875.[2]

The Political Situation

When Aleksander and Henryeta arrived in Paris, France was under Napoleon III's authoritarian government, known as the Second Empire. Civil rights were restricted, and an attempt by the Italian revolutionary Felice Orsini (1819–1858) to assassinate the emperor in 1858 led to a general security law that increased the pressure on individual liberties, authorizing, for example, the deportation of condemned political activists.

Although political expression was extremely restricted, efforts were made to liberalize commerce and encourage free enterprise, which helped to create a flourishing economy, although it left a great part of the working class behind. After 1860, when Napoleon III gave limited powers to the Chamber of Deputies, some progress was also made in increasing political liberties. The first decisions dealt with initial steps toward workers' emancipation and the emergence of a relatively free press. A strong republican opposition found its voice in the 1869 general election, and strikes became more and more frequent in 1869–70.

To some extent, the basic class conflicts that had led to the French Revolution ninety years before had not yet been resolved, and this produced increasing social conflict within a general European climate of revolution. Despite the fact that a true parliamentary regime was introduced after the plebiscite of 1870, discontent was rampant. This was especially true among the working class, owing to the widening gap between rich and poor.

The Franco-Prussian War, which started in July 1870, turned out disastrously, with the capture of Napoleon III in the Battle of Sedan on September 2

Bonaparte (Archives of the Préfecture de Police of Paris) and finally to 170 bis boulevard Haussmann.

[2] Letter from the headmaster of the lycée to the chief education officer in October 1870: "I have learned of Mr. Babinski's request; taking into account the information I have on his character and honorableness, I recommend strongly that his two sons be exempted from fees."

marking the end of the empire. A republic was proclaimed on September 4, but the war itself had not ended. Paris was under siege for months, and the repercussions of the defeat and the extremely difficult economic conditions caused by food and fuel shortages exacerbated a widespread perception of government incompetence.[3] Nevertheless, the citizens of Paris were determined to resist, and by January 1871, when an armistice was signed, a civil militia, called the National Guard, had been created to defend Paris against a Prussian attack and to support the Republic, which was menaced by a possible royalist restoration. Numerous incidents fired the animosity between the newly official government and the Central Committee of the National Guard, leading Paris to rebel against the government, the members of which were forced to retreat from Paris to Versailles in November 1870. For a two-month period in mid-1871, the Central Committee, or "Communal Council," became the administration in Paris; it included a high proportion of skilled workers and intellectuals, such as journalists and doctors. The painter Gustave Courbet (1819–1877) was responsible for culture; Camille Pissaro (1830–1903) and Arthur Rimbaud (1854–1991) were active propagandists. Strong support also came from the foreign community of political refugees in Paris. This pivotal period in the history of France is known as the Paris Commune, recalling the events of 1792, when power was deemed to come from the people.[4]

The possible role of Aleksander, Joseph's father, in the events leading up to the Paris Commune will be discussed in chapter 3. But it is certain that several Polish immigrants were centrally involved, such as Jaroslav Dombrowski (1836–1871), a fervent nationalist, who became one of the leading generals of the Commune army.

Several positive social measures were adopted, some reflecting the general philosophy of the movement (for instance, separation of church and state, the vote for women), and others very specific, such as the abolition of night work in Parisian bakeries.

The official, conservative government could not tolerate this rebellion, which threatened the central power. In March 1871, the army began to attack the insurgents, who had set up a series of barricades behind which the National Guard volunteers gathered with their limited arms. They were

---

[3] Living conditions were so extreme that by December 1870, Parisians had sacrificed the animals in the zoo, and the trees in public areas were totally destroyed, including, in January 1871, those on the Champs Elysées (J. Willms, *Paris, Capital of Europe, from the Revolution to the Belle Époque* [New York: Holmes and Meier, 1997], 309).
[4] The basic idea of the Paris Commune was to create a decentralized power, nonviolent and antiauthoritarian, that would federate cooperative municipalities (*communes*) in which private property would be permitted only if not used to exploit the people.

defeated after two months of conflict, and the army entered Paris at the end of May. Repression was ferocious, culminating in the "Bloody Week" (May 22–28), with the last resistance taking place in the Père Lachaise cemetery. The number of Parisians who died in fighting or were executed is estimated at between 20,000 and 30,000, out of a total population of 1.8 million. These few months left a lasting impression on Joseph Babinski, who was convinced that the authorities, and especially Adolphe Thiers, had gone much too far in their retaliation.

Medicine and Science at That Time

In medicine and science, two great names marked this period in France. Claude Bernard (1813–1878), the founder of experimental medicine, was named professor at the Collège de France in 1855; four years earlier, his discovery of the vasomotor nerves had allowed him to demonstrate the role of sympathetic nerves in controlling blood flow. In 1865, he published his monumental work *Introduction to the Study of Experimental Medicine*. Louis Pasteur (1822–1895) showed that microorganisms were responsible for the process of fermentation, and disproved the theory of spontaneous generation. Pasteur's discoveries inspired many scientists, including the Englishman Joseph Lister (1827–1912), who introduced phenol as a disinfectant in surgery, radically improving the survival rate. Around the same time, the German Rudolph Virchow (1821–1902) published his *Cellular Pathology*.

In basic sciences, two new principles dramatically changed humankind's perception of itself: in 1859, Charles Darwin (1809–1882) published his fundamental work *The Origin of Species*, and in 1865 the Austrian monk Gregor Mendel (1822–1884) announced the results of his experiments on hybridization in peas, shedding much light on heredity.

Even if neurology was not yet considered as an independent field, this period also saw important progress in the understanding of the nervous system. Pierre Paul Broca (1824–1880) published a paper in 1861 in which he claimed that the inferior frontal gyrus of the left hemisphere was more developed than that on the right side and was the center for articulate speech. A new step in cerebral localization came in 1864 when the physician Hughlings Jackson (1835–1911), while studying cases of epilepsy at the London Hospital, concluded that movements were represented or coordinated in certain special regions of the cerebral cortex.

In France, two years before Babinski's birth, Guillaume Duchenne (1806–1875), who had begun his career as a modest general practitioner in Boulogne and studied electrotherapy and neurology almost as a hobby, published his pioneer work *De l'électrisation localisée* (Localized faradization). Having access to Jean-Martin Charcot's patients, he described independently from Moritz Heinrich Romberg (1795–1873), whose work he did not know, tabes dorsalis lesions on the dorsal columns of the spinal cord and their syphilitic origin. Charcot (1825–1893) became very enthusiastic about Duchenne's discoveries and, continuing on the same subject, described in 1868 the neurological conditions associated with syphilis and, with Charles Bouchard (1833–1899), the lightning pain observed in tabes dorsalis.

Besides Charcot, Alfred Vulpian (1826–1887) was the other great name at the Salpêtrière at that time. A pupil of Pierre Flourens (1794–1867), he discovered adrenaline in 1856, was made a professor of pathological anatomy in 1866, and worked with Charcot for several years, especially on multiple sclerosis.

Charcot, named an associate professor in 1860, took over one of the departments of general medicine at the Salpêtrière in 1862. In 1865 he was the first to describe amyotrophic lateral sclerosis, and in 1873 he published the first volume of his *Leçons sur les maladies du système nerveux* (Lessons on Diseases of the Nervous System), a series that would continue to appear until 1882.

Various technical developments had a profound influence on the advances in histopathology, including invention of the microtome and new staining methods such as that of Camillo Golgi (1843–1926), who in 1873 used silver chromate to impregnate the nerve elements, allowing the tracing of individual fibers through much of their paths.

Parallel to these important developments in basic science and medicine, journals devoted exclusively to the publication of scientific papers began to appear: in 1868 the *Archives de Physiologie Normale et Pathologique* was founded in Paris by Charles Brown-Séquard (1817–1894), Charcot, and Vulpian. Five years later, Désiré-Magloire Bourneville (1840–1909) created *Le Progrès Médical*, which would be an important avenue of publication for Charcot.

The emergence of neurology as an independent field had significant consequences for the treatment of insanity as it was developing in different centers around the world, especially in Great Britain, Germany and the United States (see chapter 16).

Art and Literature In painting, the mid-nineteenth-century progressive opposition to academic and classicism in art and literature was first expressed by the painter Gustave Courbet—who launched the movement toward realism by his technique and choice of outdoor sites and his refusal in 1855 to bow to the academic conventions of the official "Salon" which refused him the right to exhibit. Courbet was a source of inspiration for Eugène Boudin (1824–1898), with whom he worked in 1859 in—Honfleur, in the Seine valley, and for the young Claude Monet (1840–1926), whose embrace of his new way of painting led to his famous "Impression, Sunrise" (1873), the title of which gave its name to the new school of impressionism. Other painters such as Edouard Manet (1832–1883), though influenced by Monet and the impressionists, remained more individualistic and refused to participate in the impressionists' exhibitions, the first of which, in 1874, was considered a scandal in Parisian intellectual circles.

In literature, the Romantic period gradually faded away. In 1856 Victor Hugo (1802–1885) published *Les contemplations*, a collection of poems that stands as a monument to his lyrical genius. In the year of Babinski's birth appeared *Les fleurs du mal* by Charles Baudelaire (1821–1867) and the famous novel *Madame Bovary* by Gustave Flaubert (1821–1880), torn between Romanticism and disillusioned realism.

In music, Jacques Offenbach (1819–1880) had a series of huge successes with his operettas *La belle Hélène* (1864) and *La vie parisienne* (1866). In 1875 *Carmen*, by Georges Bizet (1838–1875), had its triumphant premiere at the Opéra Comique. In that same year, after thirteen years of construction, opened the new Palais Garnier, perhaps better known as the Paris Opéra. This second home for Joseph Babinski, where he would go so regularly to relax, was part of the large-scale renovation of Paris and its architecture carried out over several decades by Georges Eugène Haussmann (1809–1891).

Education and Beginning of His Career (1875–1901)

A Medical Student Becomes Head of a Department (Fig. 1-1) On November 4, 1875, Joseph Babinski registered for the first time at the Faculté de médecine de Paris, while his brother Henri was admitted to the prestigious École des mines de Paris, where he would receive his diploma in 1878.[5] Joseph attended the Faculté de médecine for four years, finishing in July 1879. He spent the rest of 1879 in a temporary position and participated in the selective hospital competition, obtaining first a position of *externe* (nonresident student) and then that of *interne* (full resident) in 1880. In 1881

---

[5] Proceedings of the Council of the École des Mines, Library of the École des mines de Paris.

I. BABINSKI'S LIFE AND TIMES 9

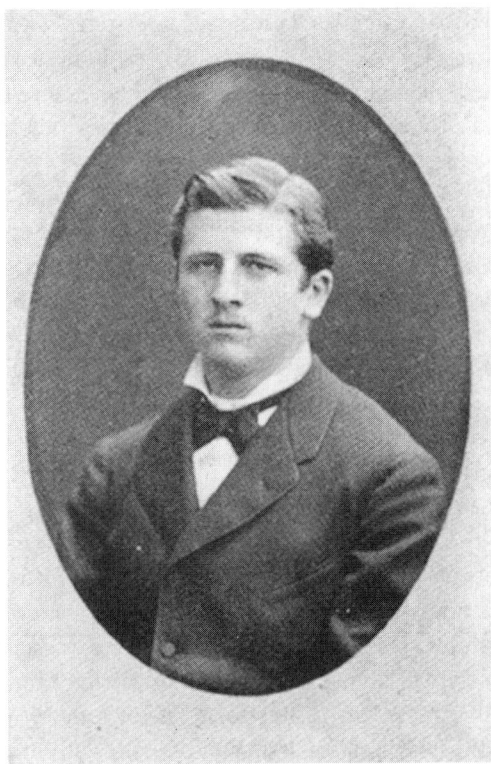

Figure 1-1 Joseph Babinski at the age of eighteen, in 1875. (*Source*: From Albert Charpentier, *Un grand médecin, J. Babinski* [Paris: Typographie François Bernouard, 1934].)

he chose a year of voluntary military service.[6] He was then free to carry on his residency program, working successively under Victor Cornil (1882), Alfred Vulpian (1883), and Jules Bucquoy (1884).[7] The public health administration awarded him a Silver Medal for his exceptional service during the cholera epidemic of 1885, which, although of great concern to the population, had been less lethal than previous ones.[8] He defended his medical thesis,

---

[6] A one-year period of voluntary service allowed medical students to avoid the normal three-year military service. A. Plichet, "Babinski (1857–1932)," in R. Dumesnil and F. Bonnet-Roy, eds., *Les médecins célèbres* (Genève: Éditions d'Art L. Mazenod, 1947), 250–251.

[7] During his residency, his closest friends were Darier, Guignard, Suchard, and Vaquez (see chapter 4).

[8] The mortality rate had reached 22 per 1,000 in 1832 before decreasing in 1854, 1865, and again in 1885, no doubt due to improvements in sanitation.

"Étude anatomique et clinique de la sclérose en plaques" (An anatomical and clinical study of multiple sclerosis), in 1885, receiving a special mention.[9] The same year the Babinski brothers gallicized their first names,[10] Henri (for Henrik) and Joseph (for Josef), and the family moved to better accommodations on rue Bonaparte in the Sixth Arrondissement.

In addition to his work on multiple sclerosis, Joseph Babinski began to document his findings on other subjects and published several papers, mainly on pathological anatomy, first through the Société anatomique (between 1882 and 1886) and then through the Société de biologie, of which he became a full member in 1887.[11]

October 1885 marked a turning point in his career, when he was appointed *chef de clinique* (chief resident) under Charcot and began his clinical neurological work, remaining with Charcot until the latter's death in 1893 (see chapter 5) In accepting this position, he set aside his first interest in pathological anatomy, a field where, except for this unexpected opportunity, he probably would have remained (Fig. 1-2).

The first twenty years of Babinski's medical career, through 1895, were particularly influenced by his mentor, Jean-Martin Charcot, who was then at the peak of his fame. During this period, Babinski was a candidate for the Bureau central of the Paris hospital system, permitting him, if successful, to apply for a position as head of department. After four unsuccessful candidacies, he was admitted in 1890. Unfortunately, his 1892 candidacy for an *agrégation* (associate professorship) met with failure and he would never try again, thus blocking all possibilities of becoming a member of the Faculté de médecine as a professor (see chapter 5). Because of this, Babinski would carry out his medical practice and research in a department of general medicine. In 1894, he took over the direction of a small medical department at the hospital of the Porte d'Aubervilliers before moving the next year to La Pitié, where he would stay until his retirement in 1922 (see chapter 8).

The turn of the century was a crucial period in his work, as it was at this time that he published the first two descriptions of the toe phenomenon (1896 and 1898) and his personal conception of hysteria (1901), marking

---

[9] J. Babinski, *Étude anatomique et clinique sur la sclérose en plaques* [Anatomical and clinical study of multiple sclerosis] (Paris: Masson, 1885). Babinski's degree was registered at the Seine Prefecture on February 22, 1886.

[10] On November 25, a notarized certificate formally changed their first names, and these modifications were later added to their birth certificate on August 28, 1873, in accord with the law of February 12, 1872.

[11] At the meeting on July 9, 1887, Babinski was elected with thirty-three votes out of thirty-six. *Comptes-rendus Hebdomadaires des Séances et Mémoires de la Société de Biologie* 1887 (IV): 460.

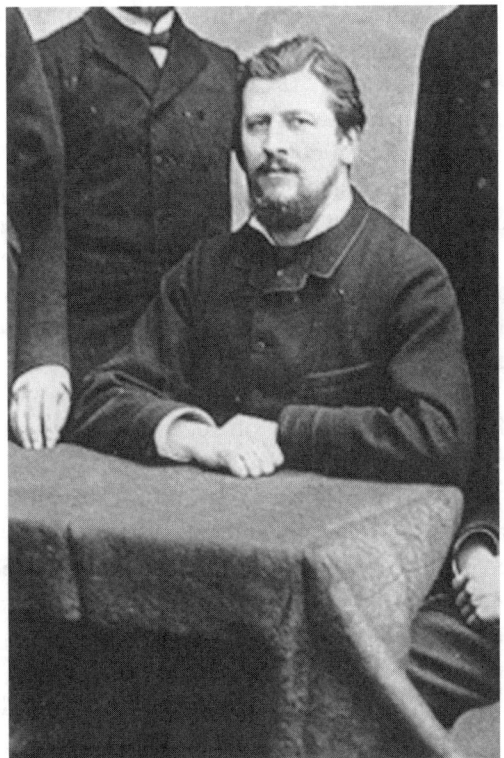

Figure 1-2 Joseph Babinski, chief resident, in 1887. (*Source*: Personal collection, J. Poirier.)

a definitive rupture with Charcot's postulates (see chapter 15). In 1899 he was one of the founding members of the Société de neurologie de Paris, which aimed to bring together physicians working on diseases of the nervous system (see chapter 10). At the same time his personal life was deeply affected in 1897 by his mother's death, in their new apartment on boulevard Haussmann. His father would die two years later, after having suffered for many years from Parkinson's disease.

The Chair for the Study of Diseases of the Nervous System Created in 1882 especially for Charcot, the chair gave him an ideal institutional basis, including a wide and diverse patient population, for his research on nervous system diseases. He soon became intrigued by the study of hysteria and hypnotism, furthered by a four-month visit by Sigmund Freud (1856–1939) to the Salpêtrière in 1885. In a departure from his traditional association of hysteria with female problems, Charcot began also to study traumatic hysteria and hysteria in men, a research interest he would continue working on until 1891. In 1888 he directed the publication of *La nouvelle iconographie de la Salpêtrière* by Paul Richer (1849–1933), Georges Gilles de la Tourette (1857–1904),[12] and Albert Londe (1858–1917). In 1890 he organized the first annual meeting on mental medicine and created a laboratory for Pierre Janet (1859–1947). In 1892 he published his last paper, on faith healing.

After the death of Charcot in August 1893, the chair was temporarily held by Edouard Brissaud, then by Fulgence Raymond in 1894 (see chapter 16).

Brown-Séquard succeeded Claude Bernard as Professor at the Collège de France in 1879, while Vulpian died in 1887. In 1893 the *Revue Neurologique* was founded (see chapter 10).

Progress in Medicine The study of infectious diseases took significant steps forward in the 1880s with the work of Robert Koch (1843–1910) and Louis Pasteur. After having isolated the anthrax bacillus in 1876, Koch demonstrated in 1882 the origin of tuberculosis (the tubercle bacillus) and in 1883 discovered the cholera vibrio. Without knowing of Koch's work, Pasteur developed in 1881 a vaccine against anthrax and in 1885 one against rabies. The Pasteur Institute was inaugurated in 1888.

Medical technology would be completely transformed by two discoveries, the consequences of which are still being felt today. In 1895, Wilhelm Roentgen (1845–1923) discovered X-rays, and in 1898 Pierre Curie (1859–1906) and Marie Curie (1867–1934) identified—radioisotopes.

The Political Situation in France After the bloody episode of the Paris Commune, the political situation in France became relatively calm, even if certain tensions persisted due to the ongoing jockeying for power between monarchists and republicans and between traditional elites and the emerging middle class. The proletariat also began to organize into labor unions to defend their wages and improve working conditions. Despite several political crises between 1880 and 1890, the Third Republic, in the last decade of the century, can be considered relatively stable.

---

[12] Georges Gilles de la Tourette succeeded Babinski as chief resident of Charcot and defended his thesis in 1886; named *médecin des hôpitaux* in 1893, he became associate professor of internal and forensic medicine in 1895, after having failed at the *agrégation* in 1892. He would die in 1904 of paralysis of the insane. His name remains associated with *maladie des tics*. F. Huguet, *Les professeurs de la faculté de medicine de Paris. Dictionnaire biographique 1794–1939* [Professors of the faculty of medicine in Paris: Biographical dictionary, 1794–1939] (Paris: CNRS, INRP, 1991), 568–569.

Two major upheavals, however, shook the government and state structures. In 1892, the Panama scandals, in which government officials took bribes to cover up the financial troubles of the Compagnie Universelle de Panama, involved in building the canal, resulted in an important lack of confidence in politicians.[13] Much more serious was the Dreyfus affair, in which a young French artillery officer was framed for treason. Erupting in 1894, the matter would deeply divide French society for twelve years.[14] It does not appear that Babinski expressed a personal opinion on the Dreyfus affair, though many other intellectuals were deeply concerned and involved (see chapter 2) The best illustration was certainly the famous open letter of Émile Zola (1840–1902) addressed to the president of the Republic and published in the newspaper L'aurore (The dawn) on January 13, 1898, with the provocative title "J'accuse" (I accuse).[15]

Despite such political tensions, the economic situation for the country as a whole was improving and the general optimism was exemplified by the 1889 World Fair which celebrated the centennial of the 1789 Revolution and dedication of the Eiffel Tower. There was nevertheless deep social unrest among the working classes whose living conditions, especially in large cities such as Paris, were often very difficult. Urban planning by Haussmann and his successors had significantly modified the city's architecture, but public hygiene progressed more slowly: typhoid was endemic, and severe cholera epidemics occurred in 1884 and 1892. It was only in 1894 that a law mandated the type of sewage system long since used elsewhere: even so, the resistance of property owners was an important obstacle to rapid application of the legislation.

---

[13] Following the bankruptcy of the Compagnie Universelle de Panama in 1888 and the financial ruin of eighty-five thousand subscribers, the true scandal broke out in 1892. According to the popular press, leading political figures had been paid to give their support to the continuation of the company; some of the businessmen involved fled the country to avoid arrest. Among them was Cornelius Hertz, whose extradition from England was demanded by the French; he was declared unfit to travel by a group of experts that included Charcot. There is no indication of any participation by Babinski.
[14] Sentenced for spying, this French officer was demoted and sent to the infamous penal colony in French Guyana. After numerous incidents, he was finally rehabilitated in 1906 and reintegrated into the French army.
[15] "As they have dared, so shall I dare. Dare to tell the truth, as they have pledged to tell it, in full, since the normal channels of justice have failed to do so. My duty is to speak out." The article caused a scandal, and Zola was sued. His sentencing caused riots in the streets and created the basis for the public and political impact of what became known as the Dreyfus Affair.

The Belle Époque In the emerging society of consumption and mass culture, there developed a thirst for places of inexpensive and pleasant entertainment. The new wave of *café-concerts* and *cabarets artistiques* (the famous Moulin Rouge opened in 1889 in Montmartre) were a source of inspiration for novelists such as Guy de Maupassant (1850–1893) and painters such as Henri de Toulouse Lautrec (1864–1901). It was the beginning of the Belle Époque, a period of optimism that would only end with World War I.

France was a vibrant laboratory for new expression in painting. In addition to Monet, Auguste Renoir (1841–1919) and Paul Cézanne (1839–1906) would exert a considerable influence on the art of the twentieth century, although their approach would not be immediately appreciated. Vincent Van Gogh (1853–1890) was also influenced by impressionism but rapidly went beyond it to his own highly individualistic approach, inspired by the Japanese style and use of blazing colors.

While there was a relatively coherent evolution in the art world, this was not the case in the movement of ideas against the positivist school of thought that had first arisen in France in the mid-nineteenth century through the writings of Auguste Comte (1798–1857). Rationalism, which had been a basic characteristic of French intellectual society since René Descartes (1596–1650), was placed in doubt. In 1889 the philosopher Henri Bergson (1859–1941) wrote *Essai sur les données immédiates de la conscience* (Time and free will: an essay on the immediate data of consciousness), opposing scientific realism to intuition, which he thought was the only path to full reality. This movement, limited at the beginning to intellectual circles, extended rapidly to a larger part of the French population, where the superficial gaiety of the Belle Époque contrasted with a general sense of unrest due to increasing economic disparities between the rich and the poor. It became increasingly popular to think that scientific and technical progress might be responsible for the difficult living conditions of the working class. Likewise, the conviction that, despite the plethora of discoveries and inventions, science could not provide answers to all questions explained the great popular interest in paranormal phenomena. The use of hypnotism was not limited to physicians, who were investigating it in an attempt to provide a rational explanation for extraordinary phenomena, but intrigued people at all levels of society because of the mysteries surrounding the mind-body relationship. The revolution represented by psychological studies was on its way.

During this period several works appeared on hysteria and hypnotism. In 1889, Hippolyte Bernheim (1840–1919) published a new edition of *De la suggestion et de ses applications à la thérapeutique* (Suggestive therapeutics: a treatise on the nature and uses of hypnotism); Pierre Janet, whose case studies were drawn from Charcot's patients, wrote on psychological automatisms, while Gilles de la Tourette lectured in psychotherapy, hysteria, and hypnosis and wrote *L'Hypnotisme et les états analogues au point de vue médico-légal* (Hypnotism and analogous conditions in forensic medicine).

The Last Two Decades of Babinski's Career

The Semiologist The period from the start of the twentieth century to the beginning of World War I represents the most active years of Babinski's career. Having clearly demonstrated his rupture with what was then accepted as the correct conceptual approach to hysteria, he would devote himself to three main tasks: the development of cerebellar semiology (1902–1903), the study of tendon and bone reflexes (the conclusions of which were published in 1912), and treatment for his patients, opening the way to neurosurgery in France (1910–1912) (Fig. 1-3).

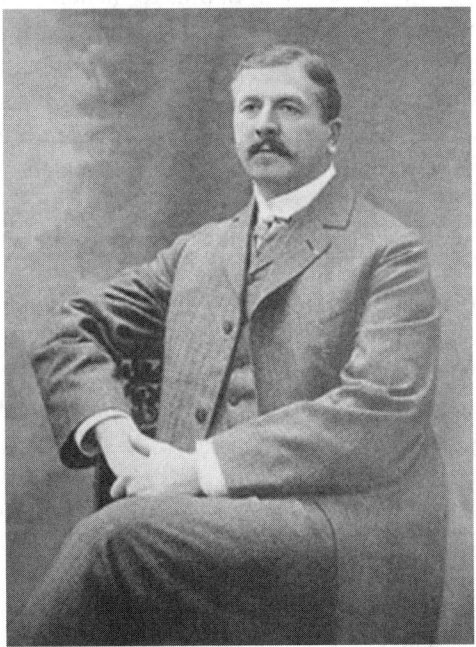

Figure 1-3 Joseph Babinski in 1904, at the age of forty-seven. (*Source*: Archives de l'Académie nationale de médecine, Paris.)

In the first decade of the century, the quarrel on hysteria had not completely died down, and fiery debates opposed Babinski to Bernheim, Raymond, and Jules Dejerine (1849–1917). The uproar disappeared at the Salpêtrière with the arrival of Dejerine, who isolated the last of the hysterical cases from other patients to prevent any "contamination" by communication between the two groups.

During this period Babinski's work was recognized by several distinctions: he was elected vice president of the Société de neurologie in 1906, becoming president in 1907, and was named a member of the advisory committee for the *Revue Neurologique*.[16] A few years later, in 1913, he received a standing ovation at the Seventeenth International Congress in London for his work on the cerebellum, and he was elected with a nearly unanimous vote to the Académie de médecine. He also received the Legion of Honor in 1905, becoming a commander in the order in 1921.[17] During World War I, he remained very active, studying with Jules Froment (1878–1946) the relationships between hysteria, pithiatism, and neurology in combat conditions (see chapter 15) (Fig. 1-4).

Joseph Babinski officially retired on December 31, 1922, having reached the age limit for a *médecin des hôpitaux*; thanks to the long-standing friendship with his successor Henri Vaquez (1860–1936), however, he was able to maintain an outpatient practice for several years. He was named an honorary member of the American Neurological Association in 1924 and of the Royal Society of Medicine in 1925. Although he refused a professorship in neurology offered by the University of Warsaw, he maintained close relationships with Poland, being accepted as an honorary member of the Warsaw School of Medicine and of the Warsaw Neurological Society (Fig. 1-5).

Progress in Medicine and Basic Sciences Sigmund Freud's studies, notably *The Interpretation of Dreams* (1900) and *The Psychopathology of Everyday Life* (1904), showed that the boundary between the normal and abnormal was indeterminate, and marked the emergence of psychology and psychiatry as important disciplines.

In France, Pierre Janet founded the *Journal de Psychologie Normale et Pathologique* (1904), while the *British Journal of Psychology* appeared in the same year, as did the *Psychological Bulletin* in United States. Pierre Janet

---

[16] His inaugural speech as president of the Société de neurologie was given on January 10, 1907, and was published in *Rev Neurol (Paris)*, 1907 (15): 78.

[17] Babinski had wished to be introduced by Count Maurice Zamoyski, plenipotentiary minister of the Polish Republic in Paris (see chapter 3), but this was administratively impossible. His friend Émile Picard, perpetual secretary of the Académie des sciences, was then asked to do so.

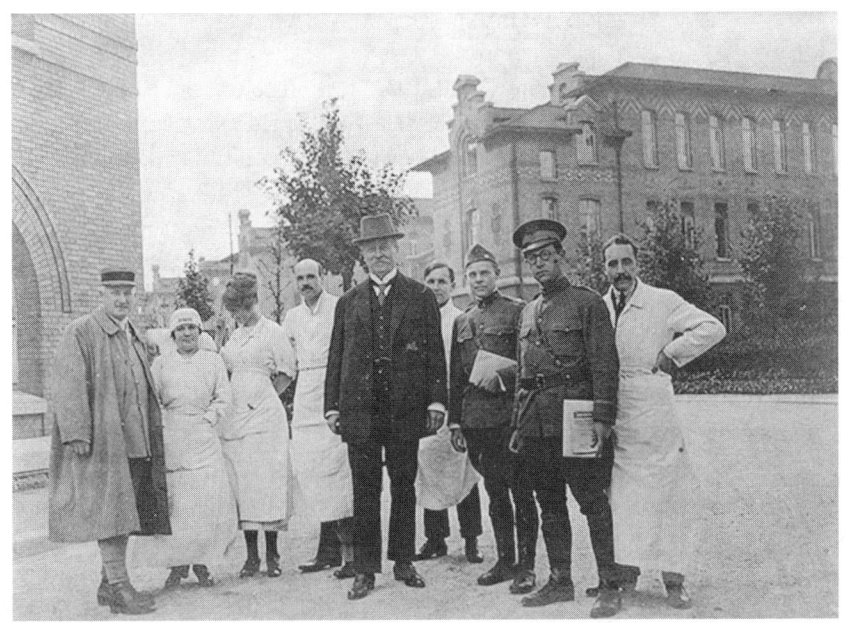

Figure 1-4 Joseph Babinski at the Pitié hospital at the end of World War I. (*Source*: Courtesy of Aude Boisaubert.)

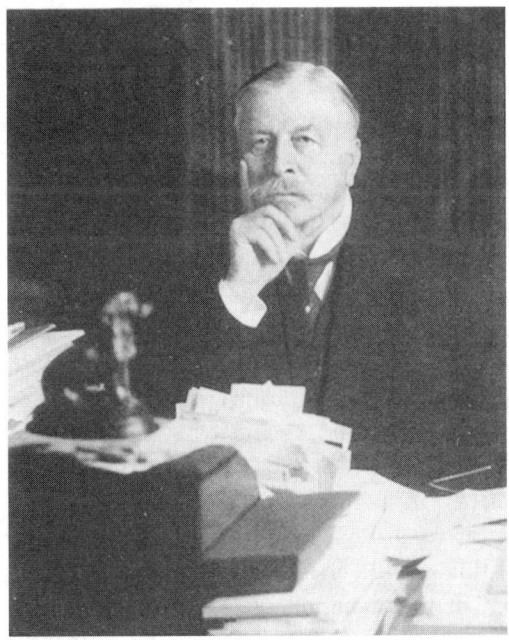

Figure 1-5 Joseph Babinski later in his life. (*Source*: From J. Babinski, *Oeuvre scientifique: recueil des principaux travaux* [Paris: Masson et Cie, 1934].)

corresponded with Ivan Pavlov (1849–1936), who received the Nobel Prize in 1904 for his work on the physiology of digestion, as they were both interested in experimental neurosis. Pavlov's description of conditioned reflexes was close to the work being done at the same period by Sir Charles Sherrington (1857–1952). The American Harvey Cushing (1869–1939) was creating the new discipline of neurosurgery, and would be a guiding light for the next twenty years (see chapter 16). Although Babinski had no direct contact with him, his pupil and former associate Clovis Vincent traveled to Boston in 1927 and came back full of enthusiasm after his visit, trying to apply in France the new techniques he had observed in Cushing's department.

Outside neurology, during the second half of Babinski's life progress in medicine was marked by several important discoveries. In 1902, Charles Richet (1850–1935), professor of physiology, described the phenomenon of anaphylaxis, for which he would receive a Nobel Prize in 1913. Paul Ehrlich (1854–1915), who also was a Nobel Prize laureate in 1908, was recognized for his work on immunity, oriented toward the search for synthetic substances that acted on specific microorganisms; after several years of trials, he found that an arsenic compound was active against *Treponema pallidum*, which causes syphilis, and he used it for the first time on humans in 1911 (see chapter 10).

At the Pasteur Institute, Ilya Metchnikoff (1845–1916), a scientist of Russian origin, continued his work on the phagocytic theory of immunity; he was co-laureate of the Nobel Prize with Ehrlich in 1908. Émile Roux (1853–1933), successor to Pasteur as the director of the Pasteur Institute, discovered that diphtheria symptoms were due to a toxin circulating in the blood; Alexandre Yersin (1863–1943) participated in this research, was later named director of the Pasteur Institute in Annam (Indochina), and discovered the plague bacillus.

Pierre and Marie Curie confirmed the importance of radioactive elements in the treatment of some pathologies such as lupus and malignant diseases. Albert Einstein (1879–1955) published in 1905 his famous treatise on special relativity, which would revolutionize physics and our conception of the universe throughout the century.

Political Climate In France, the repercussions of the Dreyfus affair meant that there was still a profound division between left and right. The consequences of this would persist for years with the formation of a leftist-oriented government, the main purpose of which was to defend the Republic against those who were perceived as threatening it, namely, the army and the church. In 1901, Parliament passed legislation banning the creation of new religious associations without authorization. This trend continued in 1905 with a law completely separating church and state, creating severe irritation among the Catholics and a conflict with the Pope.

Social protests increased with violent strikes in 1906–8, and the extreme positions of revolutionary labor unions and antimilitarist groups engendered strong nationalist sentiment in opposition. This was signaled by the debut in 1908 of the right-wing daily newspaper *L'Action Française,* of which journalist and novelist Léon Daudet (1867–1942) was one of the founders. Reinforced by a treaty of alliance with Great Britain (the Entente Cordiale) in 1904, France became progressively opposed to German politics, an atmosphere that set the scene for the World War I.

After the assassination of the Austrian archduke Franz Ferdinand in June 1914, the war broke out in August, with its most important battles in Verdun (February–December 1916) and on the river Somme (July–November 1916). American troops arrived in April 1917, while Russia after its revolution signed a separate peace treaty with Germany in March 1918. The general armistice was signed in November 1918. The war was responsible for almost 4 million casualties in France (civilian and military deaths and wounded), 15 percent of the total population one-tenth of the country's active population; following close on its heels came the global influenza epidemic (aka *Spanish flu*), which affected practically the whole world in 1918 and 1919 and caused the death of between 20 million and 40 million people.[18]

Art and Literature In tandem with the political instability of the beginning of the century, a deep reaction against rationalism appeared first in philosophy and literature and gradually reached other forms of fine arts. Painters did not want to copy reality but rather used it as an inspiration to express their emotion. After the death of Cézanne in 1906, and directly inspired by him, a new way of painting developed between 1907 and 1913, becoming known as cubism and represented by Pablo Picasso (1881–1973) and Georges Braque (1882–1963).

The revolution in music would move in a similar direction. Claude Debussy (1862–1918) was the first to follow the general climate of the time: his opera *Pelléas et Mélisande* caused a musical scandal in 1902 because of its rupture from the classical melodic line. Seeking to bring different art

---

[18] At first (June and July 1918), it was not generally fatal. But by the end of 1918, pulmonary complications appeared that caused death in a few hours, especially in children and young adults. C. Singer and E. Ashworth Underwood, *A Short History of Medicine* (New York: Oxford University Press, 1962), 735.

forms together, Debussy transcribed Mallarmé's poetry into music with his *Après-midi d'un faune*. The arrival in Paris in 1909 of Sergei Diaghilev's Ballets Russes, in which composers, choreographers and dancers, and painters all collaborated, reflected a similar departure from tradition. It was at this time that French audiences discovered Russian music; in 1913, Igor Stravinsky's (1882-1971) *Sacre du Printemps* caused yet another Parisian intellectual scandal.[19]

In French literature, the greatest name of this period was certainly Marcel Proust (1871-1922), who wrote at the end of the nineteenth century and the first twenty years of the twentieth, the last parts of his most famous novel, *À la recherche du temps perdu* (Remembrance of things past) being published after his death in 1925. His chronic illnesses were responsible for his frequent visits to doctors, particularly neurologists, one of whom was Babinski.[20]

After World War I, French intellectual life once again became very active, though it was limited to the bourgeois elite. A new generation of writers, including André Breton (1896-1966), disappointed by society's failure to avert the war and its terrible consequences, completely refused that same society's traditional artistic precepts, giving birth to surrealism.[21]

It was only with the introduction of motion pictures that the general population began to become active consumers of culture. Following a modest success in the beginning with the Lumière brothers, Auguste (1862-1954) and Louis (1864-1948), cinema gradually made its mark as a new form of entertainment and storytelling, with its biggest successes coming from the adaptation of popular novels. It seems likely, however, that Babinski remained faithful to his beloved opera.

His final years, in which his health progressively deteriorated as a result of Parkinson's disease, were affected by the death of his friend and longtime associate Jean Jarkovski (1880-1929) and more deeply by that of his brother in 1931.[22] Vaquez wrote in 1932: "He was no longer interested in medicine and we understood that life was slowly fading away." Haunted by sadness and anxiety, he died quietly, without any suffering, but in a solitude

---

[19] His ballet *L'Oiseau de feu* was created at the Paris Opéra on June 25, 1910.

[20] J. Bogousslavsky, "Marcel Proust's Lifelong Tour of the Parisian Neurological Intelligentsia: From Brissaud and Dejerine to Sollier and Babinski," *Eur Neurol* 2007 (57): 129-136.

[21] For his relationships with Babinski and Freud, see chapter 4.

[22] On August 1, 1929, Babinski wrote to his friend Egas Moniz concerning the foreword he should write for his book: "I have been unwell and had to stay in bed for two weeks. I feel better to-day. To-morrow I am leaving Paris and shall return in mid-September." On Jarkovski's death, see chapter 3.

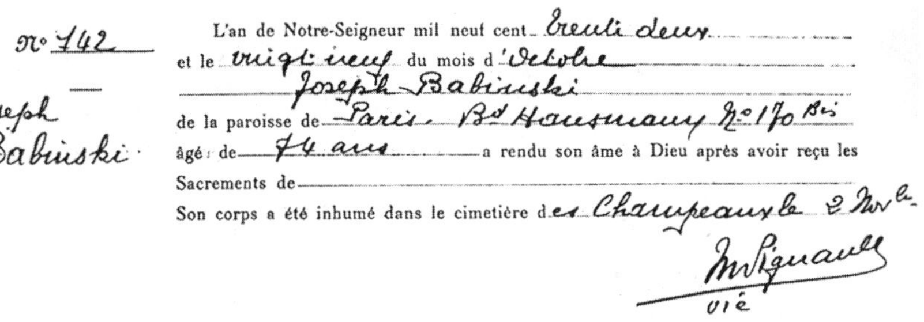

Nº 142

Joseph Babinski

L'an de Notre-Seigneur mil neuf cent trente deux
et le vingt neuf du mois d'Octobre
Joseph Babinski
de la paroisse de Paris, Bd Haussmann Nº 170 Bis
âgé de 74 ans a rendu son âme à Dieu après avoir reçu les
Sacrements de
Son corps a été inhumé dans le cimetière des Champeaux le 2 Nov.

Figure 1-6 Register of burial services in Montmorency Parish for the year 1932. (*Source*: Archives of the Pontoise Bishopric.)

relieved only by his closest pupils.[23] He was buried in the Polish cemetery Des Champeaux, near Montmorency, in the same tomb as his parents and brother (Fig. 1-6).

[23] R. Moreau, "Hommage à la mémoire de Joseph Babinski à l'occasion du 100è anniversaire de sa naissance" [Homage to the memory of Joseph Babinski on the occasion of the 100th anniversary of his birth], *Bulletins et Mémoires de la Société Médicale des Hôpitaux de Paris* 1958 (74): 449–457.

··· *two* ···

A Complex and Captivating Personality

According to those who knew him, Babinski's appearance attracted particular attention and left no one indifferent.[1] Well over six feet tall, he had a sepulchral voice combined with a gentle expression, both accompanied by an unforgettable Slavic charm. As described by his friend Vaquez, "At the height of his powers, Babinski was a fine-looking man; his majestic presence, his glance, at the same time tender and piercing, made him one of the elite."[2] Léon Daudet, who usually wrote with a scathing pen, fired off none of the unpleasant comments he habitually used with the other pupils of Charcot: "His very tall height, his open face, his rapid look, piercing glance, his strong voice, his clear laughter made him likeable to all."[3]

---

[1] P. Bailey, "Joseph Babinski (1857–1932)," *World Neurology* 1961: 134–140; H. Baruk, *Des hommes comme nous* [Men like us] (Paris: Robert Laffont, 1976), 28–32; A. Charpentier, *Un grand médecin. J. Babinski (1857–1932)* [A great physician: J. Babinski (1857–1932)] (Paris: Typographie François Bernouard, 1934); A. Charpentier, "Babinski (Joseph)" in M. Genty, ed., *Les biographies médicales* [Medical biographies], vol. VI (Paris: Librairie J. B. Baillière et fils, 1937-39), 17–32; C. Vincent, "J. Babinski (1857–1932)," *Rev Neurol (Paris)* 1932 (2): 441–446.
[2] H. Vaquez, "Joseph Babinski (1857–1932)," *Bulletin de l'Académie de Médecine*, séance du November 22, 1932, no. 35.
[3] L. Daudet, *Les oeuvres dans les hommes* [Men as seen through their works] (Paris: Nouvelle Librairie Nationale, 1922), 197–243.

Babinski's silence was remarked on by everyone who saw him regularly in his department.[4] He was not talkative with students, residents, or associates, and his patients might not hear one word spoken during their examination. He delighted in being silent, as did his master Charcot.[5] As said with admiration by Albert Charpentier, Joseph Babinski was "a blond giant with blue eyes... and obstinately mute."[6]

Addiction to Work

Babinski was addicted to work, as were many of his contemporaries: Alfred Vulpian (1826–1887), Jules Dejerine (1849–1917), Victor Cornil (1837–1908), Charles Bouchard (1837–1915), Pierre Marie (1853–1940), Gustave Roussy (1874–1948), Maxime Laignel-Lavastine (1875–1953), Eugène Gley (1857–1930), and Charles Robin (1821–1885) were all workaholics.[7] Babinksi's daily life was

---

[4] A. Tournay, "Babinski dans la vie" [Babinski in everyday life], *La Presse Médicale* 1958 (66): 1485–1489; Charpentier, *Un grand médecin*; Vincent, "J. Babinski"; R. Moreau, "Hommage à la mémoire de Joseph Babinski à l'occasion du 100è anniversaire de sa naissance" [Homage to the memory of Joseph Babinski on the occasion of the 100th anniversary of his birth], *Bulletins et Mémoires de la Société Médicale des Hôpitaux de Paris* 1958 (74): 449–457; L. Rivet, "Joseph Babinski (1857–1932)," *Bulletins et Mémoires de la Société Médicale des Hôpitaux de Paris* 1932 (34): 1722–1733; V. Neri, "Centenaire de la naissance de J. Babinski" [Centennial of the birth of J. Babinski], *Rev Neurol (Paris)* 1958 (98): 654–657.

[5] Rivet, "Joseph Babinski."

[6] Charpentier, "Babinski (Joseph)."

[7] In his obituary at Vulpian's funeral, Charcot reported: "Some time after the death of his mother, to whom he was deeply attached, I tried to boost his morale, temporarily at a low ebb. He said: 'I hope to recover with work. We are so fortunate to have such a cure!' Yes, work, always work! That was his ultimate refuge." Dossier Alfred Vulpian, Archives de l'Académie des sciences. On Dejerine: "The master needed to work, to work feverishly and with passion. An important task seems to condition his morale.... Regarding that, the correspondence of J. Dejerine with his mother is especially conclusive: 'We shall have always enough time to rest, we must work, always work.... Nothing is worth more than the enjoyment that work and particularly science gives to us.'" E. Gauckler, *Le professeur J. Dejerine (1849–1917)* (Paris: Masson, 1922), 12–13. On Cornil: "His life has been only one immense job.... You will always find Cornil working." Georges Millian, "Le Professeur V. Cornil 1837–1908," *Le Progrès Médical* 1908 (XXIII): 199—200. Bouchard had "an extraordinary ability to work." "Roger H. Bouchard (1837–1915)," *La Presse Médicale* 1915 (53 supplement): 402–406. Marie was a "tireless worker." *Le Progrès Médical* 1907 (XXIII): 884–885. On Roussy, see "Discours du Professeur Cornil (Marseille) aux obsèques de Gustave Roussy" [Cornil's speech at Roussy's funeral], Dossier Gustave Roussy, Archives de l'Académie des sciences. On Laignel-Lavastine: "For more than fifty years, he never stopped working." R. Moreau, "Maxime Laignel-Lavastine," *Rev Neurol (Paris)* 1953 (89): 274–276. Gley, a professor

mainly devoted to work, mornings at the hospital and afternoons at his private practice.[8] In the evening he worked on papers for publication, or sometimes relaxed at the opera, where he was one of the attending physicians. The same was true for his brother, of whom it was said that "he rested mainly by working."[9] One is justified in thinking that for Babinski, as for Charles Féré (1852–1907), "working personifies happiness, and any physical or intellectual work is a major contribution to the happiness of mankind."[10] At the end of his eulogy of neurologist Alix Joffroy (1844–1909), Maurice Klippel urged that all resume their normal activities, "trying if possible, to lessen our sorrow by work."[11]

"The Illness of Doubt"

Rather than seeing Babinski as cold and distant, his friend Henri Vaquez depicted him as being reserved and quite shy.[12] "Romantic by nature, with a touch of mysticism and tormented by doubt, he had the complex and subtle psychological profile of a gentle and loving individual who, in giving of himself often suffered from life's cruelties, enheartened for a short time by the certitude of being loved without ever completely satisfying him."[13] All who knew him drew attention to his "illness of doubt."[14] Extremely scrupulous, perfectionistic, finicky, demanding, meticulous, and overly conscientious, Babinski constantly needed to verify what he did; he would start something over and over again, whether examining a patient, looking for a single clinical sign, preparing a paper, or even writing a simple prescription. He would hesitate, begin again, make small changes, repeat, double-check with extreme

---

of physiology at Paris University and at the Collège de France, was described as a "tireless worker" in his biography in *Le Progrès Médical* 1903 (XVII): 97. Robin "is an extraordinary worker, a tireless researcher." J. Jolly, "Louis Ranvier (1835–1922). Notice biographique," *Archives d'Anatomie Microscopique* 1922 (XIX): 1–72.

[8] Vaquez, "Joseph Babinski"; Vincent, "J. Babinski."

[9] Alexis Rey, École des mines de Paris, class of 1876, "Nécrologie d'Henri Babinski" [Obituary of Henri Babinski], *Bulletin de l'Association des Anciens élèves de l'École des mines de Paris*, 1931; available at http://www.annales.org/archives/x/babinsky.html.

[10] "Analyse de l'ouvrage *Travail et plaisir*" [Review of *Work and pleasure*, by Charles Féré], *Le Progrès Médical* 1904 (3): 107.

[11] M. Klippel, "Hommage à M. le professeur Joffroy" [Homage to Professor Joffroy], *Rev Neurol (Paris)* 1908 (XVI): 1326–1327.

[12] Vaquez, "Joseph Babinski."

[13] Charpentier, "Babinski (Joseph)."

[14] For the phrase "illness of doubt" (*maladie du doute*), see A. Charpentier, *Un grand médecin*. Babinski has also been nicknamed the "constructive doubter"; see M. Dupont, *Dictionnaire historique des médecins dans et hors de la médecine* [Historical dictionary of physicians inside and outside medicine] (Paris: Larousse, 1999).

care, delete, and look endlessly for the exact word, with an etymological dictionary at hand; everything was reworked again and again.[15] He dreaded delivering a speech and indeed was not a good speaker, having a slow and somewhat jerky style. He could examine a patient for hours without saying a word, dictate to a resident a banal prescription for a bromide, and then sign it himself after having slowly reread it and eventually touched it up.[16] That evening, he might well call back the colleague who had asked him for a consultation in order to clarify certain details of the patient's symptomatology or to verify once again the prescription he had written (Fig. 2-1).[17]

Babinski was permanently tormented by doubt, "not the destructive one leading to skepticism and negation, but the constructive one."[18] It is interesting to note that two words used consistently by his biographers are *scruple* and *doubt*. Without speaking of a true neurosis, it is certain that Babinski's personality presented a few character traits that might be considered as obsessional.

He did not like traveling and would gladly have remained always in Paris. When his colleague Louis Delherm announced that he was going on a honeymoon to Monaco, Babinski answered mischievously that he had always been happy inside the Paris city limits.[19] During the summer months he took some vacation, at first for only a short time, then later for several weeks; at the beginning, he did not leave France, going to Font-Romeu in the Pyrénées or to the coast at Deauville. Wherever he went, he needed to be assured of finding a bed of exceptional size, in order that he not be obliged to sleep curled up.[20] Henri Vaquez eventually convinced him to travel in Europe with his brother and even to some countries in the Americas.[21] Vaquez said that he was "a nice travel companion, who spoke very little but accepted easily all proposals for excursions, on the condition that there were no initiatives to

---

[15] "I shall not insist on the difficulty he had in writing his papers. That came from his innate sense of doubt, which is the prerogative of a great intelligence and of his artistic desire to attain perfection." Vaquez, "Joseph Babinski." See also Charpentier, *Un grand médecin*; A. Tournay, *La vie de Joseph Babinski* [The life of Joseph Babinski] (Amsterdam: Elsevier, 1967), 111.

[16] Baruk, *Des hommes comme nous*, 28–32.

[17] "He was always phobic about dosage, leading him to constantly verify his prescriptions." Rivet, "Joseph Babinski."

[18] Vaquez, "Joseph Babinski."

[19] R. Khalil, "Vie et oeuvre de Babinski" [The life and work of Babinski], in *Conférences lyonnaises d'histoire de la neurologie et de la psychiatrie* (Lyon: Documentation médicale Oberval, 1982), 255–280.

[20] Tournay, "Babinski dans la vie."

[21] Rivet, "Joseph Babinski."

2. A COMPLEX AND CAPTIVATING PERSONALITY

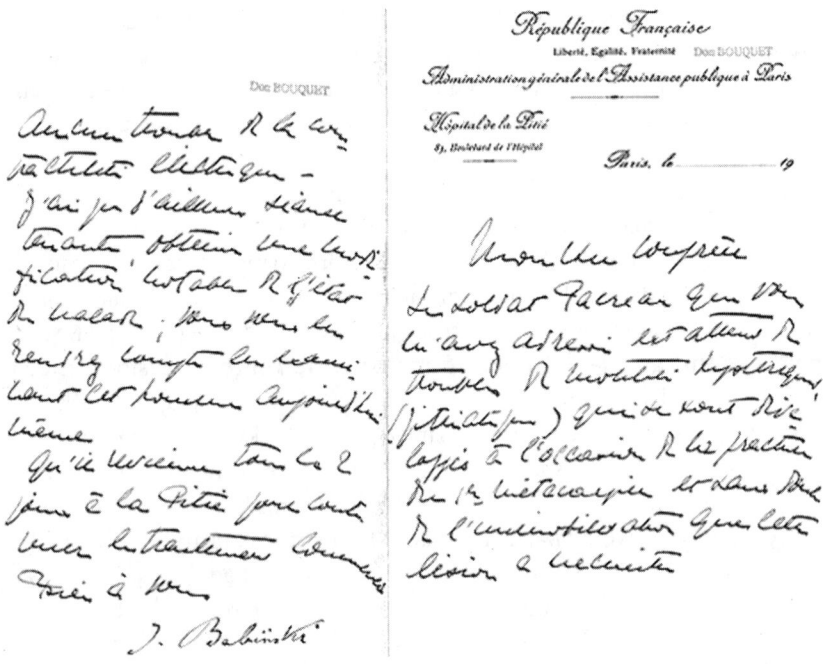

Figure 2-1 Letter from Joseph Babinski during World War I. (*Source*: Archives de l'Académie nationale de médecine, Paris.)

take."[22] In his later life, a photograph shows him relaxing in Guétary in the Basque countryside.[23]

One may wonder if his refusal to attempt the *agrégation* for a second time after his failure in 1892 could have been related to his excessive shyness and introverted personality (see chapter 5). Babinski also displayed a certain phobia in regard to illness. He could not bear to examine patients with Parkinson's disease, perhaps because his father died of it and he himself feared becoming afflicted with the same disease (which, unfortunately, proved to be the case during the last three years of his life).[24]

Babinski coined a number of neologisms, the majority of them now commonly used in everyday medical language: *anosognosia, anosodiaphoria, cerebellar asynergy, diadococinesia, cerebellar catalepsy, volitional equilibrations, hypermetry, pithiatism, thermal asymmetry, spondylotic pseudo-tabes,*

---

[22] Ibid.
[23] Because Albert Charpentier retired to Guétary, it is logical to suppose that Babinski was visiting his house.
[24] Rivet, "Joseph Babinski."

physiopathic disorders.[25] What might have lain behind this need to create new and more specific words rather than using the existing vocabulary? This may well be again a symptom of his obsessional need to give a precise, exact, and definitive place to each phenomenon he had observed, in order to avoid any possible misinterpretation.

There is a good deal of evidence suggesting that Babinski was not devoid of humor, though it was often caustic and sometimes in doubtful taste. There are several anecdotes on this subject. While preparing his candidacy for the Academy of Medicine, he spoke of "joining the toothless," because of the great age of the members of this prestigious assembly.[26] Leaving the hospital one day with Jean Alexandre Barré and Auguste Tournay, he stood aside to let pass "a nice lady, allowing her to climb up first onto the upper deck of an omnibus; his scientific curiosity permitted him, looking upward, to catch a glimpse of an intimate aspect of the beautiful traveler: he exclaimed, 'What nice skin underwear!'; he was a good enough loser and the first to laugh when the lady pertly answered back: 'I've had it for thirty years and it has only two holes in it.'"[27] He was easily moved to laughter: he had "sometimes fits of youthful blithness, bursting out laughing when confronted by triviality."[28]

[25] J. Babinski, *Oeuvre scientifique: recueil des principaux travaux* [Scientific work: selection of main papers], edited by J. A. Barré, J. Chaillous, A. Charpentier, et al. (Paris: Masson et Cie, 1934), 114 (anosognosia); J. Babinski, "Contribution à l'étude des troubles mentaux dans l'hémiplégie organique cérébrale (anosognosie)" [Contribution to the study of mental disorders in organic cerebral hemiplegia (anosognosia)], *Rev Neurol (Paris)* 1914 (XXVII): 845–848 (anosodiaphoria); J. Babinski, "De l'asynergie cérébelleuse" [On cerebellar asynergy], *Rev Neurol (Paris)* 1899 (VII): 806–816 (cerebellar asynergy); J. Babinski and A. Tournay, "Les symptômes des maladies du cervelet et leur signification" [Signs of cerebellar diseases and their meaning], *Congrès International de Médecine de Londres*, August 1913 (diadococinesia ["Considering the word adiadococinesia proposed by Bruns and commonly used in observations, it expresses by the addition of a privative *a* the loss or alteration of this function"], cerebellar catalepsy, volitional equilibrations); J. Babinski, "Quelques documents relatifs à l'histoire des fonctions de l'appareil cérébelleux et de leurs perturbations" [Some documents concerning cerebellar functions and their disturbances], *Revue de médecine interne et de thérapeutique* 1909 (1): 114–129 (hypermetry); J. Babinski, "Définition de l'hystérie" [Definition of hysteria], *Rev Neurol (Paris)* 1901 (IX): 1074–1080 (pithiatism); J. Babinski, "Thermo–asymétrie d'origine bulbaire" [Thermal asymmetry of brain stem origin], *Rev Neurol (Paris)* 1905 (XIII): 452, 568–572 (thermal asymmetry); J. Babinski, *Exposé des travaux scientifiques* [Presentation of scientific papers] (Paris: Masson, 1913) (spondylotic pseudo-tabes); J. Babinski, *Hystérie-pithiatisme et troubles nerveux d'ordre réflexe en neurologie de guerre* [Hysteria or pithiatism and reflex nervous disorders in the neurology of war] (Paris: Masson et Cie, 1917) (physiopathic disorders).
[26] Tournay, "Babinski dans la vie."
[27] Khalil, "Vie et oeuvre de Babinski."
[28] Rivet, "Joseph Babinski."

2. A COMPLEX AND CAPTIVATING PERSONALITY

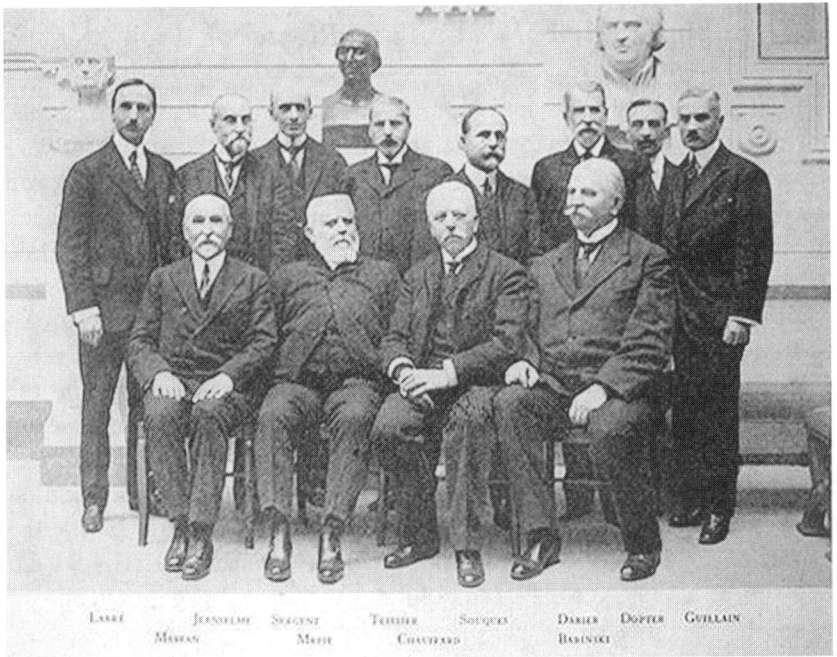

Figure 2-2 Joseph Babinski in 1920, during the centenary of the Académie de médecine. (*Source*: From *Livre du centenaire de l'Académie de médecine: 1820–1920.*)

"He laughed in a childish way and could be heard at the end of the corridor when, having put on his coat and hat while standing at the entrance of his consulting room, he had just told a Jewish story or described a drawing of a cartoonist like Forain."[29] Once, when consulting with Fernand Widal and Jean Sicard in an old castle, he saw a suit of armor with a superb helmet. "He picked up [the helmet] and jokingly put it on his head. When the pawl worked and the visor closed up Babinski, who had started out by laughing, began to get rather anxious (Fig. 2-2)."[30]

---

[29] Charpentier, *Un grand médecin*. Jean-Louis Forain (1852–1931) was a painter, pastelist, engraver, drawer, illustrator, cartoonist, and famous poster designer (see E. Bénézit, *Dictionnaire des peintres, sculpteurs, dessinateurs et graveurs*, new ed. [Paris: Gründ, 1999]; "Have you looked at the last Forain?" *La Presse Médicale*, supplément to no. 5, February 4, 1915). Politically situated on the very right wing, Forain was hostile to anarchists, socialists, and labor union members. He was violently against Dreyfus; he created in 1898, with Caran d'Ache, the weekly anti-Semitic journal *Psst*.
[30] Martin G., "La médecine anecdotique," *Le Progrès Médical*, August 30, 1930.

Babinski, Man of Reason and Righter of Wrongs

Babinski could be at times peremptory or even sententious. For example, in a June 26, 1898, letter to the famous Belgian neurologist Arthur Van Gehuchten (1861–1914), he wrote: "It was a pleasure to see the efforts you made to verify the facts I had announced and that you have confirmed them. But let me draw your attention to the fact that, contrary to what you think, my research was not exclusively related to hemorrhage of brain origin." Van Gehuchten made amends.[31] Professor Oppenheim, a well-known neurologist from Berlin, wrote to the *Revue Neurologique* to claim priority concerning Babinski's report on November 9 at the Société de Neurologie on the electric hyperexcitabiliy of the facial nerve in facial palsy, "a phenomenon to which he thought to have been the first to draw attention." "On several occasions, I have described this phenomenon and gave to it a signification grossly similar to that given by M. Babinski." Babinski answered back. "The letter of M. Oppenheim surprised me. Contrary to what he declared, I did not assert to have been the first to point out the electric hyperexcitabiliy of the facial nerve in facial palsy; by the way, in this respect, priority does not belong to M. Oppenheim either. He will always find us ready to give him his due; but his claim has to be justified."[32] At the Réunion Neurologique Internationale of 1924, regarding the analogies between multiple sclerosis lesions and those of the periaxile nevritis of Gombault, he declared: "I think I have been the first to have made this connection."[33] He argued with Rabiner about the reflex hammer.[34] He argued again, even if in a more friendly way, with Pierre Marie on tabes.[35] On several occasions during medical society

---

[31] A. Van Gehuchten, "Le phénomène des orteils" [The toe phenomenon], *Journal de Neurologie* 1898 (III): 153–155; A. Van Gehuchten, "A propos du phénomène des orteils," *Journal de Neurologie* 1898 (III): 284–286. In the paper of Van Gehuchten cited above http://www.md.ucl.ac.be/histoire/vangeA/ilvangeA.htm.

[32] J. Babinski, "À propos du procès-verbal de la séance du 9 novembre 1905 de la Société de Neurologie de Paris, au sujet de la communication de M. Babinski sur l'hyperexcitabilité électrique du nerf facial dans la paralysie faciale" [Concerning the minutes of the November 9, 1905 meeting of the Paris Neurological Society on the subject of M. Babinski's report on the electrical hyperexcitability of the facial nerve in facial palsy], *Rev Neurol (Paris)* 1906 (XIV): 79.

[33] J. Babinski, "Sur la démyélinisation dans la sclérose en plaques" [On demyelination in multiple sclerosis], *Rev Neurol (Paris)* 1924 (I): 739–740.

[34] J. M. S. Pearce, *Fragments of Neurological History* (London: Imperial College Press, 2003).

[35] J. Babinski, "Sur les scléroses systématiques, dites primitives, de la moelle" [On systematic sclerosis, known as primitive, of the spinal cord], *Bulletins et Mémoires de la Société Médicale des Hôpitaux de Paris* 1894 (XI): 21–30, abstract in *Le Progrès Médical* 1894 (XIX): 66.

meetings, he gave his definition of hysteria and strongly criticized reports of disorders presented as hysteric in origin that he did not consider as such—for example, a supposed hysterical presence of albumin in urine.[36]

His Italian pupil Vincenzo Néri described him during some memorable sessions of the Société de neurologie de Paris as "alone against everybody, admirable to see and to listen to, with the precision of a beautiful gladiator" destroying one by one the arguments of his colleagues, and concluding by presenting his own concept of hysteria.[37] Georges Shaltenbrand (1897–1979) reported that when he told Babinski that a case was one of "pseudo-sclerosis," Babinski answered: "A neurologist who lays down the diagnosis of pseudo-sclerosis is not a neurologist but a pseudo-neurologist."[38] Shaltenbrand supposed that "this severity and exactness constituted an essential trait of his character and that these same traits led to his everlasting discoveries." In honor of the centennial of Babinski's birth, when everyone made speeches in praise of him, Schaltenbrand was the only one to offer a sarcastic remark: "In all his work, one may find an extreme distrust or mistrust of himself, but also of others. That could be the reason why his interest in the findings of others diminished. But what can you expect? So he was. Among immortals, you may also find imperfection. Babinski belongs certainly to the immortals."[39] Babinski explained it thus: "I do not rate cases according to whether they are reported out of Paris or by foreigners, far from it; but it is not sufficient to accept them because they are coming from a distance. I am not satisfied with affirmations, but only facts that can be verified here. Given the countless mistakes made in this matter, my request is purely of a scientific nature, whatever M. Raymond may think (Fig. 2-3)."[40]

This distrust—of himself, other neurologists, and even his patients—explains why he needed to start again so often and repeat indefinitely the same gesture, his lack of belief in the neurological examinations of others, and the low opinion he had of patients' descriptions of their symptoms.

Henri Baruk (1897–1999), formerly chief resident under Henri Claude at Sainte-Anne, described a presentation of a patient made by Tinel, Lamache,

---

[36] *Le Progrès Médical* 1904 (XIX), reporting on the December 11, 1903 meeting of the Société médicale des Hôpitaux de Paris.

[37] V. Néri "Centenaire de la naissance de J. Babinski" [Centennial of the birth of J. Babinski], *Rev Neurol (Paris)* 1958 (98): 654–657.

[38] G. Shaltenbrand "Centenaire de la naissance de Babinski," *Rev Neurol (Paris)* 1958 (98): 640–656.

[39] Ibid.

[40] J. Babinski, "À propos du procès-verbal 'Sur la fièvre et les troubles trophiques attribués à l'hystérie'" [Concerning the minutes on "Fever and trophic disorders attributed to hysteria"], *Rev Neurol (Paris)* 1909 (XVIII): 207–209.

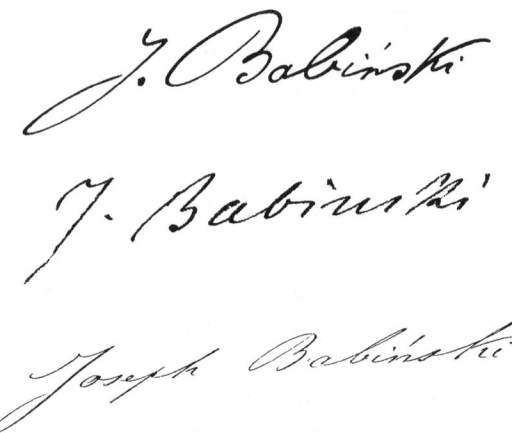

Figure 2-3 Signatures of Joseph Babinski. (*Source:* Archives nationales, Paris.)

and Baruk at a session of the *Société Médicale des hôpitaux*. Claude claimed that their patient, a young female, showed signs of a functional mesencephalic disorder, an idea that Babinski vigorously refuted: "the two exchanged rough words." An appointment was made so that Babinski could examine the patient. "During an entire morning, Babinski conducted his examination, turning her over in every angle, placing her in extraordinary positions, checking the reflexes, putting the head up and down. Finally, he said, 'I do not observe any mesencephalic dysfunction.'"[41]

There are many examples of his caustic comments at meetings of the Société de neurologie. To Dejerine and André Thomas, he said: "The absence of voltaic vertigo would not have any diagnostic value. If that is truly your opinion, I think you are wrong."[42] To Dejerine at another time: "I consider

---

[41] The description of the confrontation is in Baruk, *Des hommes comme nous* (Paris: Robert Laffont, 1976), 28–32. For Babinski's analysis of the patient, see his "Hystérie-pithiatisme. À propos du procès-verbal (à propos de la communication de MM. Tinel, Baruk et Lamache: crise de catalepsie hystérique et rigidité décérébrée)" [Hysteria and pithiatism: Concerning the minutes on the paper presented by MM. Tinel, Baruk and Lamache with the title "Hysterical catalepsy attack and decerebrate rigidity"], *Bulletins et Mémoires de la Société Médicale des Hôpitaux de Paris* 1928 (LII): 1507–1521. On Baruk, see the article written by J.-Y. Nau in *Le Monde*, June 20–21, 1999.

[42] J. Babinski, "À propos de la communication de M. Dejerine et André Thomas, 'Présentation d'un malade atteint de surdité verbale pure, de troubles de l'équilibre et de la vue'" [Concerning the paper of M. Dejerine and André Thomas, "Presentation of a patient with pure verbal deafness as well as equilibrium and sight disturbances"], *Rev Neurol (Paris)* 1902 (X): 532; J. Babinski, "À propos de la communication de M. Dejerine, 'Présentation d'un malade atteint de surdité verbale pure, de troubles de l'équilibre et de la vue'" [Concerning the paper of M. Dejerine, "Presentation of a patient with pure

that the presentation by M. Dejerine is far from convincing."[43] To Grasset and Calmette: "In summary, MM. Grasset and Calmette confirm partly what I have written...and do not invalidate any ideas I have expressed; they refute only an opinion, which, as a matter of fact, is not exact, and which I have never maintained."[44] To Leredde, on the treatment of parasyphilitic disorders with mercury: "All that said by M. Leredde is old hat. What could be new would be to obtain a true recovery, as admitted by M. Leredde;...but he fails to bring forward any convincing facts to support his statements."[45]

To Pierre Marie he commented, "I should point out to M. Pierre Marie that the case he presented is not in complete opposition to my ideas on the toe phenomenon....This one allows us to assert a disorder in the pyramidal system; it seems it is a law. But I have never pretended that all pyramidal disorders are accompanied by the toe phenomenon: to tell the truth, it is generally the case, but is only a rule, which, as all other rules, may present some exceptions, as I pointed out in my first papers on the subject."[46] To Vires and Calmette he said: "The reports of MM. Vires and Calmette confirm my own and I am pleased with this, but I confess that I am surprised by their conclusions. In fact, after having recognized that the toe phenomenon is characteristic of a disorder of the pyramidal system and that it can be the only expression, they declare that its significance has only a minor importance. This deduction seems very illogical to me." And at the end of a paper by M. Noïca, from Bucharest, on spasmodic paralysis with flexed spasm, Babinski noted: "M. Noïca declares that in his study he drew the

---

verbal deafness as well as equilibrium and sight disturbances"], *Rev Neurol (Paris)* 1902 (13): 628.

[43] Referring to J. Dejerine, "Sur l'abolition du réflexe cutané plantaire dans certains cas de paralysies fonctionnelles accompagnées d'anesthésie (hystéro-traumatisme)" [On the abolition of the cutaneous plantar reflex in some cases of functional paralysis with anesthesia (hysterical-trauma)], *Rev Neurol (Paris)* 1914–15 (XXVIII): 521–529.

[44] J. Babinski, "À propos de la communication de Grasset et Calmette (de Montpellier), communiqué par Pierre Marie, 'De la flexion du tronc dans le décubitus dorsal (acte de se mettre sur son séant)'" [Concerning the paper by Grasset and Calmette (of Montpellier), presented by Pierre Marie, "On trunk flexion in the prone position (action of sitting up)"], *Rev Neurol (Paris)* 1901 (IX): 1207–1212.

[45] J. Babinski, "A propos de la communication de M. Leredde, 'Sur les affections parasyphilitiques et leur traitement'" [Concerning the paper of M. Leredde, "On the parasyphilitic diseases and their treatment"], *Rev Neurol (Paris)* 1902 (X): 466–467.

[46] J. Babinski, "À propos de la communication de Pierre Marie, 'Un cas de ramollissement ancien énorme dans le domaine de la sylvienne. Absence d'hémianesthésie. Réflexe plantaire en flexion'" [Concerning the paper presented by Pierre Marie, "A case of an old, massive softening in the middle cerebral artery territory. Absence of hemianesthesia. Cutaneous plantar reflex in flexion"], *Rev Neurol (Paris)* 1902 (X): 271–272.

same conclusions as mine, which means that I would have simply confirmed his own results. Our colleague is obviously wrong, as our conclusions have nothing in common; it is easy to be convinced of that by comparing each of them."[47]

This is but a sample of the way Babinski defended his premises and conclusions. The tone was always polite and courteous, but there was never any concession on the content. It happened sometimes that in his insistence on persuading his colleagues that he was always right, he drew snide remarks, as this one by Fulgence Raymond: "One can be courteous, even very courteous in regard to the work of a colleague, but that does not mean that we adopt his ideas or his option concerning hysteria."[48]

On the other hand, when he was able to verify that another researcher had in fact made the same discovery as himself, Babinski had the courtesy to acknowledge it in public. For example, in regard to the disappearance of the toe phenomenon under the influence of prolonged compression by an Esmarch bandage, he wrote in the *Revue Neurologique*: "It is my duty to note that Dr. Onorio de Almeida has already observed this fact. He reported and analyzed it in an issue of the *Brazil Medico* that I have just examined but which was published before my own report."[49]

Fascinated by Paranormal Phenomena

Babinski was preoccupied and fascinated by paranormal phenomena, including telepathy and mediums. In 1886 he showed that some mental images might be transferred at a distance from one subject to another, under the influence of a magnet, though he probably repudiated these early works very rapidly.[50] In fact, in his *Notice sur les travaux scientifiques* of 1892, they are

---

[47] D. Noïca, "À propos de l'article de M. Babinski, 'Paralysie spasmodique organique avec contracture en flexion et contractions involontaires'" [Concerning the paper by M. Babinski, "Spasmodic paralysis with flexed contracture and involuntary contractions"], *Rev Neurol (Paris)* 1911 (XXII): 173–178.

[48] Babinski, "À propos du procès-verbal 'Sur la fièvre et les troubles trophiques attribués à l'hystérie.'"

[49] J. Babinski, "Modification des réflexes cutanés sous l'influence de la compression par la bande d'Esmarch (à propos d'un travail du docteur Onorio de Almeida)" [Modification of the cutaneous reflexes after compression by Esmarch bandage (concerning the work by Dr. Onorio de Almeida)], *Rev Neurol (Paris)* 1912 (XXIV): 147.

[50] J. Babinski, "Recherches servant à établir que certains phénomènes nerveux peuvent être transmis d'un sujet à un autre sous l'influence de l'aimant" [Research to demonstrate that some nervous phenomenon may be transmitted from a patient to another under the

listed as references in the bibliography but, unlike others, were not analyzed; neither do they appear in the *Exposé des travaux scientifiques* of 1913, nor in the *Oeuvre scientifique* of 1934.[51]

Albert Charpentier recounted Babinski's meeting with the famous Italian medium Eusapia Palladino (sometimes spelled Paladino; 1854–1918).[52] Born in the Abruzzi region of Italy, Palladino became known as a medium at an early age.[53] Starting in 1891, she began an international career, appearing in large cities in Europe and the United States, giving rise to a circle of believers. Leading scientific experts—such as the criminologist Cesare Lumbroso (1836–1909); Professor Charles Richet, who won the Nobel Prize for his works on anaphylaxis; the astronomer Camille Flammarion (1842–1925); and the Polish physician Julian Ochorowicz (1850–1917)—all tried to find a scientific explanation for the phenomena observed.[54] Eusapia Palladio was studied in renowned laboratories in Cambridge by William Crookes (1832–1919), in Saint Petersburg, and in Paris by a committee set up by

---

influence of a magnet], *Comptes-rendus Hebdomadaires des Séances et Mémoires de la Société de Biologie* 1886 (III): 475–477, abstract in *Le Progrès Médical* 1886 (IV): 996; J. Babinski, "Recherches servant à établir que certaines manifestations hystériques peuvent être transmises d'un sujet à un autre sujet sous l'influence de l'aimant" [Research to demonstrate that some hysterical manifestations may be transmitted from a patient to another under the influence of a magnet], *Le Progrès Médical* 1886 (IV): 1010–1011, abstract in *Annales Médico-Psychologiques*, 1891 (I): 144–145.

[51] J. Babinski, *Notice sur les travaux scientifiques* [Note on scientific papers] (Paris: Masson, 1892); J. Babinski, *Exposé des travaux scientifiques* [Presentation of scientific papers] (Paris: Masson, 1913); J. Babinski, *Oeuvre scientifique*.

[52] Charpentier, *Un grand médecin*.

[53] Harry Morgan, "Touchez pas au pèse-cocon: La vie trépidante d'Eusapia Palladino" [Don't disturb the delicate balance: The hectic life of Eusepia Palladino], http://www.sdv.fr/pages/adamantine/eusapiapalladino.htm.

[54] Richet intended to create a new science, which he called "metapsychic," dealing with all the paranormal phenomena; his *Traité de métapsychique* [Treatise on metapsychic] was published in 1922. Ochorowicz was a Polish philosopher and psychologist who graduated from Warsaw University and was a professor at Lvov. He invented an apparatus, named the "hypnoscope," used to determine an individual's sensitivity to hypnosis; "it was constituted, among other things, by powerful magnets, between which the patient put his finger." In the spring of 1893, Ochorowicz went to Rome, where, in the house of his friend H. Siemiradzki, the Polish painter, he carried out experiments with Palladino. Ochorowicz claimed he found no conscious cheating, but only unconscious attempts to manipulate the results, particularly when she was exhausted. Other scientists expressed more reservations about Palladino's practice, and finally she was unmasked as a fraud. C. W. Domanski, "Julian Ochorowicz (1850–1917) et son apport dans le développement de la psychologie du XIXè siecle" [Julian Ochorowicz (1850–1917) and his contribution to the development of psychology in the nineteenth century], *Psychologie et Histoire* 2003 (4): 101–114.

Pierre Curie at the Institut général psychologique (where Marie Curie, Jean Perrin [1870–1942], Edouard Branly [1844–1940], and Henri Bergson also worked), which led to her being nicknamed "the diva of the scientists."[55] The idea of a "fluidic body" or a "fluidic thread" emerged as an explanation for the manifestations. In reality, however, her illusions were created with the help of an impressive array of equipment under her clothes (lever, false hands, false beard, folding yardsticks, spring-driven hammer, masks, and dark silk brocade); the voices were created by ventriloquism, and so forth. In 1912, when Eusapia was at the end of her career, Joseph Babinski, with his brother, Henri, and Albert Charpentier, went to Naples to "cautiously screen" the famous medium. The cheating was discovered; Babinski became terribly angry and flew into a towering rage, the only one that Charpentier ever witnessed.[56]

Absence of Political or Religious Commitment, but an Unfailing Patriotism

The Dreyfus affair (1894–1899) took place during the same period when Babinski was making his first reports on the toe phenomenon. Though in 1899 the physician Edouard Brissaud, Charcot's former pupil, was "an ardent supporter of Dreyfus," Babinski's name was never mentioned in a document related to the Dreyfus affair.[57] He is absent from the index of the book *L'Affaire* by Jean-Denis Bredin.[58] (By the way, except for Léon Daudet, none of Babinski's closest friends—Crouzon, Vaquez, Darier, Laubry, Charpentier, Clovis Vincent, Jean Alexandre Barré, Pierre Bazy, Émile Picard—appeared either.) This, however, is not sufficient grounds to determine his opinions or his commitments, as Désiré-Magloire Bourneville, who was a fervent supporter of Dreyfus, was absent as well. Babinski liked to read Anatole France (a supporter of Dreyfus), but he also had Léon Daudet (who was against Dreyfus) to dinner and appreciated the cartoons of Forain (strongly against him). We have no documentation that allows us to know his exact position on the matter; his hagiographers did not mention the Dreyfus affair. The

---

[55] C. Blondel, "Eusapia Palladino: la méthode expérimentale et la 'diva des savants'" [Eusapia Palladino: the experimental method and the "scientists' diva"], in B. Bensaude-Vincent and C. Blondel, eds., *Des savants face à l'occulte, 1870–1940* (Paris: Éditions de la Découverte, 2002), 143–171.
[56] Charpentier, *Un grand médecin*.
[57] Daudet, *Les oeuvres dans les hommes*, 197–243.
[58] J.-D. Bredin, *L'Affaire* (Paris: Julliard, 1983).

only element regarding his political leanings we have is drawn from an article that Léon Daudet wrote after Babinski's death. He recounted the extreme indignation of the Babinski brothers when the murderer of Marius Plateau (executive editor of the right-wing newspaper *L'Action Française* and chief of the right-wing party of the same name) was released, and noted that "every year, Ali-Bab [Henri Babinski] gave me, in his name and that of his brother, a generous contribution to the A.F.... They were both very independent and abhorred any hint of Germanophile feelings. That did not prevent them giving to German science its just due, but they were repulsed by pedantry, wherever encountered."[59]

In France around that time, many physicians were elected as local or regional councilors, mayors, congressmen, or senators.[60] From 1877 to 1914, they represented, on average, 10 to 12 percent of the legislative corps. Twenty-eight were ministers.[61] In 1885, Charles Robin, Victor Cornil, and other physicians were elected to the Senate.[62] On a list of doctors in Parliament compiled early in 1901 were forty-two senators and fifty-three congressmen.[63] In the general elections on May 4, 1896, all the physicians who were local councilors were reelected.[64] Among them was Émile Duclaux (1840–1904), professor of biological chemistry at the Sorbonne, member of the Académie des sciences and of the Académie de médecine, director of the Pasteur Institute in 1895 after Louis Pasteur; he took an important part in the campaign in favor of Dreyfus, on the same side as Émile Zola and Francis de Pressensé. Duclaux participated in the founding of the Ligue

---

[59] L. Daudet, "Babinsky" [sic], *L'Action Française*, October 30, 1932. L'Action Française was a right-wing nationalist and antirepublican movement, founded in 1898 and particularly influential through 1926, when Pope Pius XI condemned it.

[60] J. Leonard, "Le corps médical au début de la IIIè République" [The medical profession at the beginning of the Third Republic], in J. Poirier and J.-L. Poirier, eds., "Médecine et philosophie à la fin du XIXè siècle," special issue of *Cahier de l'Institut de Recherche Universitaire d'Histoire de la connaissance, des idées et des mentalités*, Créteil, Université de Paris XII, 1978 (2): 9–21; J. D. Ellis, *The Physician-Legislators of France: Medicine and Politics in the Early Third Republic, 1870–1914* (Cambridge: Cambridge University Press, 1990).

[61] I. Durand, "Les médecins-ministres dans les gouvernements français de 1871 à 1958" [Physician-ministers in French governments from 1871 to 1858], thèse de doctorat en médecine, Faculté Necker-Enfants-malades, Paris, 1985; "Les médecins ministres" [Physician-ministers], *Le Progrès Médical* 1905 (4): 60.

[62] Anonymous, "Les médecins du Sénat," *Le Progrès Médical* 1885 (5): 95.

[63] Anonymous, "Le groupe des médecins du Parlement" [The physician group in Parliament], *Le Progrès Médical* 1901 (14): 253.

[64] Anon, "Les médecins conseillers municipaux de Paris," *Le Progrès Médical* 1896 (III): N° 18, 301–302.

des droits de l'homme, the Universités populaires, and the Ecole des hautes études en sciences sociales.[65]

Unlike Bourneville (a freethinker, Mason, local councilor in Paris, and congressman from the Département de la Seine), Cornil (a Mason and a senator from the Départment de l'Allier), and many other physicians of that time (including Charles Robin, a senator; Jacques-Joseph Grancher (1843–1907), mayor in Cambo-les-Bains and president of the administrative council of the Pasteur Institute; and Ferdinand Darier, mayor in Longpont-sur-Orge), Babinski was not a political activist; nor were Dejerine, Marie, and many others.

Without being politically engaged, Joseph Babinski was nevertheless a convinced republican and democrat.[66] He had bad memories of the Paris Commune, which he had lived through when he was fourteen years old, and later he expressed "a deep antipathy toward Adolphe Thiers and the way he used force to cope with the insurrection."[67] "Never has a man proved to be less favorable to revolutionary ideas; he dreamed of a republican government strong and fair, where the moral value of the elites would run and correct the impulsiveness of the masses."[68] Babinski held a moralistic, traditional position that can be seen in a letter addressed to his disciple Egas Moniz on June 26, 1918, before the end of World War I, where he questioned the benefits of science, contrasted the powers of good and evil, and spoke highly of the virtues of work inspired by charity:

> In the present circumstances, in the middle of so many tragic events, one may also wonder if science deserves to be object of a cult. The most admirable creations of the human mind, contrary to all expectations, have had as their main effect destruction and massacre; with a bit of pessimism, one may curse advances in knowledge and fear that someday some discovery might have as a consequence the destruction of mankind. I hope, however, that the powers

---

[65] J. Noir, "Nécrologie. Émile Duclaux, Membre de l'Institut et de l'Académie de Médecine" [Obituary: Émile Duclaux, member of the Institute and the Academy of Medicine], *Le Progrès Médical* 1904 (XIX): 316–317.

[66] "Jozef Babinski inherited in this way the democratic traditions which he cultivated throughout his life. He was the friend of a minister and then prime minister, the French radical Waldeck-Rousseau. But at the same time, when my father presented to him the photocopy of a title in 1909, restored to the Babinski family in 1853 by the Heraldic Society of the Polish Kingdom, he was delighted." L. Babinski, "Sylwetka Jozefa Babinskiego na tle jego zycia codziennego" [Josef Babinski from day to day], *Neurol Neurochir Pol* 1969 (III): 543–546. An extract from this article is an appendix at the end of this chapter.

[67] Charpentier, "Babinski (Joseph)."

[68] L. Babinski, "Sylwetka Jozefa Babinskiego."

of good will finish by winning out over those of evil and that work, helped by charity, will succeed in drying the sources of tears too profuse today. We could thus reach a new era, which will not be too far away, if man wanted to improve.[69]

This Manichaeism can be found as a guiding direction in most of Babinski's works. Separating the organic from the functional, neurological symptoms from psychological ones, brain lesions from malingering or psychic, hysterical, or pithiatic symptoms—in brief, distinguishing between good and evil, true and false, wheat and chaff—was both his obsession and the guiding force behind his accomplishments.

Like many Slavic people, Babinski was marked by a certain mysticism, but, in contrast to others of the same heritage, he was not religious. He respected the convictions of his patients and never advised those with a serious illness against going on a pilgrimage to Lourdes. "He held in abhorrence the narrow-minded, inquisitors, or Masons. He aspired to a world where the blossoming of love and charity, the spiritual waves that light too-short periods, should be always favored."[70] The stone covering the family burial vault in the Polish cemetery in Montmorency that contains the remains of his father, mother, brother, and himself shows no religious symbol, no freethinker or Masonic sign. However, he had, as did his brother a year before, a religious funeral in the Montmorency church.[71]

Babinski's unwavering patriotism applied equally to his parents' two homelands: France, their adopted country, and Poland, the land of their ancestors (see chapter 3).

Backstage

Babinski adored the Paris Opéra, where he was a consulting physician and was regularly on duty.[72] "For a long time, he has been a House regular.

---

[69] E. Moniz, "Dr Joseph Babinski," *Lisboa Médica* 1932 (IX): 1065.
[70] Charpentier, *Un grand médecin*.
[71] Archives de l'Evêché de Pontoise, Registres des actes de sépulture, Paroisse de Montmorency, années 1897, 1899, 1931, 1932 [Archives of the Pontoise bishopric, register of burial acts, Montmorency parish, for the years 1897, 1899, 1931, and 1932]; Rivet, "Joseph Babinski."
[72] Archives de la bibliothèque de l'Opéra de Paris: Service médical. Arrêtés de nomination des médecins de l'Opéra. [Paris Opéra library archives: medical service decree naming physicians on duty at the Opéra], 1880–1900, 1912. Specifications set in 1879 by Jules Ferry, Minister of the Department of Education and Fine Arts, in his article 55,

He has a reserved seat, from where he can be called if necessary. He appreciates music and singing. He likes dance, on the stage and in the Foyer [de la Danse]."[73] It seems that he had a special admiration for the corps de ballet, which was reciprocated.[74] "According to some accounts, Babinski was quite popular in the Paris Opéra milieu; it has been said that on some ballet paintings by Degas it is possible to recognize Babinski's features."[75] While he was an admirer of Frédéric Chopin (1810–1849), Babinski's preferences tended toward lyrics and great voices, like that of the famous tenor Enrico Caruso (1873–1921). From the Opéra, he sometimes returned home "walking, his cane in his hand, striding along the Boulevard Haussmann, rocking from one side to the other, and it was possible to hear him humming: *Adieu, superbe enfant!*"[76] His cousin, Léon Babinski, always well informed, wrote that the son of the famous dancer Mistinguett (1875–1956) had been Babinski's student.[77]

Babinski's passion for music did not prevent him from liking poetry, literature, paintings, and sculpture. He was particularly fond of Victor Hugo (1802–1885), many of whose works he knew almost completely by heart, such as the poems "Ode à la Colonne" and "Mazeppa" and the play *Hernani*. He was a faithful reader of Ernest Renan (1823–1892) and Anatole France (1844–1924). He was a frequent visitor to art galleries, and Léon Babinski recalls that Babinski was present at the private viewing of the Chauchard Collection, given to the Louvre around 1910.[78] He went willingly for a stroll at the Musée du Louvre if he did not leave the hospital too late, returning often to "La Source" by Ingres, the nudes by Corrège, the Venus de Milo, and a painting by Lesueur in which, Babinski is reported to have said, the Virgin Mary is portrayed as "the perfect personification of the beautiful Polish woman (Figs. 2-4 and 2-5)."[79]

---

stipulated that "physicians participating in medical duty at the Opéra will be nominated by the minister, after presentation by the director or after proposition of the Fine Arts department." Carton EB/96, Archives de la Préfecture de Police de Paris.

[73] Tournay, "Babinski dans la vie."

[74] Rivet, "Joseph Babinski."

[75] Babinski, "Sylwetka Jozefa Babinskiego."

[76] Charpentier, *Un grand médecin*.

[77] Babinski, "Sylwetka Jozefa Babinskiego." See also chapter 3.

[78] Ting Chang, "The Limits of the Gift: Alfred Chauchard's Donation to the Louvre," *Journal of the History of Collections* 2005 (17): 213–221.

[79] Charpentier, *Un grand médecin*.

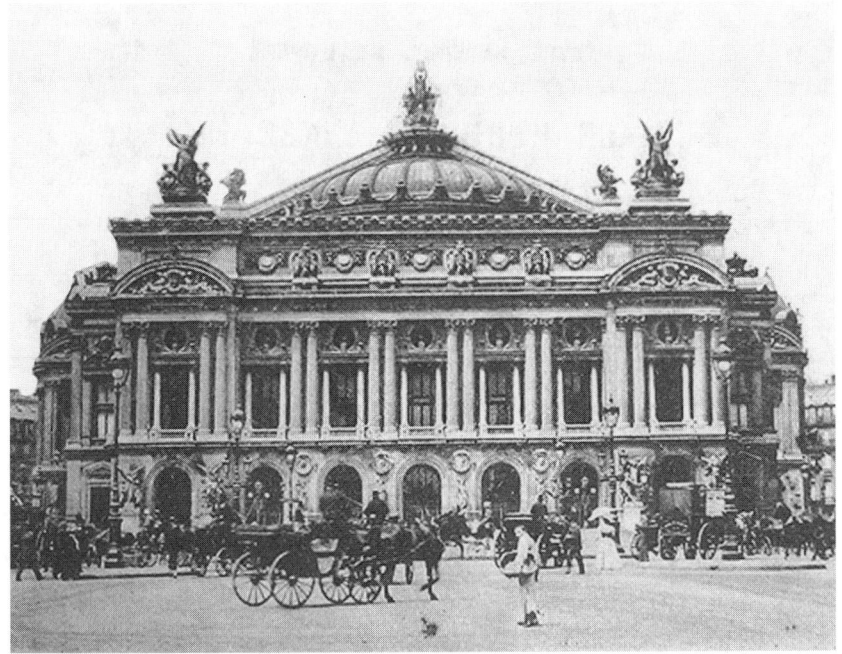

Figure 2-4 Postcard of the Opéra Garnier, Paris, 1898. (*Source*: Personal collection, J. Poirier.)

Love Combined with Admiration

Babinski's charisma explains the friendship and admiration he inspired, which are clearly reflected in the existing biographies.[80] Information about his love affairs is rare, however. The official historiography by his associates and friends mentions that Babinski adopted two or three penniless orphans, daughters of his best friend, and for whom he had given up founding a family in order to provide adequate support.[81] "Babinski, who was a good and affectionate man, certainly would have liked to create a family, as he loved small children, and his friends knew the kind of consideration he showed when taking care of two orphans, daughters of a physician friend."[82]

---

[80] Ibid.
[81] Charpentier, "Babinski (Joseph)"; Charpentier, *Un grand médecin*.
[82] Rivet, "Joseph Babinski."

THÉATRE NATIONAL DE L'OPÉRA

SERVICE MÉDICAL - ANNÉE 1912

MÉDECINS TITULAIRES

Paris-Vendôme. — Imp. H. JARDIN - 31096

1912	BABINSKY F. BOUCHUT ABADIE		FLORANT GUERRIER DE PEZZER		DEBOVE Paul REDARD DEHENNE		LEUDET CHERVIN LELONGT	
Janvier	3	29	8		15		22	
Février	26		5		12		19	
Mars	26		4		14		18	
Avril	22		[illegible]	26	15		17	
Mai	20		27		[illegible]		13	
Juin	17		24		2		16	
Juillet	15		22		[illegible]	28	[illegible]	
Août	12		18		25		15	
Septembre	9		16		28		2	30
Octobre	7		14		28		28	
Novembre	[illegible]		[illegible]		[illegible]		[illegible]	
Décembre	[illegible]	[illegible]	[illegible]		10		28	

Chirurgien : M. VIDAL

Service de Scène : M. MAIN, 17, rue Chaplal

Figure 2-5 List of the Opéra's attending physicians, 1912. (*Source*: Archives de la Bibliothèque du Théâtre National de l'Opéra de Paris.)

"He was extremely devoted to two orphans, whom he surrounded with an extreme solicitude."[83]

Without giving his sources, Khalil said that he had good reason to think that these children were the daughters of Henri Parinaud (1844–1905).[84] This supposed friendship between Babinski and Parinaud is not confirmed;

[83] R. Mainot, "Babinski," *La Vie Médicale* 1932 (22): 977.

[84] Khalil, "Vie et oeuvre de Babinski."

Parinaud, an ophthalmologist associated with Charcot, did not work with Babinski, and Parinaud's biographers do not mention Babinski.[85]

Léon Babinski proposed another version, less politically correct, in which the children were Joseph's out-of-wedlock daughters: "The mother was of Norwegian origin; she lived with her three girls near Paris."[86] Others added that, without recognizing them officially, Babinski played the role of a father.[87] Albert Charpentier, whom it is difficult to suspect of not having deference for his master, noted that Babinski had said: "If I were to discover that a man at the height of his glory had never loved, either by disability or bad luck, I would be deeply sorry for him; what an unhappy man." Charpentier also related that Babinski was able to inspire passion: "I know a most superior woman, a great artist who, far away from him, breathed her last looking at his picture."[88] Might she have been the mother of his daughters?

Finally, the moderate and cautious, even mysterious, words of Auguste Tournay tend to confirm Léon Babinski's version: "In the private life of Joseph Babinski a part belongs to him alone; he did not like to confide, and those who have spoken of this part are probably those who know the least. Let us follow his life, either public or private, in those aspects where there was no secret."[89]

Olaf and Les détraquées: *The Connection with André Breton*

Les détraquées (The mad ones) was a drama written under the names of Olaf and Palau. The two-act play was presented for the first time at the Deux-Masques theater on February 15, 1921.[90] The drama takes place in a private girls' boarding school. At the end of the year, Madame de Challens, head teacher, regularly calls to her office Mademoiselle Solange, professor of dance; both of them, obviously lesbian, subject a young pupil to their cruel perverted tastes, leading to the death of the poor girl.

---

[85] J. M. S. Pearce, "Parinaud's Syndrome," *J Neurol Neurosurg Psychiatry* 2005 (76): 99.
[86] Babinski, "Sylwetka Jozefa Babinskiego."
[87] A. Gasecki and V. Hachinski, "On the Names of Babinski," *Canadian Journal of Neurological Sciences* 1996 (23): 76–79.
[88] Charpentier, *Un grand médecin*.
[89] Tournay, "Joseph Babinski."
[90] In 1986, a movie was made by Jacques Baratier from this play: *L'araignée de satin*, with Catherine Jourdan, Ingrid Caven, Alexandra Sycluna, Michel Albertini, Daniel Mesguich, and Topor.

None among the friends or pupils who knew Babinski and wrote either biographies or obituaries referred to *Les détraquées*.[91] Pierre Palau (1885–1966), who was known by several other pseudonyms besides the single name Palau, was an actor, an author of dramas and comedies, a film director, and a TV series producer.[92] The identity of Olaf was disclosed by André Breton in 1956, in the first issue of his review *Le Surréalisme, même*: it was Joseph Babinski.[93] To carry out his project, Pierre Palau needed the input of a physician who was a specialist in nervous diseases; the surgeon Paul Thiéry put him in touch with Babinski, who agreed to collaborate.[94] Olaf was the first name of many Norwegians and especially of several kings of Norway: Olaf I Trygvason (963–1000); Olaf II Haraldsson of Norway, king and patron saint of Norway (995–1030); Olaf Kyrre, king from 1068 to 1093.[95] The description of this last Olaf corresponds quite well to the portrait of Babinski:

> Olaf was a stout man, well grown in limbs; and every one said a handsomer man could not be seen, nor of a nobler appearance. His hair was yellow as silk, and became him well; his skin was white and fine over all his body; his eyes beautiful, and his limbs well proportioned. He was rather silent in general, and did not speak much even at Things.[96]

It is tempting to find in the choice of this pseudonym an indirect confirmation of the words of Léon Babinski, repeated by Gazecki and Hachinski, regarding the alleged daughters of Babinski and the Norwegian origin of their mother.[97]

Fascinated by mental pathology and attracted by the intensity of attacks in the press against *Les détraquées*, André Breton went to see the play.[98] He was captivated by the actress Blanche Derval, saying that he had been deeply

---

[91] Of his subsequent biographers, only Khalil, in *Vie et oeuvre*, mentioned the play.

[92] Among his pseudonyms were Frederic Brunet, Brunet Pous i Palau, Pierre Palau, Brunet Pous, and Josep Pous. See http://www.imdb.com/name/nm0657404.

[93] *Le Surréalisme même* [Surrealism itself], no. 1, October 1956.

[94] A. Pierron, ed., *Le Grand Guignol, le théâtre des peurs de la Belle Epoque* (Paris: Robert Laffont, 1995), 808–809.

[95] See http://www.scandinavica.com/culture/history/olaf.htm.

[96] From "The Saga of Olaf Kyrre," http://sunsite.berkeley.edu/OMACL/Heimskringla. See also http://www.sepo.net/books/heimskringla/saga-of-olaf-kyrre.

[97] Babinski, "Sylwetka Jozefa Babinskiego"; Gasecki and Hachinski, "On the Names of Babinski" ("Both brothers were unmarried but Joseph had three daughters out of wedlock by a woman of Norwegian origin. Even though Joseph fathered the daughters, who lived and were raised on the outskirts of Paris, he never gave them his name").

[98] M. Antle, *Cultures du surréalisme: les représentations de l'autre* [Cultures of surrealism: representation of the other] (Paris: Acoria, 2001). See also Richard Spiteri's review of the Antle book at http://www.cavi.univ-paris3.fr/Rech_sur/cult_surr.htm.

2. A COMPLEX AND CAPTIVATING PERSONALITY 45

moved and had had one of the greatest theatrical experiences of his life.[99] In 1928, Breton discussed it at length in *Nadja*.[100]

The relationship of André Breton with medicine and especially with psychiatry is unclear and ambivalent, mixing admiration, a fascination with mental disease and perversions, and the denigration of psychiatric practices, particularly in the mental hospitals.[101] In 1913, he began medical studies. Drafted in 1915, Breton first served as a medical orderly at Nantes, then in 1916 was assigned as a resident at the neuropsychiatric center of the Second Army at Saint-Dizier, where he worked under Dr. Leroy, former associate of Charcot. There he studied psychiatric literature and discovered Freud's work; he was especially intrigued by the experience of free association and the story of dreams. In November 1916 he was a stretcher bearer near Verdun; in January 1917 he became a nonresident student at the Neurological Center of La Pitié in Babinski's department.

On November 18, he declared to Théodore Fraenkel: "I may be at the point of feeling a strange and, as usual, resounding admiration for Dr. Babinski. I examine with self-satisfaction the progress in my will. I've asked one of my friends to accord me the vacant position at the neurological department at la Pitié. I shall know in this way if I like it."[102] The result must have been positive, as in 1917 Breton was given the position. In 1962 he wrote in a note to the reedited *Nadja* that he had "great memories" of this period: "I am proud of the liking he showed to me—even if this in no way induced him to predict for myself a grand future in medicine!—and in my own way, I think I have taken advantage of his teaching, to which the end of the first *Manifeste du surréalisme* paid tribute."[103]

---

[99] Pierron, ed., *Le Grand Guignol*, 1376.
[100] A. Breton, *Nadja* (Paris: Gallimard, 1928), 47–62.
[101] C. Drèze, "André Breton, de la médecine et la psychiatrie à la surréalité" [André Breton: from medicine and psychiatry to surrealism], *Louvain Médical* 2003 (122): 367–374. All his remarks on psychiatry and criticism of the mental hospitals appeared in *Nadja*.
[102] Medical student, friend of André Breton, Dadaist, then Surrealist, Fraenkel (1896–1964) studied under Babinski from March 3, 1921, to February 28, 1922, and received the grade of "Very good" from Babinski and "Very good student" from the director of the Pitié. He resigned from his position on May 2, 1922 (Carton 774 FOSS-15, Archives de l'Assistance publique-Hôpitaux de Paris). Théodore Fraenkel published *Carnets de guerre 1916–1918* (Paris: Éditions des Cendres, 1990); see http://entretenir.free.fr/breton69.html.
[103] M. Bonnet, *La rencontre d'André Breton avec la folie, Saint-Dizier, Août-novembre 1916* [André Breton's encounter with insanity, Saint-Dizier, August–November 1916], http://entretenir.free.fr/breton3.html. Breton wrote: "I saw the inventor of the plantar cutaneous reflex at work; he manipulated the patient's body continuously; it was not really an exam that was practiced, it was clear that he did not follow any particular plan. Here and there, he made a remark, far away, without putting down his pin, while his hammer remained active. He left to others this trivial task, patient's treatment.

André Breton's library contained copies of Babinski's works that Babinski had inscribed to his young student.[104]

André Breton was interested and fascinated by Freud, to whom he wrote several times and whom he met in Vienna.[105] However, Freud remained relatively impervious to surrealism, which he did not understand.

> In October 1921, André Breton went to Vienna in order to meet the "greatest psychologists of the time," but came back very disappointed by his contact with "one of the most prosperous manipulators of the modern racket." Instead of a hoped-for God, he had only found a little old man without any stature who receives his patients in an office worthy only of a poor local doctor. Ah, he does not like France very much, where they have remained indifferent to his work.... I tried to start him talking, introducing the names of Charcot and Babinski in the conversation; but either because these memories were too distant or because of his hesitation in the presence of someone unknown, I could not get a word from him other than generalities.[106]

In a letter dated December 26, 1932, Freud wrote to Breton:

> And now a confession which you must accept with tolerance! Although I have received so much evidence of the interest which you and your friends show toward my research, for myself I am not in the position to explain what Surrealism is and what it is after. It could be that I am not in any way made to understand it; I am at such a distance from art.[107]

At the end of World War I, while assigned to the Val-de-Grâce in a psychiatric department, André Breton met Louis Aragon (1897–1982), the future poet and novelist, who became his friend.[108] By early 1920, Breton had definitively left his medical studies.

He was only concerned by this sacred excitement." A. Breton, *Manifeste du surréalisme* [Manifesto of surrealism] (Paris: Éditions du Sagittaire, 1924).

[104] Ibid.

[105] André Breton's book *Les vases communicants* was dedicated to Freud.

[106] A. de Mijolla, "La psychanalyse en France (1893–1965)" [Psychoanalysis in France (1893–1965)], in R. Jaccard, ed., *Histoire de la Psychanalyse* (Paris: Hachette, 1982), II:9–105; see the section "La psychanalyse en France (1893–1965)," available at the Société Psychanalytique de Paris Web site, http://www.spp.asso.fr/Main/HistoirePsy/Histoire/Items/3.htm.

[107] F. B. Davis, "Three Letters from Sigmund Freud to André Breton," *J Am Psychoanal Assoc* 1973 (21): 127–134.

[108] P. Robert, A. Rey, and J. Rey-Debove, eds., *Le grand Robert des noms propres: dictionnaire universel alphabétique et analogique des noms propres* [The great Robert dictionary of proper names] (Paris: Le Robert, 1980, 1989).

APPENDIX

Jozef Babinski: From Day to Day

Léon Babinski[109]   I met Jozef Babinski in 1905 at Zakopane, where he visited when I was there with my parents. But it was only at the time of my studies in Paris during the years 1909–14 that we kept up a more steady contact, which was maintained during my journeys between Warsaw and Paris from 1922 to 1932. Even if Jozef Babinski was not a close relative, our relationship was very cordial; with no other person of his family, did he have the same kind of relationship. Aleksander Babinski—Jozef's father—would have been the son of an administrator of one the great wealths of the magnats [*magnat* was a title given to the true nobility]. He was a "professional" revolutionary, having participated in many different movements in the Principality of Poznan in 1846, in Hungary in 1848, then in the insurrection of 1863, and eventually in the Paris Commune in 1871. He may have been condemned to exile, explaining his departure to Peru. He stayed there for nearly twenty years, working as an engineer on a railway building site. A statue was erected to his memory in Lima. Aleksander Babinski's brother was the emissary of La société démocratique polonaise and was shot by the Germans in 1846 at Poznan.

Jozef Babinski inherited in this way many democratic traditions, which he cultivated during his whole life. He was a friend of a minister, then prime minister, the French radical Waldeck-Rousseau. But at the same time, when my father presented to him in 1909 the photocopy of a title, restored to the Babinski family in 1853 by the Heraldic Society of the Kingdom of Poland, he was most delighted....

As for my personal memories, I would start by recalling my first visit to Jozef Babinski's apartment, located at 170 bis Boulevard Haussmann. It was during the autumn of 1909 and I remember that it was Jozef Babinski himself, very good-looking, who welcomed me warmly. The apartment was large, composed of seven rooms; after the entrance hall, you entered a small study room, which was used as an office for Henryk, Jozef's brother.

On the walls were hung photographs of some famous patients of Jozef Babinski, such as the King of Spain, Alfonso XIII, or Marshal Pétain—at that time a living god of the French and hero of the battle of Verdun. In a corner was a knight's armor. In the middle of a large living room was placed a large

---

[109] Babinski, "Sylwetka Jozefa Babinskiego na tle jego zycia codziennego," *Neurol Neurochir Pol* 1969 (III): 543–546, translated from Polish by Lucyna Haaso-Basta.

table, Louis XV style; in the corner, a Renaissance chest, and on the walls some paintings (notably "La tête" [The head], painted by Olga Boznanska), a bust of Aleksander Babinski, a photograph of Henryeta Weren-Babinska (the mother), a beautiful carpet and masses of curiosities.

The other large room in the apartment was the office of Jozef Babinski. Except for a large desk, there was only a vast bookcase. From these rooms, we proceeded to the dining room, with an elaborate decor, but at the same time very official and dark; it was not used every day. Another room, next to the bedrooms, was used for family meals.

I must also evoke the personality of Henryk, brother of Jozef. Both brothers were bachelors. Henryk took care of the family home and of the correspondence. He has written a well-known recipe book, *Gastronomie Pratique*, published under the pseudonym of Ali-Bab, which has been frequently reissued in the twenty years following its first editions. In 1967, a reproduction of this book was published by Flammarion, and in the menu of the well-known Parisian restaurant Lapérouse appeared a dish called Homard de Babinski.

The childhood and the young years of the Babinski brothers were financially difficult, but the careful education looked after by their mother, always present at their side, compensated for the financial constraints. Jozef's mother was a cultivated person who for several years taught in the notable family Baranowscy at Marszewo in the Principality of Poznan. Henryk was the first to obtain a solid financial position. An engineer, he began working at an early age to help the family. He traveled to far distant countries, conducting geological research. He said that his travels, where he was obliged to feed himself, improved his art of cooking. By the end of the century, forty-four years old, he had at his disposal enough capital to be able, as it was usual at that time, to retire from professional life. He set himself up with his brother and parents on the Boulevard Haussmann.

Jozef reached a high standard of living some years later; but his private-practice medical consultations were well paid (I heard an average of 500 francs for each). He was consulted for various diseases, not only neurological ones. The Babinski brothers were eventually rather wealthy considering the average of the French population. They were both bachelors, but Jozef had three daughters born out of wedlock. Their mother was of Norwegian origin, living with the three girls very close to Paris. According to different testimony, Jozef had great success in the circles of Paris Opéra; it has also been said that in the paintings by Degas of ballet scenes, it is possible to recognize his features.

Family meals were good occasions to meet the Babinski brothers. I was rarely invited to the official receptions, which took place in the large dining room. A smaller room was used for the "ordinary" lunches, at which I was often present; they started precisely at noon. Henryk always said that a guest who is not on time does not deserve to be invited. Usually, all three of us had lunch together, sometimes joined by the engineer-geologist Chacornac. Today I still remember the delicious lobster dish or the calf's head. Jozef Babinski personally served the meat; we drank a light white wine; at the end of his life, the doctor no longer drank wine but rather cider. I never saw anybody eat as rapidly as Jozef Babinski; it was really something phenomenal. After lunch, our host returned to work in his office, and the guests went to the small living room to have coffee and a glass of Armagnac. Afterward (it was nearly 2:00 P.M.), we took a small walk with Henryk, talking of one thing and another, recalling our family memories. Sometimes we went to a café before saying goodbye. Henryk Babinski then made his way towards the apartment of the lady of his heart—a French woman, who survived the Babinski brothers; she attended Jozef's funeral; I was never introduced to her, probably because of modesty.

Jozef Babinski, this exceptional and wise man, had other passions than his beloved medicine; he was interested in dance and music—he had a season ticket at the Paris Opéra. He admired Chopin's works particularly when performed by August Radwan, who by the way was a very good friend of the two brothers. Later, among the students of Jozef Babinski was the son of the famous dancer Mistinguett.

Plastic arts (painting and sculpture) were also subjects of interest for Jozef Babinski. He knew perfectly the art galleries in the great capitals. I remember his presence at the opening of the exhibit of the Chauchard Collection, offered to the Louvre in 1910 by a wealthy trader. Sometimes, during my walks with Henryk, we entered a museum or went to a special exhibit. Jozef Babinski's passion for the arts is reflected in his choice of his vacation destinations: Constantinople, Dolomites, Switzerland, Evian, Zakopane. During these trips, the Babinski brothers were sometimes accompanied by the famous French cardiologist Dr. Vaquez.

Finally, I must mention the question of the national feelings and the Polish traditions that Joseph Babinski held dear. He has certainly been a true and fiery Pole, educated in this sense by his parents, who safeguarded the national traditions. When a child, he frequented the Polish school of Paris, located on rue des Batignolles. The two brothers, but mainly Henryk, spoke and wrote Polish perfectly; however, on a daily basis they used French, even in talking together. When they were speaking Polish, they used out-of-date expressions, sometimes crude; speaking of their distinguished butler, they were using the word *parobek* (flunky), and somebody for whom they had no liking might be called a "fat pig."

The French sometimes forget to mention the Polish origin of Jozef Babinski; in the last edition of the Larousse dictionary in ten volumes, beside the name of Jozef Babinski was written "French physician." My brother and I promptly protested, arguing that if Chopin was qualified in the same dictionary as a Polish musician of French origin, concerning Jozef Babinski one should speak of a French physician of Polish origin. With their excuses, the editorial department admitted that, correcting the error in the next issues (Vol. 1, p. 816).

Jozef Babinski very much appreciated being an honorary member of different Polish scientific societies, such as those of Warsaw, Vilnius, and Poznan. During his career he was often assisted by Polish associates—for example, Dr. J. Jarkowski, or Dr. Karol Vecqueret—and was the associate for a long time of another Polish physician, Dr. Motz.

Everything concerning the activities of the Polish emigrant organizations was more the responsibility of Henryk than of Jozef, very busy with his daily work. For example, Henryk was a member of the administration of the Polish charity Honneur et Pain [Honor and Bread]; I met him often at informal meetings of Polonia. From a political point of view, the Babinski brothers placed themselves within the realistic approach of the more recent immigrants, denouncing the ideas of some representatives of the "old emigration," which could not accept changes occurring in the country, obstinately defending the line of the 1863 national government.

Jozef Babinski, this great scientist, whose research has been and remains a considerable contribution to advances in medicine, was a modest and hearty man in his circle, without any pretension. This was marked to such an extent that the engineer Chacornac, whom we knew, wondered in my presence if Babinski was really conscious of the importance of his work. Dr. Tournay's memoirs, mentioned in the book of Prof. Herman, seem to confirm this supposition.[110]

Even if he died more than thirty years ago, Dr. Babinski is still alive in the memory of his colleagues and within the scientific tradition. A few years ago, on the occasion of the thirtieth anniversary of his death, a street in Paris was named after him. Many hospitals in Poland have done the same.

Despite his Parkinson's disease, Jozef Babinski felt relatively well, complaining only and from time to time of digestive problems, confirming that after the age of seventy, a man feels negative changes in his state of health, particularly between seasons. It was only during the autumn of 1931, when I saw him after the death of his brother, Henryk, that I was struck by a

---

[110] This refers to E. Herman, *Jozef Babinski; jego zycie i dziela* (Warsaw: Panstwowy Zaklad Wydawnictw Lekarskich, 1965).

complete change in him. There was a slight improvement between 1931 and 1932, but not for long. In 1932, after my father's death, I had a final contact when he sent me a handwritten letter, but that was the last correspondence we exchanged.

He lies in the cemetery of Montmorency, beside his brother, Henryk, and his parents. The family vault is kept in good condition; last year, visiting the resting place of our grandfather, we saw fresh flowers lying on the grave. We placed our own by the side of those put down probably by his daughter, a pupil, or perhaps a patient.

—Written in 1967 on the occasion of the 110th anniversary of the Babinski's birth.

··· *three* ···

The Babinskis and Their Polish Roots

At the time of Joseph Babinski's birth in 1857, Poland could boast but a mere shadow of its former glory. Following three successive partitions in the late eighteenth century, it was divided between Austria, Prussia, and Russia. As delimited in 1815 by the Treaty of Vienna, the Kingdom of Poland, also named "the Congress Kingdom," comprised roughly three-quarters of the former Great Duchy of Warsaw and was ruled over by the Russian emperor. Cracow, where Joseph's father was born, became a free city and enjoyed limited autonomy. One might as well say that Poland no longer existed.

Things got worse in 1830, when reprisals for a nationalist insurrection resulted in suppression of the constitution, the Diet, and the Polish army, as well as an intensive Russianization of state institutions. With this came the first wave of Polish emigrants, some well known, such as the poet Adam Mickiewicz (1798–1855) or the musician Frederic Chopin (1810–1849).

New nationalist insurrections in 1846, 1848, and 1861 and above all in 1863 prompted more reprisals and new waves of Polish emigration, particularly to France. Such was the case in 1848 for Aleksander Babinski, Joseph's father. Polish territories occupied by Russians completely lost their autonomy and Russianization increased once again.

During World War I, numerous Polish contingents fought with the French. Following first the fall of the Russian Empire in 1917, then more specifically the German defeat in November 1918, Poland became once again an independent state with the proclamation of a republic.¹ As a result of the Treaty of Versailles (1919), Poland regained several territories; following a conflict with Russia were added those of Byelorussia, Ukraine, and Silesia.

The death of Joseph Babinski in 1932 meant that, perhaps luckily for him, he never knew what followed in the history of his native country in the years before and after World War II.

Babinski's Sentimental Attachment to His Native Country

"Without forgetting any of his Polish roots, [Babinski] always acted as a French citizen."² These words could well be inverted to read: "Always acting as a French patriot, he never forgot his Polish roots." Like many naturalized citizens who were foreign by origin but held French citizenship, the Babinskis were patriotic and almost chauvinistic, more French than those whose French-born families went back over several generations. But at the same time, they remained completely attached to their roots, becoming eventually more Polish than the Poles. This attachment to his two countries was noted by all his friends and pupils.

Joseph Babinski was French by the land of his birth and Polish by blood. As provided for in the conscription law, like many other medical students, he carried out his military service as a one-year volunteer at Lille, thereby avoiding the regular three years of duty owed by draftees.³ As he was born of Polish parents in France, Joseph had to request "his qualification as French according to article 9 of the civil code" in order to be accepted for such voluntary service.⁴

When World War I began, Babinksi was fifty-seven years old. In addition to his departmental responsibilities at la Pitié, he assumed responsibility

---

[1] "Pologne: données historiques" [Poland: historical data], http://www.tlfq.ulaval.ca/axl/europe/pologne-2histoire.htm.

[2] "He fulfilled his military duty and, without forgetting any of his origins, always behaved as a child of France." C. Vincent, "J. Babinski (1857–1932)," *Revue Neurologique*, 1932 (2): 441–446.

[3] "Military duty for medical students was essentially that of a medical orderly, but during the first two months they were trained as soldiers. They were then assigned to military hospitals, where they received specific training as orderlies; after a qualifying examination, they were named to their official functions through the end of their year of duty." *Le Progès Médical*, 1888 (VII, no. 2): 30–31.

[4] Explanatory instructions for the decree of December 1, 1872, on one-year voluntary enlistments, *Journal Officiel*, January 10, 1873, 146–150.

for the treatment of nervous system injuries at the Lycée Buffon, which had been transformed into a military hospital under the direction of Maurice Letulle (1853–1929). Jules Froment (1878–1946), coming from Lyon, became his associate; Maurice Loeper (1875–1961), who worked with him at the Lycée Buffon for several months, testified that he had learned from him all the essentials of neurology while he was there.[5] Babinski was particularly proud of the courage shown by his pupil Clovis Vincent (1879–1947) on the battlefield and was delighted to see him decorated.[6] After the Allied victory, he was touched by the prospect of seeing the Polish cavalry parade down the Champs-Elysées, and he and his brother, Henri, were especially delighted to see their homeland finally restored.[7]

Babinski's service to France was recognized by his being named a commander in the Legion of Honor. He showed his patriotism in other ways as well, for example, by subscribing five hundred francs in 1915 to the Caisse d'assistance médicale de guerre de l'Association générale des médecins de France.[8]

At the same time, he remained deeply attached to his Polish roots.[9] As we have seen, his secondary studies were at a Polish school in Paris, and he wrote and spoke Polish, even if less fluently than his brother.[10] He published medical papers in Polish scientific journals, maintained close contacts with Polish universities and scientific societies, and was a member of the editorial committee of the Polish journal *Neurologia Polska*. In 1909 he chaired the first meeting of Polish neurological, psychiatric, and psychological professionals. In 1920 his name was proposed for a neurological chair at Warsaw University; in 1925 he became an honorary professor of neurology at the University of Vilnius, and he was an honorary member of the Neurological Societies of Warsaw and Cracow and of the Medical School of

---

[5] A. Tournay, "Babinski dans la vie" [Babinski in everyday life], *La Presse Médicale* 1958 (66): 1485–1489; M. Loeper, "Babinski," *Le Progrès médical* 1932 (45): 1885.

[6] A. Tournay, *La vie de Joseph Babinski* [The life of Joseph Babinski] (Amsterdam: Elsevier, 1967); Tournay, "Babinski dans la vie."

[7] R. Moreau, "Hommage à la mémoire de Joseph Babinski à l'occasion du 100è anniversaire de sa naissance" [Homage to the memory of Joseph Babinski on the occasion of the 100th anniversary of his birth], *Bull Mém Soc Méd Hôp Paris* 1958 (74): 449–457; T. Alajouanine, "Le centenaire de Babinski" [The centennial of Babinski], *Sem Hôp Paris* 1958 (22): 1355–1364; L. Daudet, "Babinsky" [sic], *Action Française*, October 30, 1932.

[8] Professor Pitres, from Bordeaux, gave only 200 francs, and Professor Dejerine gave 300 francs, whereas Babinski and his friends Widal and Vaquez gave 500 francs. *La Presse Médicale*, 1915 (supp. to no. 56): 427, (supp. to no. 57): 438.

[9] A. Gasecki and H. Kwiecinski, "On the legacy of Joseph Babinski," *Eur Neurol* 1995 (35): 127–130.

[10] "Nécrologie d'Henri Babinski" [Obituary of Henri Babinski], in *Bulletin de l'Association des Anciens Élèves de l'École des Mines de Paris*, 1931, http://www.annales.org/archives/x/babinsky.html.

Lvov. A group of Polish professors proposed him for the Nobel Prize, but he was not selected. He missed no opportunity to show his attachment to Poland, and he asked the editor of his biography in an encyclopedia to add "of Polish origin" after "French physician."[11]

The first joint meeting of French and Polish physicians took place in Warsaw in 1921. Babinski was present, and the welcome he received clearly showed that he was considered a national hero.[12] On the occasion of the second meeting in Paris, four years later, the Académie de Médecine organized a special session on April 23, 1925, during which the presentation of papers was reserved for "scientists of Polish origin or nationality."[13] Only two French citizens made a speech: Marie Curie (1867–1934) spoke on the preparation of radioactive materials not currently used in medicine, and Joseph Babinski presented a paper on the cerebellar syndrome, studied by motion picture and histological sections.[14]

As shown by their signatures, Joseph Babinski and his brother spelled their name with an accent on the *n* (*ń*), a letter characteristic of the Polish alphabet.[15] In the same vein, quite frequently their name is incorrectly spelled "Babinsky," with a *y*.[16] In the Polish language (contrary to Russian), this name ends with an *i*. In a manuscript letter, Joseph insisted on this and on a correct Polish pronunciation.[17] The *n* in Babinski should not be pronounced with the English value of "in," as in "information,"[18] but, as pointed out by Gazecki and Hachinski, as in "cognac" or "armagnac."[19] Unfortunately, French neurologists kept the habit of writing the name without an accent on the *n* and pronouncing the *n* incorrectly.

---

[11] L. Babinski, "Sylwetka Jozefa Babinskiego na tle jego zycia codziennego" [Babinski day by day], *Neurol Neurochir Pol* 1969 (XIX): 543–546.

[12] L. Le Sourd, "Le docteur Joseph-François-Félix Babinski (1857–1932)," *Gazette des hôpitaux* 1932 (92): 1681.

[13] *Bulletin de l'Académie de Médecine* 1925 (XCIII): 415–452.

[14] Marie Curie (born Maria Sklodowska) was born in Warsaw and came to Paris to study in 1891. She became the first female professor at the Faculty of Science. Her work on radioactive isotopes, particularly on radium, was recognized in 1903 by a Nobel Prize in physics, shared with her husband, Pierre Curie, and that in chemistry in 1911.

[15] A. Gazecki and W. Hachinski, "On the names of Babinski," *Can J Neurol Sci* 1996 (23): 76–79.

[16] A. O. Orden, "Que Babinsky?" *Medicina (Buenos-Aires)* 1999 (59): 119. The incorrect spelling can be seen, for example, at the bottom of the engraving "Charcot Lesson."

[17] Archives nationales, Dossier Légion d'honneur L0085063.

[18] J. Fulton, "Joseph François Félix Babinski, 1857–1932," *Archives of Neurology and Psychiatry* 1933 (29): 168–174.

[19] Gazecki and Hachinski, "On the names of Babinski."

3. THE BABINSKIS AND THEIR POLISH ROOTS

Joseph Babinski maintained close relationships with many Polish physicians, such as Karol Vecqueret, associate to Dr. Motz.[20] Léon Babinski's father sent two of his residents from the Evangelist Hospital to him for periods of training.[21] Closest of all was Edouard Pozerski de Pomiane (1875–1964). A number of similarities exist between de Pomiane and the Babinski brothers, which no doubt reinforced their friendship.

As was the case for the Babinskis, de Pomiane had Polish parents who fled their country and found shelter in Paris; his mother had been sentenced to death during the Polish rebellion of 1863, and his father had been sent to the same concentration camp in Siberia as Dostoyevsky.[22] Following his studies at the Polish School of Paris, he decided to become a physician. To make some extra money, as a part-time job Pozerski checked on Babinski's patients.[23] After his doctoral thesis he moved on to a scientific career, taking over the direction of a laboratory at the Pasteur Institute.[24] Like Henri, he was also a gourmet and a gastronomical writer. In the spirit of their friendship, Henri wrote a preface (under his pseudonym, Ali-Bab) the first of the numerous books de Pomiane wrote on gastronomy.[25] He was also certainly a friend to Joseph, and it can be supposed that in 1917 when Joseph, demoralized and depressed, thought of abandoning neurology for a laboratory at the Pasteur Institute, the presence there of Edouard Pozerski could well have been a motivation.[26] Just like the members of the Babinski family, Edouard Pozerski is also buried in the Champeaux cemetery at Montmorency.

Born in Moscow on February 1, 1880, Jean Jarkowski (1880–1929) was of Polish nationality and held medical degrees from both the St. Petersburg

---

[20] Babinski, "Sylwetka Jozefa Babinskiego."
[21] Ibid.
[22] "Edouard Pozerski (20 avril 1875–26 janvier 1964)," *Annales de l'Institut Pasteur* 1964 (196): 813–818.
[23] E. Pozerski de Pomiane, *Souvenirs d'un demi-siècle à l'Institut Pasteur* [A half century of memories at the Pasteur Institute," typewritten brochure, n.d., Archives de l'Institut Pasteur, 56.
[24] See http://www.pasteur.fr/infosci/archives/poz1.html; "L. Edouard Pozerski (20 avril 1875–26 janvier, 1964)."
[25] E. de Pomiane, *Bien manger pour bien vivre. Essai de gastronomie théorique* [Eat well to live well: an essay on theoretical gastronomy] (Paris: Albin Michel, 1922). The preface is appended at the end of this chapter. Pomiane's reputation extends far beyond the borders of France. English translations, especially *Cooking with Pomiane*, have met with great success in the United States.
[26] A. Charpentier, "Babinski (Joseph)" in M. Genty, ed., *Les biographies médicales* [Medical biographies] (Paris: Librairie J. B. Baillière et fils, 1937–39), VI: 17–32.

and Warsaw Universities.[27] Fleeing the Russian oppression, he came to France in 1908. He became a "voluntary associate" of Joseph Babinski at La Pitié in 1908 and published numerous papers in collaboration with Babinski or his pupils, especially at the Société de Neurologie.[28] From October 9, 1914, to June 1, 1919, he served as a volunteer in the French Army with the rank of medical officer, first on the front line, then from August 14, 1918, in Babinski's neurological department. He received the Military Cross in June 1917. After the war, he defended his medical thesis at Strasburg University on Parkinsonian paradoxical kinesis. In 1925, he became an associate professor at Warsaw University but continued to publish in Paris. A member of the Société de Neurologie, he was decorated with the Legion of Honor in 1927.[29]

After Babinski's retirement, Jarkowski published on his own.[30] He died in Paris at the age of forty-nine; Babinski was deeply affected. Writing in *La Presse Médicale*, Oscar Crouzon (1874–1938) concluded Jarkowski's obituary with these words, celebrating the man's greatness: "The rare friends present in Paris during the month of August met at the Church of Notre-Dame des Champs: in the tribute paid by the Polish groups with their unfurled flags they realized how important he was not only to neurological science, but also to the revival of charitable institutions and Polish associations through the efforts made by this dedicated man, this great patriot, and great friend of France, whose premature death we deplore."[31]

When he was to be promoted to the rank of commander in the Legion of Honor, Babinski solicited as his sponsor Count Maurice Zamoyski, but this was challenged by the Great Chancellery because a foreigner, even with substantial credentials, could not endorse a French citizen. Count Zamoyski, special envoy and plenipotentiary minister of the Polish Republic in Paris,

---

[27] O. Crouzon, "Jean Jarkowski (1880–1929)," *La Presse Médicale* 1930 (14): 246; Archives nationales, Dossier Légion d'honneur L1355013.
[28] Ibid.
[29] Ibid.
[30] J. Jarkowski, "Essai d'application thérapeutique de l'osmium, en particulier dans la sclérose en plaques (Note préliminaire)" [Essay on the therapeutic use of osmium, especially in multiple sclerosis (preliminary remarks)], *Rev Neurol (Paris)* 1929 (I): 631–633.
[31] Crouzon, "Jean Jarkowski." Jarkowski served as an expert to the emigration committee of the International Labor Organization and president for social and intellectual development at the Society for Polish Workers in France, and he participated in the work of the French-Polish health commission. As part of the exceptional services noted for his candidacy to the Legion of Honor, mention is made of "promotion in favor of French medical science among Polish charitable institutions, contributing to strengthened relationships between Polish immigrants and French population." Archives nationales, Dossier Légion d'honneur L1355013.

represented the president of the Polish Republic during the signing of the Treaty of peace between the Allied and Associate powers and Turkey signed at Sèvres on August 10, 1920.[32] The Zamoyski family, among the most well-known families of the Polish nobility, owned a Warsaw mansion, the Blue Palace, where they held one of the liveliest downtown salons, at which Frederic Chopin and Alexandre Rembielinski had given several recitals, and where Chopin made his first public appearance at the age of five.[33]

Ignace Meyerson (1888–1983), who established the field of comparative historical psychology, was largely responsible for the spread of psychology to the social sciences and humanities (history, sociology, linguistics, fine arts).[34] Born in Warsaw, he had to flee to Germany after having taken part in the 1905 insurrection; he eventually arrived in Paris, where he started his scientific, philosophical, and medical studies. A nonresident student (*externe*) of Babinski's in 1911–12 and then again in 1915, he became a resident at the Salpêtrière in the departments of Philippe Chaslin and Jean Nageotte. He worked in the physiological laboratory of Louis Lapicque at the Sorbonne. He was then appointed assistant professor at the Psychological Laboratory of the Sainte-Anne hospital. Pierre Janet asked him to start up the *Journal de Psychologie*, and his success in doing so was rewarded with a prize by the Académie des sciences. Secretary of the Société de psychologie until 1939, he was named to the chair of comparative psychology at the *École pratique des hautes études* in 1951.

One may also mention Joseph Obalski (1852–1915), who graduated as an engineer from the Ecole des mines de Paris the same year as Henri and who remained a close friend, and Sophie Rosenblum, born in Poland, a nonresident student in 1912–13 under Babinski, who supervised her thesis.[35] Henri Babinski gave a speech in memory of Joseph Obalski (1852–1915), published in the *Bulletin de l'Association des anciens élèves de l'Ecole des Mines de Paris*, July and August 1915.

---

[32] See http://www.senat.cz/zajimavosti/tisky/1vo/tisky/T0225_04.htm.

[33] "Une dynastie d'ingénieurs-géographes lyonnais au XIXè siècle, les Dignoscyo-Rembielinski" [A dynasty of Lyonnais engineer-geographers in the nineteenth century: the Dignoscyo-Rembielinskis], http://www.archives-lyon.fr/old/fonds/plan-g/25.htm.

[34] On Meyerson, see http://www.univ-paris12.fr/scd/meyerson/i-meyerson-frame.htm; http://www.upsy.net/upsychologie/ancetres/meyerson.htm; http://www.pasteur.fr/infosci/archives/mey1.html.

[35] S. Rosenblum, *Du développement du système nerveux au cours de la première enfance. Contribution à l'étude des syncinésies, des réflexes tendineux et cutanés et des réflexes de défense* [Development of the nervous system during early childhood. Contribution to a study on syncinesis, tendon and cutaneous reflexes and defense reflexes] (Paris: Le François, 1915).

Babinski also had close contacts with the well-known Polish neurologists Samuel Goldflam (1852–1932) and Edward Flatau (1869–1932) not only in Poland but also at the Société de neurologie de Paris, where both of them, along with C. Orzechowski, W. Mitkus, and others, made oral presentations and published several papers in French in the *Revue Neurologique*.[36]

A Polish neurologist known mainly for the original description in 1893 of myasthenia or Erb-Goldflam disease, Goldflam attended the lectures of Karl Westphal (1833–1890) and Charcot in 1882 before returning to Warsaw. During World War I, he worked at the Jewish Hospital with his friend Edward Flatau. Considered a neurological genius, Goldflam was also an artist and a Beethoven admirer, and he helped the careers of many young artists.

Flatau is one of the best-known Polish neurologists. Trained alongside Sergei Korsakoff (1854–1900) and Alexis Kozhevnikof (1836–1902), he published in 1894 his *Atlas of the Human Brain and Description of the Course of the Nerve Fibers*, in German, English, French, and Russian, and two years later in Polish. In 1897, after clinical observations and animal experimentation, he discovered that the greater the length of the fibers in the spinal cord, the closer they are situated to the periphery (Flatau's law). His work also dealt with the neuronal anatomy and physiology and their modification under the influence of mechanical, thermal, or toxic factors; in addition, he studied child spasm distortion, spinal cord and spine tumors, migraine, disseminated epidemic encephalomyelitis (Flatau-Redlich disease), and periaxial diffuse encephalitis (Shilder disease). Chief of the neurobiological department of the Scientific Society of Warsaw, and then chief of the neurological department at the Jewish Hospital, Flatau had a recognized referral practice and was also a passionate Polish patriot who fought for democratic causes.

---

[36] On Goldflam, see http://www.whonamedit.com/doctor.cfm/1349.html; on Flatau, see http://www.whonamedit.com/doctor.cfm/318.html. See C. Orzechowski and W. Mitkus, "De la forme parkinsonienne des tumeurs de la région infundibulo-hypophysaire" [On the Parkinsonian form of tumors in the infundibulo-hypophysaire region], *Rev Neurol (Paris)* 1925(II):1–17; E. Flatau, "De la radiothérapie des tumeurs du cerveau et de la moelle" [On radiotherapy of cerebral and spinal tumours], *Rev Neurol (Paris)* 1924 (I): 23–40, 176–191; E. Flatau and B. Sawicki, "Kyste hémorragique intradural du sac spinal" [Intradural hemorrhagic cyst in the spinal sac], *Rev Neurol (Paris)* 1925 (I): 590–591; E. Flateau, "Recherches expérimentales sur la perméalibilité de la barrière nerveuse centrale" [Experimental research on the permeability of the central nervous system barrier], *Rev Neurol (Paris)* 1926 (II): 521–540; S. Goldflam, "Sur la valeur clinique du signe de Gordon. Réflexe paradoxal des fléchisseurs. Phénomène paradoxal des orteils et du mollet" [On the clinical value of Gordon sign. Paradoxical reflex of the flexor muscles. Paradoxical phenomenon of toes and calf], *Rev Neurol (Paris)* 1925 (I): 590.

While it is a supposition, one may wonder if Babinski met with the sculptor Georges Clément de Swiecinski (1878–1958), of Polish origin, who, after having come to Paris in 1902 to finish his surgical studies, became totally involved in sculpture after the war, and lived in Guéthary, a small village in the Basque country.[37] Albert Charpentier, a beloved pupil of Babinski, retired to Guéthary, and there is a picture of Joseph Babinski in Guéthary in 1930 beside an unidentified woman.

Aleksander Babinski

Born in Zwierzyniec, a suburb of Cracow, Aleksander Babinski fled Warsaw to escape the terror inflicted by the Russians after the Polish rebellion of 1848, in which he participated.[38]

In the most widely held version of Aleksander's life following his emigration to Paris, he was a civil engineer and surveyor at the Inspection des carrières.[39] He married a Polish woman, Henryeta Weren (1819–1897). He returned to Warsaw during the 1863 insurrection, in which he had an active role. Aleksander then left for Peru, where he was offered a well-paid position, allowing him to send subsidies to his wife for the support and education of their two sons. He stayed in Peru for more than eight years, and when the war with Chile began in 1879 he worked for the Peruvian defense, in recognition of which the Peruvian government placed his bust on a monument erected in Lima to the memory of Polish immigrants.[40] He returned

---

[37] See http://musee.guethary.free.fr.
[38] However, without citing his sources, R. Khalil sets his birth in Radom. R. Khalil, "Vie et oeuvre de Babinski" [The life and work of Babinski], in *Conférences lyonnaises d'histoire de la neurologie et de la psychiatrie* (Lyon: Documentation médicale Oberval, 1982).
[39] L. Rivet, "Joseph Babinski (1857–1932)," *Bull Mém Soc Méd Hôp Paris* 1932 (34): 1722–1733; H. Vaquez, "Joseph Babinski (1857–1932)," *Bulletin de l'Académie de Médecine* 1932 (35): 1264–1273; Charpentier, "Babinski (Joseph)"; Tournay, "Babinski dans la vie"; Alajouanine, "Le centenaire de Babinski"; *Josef Feliks Franciszek Babinski (1857–1932)* (Opole: Oficyna Wyd. Politechniki Opolskiej, 2000). The Inspection des carrières was created in 1777, after the impressive collapse of the rue d'Enfer three years before. Its objective was to list, map, and reinforce the underground empty spaces threatening the capital. Becoming later the Inspection générale des carrières, it continued to update a precise atlas of the Parisian underground. See http://www.troude.com/CarrieresTexte/CarrieresTexte.html-ssi.
[40] The "Habich monument" was erected in Lima in 1913 by the French sculptor Charles Perron (1862–1934). Edward Jan Habich (1835–1909), engineer and mathematician, professor of technology at Warsaw University, participated in the 1863 rebellion and was

to France around 1870, participating in the defense of Paris by joining the National Guard.

Another version, very different and probably closer to reality, can be extracted from Stefan Bratkowski's research in Polish archives.[41] According to this account, Aleksander married Henryeta in Poland and they came to France in 1849. The financial situation of the emigrants at that time was difficult, and poverty prevailed in the Polish circles in Paris. In 1852, the Babinski couple resided in what was considered cheap accommodations at the Hotel Corneille. Having attended courses at the École préparatoire (which later became the École supérieure polonaise, at 129 boulevard Montparnasse) and perhaps several at the École des mines, Aleksander found a comfortable job as an engineer-surveyor in Paris. When the Polish insurrection of 1863 broke out in January, he returned to his native land to organize the provision of weapons, leaving his sons, Henri and Joseph, under the care of his wife. Returning to Paris in 1871, he participated in the Paris Commune.[42] After the Commune, he was hired as an engineer by Pedro Galvez, the Peruvian envoy in Paris, and left to work in Peru in 1874, where he remained until 1887.[43] During his stay in South America, which encompassed the war between Peru and Chile, he earned a good reputation "because of his knowledge, tremendous activity, and very honest character (Fig. 3-1)."[44]

---

forced to emigrate to France. He then left for Peru, founding in 1876 in Lima a school of engineering studies (Universidad Nacional de Ingeniería). He was a member of the Peruvian Geographical Society and made a freeman of Peru. The town of Lima has also a public garden bearing his name and a museum dedicated to him. Edward Habich was a member of the Société Mathématique de France. *Bulletin de la Société Mathématique de France* 1885 (13): 5–12; "Exploring South America," *Warsaw Voice*, July 3, 2003, http://www.warsawvoice.pl/view/2824; http://en.wikipedia.org/wiki/Edward_Jan_Habich; http://encyclopedia.thefreedictionary.com/Universidad+Nacional+de+Ingenier%eda.

[41] S. Bratkowski, "Inzynierowie Babinscy," [Babinski engineer] *Kwartalnik Historii Nauki I Techniki* 1975 (XX): 295–311.

[42] Léon Babinski indicates that "Aleksander Babinski…was a professional revolutionary, as he participated in the revolutionary movements in the Great Principality of Poznan in 1846, in Hungary in 1848, then in the insurrection of 1863, and finally possibly in the Paris Commune in 1871, as he was afterward sent by France into exile, explaining his departure to Peru." Babinski, "Sylwetka Jozefa Babinskiego."

[43] It is legitimate to presume that Aleksander, having been recruited as an engineer, had a diploma (or equivalent) in civil engineering.

[44] "Between 1879 and 1883, the Pacific war opposed Peru and Chile for the control of the Tarapaca province, rich in nitrates. Defeated and deprived of part of their territory, ruined by years of war and internal dissensions, Peruvians tried then to reorganize themselves." See http://www.americas-fr.com/histoire/perou.html. The passage about Aleksander is quoted in Bratkowski, "Inzynierowie Babinscy."

3. THE BABINSKIS AND THEIR POLISH ROOTS 63

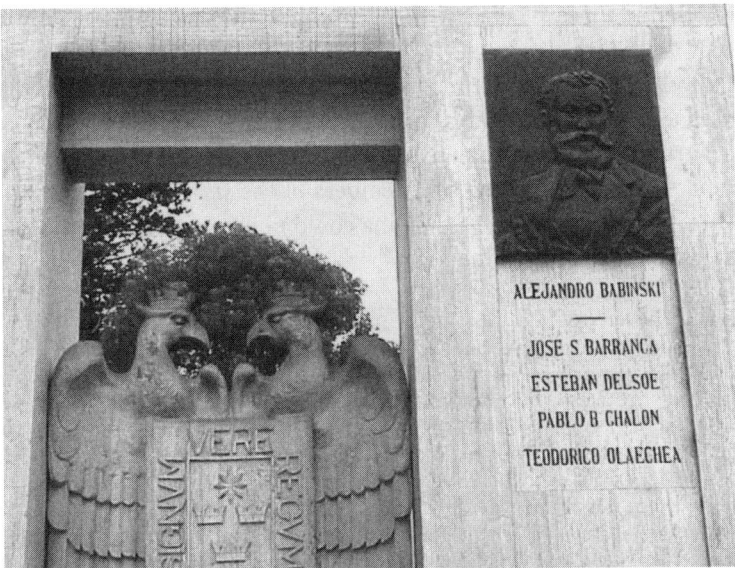

Figure 3-1 The Habich Monument in Lima, Peru, with bas-relief of the bust of Alexander Babinski, Joseph's father. (*Source*: Courtesy of Dr. Diana Rivas and Ms. Mariella Aleman.)

The participation of Aleksander Babinski in the Paris Commune is worth a closer look. In fact, it seems logical to attribute to his father's personal experiences the bad memories Joseph had from that period, when he was fourteen (see chapter 2). He professed "a true antipathy for [Adolphe] Thiers and the strong-arm tactics he used against the insurgents."[45] The extent of Aleksander's engagement in the Commune is not addressed directly by Joseph's biographers, who refer to his stint in the National Guard only as an indication of his "attachment to his adoptive country," which led him to place himself "at the service of France," "at the disposal of the Government of the National Defense."[46] In reality, as was the case for many Polish refugees, Aleksander actively participated in the Paris Commune. In the *Dictionnaire des polonais ayant participé à la Commune de Paris*, it is said only that Alexandre Babinski, living on the boulevard Montparnasse, was mentioned by Belina in his book *Les polonais et la Commune de Paris*.[47]

---

[45] Charpentier, "Babinski (Joseph)."
[46] Alajouanine, "Le centenaire de Babinski"; Charpentier, "Babinski (Joseph)"; Tournay, "Babinski dans la vie."
[47] "Dictionnaire des Polonais ayant participé à la Commune de Paris" [Dictionary of Poles who participated in the Commune of Paris], Archives nationales, carton

Indeed, Belina, fiercely against the Commune, was delighted to quote the words of the Polish newspaper *Gazeta Narodowa*, which listed thirty-seven Poles who had disappeared or been killed after having been caught carrying weapons, and the names of thirty-one other Poles "who were prosecuted in a court-martial." In this list one may find the names of Julien and Aleksander Babinski, who are also listed as "members of the International," as an allusion to communist affiliations.[48] Belina could not resist dragging these Polish communards through the mud:

> We have never stopped warning France that she was warming up vipers in her bosom that one day would viciously bite her. Today experience is the proof that our judgment was not too severe. Our expectations have been exceeded; the whole revolutionary mob had rushed into Paris and against the Parisian bourgeoisie, which had for such a long time applauded, honored, and fed them. O! philanthropists and polonophiles! What do you think of these "good Poles" who have shed French blood, burnt the city that had offered them hospitality, and spat in the full plate you have given them over so many years?... Will France finally recognize that the time has come to open her eyes to these expensive and dangerous guests and put an end to the anarchist propaganda spread by all revolutionaries in general and especially the Poles, insulting authority, breaking laws, killing French people in their streets, and even daring to write in their newspapers that they are persecuted in France?

No doubt not all the members of the National Guard who took part in the Commune were fierce revolutionaries; many of them, in fact, were more or less forced to participate.[49] Prince Czartoryski insisted on that point in his "Mémoire justificatif du Comité de l'émigration polonaise," an appendix in Belina's book.[50] Antoine Errera's "La Garde nationale sous la Commune de Paris, 1871" used three concrete examples to show that the participants' motivations were not always revolutionary.[51]

AB/XIX/3779, dossier 4; A. Mlochowski de Belina, *Les polonais et la Commune de Paris* [The Poles and the Paris Commune] (Paris: Librairie générale, 1871).

[48] The military justice archives in the Ministère de la défense contain no record of a criminal file for Alexander Babinski, nor he is in the alphabetical listing of those condemned or released. Letter from Louis de Contenson, head of the Historical Services of the Defense Ministry, June 25, 2006.

[49] See http://lacomune.club.fr/pages/Actua2003B18/pageactua/page3.html.

[50] Prince L. Czartoryski et al., "Mémoire justificatif du Comité de l'émigration polonaise" [Justifying memorandum of the Committee on Polish Emigration], appendix in Belina, *Les polonais et la Commune de Paris.*

[51] See 43 ème Concours de l'Historien de demain, Paris, Archives Nationales, May 1996, esp. the appendixes.

It is thought that upon his return from Peru in 1887, Aleksander Babinski might have found a job as a librarian at the École des mines de Paris.[52] Severely handicapped by Parkinson's disease, he died on January 31, 1899, in the apartment where he resided with Joseph.

Henryeta Weren-Babinska

The Babinski brothers' mother, Henryeta Weren-Babinksa, from the area of Wilno, was a well educated person and had taught for several years in the noted Baranowscy family at Marszewo, in the principality of Poznan.[53] In Paris, she learned French, and made many sacrifices to give her two sons a very good education. Henri and Joseph would show deep love and appreciation for their mother throughout their lives. At her death, the *Bulletin polonais littéraire, scientifique et artistique* paid tribute to "this valiant Polish woman, who had been an incomparable spouse and mother."[54]

French naturalization records make no mention of Aleksander or of Henryeta, nor is there any trace of a marriage certificate in Paris or of religious funerals at the church of Montmorency. These elements suggest that, according with some sources but contradicting others, Aleksander and Henryeta met in Poland, where they were married before coming to France, and never applied for French citizenship.

Henri Babinski

It would not be fair to let the reputation of Joseph Babinski among physicians, especially neurologists, overshadow the very interesting personality and memorable work of his brother, Henri (1855–1931). Henri, who was corpulent, was nicknamed "the big" by their closest friends and was born two years before Joseph, who was called "the young," "my little brother," or simply "Jo."[55]

---

[52] A. Plichet, "Babinski (1857–1932)," in R. Dumesnil et F. Bonnet-Roy, eds., *Les médecins célèbres* [Famous physicians] (Genève: Editions d'Art Lucien Mazenod, 1947), 250–251.
[53] "Z wilenszczyzny," *Polski slownik biogr.*; Babinski, "Sylwetka Jozefa Babinskiego," 546. Wilno is today known as Vilnius and is the capital of Lithuania.
[54] *Bulletin polonais littéraire, scientifique et artistique* 1898 (114): 31.
[55] Rivet, "Joseph Babinski."

Like his brother, he was deeply attached to his two countries: "Son of refugees, born and raised in France to which I am indebted for everything, having spent part of my life in foreign countries and going to Poland only as a place of pilgrimage, I developed a religious cult for my country of origin, being at the same time deeply attached to my adoptive country."[56] He was a member of the Polish charitable association Honneur et pain and attended the meetings of Polonia.

A Rough but Generous Man

Not as tall as his brother, Henri was high-spirited, often ironical, and his speech was accompanied by an occasional slight stutter. He tended to be frank and undiplomatic, but his classmates at the École des mines recall a joyful companion, and several families of engineers who fell on hard times could testify to his sympathy and generosity.[57] A lover of food, he became overweight around forty, happily showing off what he called "the marks of his weaknesses."[58]

Profession: Engineer

Having successfully passed a highly competitive examination, Henri entered the prestigious École des mines de Paris in 1875. During a year of preparatory studies, he had taken a position as proctor in a local high school in order not to be a financial burden for his parents.[59]

His school record, while quite acceptable, was not particularly brilliant. In his first year, he submitted a handwritten report of 72 pages on a study trip in Belgium concerning coal mining.[60] At the end of that year, he ranked fifth out of twenty-one students and was admitted to the upper class.[61] The next year, a report of 188 pages was devoted to lead mining in Pontgibaud

---

[56] *Bulletin de l'Association des anciens élèves de l'École des mines de Paris*, December 1923.
[57] A. Rey, "Nécrologie d'Henri Babinski" [Obituary of Henri Babinski], in *Bulletin de l'Association des anciens élèves de l'École des mines de Paris*, January–February 1931. http://www.annales.org/archives/x/babinsky.html; Charpentier, "Babinski (Joseph)."
[58] Ibid.
[59] Vaquez, "Joseph Babinski."
[60] Archives de l'École nationale des mines, "Comptes-rendus de voyage de MM. les élèves 1876 (1), N° 169 Babinski."
[61] Archives de l'École nationale des mines, meeting of School Council, June 13, 1876.

in central France.[62] Placing fifth out of eighteen and having passed all his partial exams, he was admitted into the next class.[63] At the end of his third year, he was again ranked fifth out of eighteen, but just missed passing two partial exams (on the railway, scoring 93 out of 100, and on legislation, with 89 out of 100); however, he was "proposed by the council for a diploma" and became a qualified mining civil engineer in 1880.[64]

As soon as he left the school, he was named director of a zinc factory and astutely organized the recovery of waste material from coal washing plants so it could be used as fuel for the foundry. He successfully supervised the relocation of the plant but was obliged to resign after a stormy meeting with the president of the company that owned the factory, Count de Lagrange, who was well known on the racetrack thanks to his famous horse Gladiateur.[65]

After working a few months in Italy, Henri was put in charge of prospecting for gold in French Guyana, along the Maroni River.[66] In 1888, he published his mission report as a sixteen-page pamphlet, concluding that Guyana was especially rich in gold deposits.[67] The future would substantiate his assertion: 207 metric tons of gold have been extracted to date, and in 2004, the Bureau des recherches géologiques et minières estimated the gold reserves in French Guyana still at 500 metric tons.[68]

Back in South America in 1893, traveling on a small rented boat, he explored Patagonia in order to verify whether gold and diamonds might be found in the extreme south of the continent, but found no trace of those.[69] On the other hand, he discovered rich coal resources and proposed creating a coal-supplying station in the Straits of Magellan for boats taking this route between the Atlantic and Pacific oceans, though the project would never materialize.

---

[62] Archives de l'École nationale des mines, "Journaux de voyage de MM. Les élèves 1877, N° 579 Babinski (J 1877/579)."

[63] Archives de l'École nationale des mines, meeting of School Council, June 12, 1877.

[64] Archives de l'École nationale des mines, meeting of School Council, June 13, 1878.

[65] Rey, "Nécrologie de Henri Babinski."

[66] Ibid.

[67] H. Babinski, *Quelques mots sur les gisements aurifères de la Guyane française et en particulier sur les recherches des filons dans cette contrée. Suivis d'une notice sommaire sur les gisements appartenant à la Société de Saint-Elie* [A few words on the gold deposits in French Guyana and, especially, on searching for lodes in this area. Followed by a brief note on the deposits held by the Société de Saint-Elie] (Paris: Imprimerie Barthe et fils, 1888).

[68] M.-P. Ferey, "La Guyane rongée par la nouvelle fièvre d'or," Agence France-Presse, October 26, 2004, http://www.jne-asso.org/dossiers_guyane.html.

[69] Bratkowski, "Inzynierowie Babinscy."

In addition to his extended studies in French Guyana and Patagonia, Henri Babinski undertook several other prospecting assignments: in the far west of the United States, in northern Italy, and in diamond and carbon mines in the state of Bahia in Brazil.

At the age of forty-four, after more than twenty years of difficult and tiring exploration assignments, Henri Babinski had accumulated enough capital to permit him to retire in peaceful comfort.[70] Nevertheless, he accepted two other important gold-prospecting jobs, one in Siberia, and the other in the Transvaal, but afterward he traveled only for pleasure.[71]

Ali-Bab, Famous Gourmet

It was soon after his parents' deaths—his mother in 1897 and his father in 1899—that Henri came back to Paris to share the apartment with Joseph. Within their bachelor quarters, Henri took the culinary lead, compensating for all the years spent in camping conditions. A new facet of his character emerged, and in 1907 he published, under the pseudonym of Ali-Bab, his only but quite famous book, *Gastronomie pratique* (Fig. 3-2).[72]

The origin of the author's pseudonym is not known. One author notes, "The rationale for the pseudonym is not known to me. Could 'ALI' stand for 'other' and 'BAB' for 'Babinski', thus making Henri the 'other Babinski'?"[73] More poetically, the pseudonym Ali-Bab could have been a polysemous finding, recalling his visits to Constantinople; apart from the obvious "Bab" for Babinski, it could recall the magic of the Orient (Ali Baba, hero of one of the tales in *One Thousand and One Nights*), the greatness of the Arabic world (the fourth caliph, Ali ibn Abu Talib, who ruled from 656 to 661, was a cousin and son-in-law of the Prophet Muhammad; in early Shiite religion, a *bab* was a high-ranking monk; Mirza Ali Muhammad, founder of Babism in 1844, proclaimed himself *bab*, meaning in Arabic "the gate leading to the knowledge of the divine will"). It could also be a mark of nostalgia for Poland and of its sweets (*baba* is the Polish word for cake, as in rum baba, baba au rhum).[74]

---

[70] Babinski, "Sylwetka Jozefa Babinskiego."
[71] Rey, "Nécrologie de Henri Babinski."
[72] Ali-Bab, *Gastronomie pratique. Études culinaires suivies du traitement de l'obésité des gourmands* [Practical gastronomy: culinary studies followed by treatment for the obesity of gourmands] (Paris: Flammarion, 1907).
[73] P. Bailey, "Joseph Babinski (1857–1932). The man and his works," *World Neurology*, 1961: 134–140.
[74] "The Polish baba, the father of all babas, is an excellent biscuit." Ali-Bab, *Gastronomie pratique* (2001 Flammarion ed.), 1099.

3. THE BABINSKIS AND THEIR POLISH ROOTS 69

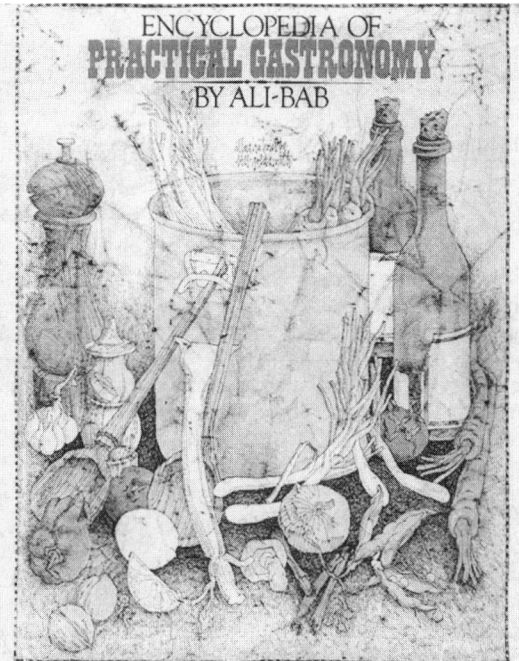

Figure 3-2 Jacket of *Encyclopaedia of Practical Gastronomy,* English translation of *Gastronomie pratique* by Ali-Bab (New York: McGraw-Hill, 1974). (*Source*: Personal collection, J. Poirier.)

Gastronomie pratique was very well received and has since met with considerable success.[75] It is considered a monument of twentieth-century gastronomy and a great classic in the art of cooking. Gérard Oberlé, a specialist in gastronomic literature, wrote:

> "one of the most famous 20th century collections of recipes. [...] Contrary to his claims in the preface, not all are up to the challenge of Mr. Babinski's dishes. One must be rather well-off to be able to afford the ingredients and well-versed in the art of cooking. Lots of truffles, fatty capons, sauterne sauces and foie gras !."[76]

Léon Daudet praised the "incomparable Ali-Bab": "The perfection of the buccal palate is the prerogative of persons of great mind."[77] The 1912 edition

---

[75] Its success was such that the book had ten successive editions by Flammarion, from 1907 to 2001, and several translations.
[76] Oberlé, G. *Les Fastes de Bacchus et de Comus ou l'Histoire du Boire et du Manger en Europe, de l'Antiquité à Nos Jours, à Travers les Livres* (Paris, Belfond, 1989), 642.
[77] L. Daudet, *Les oeuvres dans les hommes* [Men as seen through their works] (Paris: Nouvelle Librairie Nationale, 1922), 197–243; L. Daudet, *Souvenirs littéraires* [Literary

was praised in *Le Progrès Médical*: "What a good book, which speaks only of good things! Greediness is awakened when reading the loving description of so many exquisite dishes.... We have to bow down with respect in the presence of this science combined with so much conscience."[78]

When Joseph Babinski was elected to the Académie de médecine in 1914, Dr. Mathot, in the *Journal des Praticiens*, mentioned Henri in connection with the congratulations awarded to Joseph:

> But they are two... I imagine that the second is even happier than the first with this election. He, who did not become involved in neurology, reserved for himself the specialty of diet; if one brother has not yet put together his numerous works in the volume that we are waiting for, his brother has already published a second edition of an excellent treatise as thick as skillful, as complete as necessary to everybody.... He was not a pupil of Charcot, but of Frédéric.... Babinski has brought together in a cookbook under the pseudonym of Ali Bab the famous recipes of Frédéric. I think that he deserves a place beside his brother; gastronomy is an area as important to health as neurology to pathology. Let us be fair: if Dr. Babinski deserves a chair at the Académie de médecine in the pathology section, we are certain, for those of us who think that a good meal is worth a good poem, that a chair for the elder M. Babinski is already reserved in the highest, between Brillat-Savarin and Vatel... this chair is socially as important as the one granted to the finder of the [Babinski] sign.... Food is at the same time our source of customers and... the base of any well-organized society.[79]

The preface to the 2001 edition of *Gastronomie pratique* summarizes the critics' enthusiasm: "a true gourmet bible, an inexhaustible source of discoveries, of expertise, and of tasty creations, *La Gastronomie pratique* divulges the secrets of more than 5,000 recipes.... *La Gastronomie pratique*, the richness of which remains unequaled, is an initiatory and marvelous work, transforming cooking into an art and making its reading an exquisite adventure." Today food writers continue to be interested in the *Gastronomie pratique* and speak highly of its merits: "an expert guide to traditional French cuisine and how to cure the resulting obesity."[80]

---

recollections] (Paris: Bernard Grasset, 1968), 133–134. See also See J. Kother, "1927. Les savoureux conseils de Léon Daudet? Un régal!" [Tasty advice by Léon Daudet? Delicious!"] *Le Guide des Connaisseurs*, August 28, 2005, http://www.leguidedesconnaisseurs.be/article1126.html.

[78] C. Esmonet, "La gastronomie pratique" [Practical gastronomy], *Le Progrès Médical* 1912 (17): 216.

[79] Dr. Mathot, "Causerie médicale. Nouveau Palmarès. À M. Babinski, ingénieur" [Medical chat: New list of honors for M. Babinski, engineer], *Journal des Praticiens*, 1914 (CLXI). Frédéric Delair (1840–1910), known by just his first name, was for about forty years the renowned *chef de cuisine* of the famous restaurant La Tour d'Argent. See www.dininginfrance.com/tourdargent.htm.

[80] Quote from http://www.maggs.com/title/MO40768.asp. See also Margaret McArthur, "The lost worlds of Ali-Bab," *The Daily Gullet*, August 25, 2003, http://www.egullet.org/tdg.cgi?pg=ARTICLE-maggiealibab.

3. THE BABINSKIS AND THEIR POLISH ROOTS

Henri Babinski did not hide his credo: "if it is indecent to live for eating, it is suitable while eating to live to try to fulfill this task, as all others, the best you can and with pleasure."[81] Written in the first person, in a pleasant and fluent style, *Gastronomie pratique* is full of tricks of the trade, remarks, personal opinions, anecdotes, and more or less esoteric allusions, all based on a good sense of humor. It is sprinkled with erudite notes and is full of scientific, biological, physical, and even mathematical data, behind which it is easy to recognize the scientist and the engineer. Very precise, it gives for all recipes the exact quantities of each ingredient and the correct cooking time. Footnotes are numerous, which is rarely seen in cookbooks. In a certain way, this book looks like a scientific work, but it is easy and pleasant reading. The foreword to the first edition (1907, reprinted in 2001) sets forth the origin of the book in the author's long voyages around the world as an engineer. Because of the frugality and monotony of his meals in the middle of nowhere (largely based upon canned food or the products of local hunting and fishing simply boiled or grilled), he tried to find spices and other flavorful variations that might stimulate the appetite. This principle would be the basis of his future recipes.

In the first part, termed a preamble to gastronomy, the treatise begins with a historical perspective on gastronomy through the ages and in a wide range of countries. Then it tackles the dinner service, discusses cooking methods, and provides general advice on sauces, soups, edible mushrooms in France, choice of wines, organization of meals among friends, and finally a few menus typical of the author.

To give an example, here is a menu for a "small" dinner party:

Consommé de volaille *Salade de légumes*
Langouste à la parisienne *Fromage*
Salmis de bécasses *Fruits*
Chou-fleur au gratin *Soufflé glacé*
Selle de chevreuil grillée

And for a larger, more formal event:

Potage à la queue de bœuf *Pâté de cailles*
Barquettes de riz d'agneau
  Villeroi *Salade de mâche, céleri, betterave*
Omble-chevalier à la
  meunière tomatée *Fromages*

---

[81] Ali-Bab, *Gastronomie pratique*, 296 (1907 ed.).

Turban de poulet garni *Fruits*
Selle de sanglier rôtie *Glace plombière*
Purée de cerfeuil bulbeux *Gâteau au chocolat*

But consider even a private working lunch between Joseph, Henri, and their friend Egas Moniz (a disciple of Joseph Babinski and friend of the two brothers) (see chapter 9). The simple and frugal meal would

> begin with a "vol-au-vent financière," whose light pastry harmoniously mingles with the carefully orchestrated filling overflowing with the rare rooster crests so appreciated by gourmets. Follow[ed] by a Chateaubriand with puffed potatoes, which would make the head chef at the Meurice jealous. To end with, a slice of calves' liver that reminded me of the Chapon-Fin in Bordeaux. For dessert, wild strawberries from Turenne, perfumed and pulpy, with which the cream and sugar produced the creamy consistency of a precious jewel. Finally the meal was washed down by a Château-Yquem, then a Burgundy wine, and finally a marvelous port of 1845. We took together a cup of coffee in the Master's office, with a glass of cognac dating from the Empire period. The French really know how to eat.[82]

The next chapters consider all imaginable dishes and give numerous recipes, from soups to coffees and liqueurs, going also through seafood, fish, meats, vegetables, cheeses, and desserts. The last nine pages, rather exceptionally for a cookbook, are devoted to the treatment of obesity in those fond of good food; they have an autobiographical touch. Ali-Bab pointed out that his friend Professor Vaquez had honored him by publishing a summary of his method in his book.[83] In fact, in his *Précis de thérapeutique*, in speaking about the diet for those overweight, Henri Vaquez described with some detail the regime kindly passed on to him by his friend Henri Babinski:

> We report here, as an example and for teaching purposes, the diet followed by an obese man and based upon his personal observations. This bright man was able without any medical help to decrease his weight from 150 to 106 kilograms in 8 months, without incident. He is still today in good shape and has not increased his weight, as he was wise to continue to follow for himself the general rules that he prescribed.[84]

In the foreword to the fifth edition (1928), reedited in 2001, Ali-Bab humorously expresses thanks for the "eulogistic comments of the press of every country" and "the unexpected success" of the previous editions (see

---

[82] *Rev Neurol (Paris)* 1958 (98): 660.
[83] Ali-Bab, *Gastronomie pratique,* 1st ed., 281: "My friend Professor Vaquez has done me the honor of publishing a summary of my method in his excellent *Traité de thérapeutique* (published by J. B. Baillière, 1907), an honor for which I am most grateful."
[84] H. Vaquez, *Précis de thérapeutique* [Textbook of therapeutics] (Paris: Librairie J.-B. Baillière et fils, 1907).

the appendices to this chapter). He also included a parody of Du Bellay's sonnet in honor of Ali-Bab:

> *Happy is Ali Bab who took a pleasant trip,*
> *Acquired the art of preparing poultry and venison,*
> *And then returned full of practice and wisdom,*
> *Ending up cooking for the rest of his days!*
>
> *When shall he see, alas, in even the smallest village,*
> *The ham fat smoking, the salted meat cured,*
> *And plants in the garden kitchen*
> *Tomatoes, onions, parsley, and so many other things?*
>
> *The more he likes the roast tasted by his ancestors,*
> *The less he likes the daring dishes of the Palace Hotel:*
> *More than the tough chicken, he likes the sweet quail,*
>
> *More than a disappointing pâté, a nice little rabbit,*
> *More a Médoc wine than the Italian Chianti,*
> *More than mineral water a bottle of Anjou wine.*

In his *Confidences d'un chercheur scientifique*, Egas Moniz gave a humorous commentary on the full-flavored words of Ali-Bab concerning oysters.[85] He concluded by defending Portuguese oysters from Portugal, despised—unfairly, he thought—by Ali-Bab.[86]

Once a Mining Engineer, Always a Mining Engineer

Though perhaps best known as an eminent gastronome, Henri nevertheless remained a mining engineer throughout his life, deeply attached to his school and his former fellow students. He wrote several obituaries in the newsletter for former students at the École des Mines, notably those on Bertrand Joseph Jean Marie Bruno Chaumond (1853–1888), Léon Benoist

---

[85] *Confidências de um Investigador Científico* [Confidences of a scientific investigator] (Lisbon: Edições Ática, 1949), 72–73, http://mhroque.blogspot.com/2004/12/confidpicanum-jantar-ou-numa-ceia-de.html. Oysters were often found on Parisian tables: "Paris is no doubt one of the biggest necropoles for this precious shellfish. There is not a single street or neighborhood where one cannot find in the window of a local wine merchant a display more or less full of half-opened baskets giving a glimpse of tempting shells, not to speak of vendor carts overflowing with Portuguese oysters at 40 cents a dozen." *Journal de la Santé*, 1889 (VI): 260.

[86] Ali-Bab, *Gastronomie pratique*, 308 n. 1.

(1855–1906), his childhood friend Joseph Obalski (1852–1915), and Leopold Michel (1846–1919), and contributed notes to the one on Ceslas Waliszewski (1852–1897).[87]

In 1914, he wrote an article for that newsletter containing advice for young colleagues interested in foreign assignments and in which he set forth the difficulties, traps, and hazards, clearly explaining how to avoid them. He didn't hesitate to go into the details of suitable contracts, precautions to be followed, and recommended clothing, food, drugs, and equipment. The conclusion was encouraging, moral, and patriotic:

> Following this advice, the young colleagues will, as their elders, travel through the whole world in the best conditions, maintaining the excellent reputation of the French engineers. They will see many countries off the beaten track; they will have larger ideas; they will better appreciate France more than if they had never left it; and they will keep for life interesting memories. They will go over again later the pleasant episodes of their peregrinations and will recall without bitterness the difficulties they encountered because they have overcome them. *Forsan et haec olim meminisse juvabit.* That is what I hope for them, with all my heart.[88]

During a 1923 visit to Paris by engineers from the Mine Engineering School of Cracow, Henri Babinski gave a welcoming speech in Polish in which he glorified the French-Polish relationship, showing his deep attachment to his two homelands and his gratitude to France, a land of welcome.[89]

The Inseparable Brothers

Joseph and his brother, Henri, formed an inseparable pair (Fig. 3-3). In the scientifico-medical world of the nineteenth and twentieth centuries, especially in neurological circles, several other pairs are well known. Some were married couples, including Pierre Curie and Marie Curie, Jules Dejerine and Augusta Dejerine-Klumpke (1859–1927), Oskar Vogt (1870–1959) and Cécile

---

[87] *Bulletin de l'Association des anciens élèves de l'École des mines de Paris,* January–February 1888, 1907, July–August 1915; *Bulletin de l'Association amicale des anciens élèves de l'École des Mines,* January–March 1920, June 1898.

[88] H. Babinski, "Quelques conseils aux jeunes camarades qui désirent être chargés de missions" [Some advice to young friends who aspire to lead missions], *Bulletin de l'Association amicale des Elèves de l'École Nationale supérieure des Mines,* April 1914.

[89] Ceremony welcoming the Mine Engineering School of Cracow at the Association's office in Paris. Translation from Polish of M. Babinski's speech. *Bulletin de l'Association des anciens élèves de l'École des mines de Paris,* December 1923.

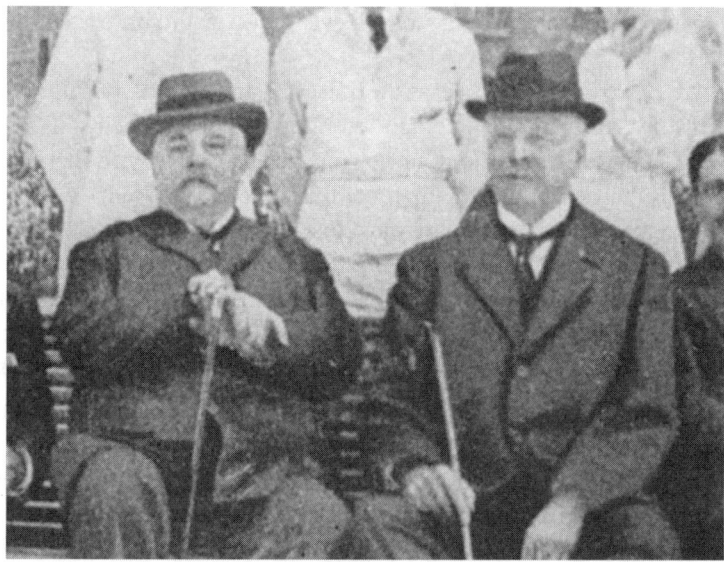

Figure 3-3 Henri and Joseph Babinski on a park bench near the Pitié hospital. (*Source*: From Albert Charpentier, *Un grand médecin, J. Babinski* [Paris: Typographie François Bernouard, 1934].)

Mugnier-Vogt (1875–1962); some were not, such as Jean-Martin Charcot and his son Jean-Baptiste Charcot (1867–1936), Thierry de Martel (1875–1940) and his novelist mother Gyp (Sibylle Gabrielle Riquetti de Mirabeau, comtesse de Martel, 1849–1932), and the Babinski brothers. In each case, it is impossible to speak of one without making reference to the other. From another point of view, the Babinskis may be compared to the famous Goncourt brothers, Edmond (1822–1896) and Jules (1830–1870); the same questions could be raised—with no definite answer—on their bachelorhood, the lack of known descendants, and the nature of their relationship to women. There were also the Wright brothers, Wilbur (1867–1912) and Orville (1871–1948), American pioneers of aviation; the Lumière brothers, Auguste (1862–1954) and Louis (1864–1948), seminal figures in the development of motion pictures; and the brothers Grimm, Jacob (1785–1863) and Wilhelm (1786–1859), linguists and collectors of fairy tales.

Henri was totally devoted to his younger brother, whom he adored "like a god."[90] Clovis Vincent described in a few words the deep relationship between the two brothers: "His brother and Joseph had for each other a true cult, which never slackened. Joseph lived for his career and for science; Henri

[90] Charpentier, "Babinski (Joseph)."

lived for Joseph. Without Henri, Joseph eventually would have accomplished much less."[91]

Even if Henri spent long years away from Paris, the two brothers never really left the family home. During their childhood, with their father absent for extended periods, they no doubt formed a close circle with their mother. Joseph shared a home with his parents until they died; Henri retired soon after, perhaps because he did not want Joseph to have to live alone (see the appendix to chapter 2). Henri took care of the family home, managed the table, and played the role of a secretary by typing papers, prescriptions, and letters; he also attended Joseph's lessons and looked after the brothers' finances.[92] In brief, he handled all the material concerns that Joseph, some say, was unable to deal with. "He listened, with his pipe in his mouth, to the successive drafts of the papers to be presented at the Neurological Society, giving wise advice on the sense of a word that Joseph immediately verified in the Littré Dictionary."[93] Henri did not hesitate to substitute for his brother "in answering passionate letters sent to [Joseph] and in avoiding romantic entanglements."[94]

> Between two missions in America, Henri Babinski returned to Paris to rest; but for such an active man, he found rest only by working. And that was why he began to study with his brother, Dr. Babinski, the construction of electrical machines to treat some diseases. His efforts were successful and he was rewarded, both as electrician and prospector, with the Legion of Honor.... [T]his long companionship of two remarkably cultivated men, of two elite personalities, of two minds open to any scientific, literary or artistic expression or movements, has certainly contributed to their mutual growth.[95]

If we accept the idea that Joseph had a tendency to be obsessional, Henri may be considered as a protective and permanent presence without which Joseph could not have worked or lived to the fullest (see chapter 2). Egas Moniz recalled that Joseph Babinski offered a gloomy presentiment a few days after his brother's death: "The end of an existence."[96] The rapid decline of Joseph after Henri's death, noted by all his biographers, confirms this hypothesis:

> Our colleague was conscious of his progressive deterioration, deeply affected by the economic situation, and continually anxious about the future. In the last months of his life, this giant was only a mere shadow of his former self, having lost weight, become bowed over, and shuffling. But the intellectual

[91] Vincent, "J. Babinski (1857–1932)."
[92] Rivet, "Joseph Babinski"; Gasecki and Hachinski, "On the names of Babinski."
[93] Charpentier, "Babinski (Joseph)."
[94] Rivet, "Joseph Babinski."
[95] Rey, "Nécrologie de Henri Babinski."
[96] *Rev Neurol (Paris)*, 1958 (98): 660.

faculties and judgment were intact. He was apprehensive about old-age disabilities, and once his work had been completed and his brother had died, he wanted to die in his turn.[97]

The Polish School of the Batignolles

In their youth, from 1863 to 1870, Joseph and Henri attended the Polish school that had opened in 1848 at 56 boulevard des Batignolles in Paris.[98] It was a private institution "founded on Polish patriotism" and dedicated to educating the children of Polish refugees.[99]

For financial reasons, the school had to move into a more modest building, 15 rue Lamandé in the Seventeenth Arrondissement, and the new school opened on October 1, 1874.[100] The director, a venerable man, enforced both discipline and hard work.[101] The inspection report of February 1876 noted that education was "based on religious principles."[102] In 1879, it was also noted that the school provided "moral and religious education, mainly patriotic," a point amplified in 1881: "love for homeland and adoptive country."[103]

As emphasized with pride by Prince Czartoryski, the attitude of the Batignolles school and of its students during the siege of Paris and the Commune was clear: "Eighty-nine former students, among whom sixteen died, fought in the French army; no current student has served under the

---

[97] Rivet, "Joseph Babinski."

[98] *Liste générale des anciens élèves de l'École Polonaise* [Alumni list for the Polish School] (Paris: Imprimerie polyglotte A. Rueff-Heymann, 1908). Courtesy of Dr. Pierre Konopka. After leaving the Polish School, Henri became a student at the École des Mines de Paris in 1875. On July 20, 1875, Joseph received his bachelor of arts, and he registered at the medical school on November 4, 1875. On April 4, 1876, Joseph received the diploma of bachelor of science.

[99] Inspection notice of June 1875, Archives nationales, AJ/16/4733. The early beginning of the École polonaise dated from the May 16, 1841, with the creation of the Conseil des fondateurs de la Société de l'Éducation nationale, six days before those of the Association des pères de famille polonais en émigration, and the opening of the École nationale polonaise, for the year 1842–43 at Chatillon, with twenty students. E. Pozerski, *L'école polonaise ou l'esprit de 1830*, 13–15, Archives de l'Institut Pasteur, carton POZ.

[100] L'école polonaise des Batignolles still exists at the same address in Paris.

[101] Inspection notice of June 1875, Archives nationales, AJ/16/4733. The director was Stanislas Malinowski, with a double baccalaureate from the Warsaw University. Archives nationales, AJ/16/4699.

[102] At this date, all students were Catholics.

[103] Inspection notices of May 14, 1878, and June 1879, Archives nationales, AJ/16/4733; inspection notice of April 11, 1881, Archives nationales, AJ/16/4733.

Commune." It was the same for the other Polish school in Paris: "All the students of the Montparnasse School, numbering fifty, served in infantry battalions; four were killed during the siege; no student joined the Commune."[104]

It is clear that the École polonaise des Batignolles helped inculcate in the Babinski children patriotism toward both Poland and France, with a spirit particularly hostile to the Commune. One day, in the presence of Henri Babinski, a former student recalled with emotion his memories of the Polish School, saying that it had been his spiritual mother. Henri, whose adventurous and independent spirit didn't fit very well into the strict discipline of the French educational system, replied: "The school was like forced labor."[105]

The association of the Polish school's former students was always ready to demonstrate its double allegiance toward France and Poland.[106] The group started a fund to benefit wounded members of the French armed forces.[107] And the association's secretary gave a speech in 1867 in which he said:

> Sons of emigrants, here is our name; exile has been our nationality, and if there be duties related to this painful nationality, we have to understand and accomplish them. We know that our duty is to work for Poland, which needs all our efforts, but to work for it through France, which has opened to us all its sources of enlightment and riches.[108]

In 1870 another member said:

> Confronted by the sad news that affects us so deeply, let us swear to defend Paris at the front ranks, if the Prussians arrive as far as here. I ask therefore, before any debate, that we affirm our dedication to the freedom of France and Poland, giving three cheers for France and three more for Poland.[109]

In a brochure on the school's history, Edouard Pozerski wrote:

> The Polish School has given to France and to the world first rank citizens: engineers…[including Henry] Babinski…; mathematicians…; explorers …; diplomats…; sculptor Cyprien Godebski; the famous physician Joseph

---

[104] Czartoryski et al., "Mémoire justificatif."

[105] Pozerski E. The Polish School, or the spirit of 1830 [L'école Polonaise ou l'esprit de 1830], Paris, edited by the Alumni Association of the Polish School, 15 rue Lamandé, p. 48 (Archives of the Pasteur Institute, cardboard POZ).

[106] *Association des anciens élèves de l'école polonaise. Procès-Verbal 1865–1897. Bulletin littéraire et scientifique*. This monthly Polish bulletin "was telling France that Poland still existed, was living and working for its revival and the whole world." See www.mairie17.paris.fr article Ecole polonaise des Batignolles.

[107] Minutes of the General Assembly, August 7, 1870.

[108] Speech by the secretary, W. Gasztowtt, minutes of the General Assembly, August 4, 1867.

[109] Speecy by Armand Zagrodzki, minutes of the General Assembly, August 7, 1870.

Babinski, the greatest clinician in France since Laënnec. Students from the Polish school shed their blood for Poland and France, their two homelands.

He also recalled that "the Polish school was present at Victor Hugo's funeral; it walked behind the 'hearse of the poor.'"[110]

Henri and Joseph Babinski were members of the association in the second semester of 1873 and probably retroactively to 1870.[111] The two brothers regularly paid their dues and often contributed to funds for the school and for apprentices; however, between 1876 and 1888, neither of them was present at the association's General Assembly nor the banquet that followed.[112] In August 1890, Joseph was elected to the association's committee.[113] At the same meeting reference was made to the transfer of the ashes of Adam Mickiewicz from the Montmorency cemetery in France to the Wavel castle in Cracow on June 28, 1890, and the funeral of Stanislas Malinowski, director of the Polish School of Paris, on July 5, 1890. In his speech during the banquet offered to the delegates of the Diet of Galicia, Jules Jasiewicz cited, among other former famous students, "Dr. J. Babinski, who in the near future will receive new laurels."[114] As of 1892, Henri became more involved in the association; he was present at the General Assembly and the annual banquet, and he was elected twice to the Committee, spoke at the assembly, led meetings, and attended dinners at which he talked humoursly about his travels.[115] Joseph, often absent from the General Assembly, frequently attended the banquets with his brother.

---

[110] Pozerski, *L'école polonaise ou l'esprit de 1830*.

[111] They are included among the members in the minutes of the General Assembly, February 1, 1874. List of the members in August 1879: "Henri Babinski, engineer at the Society of Zinc Factories of the Bousquet d'Oebn near Bédarieux, Hérault, member since 1870. Joseph Babinski, medical student, 151 bis boulevard du Montparnasse, Paris, member since 1870." Members in July 1893: Henri Babinski, "mining civil engineer, 54 rue Bonaparte, member since 1870." Joseph Babinski, "medical doctor, *médecin des hôpitaux*, 54 rue Bonaparte" (at this date Joseph Galezowski, Xavier Galezowski, ophtalmologists and Edouard Habich were honorary members). List of the members in July 1894: Henri Babinski, "mining civil engineer, 54 rue Bonaparte, member since 1870." Joseph Babinski, "medical doctor, *médecin des hôpitaux*, 54 rue Bonaparte" (this list included Edouard Pozerski, 16 rue Lacroix, member since 1892).

[112] Minutes of the General Assembly, February 1895.

[113] Minutes of the General Assembly, August 3, 1890.

[114] Ibid.

[115] Minutes of the General Assembly, July 30, 1893. At one meeting Henri defended the project of having two different banquets, one with members, the other with their families. Minutes of the General Assembly, February 3, 1895.

The Babinski Vault at the Polish Cemetery of Montmorency

Joseph Babinski was buried with his father, mother, brother, and a cousin of his mother in the Champeaux Cemetery in Montmorency, which "has become the most prestigious cemetery for the Polish immigrants in France" and is often named "the Pantheon of the Polish emigration" and "of the Polish insurrections of the nineteenth century, of the world wars (Fig. 3-4)."[116] Contrary to the Polish burial vaults in the Montmartre and Père-Lachaise cemeteries, which are in the main beautiful artistic monuments, the Babinski gravesite is extremely simple, with just an engraved tombstone.[117] Only Henri and Joseph appear on the burial registers of the Montmorency parish, giving proof of a religious ceremony; their parents are not mentioned in these registers.[118]

Vaquez, Joseph Babinksi's close friend, ended his obituary with these words:

> As for the man, he lies forever with his Polish ancestors, in eternal rest in this little cemetery of Montmorency, close to the forest that reminded Mickiewicz of the woods of his lost country. He lies there, in French soil, with his family brought together by death, taking away in his heart the image of his beloved restored Poland: everything he has loved, everything about which he has dreamed!"[119]

Other Babinskis

Besides Joseph, his father, his mother, and his brother, several other Babinskis appear in different sources.

It is logical to think that Antoni Babinski (also known as Alojzy Boguslawski, 1812–1847) was a brother of Alexander Babinski.[120] We have found in the Polish encyclopedias and dictionaries we consulted only one entry concerning him.[121] Here one learns only the dates of his birth and

---

[116] In the Montparnasse cemetery in Paris there is also a "collective grave for Emigration, a true Polish Pantheon." Pozerski, *L'école polonaise ou l'esprit de 1830*, 74. See also http://www.mission-catholique-polonaise.net/histFR.htm.

[117] Société pour la protection des souvenirs et tombeaux historiques polonais en France, http://www.pologne-opportunites.com/polonite/montmorency.htm.

[118] Registers of burial acts, Montmorency Parish, Archives de l'Evêché de Pontoise.

[119] Vaquez, "Joseph Babinski."

[120] Babinski, "Sylwetka Jozefa Babinskiego."

[121] *Nowy leksykon PWN* (Warsaw: Wydawnictwo Naukowe PWN, 1998).

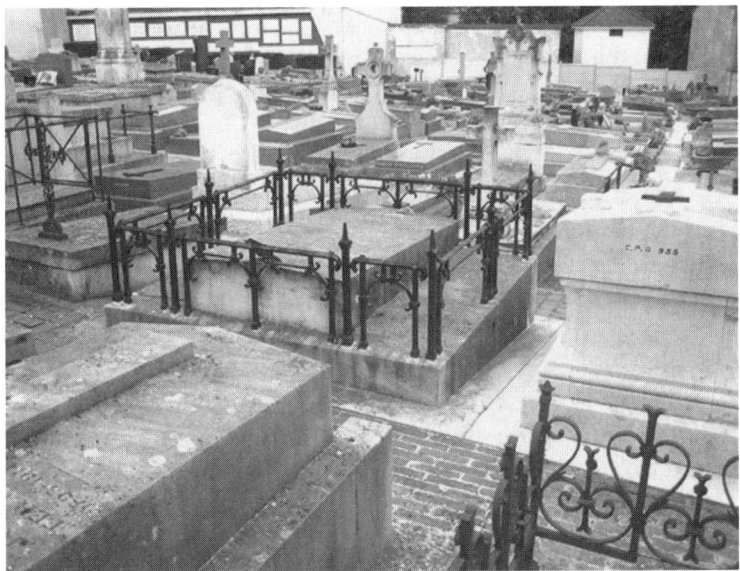

Figure 3-4 Babinski family tombstone in the Champeaux Cemetery, Montmorency, near Paris. (*Source*: Personal collection, J. Poirier.)

death, the fact that in 1847 he was the emissary of the Association démocratique polonaise for the principality of Poznan, and that he was a revolutionary activist, condemned to death and shot by the German in Poznan after having killed a Prussian policeman.[122]

Born in 1891 in Warsaw, Léon Babinski (1891–1973), a distant cousin of the brothers, became a legal expert, specialist in international law, and professor at the Business School of Warsaw (1938–1939), Poznan University (1945–1950), and then at the Polytechnical School of Szczecin (1955–1961).[123] He also taught at the Academy of International Law at the Hague and was a member of the International Law Institute from 1947. He wrote several university textbooks and monographs on international law. Moreover, he published an article in Polish on Joseph Babinski.[124] Another cousin, Waclaw (1887–1957), diplomat in the Hague, represented Léon at Joseph's burial, as cited in the obituary published by the newspaper *Le Figaro*, on November 3. Other than this reference, we have found no trace of direct

---

[122] See also *Polski slownik biogr.*, 1:194.
[123] *Wielka encyklopedia powszechna PWN* (Warsaw: Panstwowe Wydawnictwo Naukowe PWN, 1978–1993); *Nowy leksykon PWN*; *Wielka encyklopedia polski* (Krakow: Wydawnic two Tyszard Kluszczynski, 2004).
[124] Babinski, "Sylwetka Jozefa Babinskiego."

contact between the cousins, although Léon and Waclaw no doubt met regularly through their representatives functions at the Hague. Waclaw had a long diplomatic career, first as ambassador of Poland to Yugoslavia (1929–1931) and then to the Hague (1931–1943). He presumably joined the Polish government in exile in London during the war and was then appointed their representative to Canada (1943–1945). A fierce patriot, he played a key role in hiding the treasures of the royal collection of Wavel Castle, resisting their return to the communist regime of Poland after the war. He retired in Canada and died in 1957. In the encyclopedias and Polish dictionary, entries on Jan Josef Babinski (1873–1921), a chemical engineer specializing in sugar products and director of the Central Sugar Laboratory in Warsaw, do not indicate whether there was any family relationship with Joseph.[125]

With the exception of Stanislas A. Babinski, an engineer living in Montréal and a distant relative of Joseph Babinski, there is no information about any relationship to Joseph Babinski's family.[126] In France in 2005, the Babinskis were very few, with most of them living in the north region.[127] Barring any error or omission, it can be said they are not related to Joseph Babinski.

APPENDIXES

Foreword to Bien manger pour bien vivre by Edouard de Pomiane (1922)

Ali Bab (Henri Babinski) I little trust treatises on gastronomy written by scientists; I always fear to find therein the formula of the famous synthetic pill with which they have threatened us, a pill that, offering every day our food ration theoretically calculated, leads to eliminating the taste of bread and "saving" time devoted to our meals. What a truly delightful prospect!

But knowing my friend de Pomiane for a long time, I was reassured on this point and accepted with pleasure the honor he accorded to me to introduce himself and to present his book.

De Pomiane is above all a biological scientist, but he is also a physician, and generally physicians do not fear anyone in regard to greediness. Furthermore,

---

[125] S. Lama, ed., *Ilustrowana encyklopedja trzaski, everta i michalskiego* (Warsaw: Nakladem Ksiegarni Trzaski, Everta i Michalskiego, 1927); *Mala encyklopedia powszechna PWN* (Warsaw: Wydawnictwo Naukowe PWN, 1997); *Nowy leksykon PWN*.
[126] C. Belanger, "What do you know about Joseph Babinski?" *Can J Neurol Sci* 1989 (16): 4–7.
[127] We have identified a dozen and thank them for having answered our genealogical inquiry.

he is an experienced cook and an accomplished physician; nobody is more qualified than he is to write about the *science de gueule*. I spent an excellent evening reading his work.

He had the difficult task of explaining to the uninitiated the principles of *gastrotechnie*; he has made it pleasant to delve into the deep knowledge he has of the subject in a way that anyone can understand. He gives precise and precious indications on the nutritional value of different foods, their digestibility, the fundamental methods of their preparation; he tries to bring into the cult of good and healthy French cooking those who should be tempted to reduce the pleasure of eating under the pretext of diet.

Eat Well to Live Well is a charming book, witty, very instructive; it has been written in a lively style; it is worth reading, rereading, and meditating upon.

I wish readers the jovial mood and hearty appetite of the author, following in the glorious steps of our Master [Brillat-Savarin], the immortal author of *Physiologie du Goût*.

Preface to the Fifth Edition of Gastronomie pratique *(1928)*

Ali Bab (Henri Babinski) If a diviner had predicted twenty years ago that the first edition of my very small book would one day become a huge volume, I would have doubted his lucidity. This unexpected success may be related to the fact that this book is faithful to its title and that a new craze for cooking is coming into in vogue; but it is also due, without any doubt, to a great extent to the eulogistic reports in the press in many countries.

Critics, in turn, have wanted to see me as a man of letters, an erudite, an historian, a philosopher, a humorist, a great priest in the art of cooking; and in the *Gastronomie pratique* a masterpiece, an encyclopedia, a profane bible, a compilation of psalms, which even has been compared—sacrilege!—to the work of St. Thomas Aquinas. The Muses also were asked to participate, and a poet has cleverly parodied, in honor of Ali Bab, the immortal sonnet of Joachim du Bellay.

All that incense burned on my altar has not clouded my eyes; it has not masked the imperfections and weaknesses of a work conceived without any ambitious design and which has been just a hobby—certainly quite pleasant. Recalling Boileau's advice, I turn back again to my loom. I present it for the fifth time, enriched by many contributions and new formulas.

I hope that the readers will maintain their kind welcome.

···*four*···

The Babinski Circle

Joseph Babinski's personal relationships help to shed light on his character and personality. Family is the innermost circle, composed of his parents and brother, with whom he shared living space and meals throughout his life, beginning on boulevard Montparnasse, where the brothers were born, on rue Bonaparte, and finally on boulevard Haussmann, where all the family members successively passed away.

A second circle was made up of a small number of close and intimate friends, carefully selected, all of whom were about the same age, and who were regular guests at Sunday luncheons.[1] This group included Henri Vaquez, Jean Darier, Pierre Bazy, Émile Picard, and Fernand Widal.[2] Except for Picard, they were all physicians, but not neurologists, and of high social and cultural standing: physicians in chief in the Parisian hospital system, university professors, members of the national academies, and recipients of the Legion of Honor.

[1] L. Rivet, "Joseph Babinski (1857–1932)," *Bull Mém Soc Méd Hôp Paris* 1932 (34): 1722–1733; O. Crouzon, "Discours d'ouverture de la Chaire d'assistance médico-sociale" [Speech at the inauguration of the chair for medical and social welfare], given November 22, 1937, at the Medical School of Paris.
[2] "Babinski, Vaquez, Darier: how could one speak of these three leading figures of contemporary medicine without referring to them together? Theirs was a friendship where joy and loyalty were the source of continual renewal. Nothing and no one could destroy it. Such a friendship can never be truly explained, but is certainly founded on a shared appreciation of a set of common values and a similar, high, and noble character." G. Roussy, "Nécrologie de M. Jean Darier (1856–1938)," *Comptes-Rendus de l'Académie de Médecine*, meeting of June 28, 1938, 737–742.

A third circle includes slightly more distant friends: Albert Charrin, Léon Daudet, Edouard Enriquez, Charles Féré, Charles Laubry, Félix Lejars, Eugène Suchard—all doctors, but still no neurologists.

The last and largest group included his former students, forming a kind of royal court around their mentor (see chapter 6). To this group René Moreau added the names of Jules Séglas, Jacques Bainville, and F. Strowski, whereas John F. Fulton (1899–1960) included those of Leon Guignard and Léon Babinski, the Radical government minister Pierre Waldeck-Rousseau (1846–1904), and the engineer-astronomer Chacornac.[3]

This was indeed quite a fashionable Right Bank society. In Babinski's time, all the hospitals that specialized in neurology (Salpêtrière, Pitié, Bicêtre, Ivry, Paul-Brousse, Saint-Joseph, Sainte-Anne) were located on the Left Bank of the Seine River, while the leading physicians (with the exception of Pierre Marie, Achille Souques, and Georges Guillain) all had their private homes, and therefore their private practices, on the Right Bank, mainly in the Monceau area.[4] The Babinskis were part of this general trend, a result of Haussmann's massive restructuring of Paris, in which a large section of the bourgeoisie moved from the Latin Quarter, the traditional intellectual center, to the more modern Right Bank.

The Intimate Friends

In his own words, Vaquez "had close and reciprocal relations with Babinski for 45 years, a friendship that only death could end."[5] Resident, *médecin des*

---

[3] R. Moreau, "Hommage à la mémoire de Joseph Babinski à l'occasion du 100è anniversaire de sa naissance" [Homage to the memory of Joseph Babinski on the occasion of the 100th anniversary of his birth], *Bull Mém Soc Méd Hôp Paris* 1958 (74): 449–457; J. F. Fulton, "Science in the clinic as exemplified by the life and work of Joseph Babinski," *Journal of Nervous and Mental Diseases* 1933 (77): 121–133; L. Babinski, "Sylwetka Jozefa Babinskiego na tle jego zycia codziennego," *Neurol Neurochir Pol* 1969 (III): 543–548.

[4] From the early Renaissance, with the creation of the Sorbonne in 1257, the Left Bank of the Seine was considered as more intellectual than the right. This changed with Haussmann's transformation of Paris in the latter part of the nineteenth century. In 1927, the physicians residing on the Right Bank included Albert Charpentier, Henri Claude, Ferdinand Darier, Edouard Enriquez, Joseph Jumentié, Maxime Laignel-Lavastine, André Léri, Jean Lhermitte, Thierry de Martel, Gustave Roussy, André Thomas, and Clovis Vincent. Marie was at 76 rue de Lille, Souques was at 17 rue de l'Université, and Guillain was at 215 bis boulevard Saint-Germain, all in the Seventh Arrondissement. *Rev Neurol (Paris)* 1927 (I): 42–43; 1933 (I): 49–51.

[5] H. Vaquez, "Joseph Babinski (1857–1932)," *Bulletin de l'Académie de Médecine* 1932 (35): 1264–1273. For more on Vaquez, see F. Huguet, *Les professeurs de la faculté de*

hôpitaux (1895), associate professor (1898), professor of a chair in clinical medicine (1918), member of the Académie nationale de médecine, Vaquez described polycythemia vera (later known as polyglobuly or Vaquez disease), the clinical description of which would later be made by William Osler (1849–1919). Under the influence of Professor Carl Edouard Potain (1825–1901), he specialized in heart disease and published several papers on heart rate disorders and arterial hypertension. He founded and edited the *Archives des Maladies du Coeur, des Vaisseaux et du Sang*. Henri Babinski was a witness at his marriage.[6] He had close artistic contacts, for example with the poet and dramatic author André Rivoire (1872–1930) and the painter Edouard Vuillard (1868–1940) (Fig. 4-1).[7]

Born in Pest (Hungary), in a French Protestant family exiled in the seventeenth century after the revocation of the Edict of Nantes, Jean-Ferdinand Darier (1856–1938) followed a medical career similar to that of Babinski: nonresident student in 1878, resident of the Paris hospitals in 1880, he defended his thesis in 1885.[8] From 1884 to 1903, he was a demonstrator in the histological laboratory of the Collège de France under Ranvier and from 1885 to 1894 directed the laboratory of pathological anatomy at the Saint-Louis Hospital. He first became *médecin des hôpitaux* in 1894 and served successively at La Rochefoucauld, La Pitié, Broca, and finally at Saint-Louis, where he remained from 1909 to 1922. Like Babinski, he was not a university professor. Elected to the Académie nationale de médecine in 1919, Darier was one of the most brilliant dermatologists of his time, not only at a clinical level but also because of his histological expertise. He founded the Saint-Louis Hospital museum. One of the five great names in his discipline at the turn of the century, he made French dermatology known worldwide, along with Ernest Henri Besnier (1831–1909), Louis-Anne-Jean Brocq (1856–1928), Raimond Sabouraud (1864–1938), and Alfred Fournier (1832–1914). He was the originator of the cutaneous biopsy. His name was given to several cutaneous diseases that he described (dermatofibrosarcoma protuberans of Darier-Ferrand, Darier-Roussy's hypodermic sarcoids, and Darier-White syndrome) and also the Darier sign in urticaria pigmentosa.

---

médecine de Paris. Dictionnaire biographique 1794–1939 [Professors at the Paris Medical School. A biographical dictionary 1794–1939] (Paris: CNRS, INRP, 1991).

[6] Huguet, *Les professeurs*.

[7] In 1896, Vaquez commissioned from Edouard Vuillard four panels for his study. J. L. Binet, "Edouard Vuillard et Henri Vaquez," paper presented at the Académie des beaux-arts, meeting of December 15, 2004, 69–75.

[8] M. P. Ledoux and G. Ledoux, *Un homme, une œuvre: Ferdinand-Jean Darier (1856–1938)* [A man and his work: Ferdinand-Jean Darier (1856–1938)] (Longpont-sur-Orge: Société historique, 1987); see also http://www.whonamedit.com/doctor.cfm/514.html.

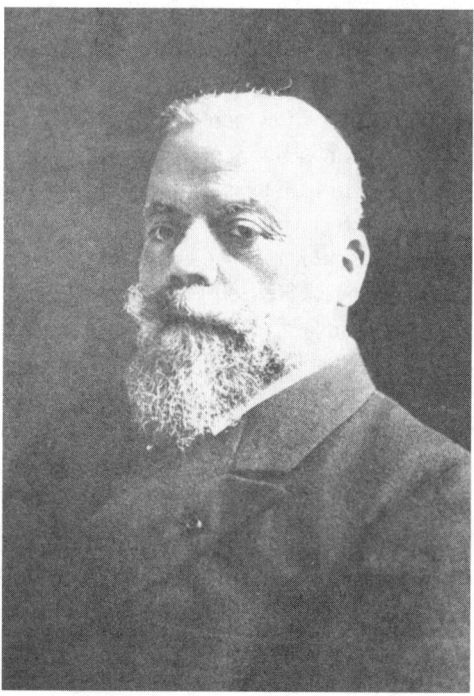

Figure 4-1 Professor Henri Vaquez. (*Source*: Archives of the Académie nationale de médecine, Paris.)

His textbook on dermatology, first published in 1909, was translated into several languages and referred to internationally. In 1936, Darier was asked to be editor in chief of *Nouvelle pratique dermatologique*, a truly comprehensive eight-volume encyclopedia. After his retirement, he was mayor of Longpont-sur-Orge, a village near Paris, from 1925 to 1935. Darier was decorated with the Legion of Honor; as knight in 1908, his application was signed by Georges Clemenceau (1841–1929), president of the cabinet, and his sponsor was Alfred Fournier, his former mentor.[9] When he was promoted to officer in 1917 and then to commander in 1928, his sponsor was Joseph Babinski. Known as a collector of objets d'art, Darier was highly cultivated and had a charming personality and an acute sense of humor that delighted all those who knew him (Fig. 4-2).[10]

---

[9] Archives nationales, Dossiers de la Légion d'honneur, cote LO661042.
[10] G. Guillain, "Eloge de Jean Darier" [Speech by Georges Guillain on the death of M. Jean Darier], Société médicale des hôpitaux de Paris, meeting of June 10, Semaine des Hopitaux de Paris: 1938, 1018–1020.

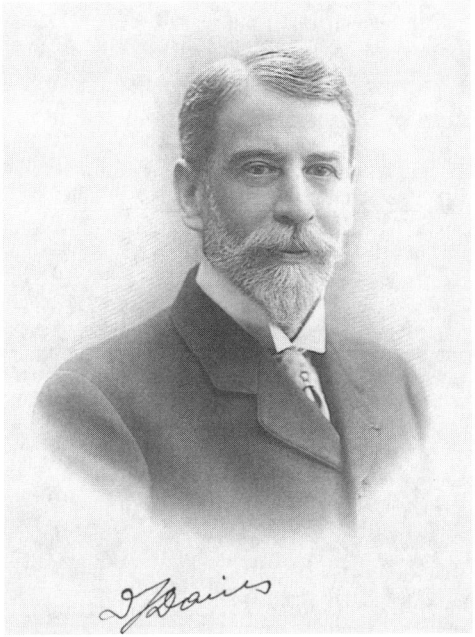

Figure 4-2 Dr. Jean-Ferdinand Darier. (*Source*: Archives of the Académie nationale de médecine, Paris.)

Pierre Bazy (1853–1934) was successively resident and surgeon in chief at Bicêtre, then at Tenon, Saint-Louis, and finally Beaujon.[11] His humane and professional qualities were widely recognized.[12] He was a member of the Académie nationale de médecine and of the Académie des sciences, and he was a commander in the Legion of Honor.[13] In collaboration with Félix Guyon, he published the *Atlas des maladies des voies urinaires*.[14] He was a close friend of Field Marshal Ferdinand Foch (1851–1929), with whom he founded a charitable institution for the children of officers killed during the war (Fig. 4-3).

Five years younger than Joseph Babinski, Fernand Widal (1862–1929) had a notable medical and scientific career.[15] He was successively resident,

---

[11] Dossier Pierre Bazy, Archives de l'Académie des sciences.
[12] On April 30, 1907, on the occasion of the inauguration of a new surgery building at the Beaujon hospital. *Journal des Praticiens* 1907 (21): 287.
[13] Archives nationales, Dossiers de la Légion d'honneur, cote LO151091.
[14] F. Guyon and P. Bazy, *Atlas des maladies des voies urinaires. Maladies de l'urètre et de la prostate* [Atlas of urinary tract, urethra and prostate diseases] (Paris: Doin, 1886).
[15] Dossier Fernand Widal, Archives de l'Académie des sciences; http://www.whonamedit.com/doctor.cfm/1004.html.

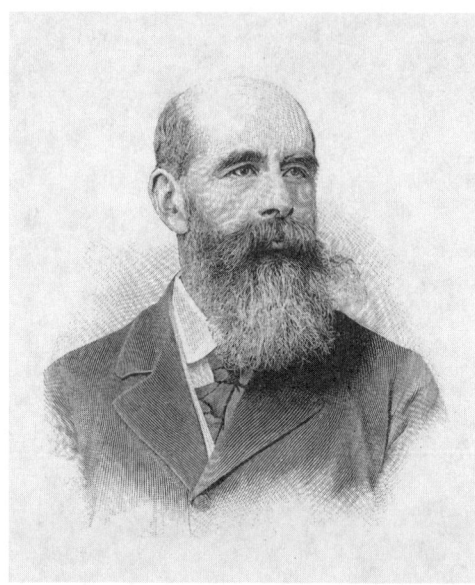

Figure 4-3 Dr. Pierre Bazy. (*Source*: Personal collection, J. Poirier.)

médecin des hôpitaux, associate professor, full professor in internal pathology, and later holder of a chair in clinical medicine, and a member of the Académie nationale de medecine and of the Académie des sciences (1919). He was trained in anatomopathology by Victor Cornil and in bacteriology at the Pasteur Institute. Apart from the writing and direction, with Roger and Teissier, of a famous textbook on internal medicine, and his works on the cytology of pleural extravasation and of cerebrospinal fluid, Fernand Widal is particularly known for his research on typhoid fever, and especially the serodiagnosic technique bearing his name. He discovered the importance of the retention of sodium chloride in kidney and cardiac edema, and the value of a salt-free diet in these pathologies. He may be considered as a pioneer of the modern clinical method, and his reputation as scientist and leader of a school of thought is widely recognized.[16] His memory was honored in 1933 by the erection of a monument inside the Cochin hospital and when the name of the Maison Dubois was changed to the Fernand Widal Hospital (Fig. 4-4).[17]

---

[16] E. Rist, *25 portraits de médecins français, 1900–1950* [25 portraits of French physicians, 1900–1950] (Paris: Masson, 1955), 87–95; "Allocution de M. Babonneix, president: A propos de la mort de F. Widal" [Allocution of the president on the death of Professor Widal], *Rev Neurol (Paris)* 1929 (I): 205.

[17] M. Hulmann, "Inauguration à l'hopital Cochin d'un monument à la mémoire du Professeur Widal" [Inauguration at the Cochin hospital of a monument to Professor Widal], *La Presse Médicale* 1933 (57): 1159–1160.

4. THE BABINSKI CIRCLE 91

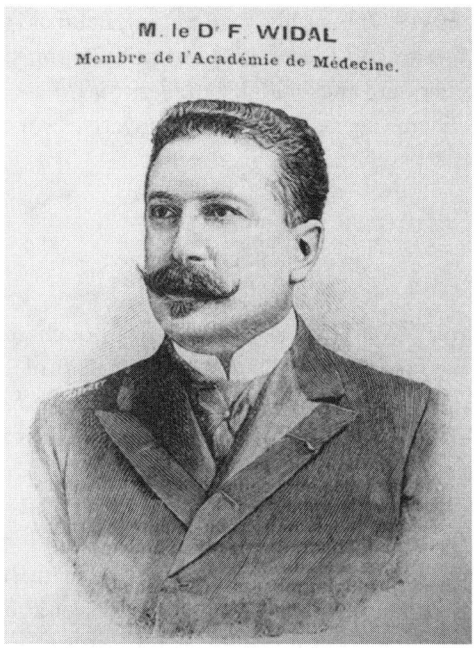

Figure 4-4 Professor Fernand Widal. (*Source*: From *Le Progrès Médical*, 1906 [29]: p. 459).

Émile Picard (1856–1941), though not a physician, was a top-rank scientist, graduating second in rank from the prestigious École polytechnique and first at the École normale supérieure, where he decided to make his career.[18] He became associate professor and lecturer there and then professor at the Sorbonne, holder of the chair in differential calculus, and then that of analysis and algebra. He also taught at the École centrale des arts et manufactures. He became a member of the Académie des sciences in 1889, its president in 1910, and its permanent secretary in 1917. Apart from his fundamental work on algebra and geometry, he also conducted applied research on elasticity and heat. His *Traité d'analyse* was for a long time a standard reference. He was also among the first to support Einstein's theories. Not only a mathematician but also a historian of science and philosophy, he was elected to the Académie française in 1926. Knight in the Legion of Honor in 1892, officer in 1900, and grand officer with Field Marshal Foch as his sponsor in 1928, he reached the highest rank in the Legion (grand cross) in 1932, with the sponsorship of the President of the Republic, Paul Doumer (1857–1932). Somewhat curiously, Babinski's name was not listed among the members of the patronage committee for the fiftieth anniversary of his academic career in 1928.

[18] Dossier Émile Picard, Archives de l'Académie des sciences.

Jules Séglas (1856–1939) is rarely cited among Babinski's closest friends.[19] However, René Moreau considered him an intimate, on the same plane as Darier, Enriquez, Vaquez, and Widal.[20] *Médecin-aliéniste*[21] *des hôpitaux de Paris* at the Salpêtrière, Séglas produced innovative works in the clinical, epistemological, and psychopathological fields.[22]

The Friends

Former resident and brilliant student of Charles Bouchard, Albert Charrin (1856–1907) became *médecin des hôpitaux*, associate professor, officer of the Legion of Honour, and assistant to and substitute teacher for Jacques-Arsène d'Arsonval (1851–1940) at the Collège de France, then professor of general and comparative pathology at the same institution.[23] His works concern bacteriology and microbial diseases, and he collaborated with Babinski on pyocyaneus infection.

Félix Lejars (1863–1932) first came into contact with Babinski when he operated on him for appendicitis.[24] Associate professor and surgeon in chief at Tenon and later at Saint-Antoine, he was professor of external pathology and finally professor of a surgical clinic chair at Saint-Antoine in 1919. He published several textbooks, the most popular being the *Traité de chirurgie d'urgence* (Treatise on surgical emergencies).[25] Lejars was a member of the Académie nationale de médecine and a commander in the Legion of Honor.

---

[19] T. Haustgen and M. L. Bourgeois, "Dr Jules Séglas (1856–1939), president de la Société médico-psychologique, sa vie et son oeuvre" [Dr. Jules Séglas (1856–1939), president of the Société médico-psychologique, his life and work], *Annales médico-psychologiques* 2002 (160): 701–712.

[20] Moreau, "Hommage à la mémoire de Joseph Babinski."

[21] At the time, when psychiatry was emerging as a new specialized discipline in France, a distinction was made between a "médecin-aliéniste" who held a position in the Paris hospital system and treated a wide spectrum of mental disturbances and the "aliénistes" who worked in the asylums and whose patients were restricted to those already diagnosed as being insane.

[22] Haustgen and Bourgeois, "Dr Jules Séglas."

[23] He was designated by a decree of the president of the Republic on April 1, 1903. Dossier Albert Charrin, Archives du Collège de France; *Le Progrès Médical* 190 (XXIII): 332.

[24] R. Dumesnil, *Histoire illustrée de la Médecine* [Illustrated history of medicine] (Plon: Editions Histoire et Art, 1935, 1950); Huguet, *Les professeurs*, 568–569; Rivet, "Joseph Babinski."

[25] F. Lejars, *Exploration clinique et diagnostic chirurgical* [Clinical exploration and surgical diagnosis] (Paris: Masson, 1923); F. Lejars, *Traité de chirurgie d'urgence* [Treatise on surgical emergencies] (Paris: Masson, 1901).

Charles Laubry (1872–1960) was resident on duty when Babinski was hospitalized for his appendicitis.[26] First a student of Vaquez and then the latter's favorite associate, he became *médecin des hôpitaux* and the holder of the chair of cardiology established for him at the Université de Paris, and a member of the Académie nationale de médecine and of the Académie des sciences; he was as well a grand officer in the Legion of Honor. His works dealt with arterial blood pressure and its clinical measurement with a sphygmomanometer, an apparatus designated under Vaquez's name and sometimes under his own. His findings were published in numerous treatises written with his associates on subjects such as the study of congenital heart diseases and coronaropathies, identification of myocarditis, and perfecting cardiovascular radiology. He founded the Société française de cardiologie and the Société internationale de cardiologie. His pupil Mouquin, in his obituary of Laubry, recalled that the Babinski brothers were among his close friends.[27] Laubry had a fashionable practice, having as patients Georges Clemenceau (1841–1929), who became his friend, Claude Monet, Léon Blum (1872–1950), and Edouard Herriot (1872–1957). Laubry was a celebrity in his native Yonne, where two streets are named after him—one in Flogny, his birthplace, and the other in Tonnerre.

Former resident of the Paris hospital system, supervisor of postmortem examinations in the department of Professor Carl Edouard Potain at the Charité hospital, Eugène Suchard (1852–1915) was demonstrator at the general anatomy lectures of Louis Ranvier (1835–1922) at the Collège de France and tutor in the histological laboratory of the École pratique des hautes études.[28] Suchard was an "accomplished technician whose skill exceeded eventually that of his master," whom, however, he admired to the point of copying his techniques.[29] He presented several papers to the Société anatomique, notably in 1881, 1882, and 1884, on the histological lesions of nail diseases.[30] With Victor Cornil he jointly published on the pathological anatomy of leprosy,

---

[26] Dossier Charles Laubry, Archives de l'Académie des sciences; Huguet, *Les professeurs*, 274–276; http://www.whonamedit.com/doctor.cfm/2277.html; http://www.lyonne-republicaine.fr; http://perso.wanadoo.fr/biblioflc/_private/flc/histoire.htm.

[27] M. Mouquin, "Nécrologie de Charles Laubry (1872–1960)" [Obituary of Charles Laubry], *La Presse Médicale* 1961 (69): 703–704.

[28] Dossier Suchard, Archives du Collège de France. *Le Progrès Médical*, 1901, 329; 1902, 331; 1903, 341; 1904, 330; 1905, 770; 1906, 758. Professor of the Clinical Medicine, Potain succeeded Charcot at the Académie des sciences in 1893, following the favorable report of Charles Bouchard. Dossier Carl Potain, Archives de l'Académie des sciences.

[29] J. Jolly, "Louis Ranvier (1835–1922). Notice biographique" [Louis Ranvier (1835–1922). A biographical note], *Archives d'Anatomie microscopique* 1922 (XIX): 1–72.

[30] E. Suchard, "Note sur les lésions histologiques de l'ongle incarné ou onyxis latéral" [Note on histological lesions of ingrown toe or lateral onyxis nail], *Le Progrès Médical* 1885 (II): 202.

and he wrote the chapter on the technique of clinical postmortem examination for Potain's volume of clinical lessons.[31] Suchard was inseparable from Georges Hubert Esbach (1843–1890), chief of the chemical laboratory in Potain's department, who went down in medical history as the inventor of the albuminometer, or Esbach's tube.[32] Both bachelors enjoyed the pleasures of life and were discerning gourmets, which favored their contacts with the Babinski brothers.[33]

The son of the writer Alphonse Daudet (1840–1897), Léon Daudet was designated a nonresident student in February 1888 at Necker Hospital, then at the Charité Hospital[34] He became a temporary resident in December 1890 at Cochin with Gouraud, then with Babinski.[35] Léon Daudet married Jeanne Hugo (1869–1941), daughter of Victor Hugo, in 1891. He tried once more for the position of resident, but he had too low a grade on the written exam, so he did not go to the oral session and decided not to defend his thesis. He then started a literary career, showing talent as a polemicist and pamphleteer, beginning with the publication in 1894 of the *Morticoles*, a cruel satire of university and hospital circles that created a scandal while being at the same time an immediate success.[36]

Charles Féré (1852–1907) defended under the supervision of Charcot a thesis on functional disorders of sight related to cerebral lesions (1882).[37] Alienist at Bicêtre, a fine clinician, he was also a research scientist and published through the Société de biologie several works on psychophysiology and psychopathology. After his death, Babinski, as president of the Société de neurologie, wrote a short obituary in which he described Féré as a "straightforward and high-principled man."[38]

---

[31] V. Cornil and E. Suchard, "Note sur le siège des parasites de la lèpre" [Note on the site of parasites in leprosy], *Mémoires de la Société Médicale des Hôpitaux de Paris* 1881 (XVIII): 151–154; E. Suchard, "Technique générale et sommaire des autopsies cliniques" [General techniques and review of clinical autopsies], in Carl Edouard Potain et al., *Clinique médicale de la Charité, leçons et mémoires* (Paris: Masson, 1894), 1011–1056.

[32] See the obituary of Georges-Hubert Esbach in *Le Progrès Médical* 1890 (XI).

[33] L. Daudet, *Souvenirs et polémiques* [Memories and controversy] (Paris: Robert Laffont, 1992), 166 and appendixes of Daudet book.

[34] M. Bonduelle, T. Gelfand, and C. G. Goetz, *Charcot: un grand médecin dans son siècle* [Charcot: a great physician of his century] (Paris: Éditions Michalon, 1996), 305.

[35] Ibid.; F. Broche, *Léon Daudet, le dernier imprécateur* [Leon Daudet, the last doomsayer] (Paris: Robert Laffont, 1992).

[36] L. Daudet, *Les morticoles* (Paris: Bibliothèque Charpentier, Charpentier et Fasquelle, 1894).

[37] *Le Progrès Médical* 1907 (XXIII): 298.

[38] *Rev Neurol (Paris)* 1907 (XV): 510–511.

Specialist in gastroenterology, writer of a successful medical treatise, Edouard Enriquez (1865–1928) was for many years head of a medical department close to that of Babinski at the Pitié hospital, and a great figure of French medicine at that time.[39] He had little interest in theoretical papers, and read them rarely; on the other hand, he showed at the patient's bedside a remarkable sense of observation, leading him to a very sure diagnosis.[40] In 1918, Enriquez, a member with tenure of the Société de neurologie of Paris since 1901, became its president.[41] Quite the opposite of his colleague Babinski, he was always in a good mood, happy to be alive, cheerful, full of enthusiasm, and bubbling over with energy and vitality.[42]

John Farquhar Fulton (1899–1960) and Georges Guillain (1876–1961) are the only ones to cite the name of Guignard among the friends of Babinski.[43] Although not absolutely certain, it is reasonable to think they were referring to Léon Guignard (1852–1928), pharmacist, former resident in pharmacy in Paris, professor of science at Lyon and then of botany at the School of Pharmacy in Paris, where he later became the dean.[44] Member and then president of the Académie des sciences, member of the Académie nationale de médecine, a commander in the Legion of Honor, his scientific work is substantial and dealt with several problems of plant life biology. His bust, erected in the botanic garden of the School of Pharmacy, was dedicated in 1933.

Students Who Became Friends

Among the 40 or so residents, 150 nonresidents, and numerous foreign visitors who were disciples of Babinski, some became more or less close friends (see chapter 9). In first position were the faithful Albert Charpentier, Auguste Tournay, Octave Crouzon, Clovis Vincent, Jean Dagnan-Bouveret, and, just after, all those who edited Babinski's *Oeuvre scientifique*, published

---

[39] E. Enriquez, A. Laffitte, A. Bergé, and H. Lamy, *Traité de médecine* [Medical treatise] (Paris: Octave Doin, 1909); Rist, *25 portraits de médecins français*, 57–63.

[40] G. Durand, P. A. Carrié, "E. Enriquez", *La Presse Médicale* 1928 (55): 876–877.

[41] "Allocution de M. Enriquez, président" [Speech by M. Enriquez, president], *Rev Neurol (Paris)* 1918 (I): 69–71.

[42] Rist, *25 portraits de médecins français*, 57–63 [25 portraits of French physicians, 1900–]; Durand, Carrie, *ibid*.

[43] J. F. Fulton, "Science in the Clinic as Exemplified by the Life and Work of Joseph Babinski," *Journal of Nervous and Mental diseases* 1933 (77): 121–133; G. Guillain, "J. Babinski (1857–1932)," *La Presse Médicale* 1932 (91): 1705–1707.

[44] Dossier Léon Guignard, Archives de l'Académie des sciences.

posthumously in 1934: Alexandre Barré, Joseph Chaillous, Louis Delherm, Jules Froment, Claude Gautier, Edward Hartmann, Edouard Krebs, Raymond Monier-Vinard, René Moreau, André Plichet, and G. A. Weill. Among the foreign visitors, the closest were no doubt Egas Moniz (1874–1955) and Charles Gilbert Chaddock (1861–1936).

Through this all too brief summary, one can see that Babinski drew around him an exceptional group of friends and associates. While discussion at the hospital was strictly limited to medicine, conversation in a social environment touching a wide range of subjects was no doubt stimulating to all parties.

··· *five* ···

The Competitive Examinations

Competitive examinations in both the university and hospital systems are a French peculiarity, the purpose of which is to select the "elites" based upon a series of difficult and challenging tests, both written and oral. For medicine, they were institutionalized at the beginning of the nineteenth century under the First Empire, as part of Napoleon's educational reforms. The *externat*, *internat*, and *médicat* examinations in Paris hospitals were defined by the statutes of the Health Service in 1804, while the *agrégation* dated from 1823.

The open competition of the Paris Hospital system was completely independent from that of the University, and held under the authority of the *Assistance Publique*: in French medicine, they have the highest reputation and are the most sought after.

After two years of medical school, a student may compete for the *Externat*; those who succeed are attached to a medical or surgical department where they walk the wards with senior physicians and can be assigned accomplish some simple tasks (dressing, punctures, therapeutic bleedings).

After two years, they can compete for the much more difficult *Internat* examination: grossly only one out of ten *externs* were selected. The *interne* has a key position and assumes patient care under the supervision of the department head. After four years, having defended his medical thesis, he may go into private practice or continue on in a hospital and/or university career.

In the hospital system, the next step is the very difficult competition for *Médecin* or *Chirurgien des Hôpitaux*. Once having succeeded, physicians were firstly assigned to the *Bureau Central*, a patient clearing-house for the different Paris hospitals. After a few years, depending upon the available slots and according to seniority, they took over the direction of a department (*Chef de service*). Until 1970 these positions were part-time and it was quite common to have a private practice outside the hospital.

A university career was possible only after defense of a thesis. Following the doctorat, the next academic degree is *Chef de clinique*, in general open to former residents as a two-year position, during which period he is the direct collaborator of the department head, with specific teaching responsibilities for *externes and* medical students. If he wants to continue in a university career, the next step will be the *Agrégation* (Associate professor) where he assumes a new role, that of assisting the full professor in his lectures at the *Faculté de Médecine*. There were four different fields for the *Agregation*: Anatomy and Physiology, Medicine, Surgery and Obstetrics, Physics.

Promotion to the rank of full professor, usually carrying with it the status of department head, was made by decision of the faculty, through a committee composed of full professors who voted until there was a majority. At this level, two further distinctions might be obtained, holder of a Chair or, for the selected few, Professor of a medical, surgical or obstetrical Clinic.

Written examinations had long been called for as a democratic means of, at least theoretically, avoiding favoritism and nepotism within the medical community itself, not to speak of political pressure and appointments imposed by the Minister for education. Bourneville had gone even further and recommended anonymous examinations. A series of scandals and excesses led to the call, notably in *Le Progrès Médical*, for the elimination of all such examinations, pure and simple. The examinations were accused of forcing candidates to go through a mind-numbing cramming process by which they were obliged to learn by heart the answers to standard theoretical questions and then regurgitate them in totally artificial conditions, often in a very short period of time (e.g., five minutes of thought followed by five minutes of response for the *externat* examination).

The Externat des Hôpitaux de Paris *(Part-Time Nonresident Student)*

First begun in 1802, the *externat* examination was not in the beginning difficult because the number of available positions was not very much smaller than the number of candidates (the success rate was 60 percent at the time

5. THE COMPETITIVE EXAMINATIONS

Babinski took it). It progressively became much more selective by the middle of the twentieth century.[1]

Joseph Babinski enrolled for the October 1877 examination,[2] which took place in two oral sessions in the lecture hall of the Administration of Paris Hospitals. Babinski sat for the first test, descriptive anatomy of the trapezius muscle, on October 31 and obtained the best mark of his particular session (17 out of 20). His second test, on an elementary subject of pathology or basic surgery—in his case, burns—received a score of 20 out of 20 on December 7. With a total of 37 points, Babinski came in third overall (and, for the first time, his name was misspelled with a *y*). Why did Babinski finish third with such outstanding scores? There were actually several groups of candidates at each competition. So although Babinski was first within his own group, two other candidates in other groups had an even better grade on the first examination than Babinski's 17 out of 20. Of the 414 candidates, 247 were nominated, confirmed by a decree of the general director of the Paris hospital administration, and took up their functions on January 1, 1878 (Fig. 5-1).

The Internat des Hôpitaux de Paris *(Full-Time Resident)*

After having been named to a temporary position as resident based on the results of his first *internat* examination in December 1878, where he ranked twenty-second out of twenty-five, Babinski was promoted to a permanent post following his second examination in December 1879, in which he placed fourth. The written test in anatomy concerned the testicles, and the test in pathology was on tubercular diseases of the testicles. The oral examination confirmed the results of the written examination.[3] At the general distribution of prizes, Babinski received the second honorable mention, placing him in fifth position, behind the winners of the first and second prizes and the first two honorable mentions.[4]

---

[1] A. D'Écherac (G. Dargenty), *L'Assistance publique. Ce qu'elle fut; ce qu'elle est* [Past and present of the Assistance Publique] (Paris: G. Steinheil, 1909), 355–356.
[2] Archives of the Assistance publique, Hôpitaux de Paris, 761 FOSS 10.
[3] Documents related to the competition and honor list of the residents and nonresidents (1820–1922), Archives of the Assistance publique, Hôpitaux de Paris, 680 FOSS.
[4] Decree of the general director of the Assistance publique, December 23, 1879, Archives of the Assistance publique, Hôpitaux de Paris, 680 FOSS.

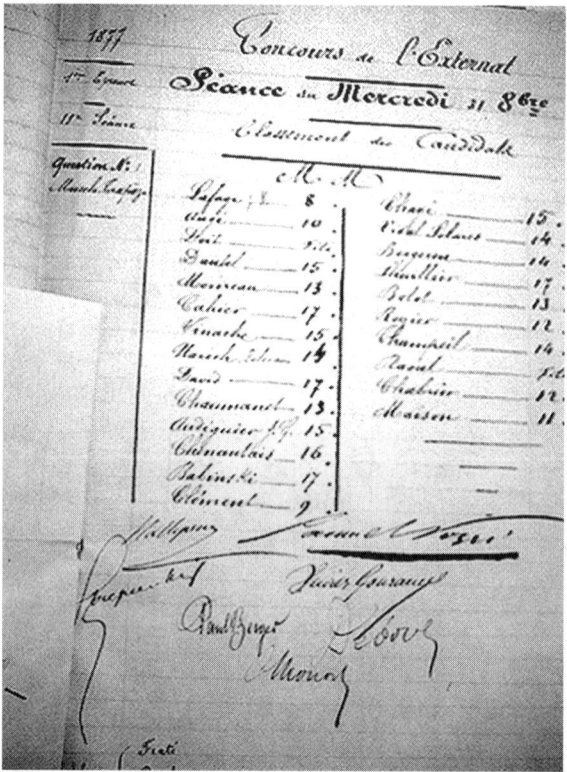

Figure 5-1 Minutes of Joseph Babinski's competition for the *externat*. (*Source*: Archives of the Assistance publique, Hôpitaux de Paris.)

The competition for the residency Gold Medal

This episode in Babinski's life was of such importance to his future career that it deserves a detailed account.[5] The Residency Gold medal was a competitive examination for the residents who had completed at least two years of the four years program. They were required to take it or risk dismissal. Babinski therefore signed up for the test in November 1882. The written examination (which lasted two hours) dealt with subjects of anatomy, physiology, and pathology on a topic chosen at random. When Babinski took the examination, the subject was the gastric mucous membrane, anatomy and physiology, and in pathology non complicated stomach ulcer. Although qualified for the oral, he was not able to make his presentation

---

[5] Residency prizes from 1879 to 1887, Archives of the Assistance publique, Hôpitaux de Paris, 761 FOSS 56.

on November 27 due to illness and was dropped from the competition, although he retained his residency post. The results were announced on December 11: no Gold medal was awarded this year; the first place (with the silver medal prize) was given to Henri Richardière, the first honorable mention (books) to Alfred Ricard, the others to Jean-Ferdinand Darier and to Paul Gallois.

This examination was also mandatory for residents who had completed their four-year program. Babinski therefore applied for the session of November 1884. The written test (two hours) dealt with two subjects: liver cells and the neurological complications of diabetes. Twelve candidates were qualified for the oral examination by the board of examiners (chaired by Professor Alfred Fournier, physician in chief at Saint-Louis hospital). Babinski obtained a score of 29 out of 30; Benoît Charrin and Richardière both received a 29 as well, and Darier got a 27. In the first oral test, which dealt with congenital hip dislocation, Babinski and Richardière both scored 16 out of 20. In the written part, the anatomical and clinical study of multiple sclerosis, Richardière, Charrin, and Babinski got 40 out of 40 and Darier 36. In the second oral test, on the effects on the nervous system of lead poisoning, Richardière was credited with 20 out of 20, Babinski and Darier 18, and Charrin 16. The results were declared on November 29, 1884: the gold medal was given to Richardière, the silver medal to Babinski, and the two honorable mentions to Charrin and Darier.

Because he had won the gold medal, Richardière was able to extend his residency for two years, whereas Babinski found himself having to apply for an appointment as chief resident. Fortunately for Babinski, Charcot had such a position available, as one of his residents had died suddenly. On the suggestion of Alix Joffroy and with recommendations from Vulpian, Cornil, Ranvier, and Bucquoy, Babinski was appointed.

The Médicat des Hôpitaux de Paris

To become a *médecin des hôpitaux* in the Paris hospital system, one had to be of French nationality and pass written and oral competitive examinations. Once having succeeded, the applicant became part of a pool called the *bureau central*, without being attached to a specific department.[6] Promotion

---

[6] The *bureau central*, located at the Hôtel-Dieu, operated as a clearinghouse where patients went for initial diagnosis and were then referred to the various Parisian hospitals according to the vacant beds, taking into account, when possible, the physician's main center of interest.

to the position of department head was then made by seniority among the physicians of the *bureau central*.

From 1886 to 1890, Babinski was obliged to go through this unpredictable and difficult obstacle course, often criticized but never abolished, which led to the selected few of the *bureau central (Médecin des Hopitaux)*.[7] For five successive years, during two or three months, he had always to be on the alert, because the order in which candidates took the examination was determined by lot and only known at the last minute. Preparation was diabolical, and one had to cram by reading many papers, often a compilation of texts such as the *Compendium*.[8] Babinski related with humor one candidate's words to the author of the book: "Sir, the *Compendium* is here: medicine is finished." Babinski remained obsessed by all this printed matter and the errors propagated therein.[9,10]

On May 10, 1886, a competitive examination was announced for two places in the *bureau central*. Babinski signed up for the first time, along with fifty other candidates, and on June 2 he took the first clinical test at the Hôtel-Dieu. The patient case—hydatid cyst of the liver, stomach dilatation—had been drawn by lot. After ten minutes of physical examination and five minutes of reflection, he gave a fifteen-minute public lecture of his findings, and scored 16 out of 20, which was not enough to qualify for the oral examination.

The following year, on April 15, 1887, a new competition was held for three *bureau central* positions. This time there were sixty-one candidates (among them Joseph Babinski, Pierre Marie, and Gilles de la Tourette). Babinski passed the clinical test on May 5, with 16 out of 20. He was among the twenty-six candidates who qualified for the oral examination (as did Gilles de la Tourette and Pierre Marie), which took place on May 31. He had to present a lecture on chicken pox, and obtained a score of 14 out of 20. Neither he, Tourette, nor Marie was definitively admitted.

On April 30, 1888, a competition began for three positions. Babinski registered for the third time, with sixty-three other candidates; among them

---

[7] Archives of the Assistance publique, Hôpitaux de Paris, 761 FOSS 30–31. See, for example, "Pour l'abolition du concours de médecin des hôpitaux" [For the abolition of competitive examination of *médecin des hôpitaux*], *Le Progrès Médical* 1914 (10): 115.

[8] Ibid.

[9] A. Charpentier, *Un grand médecin. J. Babinski (1857–1932)* [A great physician. J. Babinski (1857–1932)] (Paris: Typographie François Bernouard, 1934).

[10] Published by *La Semaine Médicale*, but not an official source-book, the Compendium contained an overview of basic clinical and therapeutic information to the medical profession as a whole. It was however not always pertinent to the competition cases studies, particularly in regard to new research findings; *La Semaine médicale*, 13è année, No. 58, October 11, 1893, p. CCXXIX.

were two future great names in neurology, Pierre Marie (who enrolled for the eighth time and was admitted to the oral test twice) and Gilles de la Tourette (who was on his second attempt). By this time the conditions of the examination had been modified: candidates had three hours to prepare a written composition on the anatomical, physiological, and semiological study of tremors which was then presented as an oral lecture. Babinski was given a grade of 27 out of 30, qualifying him for the next step. Also qualifying were Tourette (25 of 30) and Marie (30 of 30). On June 15, the first clinical examination took place at the Hôtel-Dieu; the patient case he had to discuss, drawn by lot, was aortic insufficiency of rheumatoid origin with hypertrophy of the left ventricle and pustulous disseminated acne. He obtained a grade of 18 out of 20. Moving on, as did Pierre Marie, Babinski then had to lecture for twenty minutes on narrowing of the pulmonary artery, for which he got 16 out of 20. On June 25, at the second clinical test, on gonorrheal rheumatism and aortic insufficiency of rheumatoid origin, he scored 26 out of 30, while Marie received 30 of 30. The three winners announced on July 2 were Pierre Marie, Just-Arnold Netter, and Augustin-Nicolas Gilbert.

The next year, Babinski registered for a fourth session in February 1889 and competed with sixty-five other candidates, again including Gilles de la Tourette and Darier. As in the preceding year, examination started with a three-hour written composition; the subject was heart sclerosis, and Babinski got 26 out of 30. He qualified for the second test, the clinical examination of a patient with pneumonia of the lung apex and jaundice; he scored 17 out of 20, which was not sufficient to qualify for the next stage.

In February 1890, Babinski registered for the fifth time among sixty-seven other candidates, including, once again, Gilles de la Tourette.[11] The fact that Cornil, his former faculty advisor, was on the board of examiners increased his chances of success. As in the two preceding years, examination started with a written composition. On urine albumin in scarlet fever, Babinski's composition got 30 out of 30. He qualified for the second test, clinical examination, on which he obtained 17 out of 20. He then scored a 19 out of 20 on the oral test, which was on paralysis in diphtheria. For the last clinical examination (two cases: one patient with brain disease, alcoholism, and syphilis, the other with stomach cancer), he got the maximum, with 30 out of 30. After four difficult years, Babinski was finally nominated as *médecin des hôpitaux* (Table 5-1).

---

[11] Babinski gave a new address at 54 rue Bonaparte.

Table 5-1: Babinski's five competitions for the Bureau Central

Year	Number of posts	Number of candidates	Jury	Admissibility for Babinski	Candidates nominated
1886	2	51	Hallopeau Descroizilles Landouzy Damaschino Brouardel Danlos Desprès	No	Edgar Hirtz Ernest Gaucher
1887	3	62	Cuffer Maimmer Génon-Roze Constantin Paul Hardy Robin Grancher Rendu Tillaux	Yes for the second test No for the third test	Josias Juhel-Renoy Martin
1888	3	64	Chauffard Hanot Guibout Gingeot Fernet Joffroy Labbé	Yes at the second test Yes at the third test	Pierre Marie Just-Arnold Netter Augustin-N. Gilbert
1889	3	66	Dreyfus-Brissac Dujardin-Beaumetz Desmons Labadie-Lagrave Lacombe Ferrand Th. Auger	Yes at the second test No at the third test	Dreyfous Petit Variot
1890	3	68	Constantin Paul Cornil Fournier Oulmpont S. Simon Hutinel Terrier	Yes at the second test Yes at the third test	Babinski Charrin Siredey

The 1892 Competition for the Agrégation de Médecine *(Associate Professor)*

In the French medical teaching profession, the position of associate professor (*professeur agrégé*) was created in 1823 to assist the full professors in their educational responsibilities. Who would take this major career step was determined by a national competitive examination, the board of examiners for which was designated by the Minister for education. Competition were organized in four different fields: medicine, surgery and obstetrics, anatomy and physiology, physics.

At the 1892 examination in internal medicine, Professor Charles Bouchard, a former pupil of Charcot, was in the chair (see chapter 16). In fierce and acrimonious competition with his master for leadership of the Medical School of Paris, he managed to eliminate Charcot's pupils, Babinski and Gilles de la Tourette, in favor of his own.[12] A great deal has been written about the 1892 examination. The journal *Le Progrès Médical*, under the scathing pen of Bourneville (a supporter of Charcot), reported regularly on the progress of the examination with its vicissitudes, and backed Charcot's pupils. Thirty-two years later, in his hagiographic biography, Le Gendre defended Bouchard, considering him above any suspicion of favoritism (Fig. 5-2).[13]

It must be said that the 1892 examination in internal medicine was not the only one fraught with suspicion. Protests were also voiced regarding the examination in surgery and obstetrics of June 1892, and complaints were lodged with the Minister.[14] The examination that year in physiology and anatomy, chaired by Mathias Duval, was also a subject of controversy. Because of an incident that occurred during this examination, on June 23, 1892, in the Chamber of Deputies, the Minister for education and fine arts was questioned about the rights of candidates to object to decisions made by the board of examiners.[15]

---

[12] V. Iragui, "The Charcot-Bouchard controversy," *Archives of Neurology* 1986 (43): 290–295.
[13] P. Le Gendre, *Charles Bouchard, son œuvre et son temps (1837–1915)* [Charles Bouchard, his work and times (1837–1915)] (Paris: Masson, 1924).
[14] "Encore le concours d'agrégation en chirurgie. Protestation d'un candidat de province" [Once again, the competitive exam in surgery. Protest of a provincial candidate], *Le Progrès Médical* 1892 (25): 481.
[15] *Le Progrès Médical* 1892 (15): 508–509.

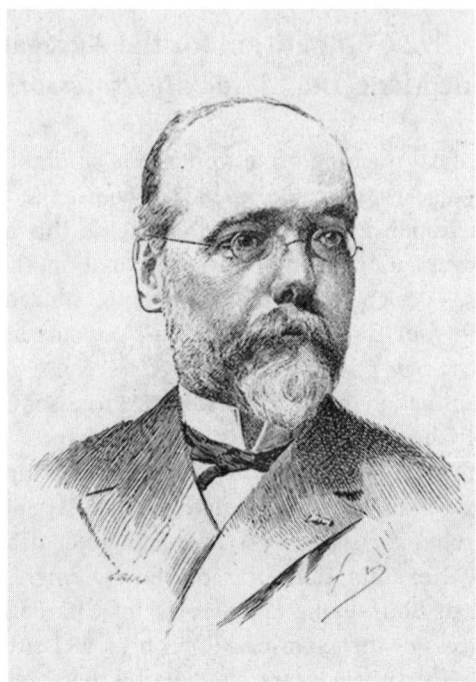

Figure 5-2 Professor Charles Bouchard. (*Source*: From Horace Bianchon, *Nos grands médecins d'aujourd'hui* [Paris: Société d'éditions scientifiques, 1891].)

Let us summarize the events of the *agrégation* of 1892:

- *The board of examiners*.[16] Selected by the Minister for education, the board was composed of nine professors. Five were from Paris: Charles Bouchard (President), Pierre Carl Edouard Potain, Germain Sée, Michel Peter, and Georges Debove. Four were from the provinces: Raymond Tripier (Lyon), Spillmann (Nancy), Mairet (Montpellier), P. Dupuy (Bordeaux).[17] Four alternates were also designated: Professors Alfred Fournier and Isidore Straus and two associate professors, Quinquaud and Victor Charles Hanot.

---

[16] "Le Concours d'Agrégation de médecine de 1892" [The 1892 competitive exam in medicine], *Le Progrès Médical* 1892 (15): 26; D. M. Bourneville, "Le concours d'agrégation en médecine" [The competitive exam in medicine], *Le Progrès Médical* 1892 (15): 223; Le Gendre, *Charles Bouchard*.

[17] Bouchard and Peter were the only jury members who also had students among the candidates. Strangely enough, the five nominated were indeed their *protégés*.

5. THE COMPETITIVE EXAMINATIONS

- *There were sixteen candidates* for five possible nominations, as seen in Table 5-2.
- *January 4, 1892*. At the first meeting of the board of examiners, Professor Germain Sée,[18] suffering from renal colic, was absent. According to the rules, President Bouchard should have asked one of the alternates, drawn by lot, to replace Sée. Rather than that, he simply declared that the session was postponed to the next day. "Why did he take such a stand? Would it not be, by chance, because he could not rely on others as much as on G. Sée to ensure the result he was seeking?"[19] Next day, Sée, still sick, was definitively unable to participate on the board. Bouchard still did not bring one of the alternates onto the board, and so the number of examiners was reduced to eight. In case of a tie the president would be the one to make the decision (Fig. 5-3).[20]
- *January 25, 1892*. Babinski took his first test, giving a forty-five-minute lecture on purulent pleuresis.[21] At the next session, Babinski lectured on peripheral neuritis.[22] Evaluation of the candidates' academic credentials and research publications was the next step.[23]
- *February 17, 1892*.[24] Babinski, on forty-eight hours' notice, gave a lecture on the severe feeling of cold in illness.[25] Then came clinical tests in the department of Professor Potain at the Charité hospital.[26]
- *March 12, 1892*. The results were declared. Charcot's two pupils were ousted, while four of the five candidates proposed for the nomination by the secretary of state were pupils of Bouchard.[27]

---

[18] Professor Germain Sée (1818–1896) became professor of medical therapeutics without having been *agrégé* (associate professor), through the influence of Empress Eugénie; he then was appointed to a chair in clinical medicine at the Charité. Member of the Académie de médecine, he founded the journal *Médecine Moderne* and published numerous papers on experimental therapeutics (*Le Progrès Médical*, 1896, 333).
[19] Bourneville, "Le concours d'agrégation en médecine."
[20] "Le concours d'agrégation en médecine d'après les journaux politiques" [The competitive exam in medicine according to the political newspapers], *Le Progrès Médical* 1892 (15): 248–250.
[21] Anonymous. *Le Progrès Médical* 1892 (15): 33.
[22] Ibid., 95.
[23] Ibid., 109. Cf. J. Babinski, *Notice sur les travaux scientifiques du Dr. J. Babinski* [Note on the scientific papers of Dr. J. Babinski] (Paris: Masson, 1892).
[24] Anonymous, 126.
[25] Ibid., 150.
[26] Ibid., 190.
[27] Bourneville, "Le concours d'agrégation en médecine."

Table 5-2: The 1892 Agrégation

Candidate 1892	Nominated 1892	Faculty advisor	Appealed	Nominated 1895
Achard, Charles		Debove		
Babinski, Joseph		Charcot		
Brault, Albert		Cornil		
Charrin, Albert		Bouchard		
Duflocq, P.				
Gaucher, P.L.E.		Bouchard		
Gilles de la Tourette, George		Charcot		
Lesage, A.				
Marfan, J.B.A.		Peter		
Menetrier, P.E.		Bouchard		
Richardiere, Henri		Brouardel		
Roger, G.H.		Bouchard		
Thibierge, G.				
Thoinot, L.H.				
Widal, Fernand				
Wurtz, Robert		Strauss		

5. THE COMPETITIVE EXAMINATIONS

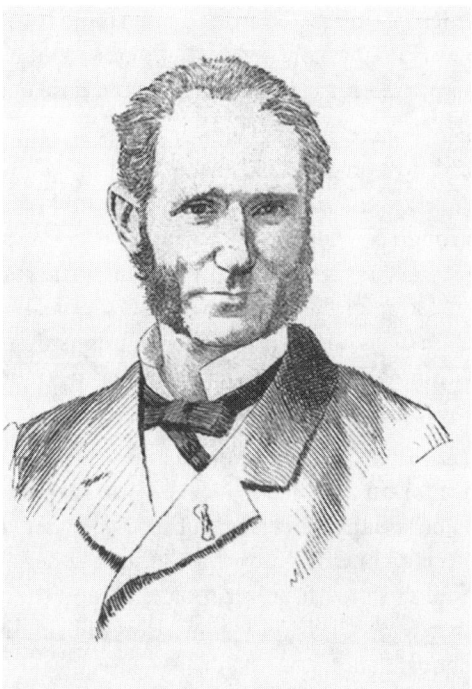

Figure 5-3 Professor Germain Sée. (*Source:* From Horace Bianchon, *Nos grands médecins d'aujourd'hui* [Paris: Société d'éditions scientifiques, 1891].)

- ·*March 17, 1892*. As reported in *Le Progrès Médical*, an anonymous contributor took advantage of Germain Sée's absence from *Médecine Moderne*, to publish in that journal an article that took the side of the unsuccessful candidates.[28] As director of the journal, Sée was furious.[29] A disclaimer rapidly appeared in *Médecine Moderne* in which he maintained that the examination had gone off normally and that the board of examiners had acted independently, even if the results had surprised some people.[30] In an interview with the newspaper *Le Matin*, Sée went so far as to say that the ousted candidates had performed poorly and that the examination had been perfectly honest and fair. However, *Le Progrès Médical* recalled that just before the examination, Sée was casually telling everyone who would listen that he had been

[28] "Le dernier concours d'agrégation" [The last competitive exam], *Le Progrès Médical* 1892 (15): 229.
[29] "Le concours d'agrégation en médecine d'après les journaux politiques."
[30] Ibid.

selected as a member of the board "to contribute toward putting an end to the power of Charcot," against whom he had a grudge for not having supported his election to the Académie des sciences.[31]

- *March 21, 1892.* Five of the thirteen unsuccessful candidates, Charles Achard, Joseph Babinski, Albert Brault, Henri Richardière, and Robert Wurtz, sent an official protest to the Minister Léon Bourgeois, through M. Lesage, an advocate attached to the Conseil d'État (council of state), and formally disputed the results of the examination.[32] Large-circulation newspapers, especially *Le Matin* and *L'Echo de Paris*, nourished the debate, publishing interviews with Charcot, Bouchard, Brown-Séquard, and d'Arsonval, the last two taking Bouchard's side against Charcot.[33]

- *March 24, 1892.* The *Tribune Médicale* maintained that there was no justification for an appeal.[34] *L'Echo de Paris* reported the words of a Bouchard confidant, referring to the rivalry between Charcot and Cornil on one hand and Bouchard on the other: "Everything stems from this: those with power took the lion's share in their turn;... In other words, it is only a question of bringing down the Salpêtrière school."[35]

- *March 26, 1892.* The *British Medical Journal* reported on the indignation created by the results of the examination and outlined the intrigues and injustices.[36] By contrast, for the *Gazette Hebdomadaire*, there had been no irregularities at any stage.[37]

- *March 29, 1892.* The *Gazette des Hôpitaux* denounced the obvious disregard for the rules, the nepotism that governed the nominations, the coteries, and the favoritism, and commented on the "thorns accumulated by generations of candidates unjustly ousted... Was this competitive examination especially unfair? Would another board of examiners, which would have nominated other candidates, other pupils, have been more commendable?"[38]

---

[31] Ibid.
[32] Ibid. The five unsuccessful candidates were introduced to Lesage by Professor Victor Cornil. Bourneville, "Le concours d'agrégation en médecine."
[33] M. Bonduelle, T. Gelfand, and C. G. Goetz, *Charcot: un grand médecin dans son siècle* [Charcot: a great physician of his century] (Paris: Éditions Michalon, 1996), 322–323.
[34] Cited in "Le dernier concours de l'agrégation en médecine."
[35] Cited in Bourneville, "Le concours d'agrégation en médecine."
[36] Cited in "Le dernier concours de l'agrégation en médecine."
[37] Ibid.
[38] Ibid.

5. THE COMPETITIVE EXAMINATIONS   111

- *March 30, 1892.* The *Journal des Débats* expressed surprised that favoritism, nepotism, plots, and other combinations had the upper hand in an examination that required such exceptional efforts from the candidates and which conferred on the lucky nominees not only substantial advantages but also heavy responsibilities.[39] *La Justice* asked for honesty and impartiality from the examiners, who should be free from the influence of the coteries and take into account only the candidates' scientific accomplishments and public lectures.[40]
- *April 25, 1892.* Georges Clemenceau, in his newspaper *La Justice*, called for the cancellation of the examination and said he was scandalized by the existence of "such haggling" in the medical world.[41]
- *May 2, 1892.* The Minister for education, Léon Bourgeois, turned down the appeal.[42] The five eliminated candidates, including Babinski, then appealed the decision by taking the case to the Conseil d'État (which would not deliver its judgment for two and a half years).
- *May 31, 1892.* The *Gazette des Hôpitaux* remarked that everybody knew that there were always candidates in the medical competitions who had mentors on the board and therefore might be nominated and others who did not have that advantage and knew in advance that they would not be chosen. The newspaper added that, recognizing this, candidates rarely presented an appeal.[43]
- *June 11, 1892.* Once more, *Le Progrès Médical* denounced the unfairness of competitive examinations in medicine.[44]
- *August 6, 1892.* The results appeared in the *Journal Officiel*, without waiting for the decision of the Conseil d'etat.[45] However, Bourgeois did not sign the controversial nominations before vacating his post. He left this doubtful honor to "his successor..., who put his noble signature at the bottom of a list, slipped in among many other

---

[39] Ibid.
[40] Ibid.
[41] Ibid.
[42] D. M. Bourneville, "Les concours d'agrégation: une série de citations" [Competitve exams: a series of quotations], *Le Progrès Médical* 1892 (15): 421–422.
[43] Cited in "À propos des concours d'agrégation" [Concerning the competitive exams], *Le Progrès Médical* 1892 (15): 458.
[44] "Technique des concours d'agrégation parisiens" [Technique of competitive exams in Paris], *Le Progrès Médical* 1892 (24): 471.
[45] *Le Progrès Médical* 1892 (33): 109. (Government decisions become formal only when published in the *Journal Officiel*.)

papers proposed to the...signature machine.... That is how the nomination of this year's associate professors has been made."[46]

- *November 12 and 16, 1894.* Two years later, the Conseil d'Etat issued its opinion: that the examination had not really begun on the first day, but only on the day after, when the whole board of examiners was present. Consequently, the facts presented in the appeal could not put in question the legality of the examination, and the appeal was rejected.[47] From a procedural point of view, the matter had to be considered as closed.

At the next competitive examination in 1895, Achard, Gilles de la Tourette, Thoinot, and Wurtz, who had failed in 1892, applied another time and were nominated. Babinski, however, did not compete in 1895 and would never apply again. This is particularly surprising since Babinski had not been discouraged by his four unsuccessful attempts for the *médicat* competition, having been nominated only the fifth time around. His decision may have been influenced by the fact that when his appeal was rejected, Babinksi was already physician in chief at the Aubervilliers Hospital, and was getting ready for a major change in his professional life: six weeks later, he would take up the post of head of a department at la Pitié, where he would remain throughout the rest of his career (see chapter 8).

Interpretations differ as to the causes and consequences of his decision not to compete again.[48] Some opinions, more or less authoritative, reflect the view that his failure was in the long run beneficial, allowing Babinski to devote more time to clinical research. For example, Vaquez thought that "this undeserved failure, which provoked in him a smile, had as a positive consequence a kind of liberation so that he could devote himself completely to neurology, which he had learned to appreciate with Charcot."[49] In the same vein, Tournay maintained that "after the initial shock, it did not take him long to recover; later, as he told some of his closest students, he appreciated this kind of freedom. In fact, it gave him the opportunity, without wasting time with

---

[46] "Un peu d'histoire ancienne à propos des concours d'agrégation en médecine" [A short review of ancient history concerning the competitive exam in medicine], *Le Progrès Médical* 1895 (1): 43–44.

[47] *Le Progrès Médical* 1894 (47): 419.

[48] O. Crouzon O. "Discours d'ouverture de la chaire d'assistance médico-sociale" [Speech at the inauguration of the chair for medical and social welfare], delivered November 22, 1937, at the Faculté de Médecine de Paris; G. Guillain, *J.-M. Charcot, 1825–1893, Sa vie, Son œuvre* [J.-M. Charcot, 1825–1893, his life, his work] (Paris: Masson, 1955), 62; M. Loeper, "Babinski," *Le Progrès Médical* 1932 (5): 1885.

[49] H. Vaquez, "Joseph Babinski (1857–1932)," *Bulletin de l'Académie de Médecine* 1932 (35): 1264–1273.

formalities or repetitive tasks, to devote himself completely to patients at the hospital or in private practice, such medical examinations giving rise to his indestructible semiology."[50] Elsewhere Tournay commented, "He always considered it an advantage not to have been invited...to participate in the official teaching sphere."[51] This retrospective rationalization seems a little superficial, however: did the positions of associate professor and then full professor prevent Charcot, Vulpian, Dejerine, Marie, Guillain, and so many others from devoting themselves totally to neurology?[52]

Rivet's version seems to us more credible:

> For a long time Babinski harbored a great bitterness about this failure and hatred for Bouchard. But he did not want to face a new examination, and later got over this failure, thinking that the position of associate or full professor would not have given him the opportunity to carry on his clinical research. He regretted being deprived of a chair only because of the influence he could have had on the future of his pupils.[53]

For Noir, the moral of the story is that one does not need to be a professor to excel in practicing medicine as a hospital physician, even without the highest university degree.[54] Bonduelle thinks "that it is more out of contempt than resentment that he abandoned the university examinations, which, however would have kept him away from neurology."[55] Is it also possible that he feared the constraints and responsibilities of a university career?

What Happened to the Competitive Examinations in Medicine?

For nearly seven decades, things stayed more or less the same, with generations of future physicians in chief spending several years of their professional careers preparing for examinations that had nothing to do with their chosen specialty.

[50] A. Tournay, *La vie de Joseph Babinski* [Life of Joseph Babinski] (Amsterdam: Elsevier, 1967).
[51] A. Tournay, "Babinski dans la vie" [Babinski in his life], *La Presse Médicale* 1958 (66): 1485–1489.
[52] Vaquez, "Joseph Babinski."
[53] L. Rivet, "Joseph Babinski (1857–1932)," *Bull Mém Soc Méd Hôp Paris* 1932 (34): 1722–1733.
[54] J. Noir, "Souvenirs évoqués par la mort de deux maîtres: Chauffard et Babinski" [Memories evoked by the death of two mentors: Chauffard and Babinski], *Concours Médical* 1932 (52): 3733–3734.
[55] Bonduelle, Gelfand, and Goetz, *Charcot: un grand médecin dans son siècle.*

After multiple vicissitudes, the separation between hospital and university functions disappeared in 1958, when only full-time positions were allowed, leading the way to a single examination.[56] The creation for the physicians of this single hospitalo-universitary function allowed the government to substantially increase the basic salary, while reducing private practice for full time hospital physicians; by decree of the Health department, private practice at the hospital was limited to 10 percent of the total activity.

In 1984, the distinction between associate and full professor was also abolished, leading to a single job title, that of *professeur des universités–praticien hospitalier*.[57] However, that the needs of hospitals were much greater than those of the university, so a special section was created for hospital physicians without any teaching functions. This group of *praticiens hospitaliers* has been considerably developed in recent years. If Babinski were practicing in our time, he would be one of them.

The series of tests to become a nonresident student (the *externat*) disappeared in May 1968, replaced by a system where all third-year medical students having passed the exam at the end of their second year have the same status (that of "hospital student" [Etudiant hospitalier]) which means, in fact, that their responsibilities have decreased. For residency, the competitive examination was modified further at the beginning of the year 2000. Everyone who passes the examination may continue with training, but those who received higher scores have first choice of available places and thus have a better chance of finding a place in their preferred specialty than those at the bottom.

Aside from what many see as blatant favoritism, to Babinski's detriment, it is important to recall that those who reached this stage of competition for the *agrégation* were all highly qualified physicians and scientists. A few of the successful candidates made no subsequent mark on medicine. However, many of the 1892 candidates went on to have brilliant careers. Ten years before the examination, Gaucher had already described in his thesis what would become known as Gaucher's disease; likewise, Ménétrier had described prior to the competition a rare gastric disorder that would carry his name. The list of syndromes and signs carrying Marfan's name is as extensive as that of Babinski, whom Marfan joined at the *Académie de médecine* in 1914, and this was the case for Widal and others as well.

---

[56] The 1908 *agrégation* competition (Bouchard was again a member of the jury) was canceled. Le Gendre, *Charles Bouchard*.

[57] "Pour l'abolition du concours de médecin des hôpitaux" [For the abolition of the competitive exam for physicians in chief], *Le Progrès Médical* 1914 (10): 115; "La crise de l'agrégation" [Competititve exams in crisis], *Le Progrès Médical* 1910: 277.

··· *six* ···

His Revered Teachers

Babinski always showed respect for his teachers, but he admired, revered, and liked some more than others. This description of his medical studies and relationships with his professors shows the breadth and depth of the curriculum as well as the high demands placed on the students at that time.

Babinski's University Medical Studies

In July 1875 Joseph Babinski received his baccalaureate degree in humanities, and in April 1876 he received one in sciences.[1] At the time, medical studies lasted four years and required a quarterly registration. Fees were 32.50 francs each quarter. His first fees was paid on November 4, 1875, for the last quarter of 1875.[2] His official address was listed as 153 boulevard

---

[1] Archives nationales, carton AJ/16/6864.
[2] A. Galinowski, "L'enseignement à la faculté de médecine de Paris au début de la 3ème République et le décret du 20 juin 1878" [Teaching at the Paris medical school at the beginning of the Third Republic and decree of June 20, 1878], Medical degree thesis, Créteil school of medicine, Université de Paris XII, 1979. To register in medical school, a student could present a baccalaureate degree in humanities; the degree of baccalaureate in sciences was required only to register for the third quarter and after, explaining why Babinski was able to register on November 4, 1875, prior to obtaining his baccalaureate in sciences on April 4, 1876. To give an idea of what the quarterly fee of 32 francs meant to the Babinski family, at that time one could rent a one-room apartment for a week in Paris with that sum.

Montparnasse, and the person in charge was his mother; this indicates that his father was not present in Paris at that time. Subsequent registrations were made regularly each quarter for the same amount of money, until the sixteenth quarter, on July 14, 1879, corresponding to the end of the fourth and final year (Table 6-1).

His university report book indicates that he became a nonresident student in January 1878 and a resident in January 1880; he passed the competitive exam for residents with distinction in 1879. As an example, for the year 1876–1877, the main subjects included in the Université de Paris medical curriculum are given in the decree signed by Vulpian, dean of the faculty; Joseph Babinski attended all of them (Table 6-2).[3]

Nonresident Student at Saint-Antoine in 1878

Babinski's first assignment as a nonresident student (*externe*) was in a department of internal medicine of Dr. Constantin Paul (1833–1896) at the Saint-Antoine hospital.[4] Associate professor and member of the Académie nationale de médecine, Constantin Paul was successively head of department at the Saint-Antoine, Lariboisière, and Charité hospitals. A pupil of Trousseau and Pidoux, Paul devoted himself to the study of heart disease and transmitted to his students a firm belief in therapeutics, "scorning sceptics who prescribe without sincerity." He considered hydrotherapy and electrotherapy as valid methods of treatment.[5] He also invented the flexible stethoscope (Fig. 6-1).[6]

Provisional Resident Under Legrand du Saulle at Bicêtre in 1879

Babinski was appointed a provisional resident (*interne provisoire*) at Bicêtre (his grade was not sufficient for him to be named to a full position) in

---

[3] Archives nationales, carton AJ/16/303/1.
[4] *Le Progrès Médical* 1896 (16): 254.
[5] Ibid.
[6] C. Paul, "Stéthoscope flexible" [Flexible stethoscope], *Le Progrès médical* 1881 (IX): 375; P. Huard, "100 years ago Constantin Paul presented his biauricular autostatic stethoscope to the Academy of Medicine," *Bull Acad Natl Méd* 1981 (165): 1117–1121.

Table 6-1: Medical studies of Joseph Babinski at the University of Paris

Type of Examination	Fees	Dates of the Examination	Result	Observations
First examination end of the year	90 F	July 20, 1876	Very satisfactory	
Second examination end of the year	90 F	July 4, 1877	Extremely satisfactory	
Third examination end of the year	90 F	July 25, 1878	Very satisfactory	
First examination for the Doctorate	Lille	July 27, 1881	Very satisfactory	By decision of the Secretary of State for Education of the 21 April 1877, M. Babinski has taken his first two examinations for the Doctorate at the Lille Medical School
Second examination for the Doctorate	Lille	November 11, 1881	Very satisfactory	
Third examination for the Doctorate	90 F	January 28, 1885	Acceptable	
Fourth examination for the Doctorate	90 F	February 3, 1885	Extremely satisfactory	
Fifth examination for the Doctorate	90 F	February 10, 1885	Very satisfactory	
Thesis: Anatomical and clinical studies on multiple sclerosis	240 F	March 9, 1885	Extremely satisfactory	President: M. Cornil Examiners: MM. Potain, Joffroy, Reynier

Table 6-2: Faculty of Medicine of Paris Scholastic year 1876–1877

Chairs	Professors
Medical Physics	Gavarret
Medical Pathology	Axenfeld, replaced by his associate professor
Anatomy	Sappey
General Pathology and Therapeutics	Chauffard
Medical Chemistry	Wurtz
Surgical Pathology	Dolbeau
Operations and Apparatus	Léon Le Fort
Histology	Robin
Medical and Surgical History	Parrot
Medical Clinic	G. Sée (Hôtel-Dieu)
	Lasègue (Pitié)
	Hardy (Charité)
	…. (Necker)
Surgical Clinic	Gosselin (Charité)
	Richet (Hôtel-Dieu)
	Broca (Hôpital des cliniques de la faculté)
	Verneuil (Pitié)
Obstetrics Clinic	Depaul (Hôpital des cliniques de la faculté)
Supplementary clinical courses	
Childhood Diseases	Blachez (Hôpital des enfants-malades)
Ophthalmology	Panas (Lariboisère and School of medicine)
Syphilis pathology	Fournier (Saint-Louis)

(continued)

Table 6-2: Continued	
Chairs	Professors
Urinary tract diseases	Guyon (Necker)
Dermatology	X......
Practical courses (winter semester)	
Dissection exercises—Course by M. SEE, Director of the Anatomical Laboratory	
1st year	Medical chemistry Medical physics
2nd year	Anatomy Histology Dissections
3rd year	Anatomy Histology Dissections Operations and apparatus Internal and external pathology Medical and surgical clinics
4th year	Internal and external pathology General pathology Practical exercises of operative technics Medical, surgical, and obstetrical clinics

January 1879 in the department of Dr. Legrand du Saulle (1830–1886). Alienist at Bicêtre and then at the Salpêtrière, physician in chief of the special infirmary for prisoners, he was a founder of the Société de médecine légale, a former president of the Société médico-psychologique, and an officer in the Legion of Honor. Legrand du Saulle published numerous papers in the *Gazette des Hôpitaux* and several books on psychiatry, especially in forensic medicine (Fig. 6-2).[7]

---

[7] H. Legrand du Saulle, *Les hystériques—État physique et état mental—Actes insolites, délictueux et criminels* [Hysterics—physical and mental condition—strange, punishable

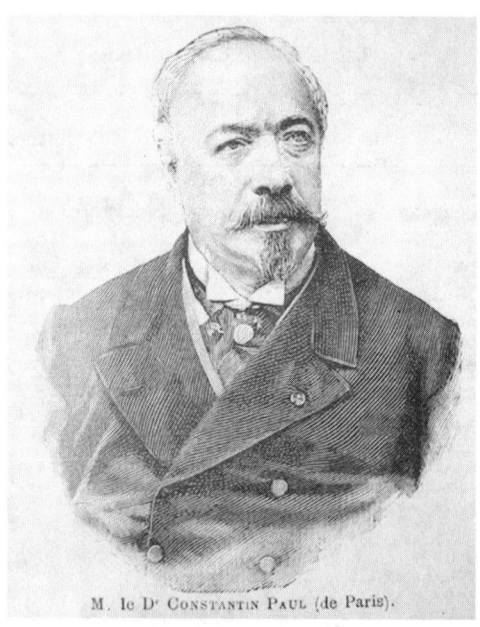

Figure 6-1 Dr. Constantin Paul. (*Source*: From Le Progrès Médical, 1908 [16]: 254.)

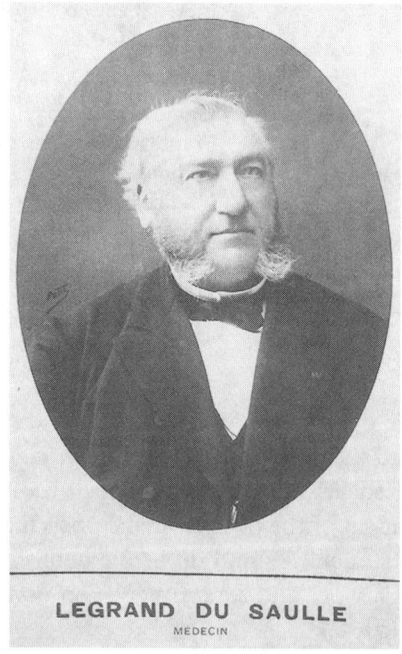

Figure 6-2 Dr. Henri Legrand du Saulle. (*Source*: Personal collection of J. Poirier.)

Resident Under Périer, Guibout, Cornil, Vulpian, and Bucquoy from 1880 to 1885

During his first half year of official residency (*interne titulaire*), from January 1 to June 30, 1880, Babinski was a resident under Dr. Charles Périer (1836–1914), surgeon at the Saint-Antoine hospital, member and then president of the Académie nationale de médecine. Périer was described a "charming old man, the most gentle, kind, affable man.... Even if he is not one who will leave a personal and durable mark, he has been an excellent teacher who, during many long years, offered to a multitude of pupils daily demonstrations of practical surgery."[8] They apparently maintained a good relationship, as shown by the fact that Babinski was called in for consultation to see one of Perier's patients with a nervous pathology.[9]

From July 1 to December 31, 1880, Babinski was a resident under Dr. Eugène Guibout (1820–1895)[10] at the Saint-Louis Hospital.

With his next residency, more serious things began. Between January and December 1882, Babinski was a resident under Professor Victor Cornil[11] at La Pitié, and from January to December 1883 he was under Professor Alfred Vulpian at the Hôtel-Dieu. During these two training periods of his residency, side by side with his eminent teachers, Babinski discovered pathological anatomy and histology, fields in which he became totally immersed. The strong personality of Victor Cornil is discussed in detail in Chapter 7 (Fig. 6-3).

Alfred Vulpian began his medical studies under the influence of Jean-Pierre Flourens, famous for his experiments on the nervous system, especially on the cerebellum.[12] To pay for his tuition, Vulpian worked as a technician in the department of his mentor at the natural history museum. His thesis dealt with the origin of the third to the tenth cranial nerves. Confirmed in a post in 1857, the year of Babinski's birth, he became successively associate professor (1860) and full professor of the chair of pathological anatomy, succeeding

---

and criminal acts] (Paris: J.-B. Baillière, 1891), cited in *Le Progrès Médical* 1886 (III): 400–401.

[8] J.-L. Faure, "Charles Périer (1836–1914)," *La Presse Médicale* 1914 (81): 743.

[9] J. Babinski, *Oeuvre scientifique: recueil des principaux travaux* [Scientific work: selection of main papers], ed. J. A. Barré, J. Chaillous, A. Charpentier, et al. (Paris: Masson et Cie, 1934), 22.

[10] Décès du Dr Guibout, Médecin honoraire des Hopitaux, *Procès-verbaux du Conseil de surveillance de l'Assistance Publique* [Obituary of Dr Guibout, meeting of January 10], 1895, 246.

[11] Dossier de Légion d'honneur, Archives nationales, L0592034.

[12] Dossier Alfred Vulpian, Archives de l'Académie des sciences.

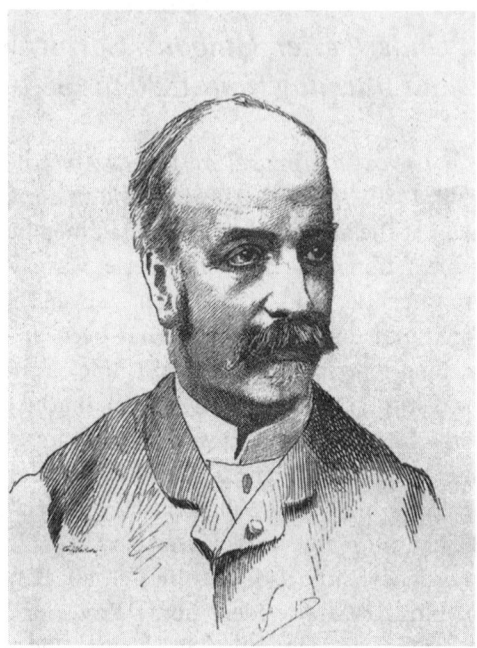

Figure 6-3 Professor Victor Cornil. (*Source*: From Horace Bianchon, *Nos grands médecins d'aujourd'hui* [Paris: Société d'éditions scientifiques, 1891].)

Cruveilhier in 1866 and preceding Charcot, who took the position in 1872. In 1862, he and his friend Charcot were named head of two different departments at La Salpêtrière. Vulpian was a workaholic. His work, even if slightly overshadowed by the glory of his pupil Dejerine and that of Charcot, is extensive in the field of clinical anatomy and physiology of nervous diseases. He was the first to demonstrate that tabes—contrary to the general opinion during his time—does not affect primarily the posterior columns of the cord. Member of the *Académie des Sciences*, he was named dean of the medical faculty in 1875, and resigned from this responsibility in 1881 (Fig. 6-4).

Some men devote their entire lives to the search of scientific truth without any other ideal or other passion. Science is for them a kind of cult, to which they belong completely and exclusively. Vulpian was that kind of man. He liked literature, he was sensible to artistic beauty, but he worked hard only for science, with his only purpose to know the truth. As Georges Hayem (1841–1933) noted after Vulpian's death, there was no doubt as to the eminent researcher's qualities.[13] A statue of Vulpian by Paul Richer (1849–1933) was unveiled in Paris on July 4, 1928.

---

[13] G. Hayem, "Professor Vulpian," *Revue Internationale de l'Enseignement*, December 15, 1887.

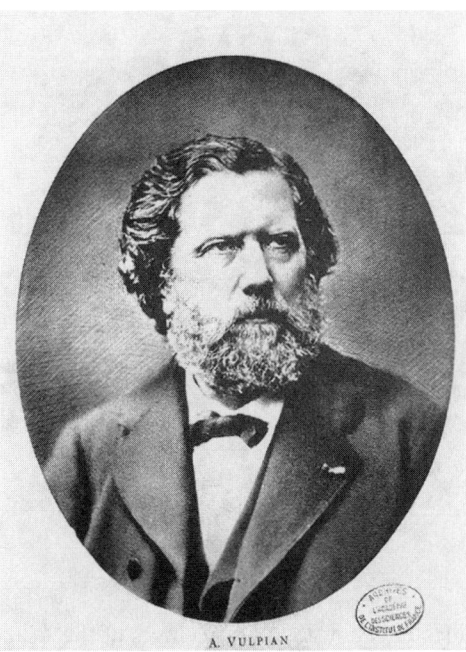

Figure 6-4 Professor Alfred Vulpian. (*Source*: Archives of the Académie des sciences, Paris.)

From January to December 1884, Babinski was a resident under Jules Bucquoy (1829–1920).[14] Bucquoy, successively head of department at the Enfants-Malades, Cochin, Saint-Antoine, and the Hôtel-Dieu, concentrated on heart, lung, and digestive tract diseases. Named a member of the Académie nationale de médecine in 1882, he became its president in 1908 (Fig. 6-5). During World War I, he gave part of his time to the *Oeuvre des prisonniers militaires* (charitable organization for prisoners of war), and in recognition of this contribution was awarded the rank of officer in the Legion of Honor. After his retirement, he devoted himself to a charitable institution, the navy sanatorium. He died at the age of ninety-one, run over by a bus. Bucquoy was as much appreciated by his pupils as by his colleagues; Babinski was greatly influenced by him and, in his later years, often recalled him Tables 6-3 and 6-4.[15]

---

[14] Mort de Mr le docteur Bucquoy, "Conseil de surveillance" [Obituary of Dr Bucquoy, meeting of July 1], 1920, 669–670; Laveran, "Nécrologie de Dr Bucquoy" [Obituary of Dr. Bucquoy], *Bulletin de l'Académie de Médecine* 1920 (27): 4–5; M. Letulle, "Bucquoy (1829–1920)," *La Presse Médicale* 1920 (48): 892–893.
[15] J. F. Fulton, "Science in the clinic as exemplified by the life and work of Joseph Babinski," *Journal of Nervous and Mental Diseases* 1933 (77): 121–133.

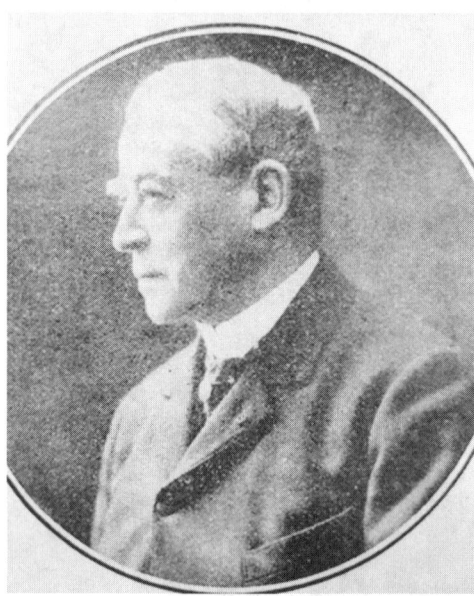

Figure 6-5 Dr. Jules Bucquoy. (*Source*: Archives of the Académie nationale de médecine, Paris.)

Chief Resident Under Charcot

Jean-Martin Charcot, head of department at the Salpêtrière from 1862 to his death in 1893, was the first holder of the chair for the study of diseases of the nervous system, which was created for him in 1882.[16] He became a member of the Académie des sciences in 1883. Among Charcot's merits, and not the least important of them, was that he knew how to surround himself with remarkable associates, some of whom are described here.[17]

Xavier Galezowski (1833–1907), born in Poland, received his first medical degree in St. Petersburg, Russia, and his second from the University of Paris in 1865.[18] He became an eminent eye specialist and was the first to use ophthalmologic examination as a routine diagnostic tool for patients with nervous diseases, preparing the way for Parinaud. His son, Jean Galezowski, followed the family tradition and in 1904 defended his thesis on the role of the retinal examination in nervous system pathology.

---

[16] M. Bonduelle, T. Gelfand, and C. G. Goetz, *Charcot, un grand médecin dans son siècle* [Charcot: a great physician of his century] (Paris: Éditions Michalon, 1996).

[17] M. de Fleury, *Le médecin* [The physician] (Paris: Hachette, 1927).

[18] "Necrologie de Mr le docteur Galezowski" [Obituary of Dr Galezowski], *Le Progrès Médical* 1907 (XXIII): 206.

Table 6-3: Joseph Babinski's teachers

	Nonresident "Externe" (1878)	Temporary Resident "Interne Provisoire" (1879)	Full Resident "Interne Titulaire" (1880–1884)	Chief-Resident "Chef de Clinique" (1885–1886)
1878	Constantin Paul (Saint-Antoine)			
1879		Legrand du Saulle (Bicêtre)		
1880			Périer (St Antoine) Guibout (St Louis)	
1881			Voluntary Military Duty (Military Hospital of Lille)	
1882			Cornil (La Pitié)	
1883			Vulpian (Hôtel-Dieu)	
1884			Bucquoy (Cochin)	
1885				Charcot (La Salpêtrière)
1886				Charcot (La Salpêtrière)

Henri Parinaud became a resident in Paris in 1872 after having started his residency in Limoges, and he wrote his thesis in 1877 on optic neuritis in childhood under the guidance of Bouchut, under whom he was a resident at the Enfants-Malades hospital. Charcot, who had been impressed by Galezowski's initial work, noticed Parinaud, and he became the permanent ophthalmologist on Charcot's staff. Parinaud also composed music under the pseudonym of Pierre Erick.

Table 6-4: Joseph Babinski's curriculum vitae during his training

Year	Hospital	Head of department	Appreciations on Joseph Babinski
Nonresidency (Externat) (ranked 3rd in his year in 1877)			
1878	St Antoine	Dr Constantin Paul	Was already in my department last year and appreciated him very much. This year he has worked to my complete satisfaction through his zeal, dependability and devoted back-up.
Temporary residency (Internat provisoire) (ranked 22nd in his year in 1878)			
1879	Bicêtre	Dr Legrand du Saulle	Very distinguished student with a great future. He is a hard worker, extremely knowledgeable and dependable.
Residency (Internat) (ranked 4th in his year in 1879)			
1880 First semester	Saint-Antoine	Dr Périer	Excellent resident whom I can only praise in all aspects.
		The Director	Has been most suitable during his stay with us.
1880 Second semester	Saint-Louis	Dr Guibout	Distinguished mind, perfect manners, remarkable intelligence; charming character, skilful clinician; exceptional resident whom I indicate to the administration as a man of first merit.
		The Director	Cold personality, quiet, serious mind.

(continued)

Table 6-4: Continued

Year	Hospital	Head of department	Appreciations on Joseph Babinski
1881	Voluntary military service		
1882	La Pitié	Dr Cornil	Zealous resident, on whom you may completely rely to manage the department, take the clinical records, make the daily rounds, etc… Good histologist, good clinician, very distinguished mind with a great future.
		The Director	Visa (indicating total agreement)
1883	Hôtel-Dieu	Dr Vulpian	Excellent resident in all aspects.
		The Director	Very serious.
1884	Cochin	Dr Bucquoy	Resident remarkable by his knowledge, by the way he combines his clinical responsibilities and the laboratory work and by the charm of his character.
		The Director	Good behavior, punctuality in his functions, excellent character, in a word exemplary resident.

Paul Richer, named as head of laboratory first with Charcot and then with Raymond, succeeded Mathias Duval (1844–1907) as professor of anatomy at the School of Fine Arts; he was a talented sculptor and medal engraver.[19] Pierre Janet joined the clinic with Charcot and remained afterward with Raymond.[20]

[19] *Le Progrès Médical* 1905 (30): 486.
[20] Conference by P. Janet, *Archives de Neurologie* 1895 (XXIX): 337.

In 1923, upon assuming the chair, Georges Guillain recalled the great merits of Charcot: "If one recalls that the associates chosen by Charcot are named Joffroy, Gombault, Richer, Debove, Raymond, Pitres, Brissaud, Gilbert Ballet, Pierre Marie, Babinski, Souques, no one could escape concluding that Charcot knew how to appreciate talent and how to increase the heritage and the brilliance of French medicine."[21] One wonders about the significance of his omission of Bourneville, Bouchard, Meige, Tourette, and Jean-Baptiste Charcot.[22]

From November 1885 to October 1887, Babinski served as chief resident (*chef de clinique*) under Charcot, with an annual salary of 1200 francs.[23] In this position, he succeeded Pierre Marie (who served from 1883 to 1885) and preceded Gilles de la Tourette (1887–1889), then Georges Guinon (1889–1891). During this two-year period (1885–1886), Sigmund Freud spent six months at the Salpêtrière, following Charcot's teaching (see chapter 2) (Fig. 6-6).

To our knowledge, no published paper was ever cosigned by Charcot and Babinski, or for that matter by Charcot and either Brissaud, Tourette, or Bourneville. On the other hand, Bouchard, Joffroy, Luys, Magnan, Marie, Pitres, Richer, Robin, Verneuil, and Vulpian all were coauthors with Charcot at one point or another. In July 1886, Babinski's name appeared on the list of contributors to the *Archives de Neurologie*, edited by Bourneville, under the direction of Charcot. Babinski authored several papers in which he paid tribute to Charcot. In "De l'atrophie musculaire dans les paralysies hystériques" and in an article describing a specific muscular deformation of the trunk in sciatica, he noted that Charcot was the first to observe this deformation and he included as an appendix a drawing made by Charcot.[24] Babinski wrote the preface to *Leçons du mardi*, edited by Blin, Jean-Baptiste Charcot, and Colin, in which Babinski in turn is cited seven times by Charcot.[25]

---

[21] "Chaire de clinique des maladies du système nerveux, leçon d'ouverture du Professeur Georges Guillain (20 décembre 1923)" [Opening speech of Professor Georges Guillain as chair of nervous system diseases, December 20, 1923], published in the January 26, 1924, issue of *Presse Médicale*. Léon Daudet wrote, "Among those who composed what was called the Salpêtrière school, the most gifted seemed to be Brissaud. I said 'seemed,' as in the final analysis the prize has been for Babinski." Daudet went on to depict Brissaud as a supporter of Dreyfus. L. Daudet, *Souvenirs littéraires* [Literary memories] (Paris: Bernard Grasset, 1968), 117.

[22] J. Poirier and F. Chrétien, "Désiré Bourneville (1840–1909)," *Journal of Neurology* 2000 (247): 481.

[23] Archives nationales, carton "Concours du clinicat 1874–1908," cote AJ/16/6350. Based on statistical records from 1900, a skilled laborer, such as a carpenter, would earn about twice the salary of a hospital physician.

[24] J. Babinski, "De l'atrophie musculaire dans les paralysies hystériques" [On muscular atrophy in hysterical paralysis], *Archives de Neurologie* 1886 (XII): 1.

[25] J. Babinski. Préface. Leçons du Mardi (Paris: Bureaux du Progrès Médical), 1–4.

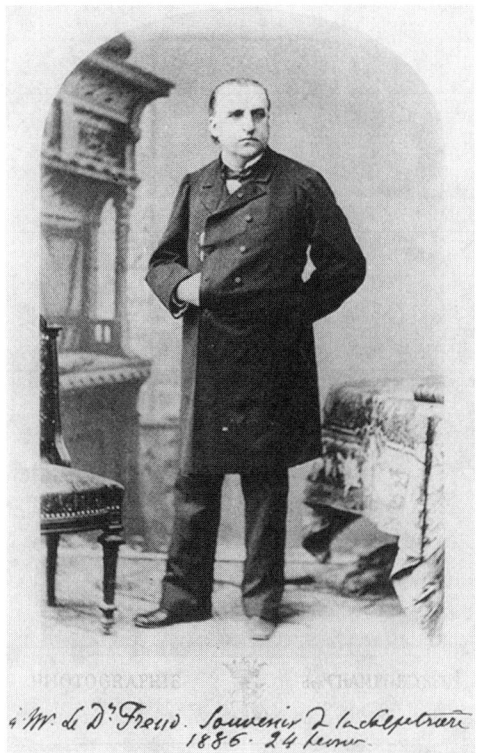

Figure 6-6 Autographed photo of Professor Jean-Martin Charcot to Freud, circa 1888. (*Source*: Courtesy of V. Leroux-Hugon.)

Needless to say, as was the case for all of Charcot's students, Babinski was a regular guest at the Tuesday evening receptions at the Charcot mansion.[26] It is clear that Charcot had a strong impact on Babinski; indeed, it is sometimes said that Babinski became the "living incarnation of Charcot."[27]

Throughout his life, starting with his chief residency (*clinicat*), Babinski took every opportunity to pay tribute and show his admiration, appreciation, and filial affection for his eminent master Charcot, to whom he would always be indebted (Fig. 6-7). In 1892, at the banquet organized in honor of Charcot at the Durand Restaurant to celebrate his being named a commander of the Legion of Honour, invitations were strictly limited to former residents, chief residents, and heads of departments working in cooperation with the clinic. Babinksi was

---

[26] Reported in G. Guillain, *J.-M. Charcot, 1825–1893, Sa vie, Son oeuvre* [J.-M. Charcot, 1825–1893, his life, his work] (Paris: Masson, 1955), 34–38.

[27] J. Fulton, "Joseph François Félix Babinski 1857–1932," *Archives of Neurology and Psychiatry* 1933 (29): 168–174.

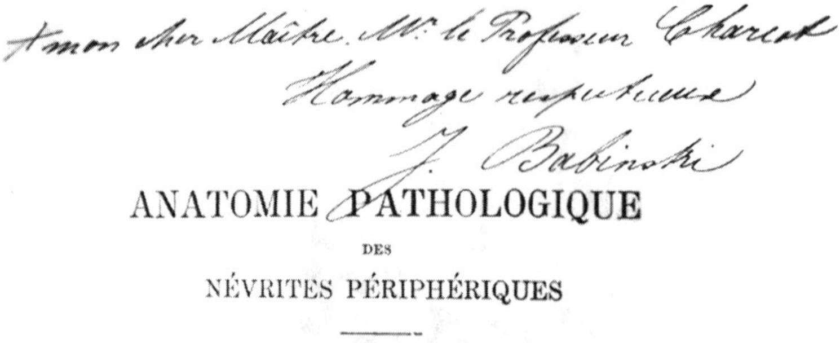

À mon cher Maître M. le Professeur Charcot
Hommage respectueux
J. Babinski

ANATOMIE PATHOLOGIQUE
DES
NÉVRITES PÉRIPHÉRIQUES

Figure 6-7 Reprint signed by Babinski for Charcot. (*Source*: From J. Babinski, *Oeuvre scientifique: recueil des principaux travaux* [Paris: Masson et Cie, 1934].)

among the invited few.[28] As the earliest of Charcot's residents, Victor Cornil gave the speech in tribute to the master. Likewise, Babinski attended Charcot's funeral and was a member of the committee to raise a monument to Charcot that was set up in 1894 under the honorary chairmanship of Pasteur and the presidency of Brouardel, dean of the faculty of medicine, and of Gréard, vice rector of the Académie de Paris.[29] Babinski was also a member of the commission appointed by the committee on May 17, 1895, to negotiate with Alexandre Falguière (1831–1900), the sculptor who had tentatively been selected to create the statue.[30] French and foreign subscribers were numerous; among the first on the list, which was begun on December 15, 1893, Babinski committed himself to 200 francs.[31] The unveiling took place on Sunday, December 4, 1898,

---

[28] The list in chronological order of Charcot's *internes* (residents) is as follows: V. Cornil (1863), Bouchard (1864 and 1866), Bourneville (1868), Joffroy (1869), Debove (1871), Gombault (1871), Pierret (1874), Raymond (1875), Pitres (1876), Oulmont (1877), P. Richer (1878), Brissaud (1879), Ballet (1880), Féré (1881), Marie (1882), Gilles de la Tourette (1884), G. Guinon (1885), Babinski (chief resident, 1885–1887), Berbez (1886), Blocq (1887), Huet (1888), Dutilo (1889), Parmentier and Souques (1890), J.-B. Charcot and Hallion (1891), Gasne, Guyon, Lamy (1892), Londe (1893), Collinet (1894), Landowski (1895). Also invited were collaborating department heads: Vigouroux (electrotherapy), Parinaud (ophthalmology), Gellé (otology), Galippe (odontology), Londe (photography).

[29] *Le Progrès Médical* 1893 (34): 144; *Le Progrès Médical* 1894 (5): 91.

[30] This commission was composed of Brouardel, Gérome, Garnier, Richer, and Babinski. Archives de Neurologie 1895 (XXIX): 493.

[31] *Archives de Neurologie* 1895 (XXIX): 493–494. The first subscription list for the committee was as follows: Pasteur (honorary president), 200 francs; Brouardel (president of the committee), 200 francs; Bourneville (secretary of the committee), 100 francs; Guinon (secretary), 100 francs; Masson (treasurer), 200 francs; Babinski, 200 francs; Baudoin, 20 francs; Gassicourt, 100 francs; Galippe, 100 francs; Tourette, 100 francs; Joffroy, 200 francs; Lereboullet, 100 francs; Londe (resident at the Salpêtrière), 20 francs; Marie,

6. HIS REVERED TEACHERS

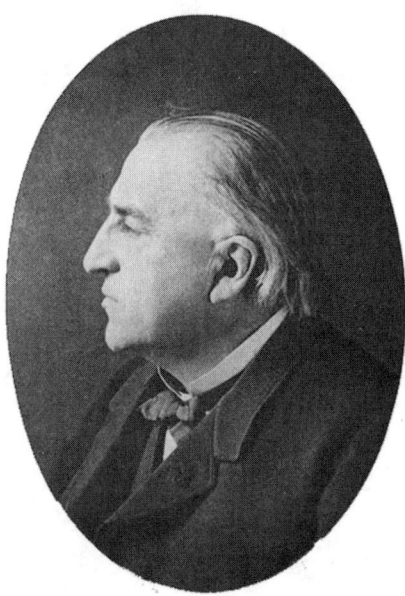

Figure 6-8 Professor Jean-Martin Charcot. (*Source*: Personal collection, J. Poirier.)

at the Salpêtrière, led by the minister of education, M. Leygues.[32] The statue, which was melted down by the Germans during World War II, was on the left side of the main entrance to the Salpêtrière. Charcot was portrayed in his professorial gown, his left hand raised as it typically was when he was demonstrating to an audience. The index finger of his right hand points to the left parietal area of the corpse that lies at his feet. In 1909, Babinski, even while tearing apart the traditional conception of hysteria, nevertheless paid a stirring tribute to Charcot and apologized for having to contradict the doctrine of his illustrious master.[33] At Charcot's centenary in 1925, the speech Babinski gave at the Sorbonne on May 26 was yet another vibrant eulogy.[34] And just prior to his death, according to Charpentier, Babinksi was still speaking with admiration of the "great Charcot" (Fig. 6-8).[35]

200 francs; Vallery-Radot, 100 francs. "Comité du Monument à élever à la mémoire de J.-M. Charcot," January 2, 1894, Charcot library at the Salpêtrière.

[32] "Inauguration of the monument to J.-M. Charcot" [Inauguration of the monument to the memory of J.-M. Charcot], *La Presse Médicale*, December 7, 1898; Le Progrès Médical 1898 (VIII): 449.

[33] J. Babinski, "Démembrement de l'hystérie traditionnelle. Pithiatisme" [Dismembering traditional hysteria. Pithiatism], *La Semaine Médicale*, January 6, 1909.

[34] J. Babinski, "Eulogie de J.-M. Charcot," *Rev Neurol (Paris)* 1925 (I): 746–756.

[35] A. Charpentier, *Un grand médecin, Joseph Babinski (1857–1932)* [A great physician, Joseph Babinski (1857–1932)] (Paris: Typographie François Bernouard, 1934).

··· *seven* ···

Babinski and the Anatomical Society

It is not clear what prompted Babinski to spend his second year of residency under Victor Cornil, or his third year with Alfred Vulpian. Some suggest his choice was influenced by the availability of residency positions, rather than personal preference, but there are no objective data to validate or refute this hypothesis.[1]

Whatever the reasons for his choice, the beginning of the residency program meant for him a career in pathological anatomy, as suggested by the title of his thesis, supervised by Vulpian and defended in March 1885: "Étude anatomique et clinique sur la sclérose en plaques" [Anatomical and clinical study on multiple sclerosis], by "Dr. J. Babinski, former resident and prize winner of the Paris hospitals, instructor in pathological anatomy at the medical school, member of the Anatomical Society" (Figs. 7-1 and 7-2).[2]

But his future changed because of the unexpected opportunity to become chief resident under Charcot. At this decisive point in his career, Babinski, student of Cornil, Vulpian, and Louis Ranvier, abandoned pathological anatomy, preferring, as reported by Clovis Vincent, "to study the living rather than the dead."[3] He would become a pure clinician interested by semiology,

---

[1] C. Belanger, "What do you know about Joseph Babinski?" *Can J Neurol Sci* 1989 (6): 4–7.
[2] Babinski was awarded a Silver Medal by the Assistance publique for his exemplary conduct during the cholera epidemic in 1884.
[3] L. Rivet, "Joseph Babinski (1857–1932)," *Bull. Mem. Soc. Méd. Hôp. Paris* 1932 (34): 1722–1733. Fulton repeated these words in "Science in the clinic as exemplified by the life and work of Joseph Babinski," *Journal of Nervous and Mental Diseases* 1933 (77): 121–133.

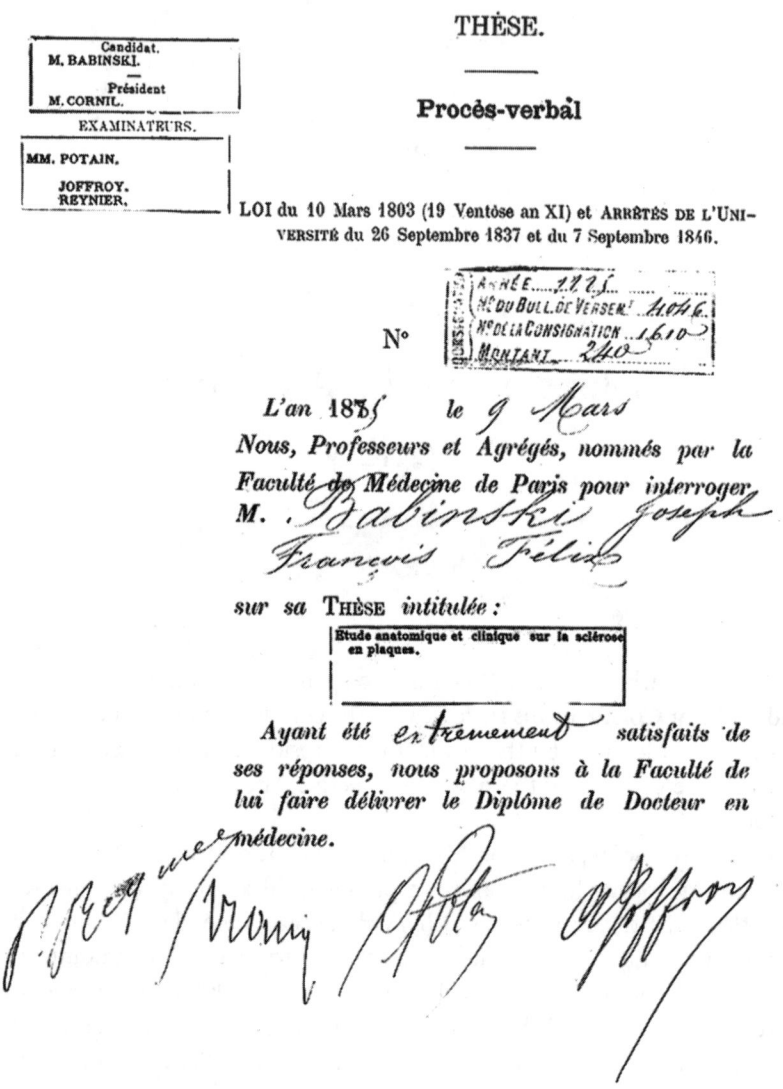

Figure 7-1 Minutes of the deliberation on Babinski's medical thesis (1885). (*Source*: Archives nationales, Paris.)

a subject far from his first interest in pathological anatomy and histology. He would never again look through a microscope, leaving this work to his associates, Jumentié and especially Jean Nageotte.[4]

This was more than a turning point in his career; it was a true rupture, a switch, a conversion that was at the same time physical (sending him in a new direction) and spiritual (giving him a new purpose). Thenceforth, the

[4] A. Tournay, "Joseph Babinski (1857–1932)," *Médecine de France* 1953 (43): 3–10.

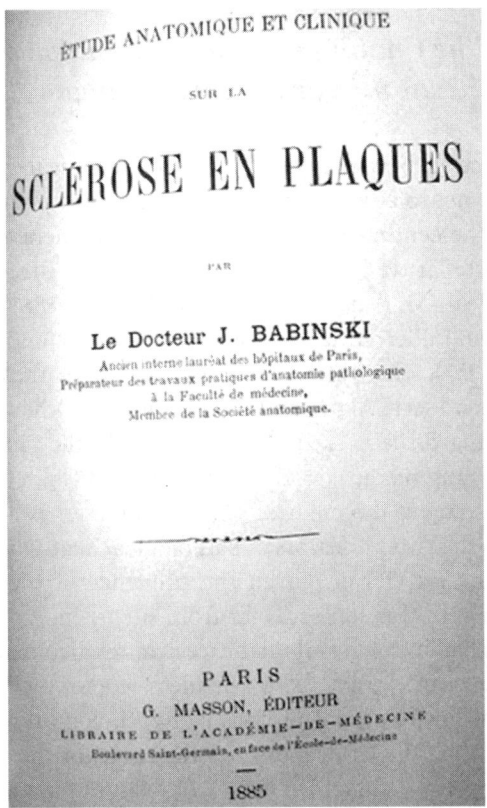

Figure 7-2 Cover page of Babinski's medical thesis (1885).

main purpose of his professional life would be to find clinical means of distinguishing organic pathology from hysteria.

However, these first years of involvement in pathological anatomy were a formative period in his intellectual and professional development, during which he acquired the skills and attention to detail that later would serve him well in his approach to semiology. During his residency and immediately thereafter, Babinski's focus was centered around his two mentors, Cornil and Vulpian. Within this microcosm there were three major poles: the chair of pathological anatomy of the medical school (held by Cornil), the Société anatomique de Paris (presided over by Cornil), and the Collège de France (where Ranvier held the chair of general anatomy). On the other hand, Babinski did not seem to have had much contact with the chair of histology of the medical school, created in 1862 for Charles Robin, whom Mathias Duval succeeded in 1886.[5]

---

[5] In 1885, the journal *Le Progrès Médical* treacherously indicated that "students who do not want to waste their time and wish to listen to more modern teaching should attend

The Chair of Pathological Anatomy at the Paris Medical School

The close interaction between the chair of pathological anatomy and the chair of clinical neurology was a particular feature of the Paris Medical School. During the century after its creation, the holders of the chair were Léon-Jean-Baptiste Cruveilhier (from 1835 to 1866), Alfred Vulpian (from 1867 to 1872), Jean-Martin Charcot (from 1872 to 1882), Victor Cornil (from 1882 to 1907), Pierre Marie (from 1908 to 1917), and Gustave Roussy (from 1925 to 1937). The only nonneurological parenthesis in this series took place between Pierre Marie and Gustave Roussy, when Maurice Letulle a specialist in lung diseases and tuberculosis held the chair from 1917 to 1924. Thus the young medical student Babinski had Charcot as professor of pathological anatomy at the medical school, and later, as a resident, had as hospital mentors the two professors of pathological anatomy before and after Charcot: Vulpian and Cornil. Given the influence of these three notable figures, his interest in this subject is far from surprising.

Victor Cornil had a successful dual career in medicine and politics.[6] The oldest among Charcot's residents, a relentless worker, he was at the same time *médecin des hôpitaux* and professor of pathological anatomy; he succeeded Charcot when the latter took over the chair for the study of diseases of the nervous system in 1882. He was a clinician but mainly a pathologist, passionately fond of postmortem examinations and of histopathology.[7] He wrote many papers, and his *Manuel d'histologie pathologique* [Handbook on pathological histology], in collaboration with Ranvier, was a wonderful and clear condensation of his observations.[8] His work with Ranvier started with the small private histological laboratory that they founded on rue Christine (in Paris's Sixth Arrondissement) and continued at the Collège de France and while he occupied the chair of pathological anatomy.

Le Progrès Médical, defender of scientific medicine, was a strong supporter of pathological anatomy and praised Professor Cornil's lectures.[9] It highlighted his skill as an educator, his clarity of expression, and the variety

---

the lectures at the Collège de France." *Le Progrès Médical* 1885 (I): 95, 100. On Duval, see *Le Progrès Médical* 1886 (III): 45.

[6] G. Milian, "Le Professeur V. Cornil 1837–1908," *Le Progrès Médical* 1908: 199; http://perso.wanadoo.fr/carteret/Noms.htm#M%e9decins.

[7] *Le Progrès Médical* 1907 (XXIII): 883.

[8] V. Cornil and L. Ranvier, *Manuel d'histologie pathologique* [Handbook of pathological histology] (Paris: F. Alcan, 1869); Milian, "Le Professeur V. Cornil 1837–1908."

[9] *Le Progrès Médical* 1888 (VIII): 412.

of the teaching methods he used, particularly the presentation of anatomical figures prepared in advance, the drawings made by hand in front of the pupils' eyes, and the projections of prepared specimens.[10]

In each of his lessons, before speaking on the subject of pathological anatomy, Cornil recalled the macroscopic and microscopic structures of the organs to be studied. He adapted his lesson to the current trends in science, especially the rapid developments in microbiology and histology. When the cholera epidemic got close to Paris in 1884, he explained the present state of knowledge about the bacillus, based mainly on the works of Robert Koch.[11] In 1887, he began his course with the study of karyokinesis and of its importance in anatomopathological processes.

For Cornil, a theoretical lecture was not sufficient and had to be complemented by practical training provided once a week at the laboratory located on rue Vauquelin. Under his direction, with the help of the director of the laboratory and instructors, students observed through the microscope the abnormalities described in the theoretical lesson.[12] In 1885, *Le Progrès Médical* regretted that Professor Cornil's course was limited to only around a hundred students. It recalled the importance of pathological anatomy, and it encouraged students to come in large numbers to the course because "they have to remember that clinical medicine is only beneficial if enlightened by examination of the cadavers."[13]

In addition to his university courses, Cornil carried out daily postmortem examinations at the hospital, pointing out to the students the major findings as they appeared.[14] All of his students emphasized the meticulousness and rigor he used at each examination. "He thought that every corpse should be autopsied; in each case, there is matter to learn from, as much from a tubercular patient as from those unusual cases which may arouse a greater interest among the students."[15] To have the opportunity to practice under the tutorship of the professor, students had to register with Babinski, the resident in the department.[16]

Under the authority of the professor were an associate professor, one or several instructors, and eventually monitors. During his last two residency years (1883–84 and 1884–85), Babinski was an instructor on Cornil's team, a position he left when he became chief resident with Charcot (Figs. 7-3 and 7-4).

---

[10] *Le Progrès Médical* 1882 (X): 912.
[11] *Le Progrès Médical* 1884 (XII): 970.
[12] *Le Progrès Médical* 1883 (XI): 933.
[13] *Le Progrès Médical* 1885 (II): 416.
[14] *Le Progrès Médical* 1884 (XII): 944.
[15] *Le Progrès Médical* 1904 (XII): 188.
[16] *Le Progrès Médical* 1882 (X): 842.

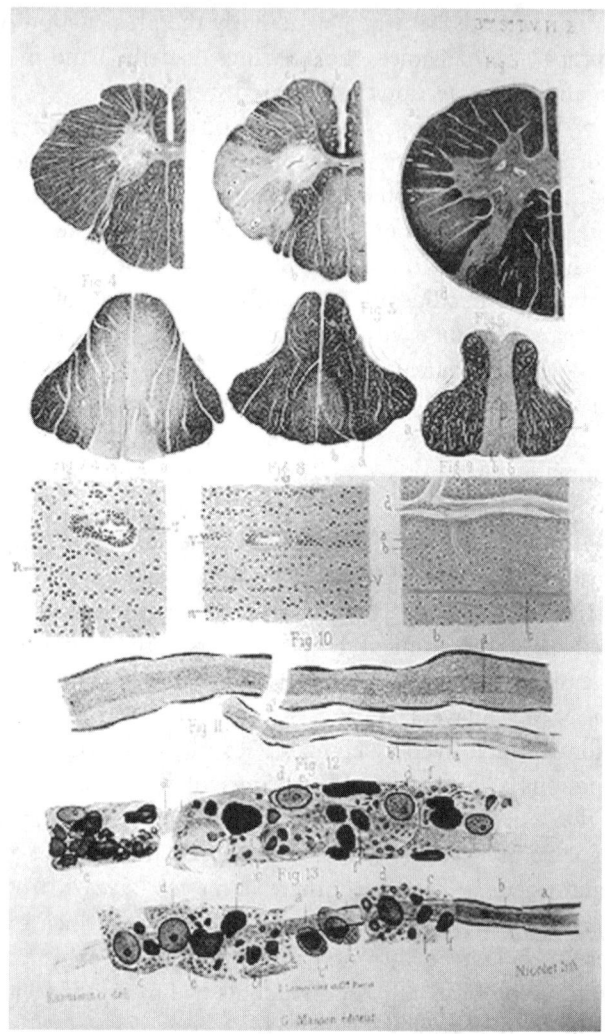

Figure 7-3 Histological sections of the spinal cord in a case of multiple sclerosis. (*Source*: Babinski's medical thesis, 1885, plate II, p. 147.)

On the political side, Victor Cornil was a congressional representative from the Allier department (1876–1882); a senator (1885–1903); mayor of his small village, Creuzier-le-neuf (1874–1897); regional councilor (1870–1871); prefect from September 6 to 24, 1870; and vice president (1871–1872) and then president (1872–1897) of the regional council in Allier. He was antimonarchist, and during the Commune he presided over the Republican League in the Sixth Arrondissement in Paris, which held its meetings in his

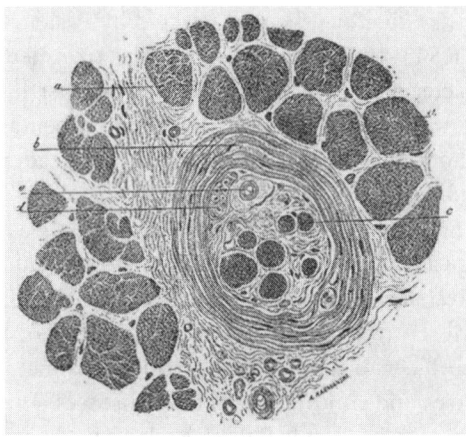

Figure 7-4 Transverse histological section of a neuromuscular spindle. (*Source*: From J. Babinski, "Sur la présence dans les muscles striés de l'homme d'un système spécial constitué par des groupes de petites fibres musculaires entourées d'une gaine lamelleuse," (On the presence in human striated muscles of special structures [neuromuscular fascicles] *Comptes-rendus Hebdomadaires des Séances et Mémoires de la Société de Biologie*, 1886 [III]: 629–631.)

private laboratory.[17] He was a member of the French committee for public health. He was made first a knight (1883) and then an officer (1903) in the Legion of Honor. Despite multiple applications from 1887 to 1906, Victor Cornil was never elected to the Académie des sciences.[18]

Beyond his roles as teacher and politician, Victor Cornil had a remarkable personality that left a deep impression on his resident Babinski. A committee composed of the main disciples of the master—Chantemesse, Babinski, Widal, Legry, Bezançon, and Bouteron—organized Professor Cornil's jubilee in 1904.[19] His medical and political life was recalled, as were his masters, Virchow, Charcot, and Hérard, and his friends, Léon Gambetta (1838–1882), Jules Favre (1809–1880), Jules Grévy (1807–1891), and Jules Simon (1814–1896).[20]

André Chantemesse (1851–1919), formerly Victor Cornil's resident, was later instructor and then associate professor in the laboratory where Babinski worked in 1883–84; he defended his thesis on tuberculosis meningitis in

---

[17] *Le Progrès Médical* 1907 (XXIII): 883.
[18] Dossier Victor Cornil, Archives de l'Académie des sciences.
[19] *Le Progrès Médical* 1904 (I): 14; (XII): 188.
[20] Milian, "Le Professeur V. Cornil 1837–1908."

adults.[21] *Médecin des hôpitaux*, he was selected by Pasteur to help Professor Joseph Grancher (1843–1907) in practicing rabies treatment. His works concerned mainly bacteriology and in particular the Eberth bacillus. A clinician and research worker, he held the chair of experimental pathology at the Paris Medical School in 1897, was a member of the Académie de médecine, and was decorated with the Legion of Honor.

Of Romanian nationality, Victor Babès (1854–1926) was successively professor of pathological histology, pathological anatomy, and then bacteriology at Bucharest University.[22] He worked with Rudolf Virchow, Robert Koch, and Victor Cornil. He was a corresponding member of the Académie de médecine and an officer in the Legion of Honor. His main work concerned tuberculosis, leprosy, and children's infectious diseases. The infection caused by an intracellular parasite (genus *Babesia*), which he discovered, was named after him (babesiosis). In 1885, with Victor Cornil, he invented, in association with Nicati and Rietsch, a shallow container used for bacteriological cultures similar to that described in 1877 by the German bacteriologist Julius Richard Petri (1852–1921), associate to Koch (the Petri dish).[23]

The Société Anatomique

Founded at the beginning of the nineteenth century, the Société anatomique (Anatomical Society) was a place where every Friday afternoon, in a room located above the Musée Dupuytren, anatomopathological cases observed in Paris hospitals were presented and discussed. As a general rule, residents presented clinical cases, and each presentation was accompanied by anatomical specimens to support the conclusions and avoid long and idle discussions.[24]

Victor Cornil, elected president in January 1883, held this position for several years. In his inaugural speech, he paid tribute to his two immediate

---

[21] "Les médecins contemporains, Le Pr A. Chantemesse" [Contemporary physicians: Prof. A. Chantemesse], *Le Progrès Médical* 1897 (V): 361–363; "Nécrologie. Professeur Chantemesse" [Obituary of Professor Chantemesse], *Le Progrès Médical* 1919 (IX): 82.
[22] http://www.whonamedit.com/doctor.cfm/367.html.
[23] V. Cornil and V. Babes, *Les bactéries et leur rôle dans l'anatomie et l'histologie pathologiques des maladies infectieuses* [Bacteria and their role in the pathological and histological anatomy of infectious diseases] (Paris: F. Alcan, 1885); summarized by the same authors and title in *Archives de Physiologie Normale et Pathologique* 1885 (6): 72.
[24] *Le Progrès Médical* 1885 (II): 370; 1886 (III): 944.

predecessors, Cruveilhier and Charcot.[25] After a rapid historical review of the Société anatomique, he recalled that it was in this place that Robin, Lebert, Follin, Broca, and Verneuil had reported their first work on pathological histology. For the young students, he had words full of hope: "May you have faith in the progress of our science and be persuaded that your personal research will be productive, as long as it remains persevering and enlightened by impartiality and the overriding desire to reveal the scientific truth."

Meeting in a formal session on December 21, 1883, the Société anatomique awarded Charcot a gold medal, commemorating his ten years as president of the society. The president-elect, Victor Cornil, recalled that when Charcot had taken over from Cruveilhier, he had given the society a new direction, and he noted that the medal was only a small token of admiration and gratitude. In his response, Charcot expressed his appreciation, offered an unqualified tribute to Cornil, and emphasized that the Société anatomique was "the true temple of the anatomoclinical method, which will always be the most powerful lever for the progress of our art through science."[26]

During the session of May 25, 1884, Maurice Letulle, in his report on Babinski's candidacy for associate membership in the society, emphasized the very special anatomopathological interest of the two epithelioma cases reported by Babinski at the Société anatomique in 1882.[27] From 1882 to 1886, Babinski reported several cases observed in the departments of his two mentors, Cornil and then Vulpian (see the table later in this chapter). In 1885 and 1886 he was treasurer of the society.

The Collège de France

Although Babinski was not directly affiliated with the Collège de France, he was often in contact with Ranvier and even more so with Nageotte; his friend Suchard was an instructor there, and Darier, one of his closest friends, was a tutor under Ranvier (see chapter 4). From the start of his medical studies, Babinski attended the teaching lectures at the laboratory of the Collège de

---

[25] *Le Progrès Médical* 1883 (XI): 70.
[26] *Le Progrès Médical* 1883 (XI): 1052–1054.
[27] M. Letulle, "Rapport sur la candidature de M. Babinski comme member associé" [Report on the candidacy of M. Babinski as associate member by M. Letulle], *Bulletins de la Société Anatomique de Paris* 1884 (VIII): 265–267. Babinski would remain an associate member before becoming an honorary member in 1894, without having been a full elected member. *Bulletins de la Société Anatomique de Paris* 1894 (VIII): 3.

France, where Ranvier carried out his research on histological lesions of multiple sclerosis, neuromuscular spindles, and modifications observed in muscles after section of their nerves.[28]

Born in Lyon, where he started his medical studies, Louis Ranvier was admitted as resident in the Paris hospital system in 1860.[29] With Victor Cornil, he founded a small private histological laboratory, attended sessions of the Société anatomique, and published their well-known textbook, *Manuel d'histologie pathologique*. Instructor at the Collège de France, then director of a histological laboratory affiliated with Claude Bernard, Ranvier became a professor at the Collège de France in the chair of general anatomy in 1875, and his teaching attracted considerable attention.[30] Ranvier followed the experimental method as taught by Bernard and always double-checked and controlled his morphological observations by physiology.[31] Among his numerous research findings were discoveries involving bone and connective tissues and also muscle histology, but he was mainly concerned with the histology of nerve fibers, their degeneration and regeneration, and nerve endings.[32] He discovered the annular constrictions of the nerve fibers (the narrowings or nodes) that were named after him, and he discovered the T structure of the axons of the sensory neurons of spinal ganglia. On the cellular nature of elements located in the bone cavities, he adopted the cellular theory of Virchow, in opposition to Charles Robin, whom he succeeded at the Académie des sciences (1887). With Edouard-Gérard Balbiani (1823–1899), he founded the *Archives d'anatomie microscopique* (1897), the first French journal dedicated to microscopic studies. Ranvier was a member of the Académie de médecine. His main associates were Charles Malassez (1842–1909), Louis-Félix Henneguy (1850–1928), Balbiani, and Justin-Marie Jolly (1870–1953); the last of these held a chair of histophysiology at the Collège in 1925. Many biologists and physicians, both French and foreign,

---

[28] H. Pieron, "Nécrologie de M. J. Babinski" [Obituary of J. Babinski], *Compte-rendus de la Société de Biologie*, meeting of November 5, 1932, 494–495.

[29] G. Vapereau, *Dictionnaire universel des contemporains* [Universal dictionary of contemporaries], 6th ed. (Paris: Hachette, 1893); Dossier Louis Ranvier, Archives de l'Académie des sciences; J. G. Barbara, "Les étranglements annulaires de Louis Ranvier (1871)" [Nodes of Ranvier (1871)], *Lettre des Neurosciences* 2005 (28): 3–5; http://www.bristol.ac.uk/neuroscience/the_node/caffeine/ranvier.

[30] *Le Progrès Médical* 1882 (X): 839.

[31] *Le Progrès Médical* 1883 (XI): 989.

[32] L. Ranvier, *Leçons d'anatomie générale sur le système musculaire* [General anatomy lessons on the muscular system], coll. by J. Renaut (Paris: Bureaux du Progrès Médical, 1880); L. Ranvier, *Leçons sur l'histologie du système nerveux* [Lessons on nervous system histology], coll. by E. Weber (Paris, 1878).

such as Babinski, Darier, Debove, Dieulafoy, Grancher, Pierre Marie, Renaut, and Zacchariadès, also worked with him.[33]

A resident in Paris hospitals, Charles Malassez worked during the afternoon in the small private laboratory founded by Cornil and Ranvier.[34] At the Collège de France, Malassez became assistant director in 1882 of the histological laboratory, and for thirty-four years he was an utterly devoted, tireless, and silent associate to his master, Louis Ranvier. He succeeded Charcot at the Académie de médecine in 1894.[35] His substantial scientific work dealt with various fields, including hematology, anatomopathology, and microbiology. He discovered *Malassezia furfur*, a yeast saprophyte of the cutaneous tissue that causes in particular pityriasis versicolor, and invented several instruments and apparatus, the best-known being the Malassez cell, permitting the counting of blood cells.

Jean Nageotte (1866–1948), also a resident in 1889, defended his thesis while at the laboratory of Professor Raymond at Lariboisière, and he thanked his hospital teachers, including Babinski.[36] After having been associate professor for anatomical research at the clinic for the study of diseases of the nervous system from 1894 to 1896, he was named *médecin-aliéniste* (psychiatrist) *des hôpitaux de Paris* at Bicêtre, then at the Salpêtrière, and in Babinski's department was responsible for anatomopathological and histological exams. He built a new brain microtome for the laboratory.[37] In the Musée de l'Assistance publique in Paris this was labeled as "Babinski's microtome," although Babinski himself never used it. Nageotte never missed the opportunity to pay tribute to Babinski, alongside whom he always found "important and most valuable specimen material as well as intellectual and moral support."[38] With Babinski, he described Babinski-Nageotte syndrome

---

[33] J. Jolly, "Louis Ranvier (1835–1922). Notice biographique" [Louis Ranvier (1835–1922). A biographical note], *Archives d'Anatomie Microscopique* 1922 (XIX): 1–72.

[34] "Les médecins contemporains. M. le Dr Malassez" [Contemporary physicians: Dr. Malassez], *Le Progrès Médical* 1894 (17): 314; M. Letulle, "Malassez (1843–1909)," *La Presse Médicale* 1909 (104): 1017–1022.

[35] "Les médecins contemporains. M. le Dr Malassez."

[36] For chronological reasons, Nageotte could not have been a nonresident student or resident with Babinski at the Pitié hospital; he probably met him at the *bureau central*.

[37] J. Nageotte, "Note sur un nouveau microtome à cerveau" [Note on a new brain microtome], *Comptes-rendus Hebdomadaires des Séances et Mémoires de la Société de Biologie* 1899: 202–203; J. Nageotte, "Présentation d'un microtome du cerveau" [Presentation of a brain microtome], XIIIth International Congress of Medicine, meeting of August 3, 1900, comptes-rendus, section de neurologie, 145–146.

[38] J. Nageotte, "Sur la nature et la pathogénie des lésions radiculaires de la moelle qui accompagnent les tumeurs cérébrales" [On the nature and pathogenesis of spinal radicular lesions observed in brain tumors], *Rev Neurol (Paris)* 1904 (1): 1.

(1902) and published on cerebrospinal fluid cytology.[39] After having been a tutor in the histological laboratory at the Collège de France from 1903 to 1912, he succeeded Louis Ranvier in the chair of comparative histology, leaving in 1937. Despite his achievements, Nageotte was not named to the Académie des sciences. In a 1911 summary of his works, he paid tribute to his teachers, especially Albert Gombault, under whom he had been a resident, Malassez, who received him in his laboratory, and Babinski.[40] Of Babinski he wrote, "For many years I found in the laboratory of my teacher and friend J. Babinski a scientific climate incredibly profitable, high ideals and precious materials."[41] Nageotte did considerable research on microscopic anatomy of the connective tissue and of the nervous system.[42] His wife helped him in his works and became a well-known pediatrician, at one time president of the Société de pédiatrie. Following an accident, Nageotte was struck down by hemiplegia and became progressively deaf (Fig. 7-5).

Henri Wallon (1879–1962)[43] was an associate professor with Jean Nageotte at Bicêtre and then at the Salpêtrière (1908–1931). A former student at the prestigious École normale supérieure, where he passed the *agrégation* in philosophy, he then obtained M.D. and Ph.D. degrees (his thesis was on the boisterous child, *l'enfant turbulent*), and opened a practice specializing in children with retardation and motor restlessness. At the same time, he was in charge of lectures on child psychology at the Faculty of Arts in Paris. Founder of a psychobiological laboratory there, he became professor of child psychology and childhood education at the Collège de France in1937; his work on sociocognitive development in childhood benefited from his dual training in philosophy and medicine. His courses were suspended by the

---

[39] http://www.whonamedit.com/synd.cfm/723.html; J. Babinski and J. Nageotte, "Contribution à l'étude du cytodiagnostic du liquide céphalo-rachidien dans les affections nerveuses" [Contribution to the cytodiagnosis of the cerebrospinal fluid in nervous diseases], *Bulletins et Mémoires de la Société Médicale des Hôpitaux de Paris* 1901 (XVIII): 537–548.

[40] J. Nageotte, *Notice sur les travaux scientifiques* [Note on scientific papers] (Paris: Imprimerie de la Cour d'Appel, 1911).

[41] Indeed, several of his papers were derived from histological examinations of patients in Babinski's department, e.g., J. Nageotte, "Note sur les fibres endogènes grosses et fines des cordons postérieurs et sur la nature endogène des zones de Lissauer" [Note on large and thin endogenous fibers of the posterior column and on the endogenous nature of the Lissauer area], *Comptes-rendus Hebdomadaires des Séances et Mémoires de la Société de Biologie* 1904, 1651; J. Nageotte, "Névrite radiculaire subaiguë. Dégénérescences consécutives dans la moelle (racines postérieures) et dans les nerfs périphériques (racines antérieures)" [Sub-acute radicular neuritis. Subsequent degeneration in the spinal cord (posterior roots) and in the peripheral nerves (anterior roots)], *Rev Neurol (Paris)* 1903 (11): 1.

[42] J. Nageotte, *La structure fine du système nerveux* [The detailed structure of the nervous system] (Paris: Maloine, 1905).

[43] http://www.upsy.net/upsychologie/ancetres/wallon.htm.

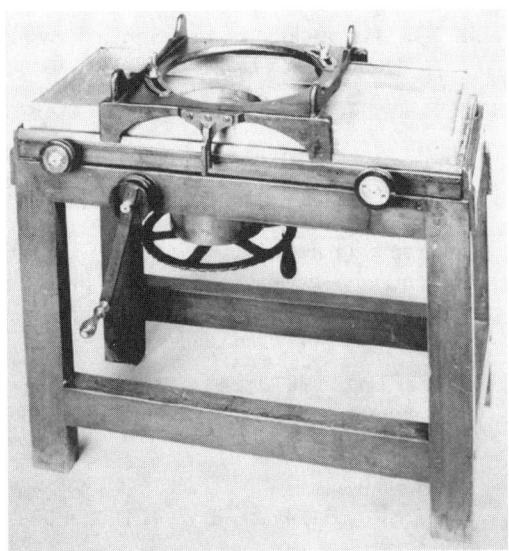

Figure 7-5 Microtome of Babinski. (*Source*: Musée de l'assistance publique, Hôpitaux de Paris.)

Vichy government, but after Liberation, the Conseil national de la Résistance named him secretary of state for education. Elected a congressman in 1946, he became vice president and then president of the committee for the reform of education, which led to the Plan Langevin-Wallon.

Babinski's Anatomopathological and Histological Papers

Under the influence of Vulpian and Cornil, and in collaboration with Ranvier, Babinski carried out several studies on normal and pathological histology. In 1883–84, with other colleagues, he edited a volume of Victor Cornil's lessons.[44] At the Société anatomique, from 1882 to 1886 he delivered thirteen papers on anatomopathology and histology. The last three he presented at the Société anatomique, in 1888 and 1889, dealt more with neurology than anatomy (Table 7-1).

---

[44] V. Cornil, "*Leçons données pendant le premier semestre de l'année 1883–1884 par M. Cornil*" [Lessons taught during the first semester of the year 1883–1884 by M. Cornil...], ed. F. Alcan (Paris: Ancienne Librairie Germer Baillière, 1884).

Table 7-1: Babinski's oral presentations for the Société Anatomique

Session	Title	Bulletins de la Société Anatomique de Paris
January 13, 1882	Anatomical parts of a patient, who, during his life has presented signs of a cirrhosis of the liver	1882, LVII year, 4th series, T. VII, p. 28
February 10, 1882	Kidney cancer developed in a woman operated on for a breast "squirrhe"	1882, LVII year, 4th series, T. VII, pp. 113
April 10, 1882	Lung tuberculosis—Tubercular tonsillitis and laryngitis Tubercular lip ulceration	1882, LVII year, 4th series, T. VII, pp. 236–238
May 4, 1882	Skin tubular epithelioma of the buttock area developed from the Malpighi mucous body	1882, LVII year, 4th series, T. VII, pp. 232–233
	Two cases of squamous epitheliomas probably originating from a dermoid ovarian cyst	1882, LVII year, 4th series, T. VII, pp. 234–236 (Analysis in Le Progrès Médical, 1884, T. XII, No. 2 (January 12), p. 29)
June 6, 1882	Liver and kidneys multiple cysts—Uraemia	1882, LVII year, 4th series, T. VII, pp. 341–344
February 16, 1883	Intestinal obstruction caused by a biliary calculus enclosed in the rectum	1883, LVIII year, 4th series, T. VIII, pp. 117–118 (Analysis in Le Progrès Médical, 1883, T. XI, No. 37 (15 September), pp.736–737)
March 2, 1883	Brain softening	1883, LVIII year, 4th series, T. VIII, pp. 140–143 (Analysis in Le Progrès Médical, 1883, T. XI, No. 39 (29 September), pp. 770–771)

(continued)

Table 7-1: Continued

Session	Title	Bulletins de la Société Anatomique de Paris
	Brain hydatid cyst	1883, LVIII year, 4th series, T. VIII, pp. 143–146 (Analysis in Le Progrès Médical, 1883, T. XI, No. 41 (October 13), p. 808)
November 30, 1883	Report on the candidacy of M. Charrin	1883, LVIII year, 4th series, T. VIII, pp. 482–484 (Analysis in Le Progrès Médical, 1884, T. XII, No. 24 (June 13), 14, p. 480)
January 23, 1885	Concerning a tumor presented by M. Ballue as a spino-cellular epithelioma of the lower maxilla, M. Babinski considers "that it that it looks more like lobulated mucous epithelioma: eleidin is scarcely present."	1885, LV year, 4th series, T. X, p. 52 (Analysis in Le Progrès Médical, 1885, T. II, 2nd series, No. 39 (September 26), p. 235)
November 6, 1885	Histological exam of the tumor presented by M. Mérigot during the last meeting	1885, LV year, 4th series, T. X, p. 464
January 8, 1886	Spinal cord sections showing a type of combined sclerosis	1886, LXI year, 4th series, T. XI, p. 17.
November 5, 1886	Report on the candidacy of M. Hallé	1886, LXI year, 4th series, T. XI, pp. 648–649.
	M. Babinski shows anatomical preparations of new structures he has found in the normal striate muscles of man	1886, LXI year, 4th series, T. XI, p. 753.

(continued)

Table 7-1: Continued

Session	Title	Bulletins de la Société Anatomique de Paris
July 1887	Report on the candidacy of M.Guillet	1887, LXII year, 5th series, T. I, pp. 496–497.
October 1887	Arthropathies of the tabetic patients	1887, LXII year, 5th series, T. I, pp. 624–626.
November 11, 1887	Locomotor ataxia Tabes arthropahies Chronic rheumatism	1887, LXII year, 5th series, T. I, pp. 669–672.
July 12, 1889	Pyocyanic disease Experimental arthropathies	1889, LXIV year, 5th series, T. III, p. 468.

In a paper at the Société de biologie, Babinski made an excellent histological description of special structures of the striated muscle that he called neuromuscular fascicles and that would later be named neuromuscular spindles, shown perfectly by his drawing.[45] (Fig. 7-4). He was thought to have been the first with this observation, but three years later, he noted that his recent bibliographical research had demonstrated that others had drawn the same conclusions before he did, particularly Golgi. However, he thought that his work had not been useless, as it had been able to show that "at least the neuromuscular fascicles constitute a normal structure, a fact little known by anatomopathologists, no more in France than abroad."

Beyond his strictly morphological works, he also carried out research on experimental palsy in diphtheria, examining the nerves corresponding to the paralyzed muscles and finding them completely normal.[46] He cut the sciatic

---

[45] J. Babinski, "Sur la présence dans les muscles striés de l'homme d'un système spécial constitué par des groupes de petites fibres musculaires entourées d'une gaine lamelleuse" [On the presence in human striated muscles of special structures (neuromuscular fascicles)], *Comptes-rendus Hebdomadaires des Séances et Mémoires de la Société de Biologie* 1886 (III): 629–631; J. Babinski, "Faisceaux neuro-musculaires" [Neuromuscular fascicles], *Archives de médecine expérimentale*, May 1, 1889.

[46] J. Babinski, *Notice sur les travaux scientifiques* [Note on scientific papers] (Paris: Masson, 1892).

nerve in rabbits, and six weeks later took samples of the innervated muscles. After fixation and coloration, he observed the atrophy of the contractile part: "Suppressing the function leads to the disappearance of the morphological differentiation, the structure returning to an embryonic state."[47]

---

[47] J. Babinski, "Des modifications que présentent les muscles à la suite de la section des nerfs qui s'y rendent" [Modifications observed in muscles following section of their nerves], *Comptes-rendus de l'Académie des Sciences*, January 7, 1884.

··· *eight* ···

Babinski, Head of a Department at La Pitié

Speaking on behalf of the *Académie de médecine* at the funeral of Dr. Duguet in 1914, Babinski gave an eulogy that could well have been written with himself in mind:

> It was to the hospital that he devoted the best of his intellect, to this hospital which apparently took up a very large place in his heart; it is through his clinical teaching in the department, which he delighted to dispense, that his influence on the young generations was the best expressed and will most certainly remain. [...] Finally, he did not limit his work to the purely clinical aspects. In therapeutics, he was not afraid to adopt new methods and did not hesitate to be bold.[1]

Médecin des Hôpitaux *Before La Pitié*

On May 1, 1890, Babinski was officially named as *médecin des hôpitaux* attached to the pool of the *bureau central*, situated at the Hôtel-Dieu, within which all the physicians recently tenured in the Paris hospital system had to spend a few years before obtaining a position as the head of a department, and where all patients (except for emergencies and some specific cases) were examined before being sent to a hospital with a vacant bed. This institution,

---

[1] *Bulletin de l'Académie de médecine* 1914 (LXXII): 10–12.

much criticized, disappeared in 1895. It was during this period of his career that Babinski coped with the cholera epidemic of 1892.

On January 1, 1894, because of his seniority, Babinski was promoted to the position of head of department at the Porte d'Aubervilliers hospital. Opened in 1884, along the old defense works around the city, it was established to handle patients recovering from cholera when they were discharged from the other Paris hospitals. It was designated in 1887 as a center for smallpox and measles, to which were added in 1892 scarlet fever and erysipelas and in 1893 diphtheria. It was in this quarantine hospital, with its dilapidated wooden barracks and without an outpatient service, that Babinski took up his first duties as physician in chief.[2] He stayed there for one year, leaving no particular impact. On July 12, 1904, the director-general of the Paris hospital system, assisted by city firemen, set on fire the squalid shacks of the hospital, which was replaced on the same site by the Claude Bernard Hospital, dedicated in 1905 (Fig. 8-1).[3]

Médecin des Hôpitaux *at La Pitié: The Old One (1895–1911) and the New One (1911–1922)*

After having thought briefly of accepting a vacant position at the Tenon hospital, Babinski decided instead on La Pitié established in 1612 by Marie de Médicis, then regent for the future Louis XIII. La Pitié, one of five poor houses built to deal with the large number of vagrants in Paris, was located next to the Jardin des Plantes. In 1656, La Pitié housed the central administration for the General Hospital which was composed of three hospitals, and also served as a home for the children of those interned at the Salpêtrière. During the Revolution, La Pitié was given the name of *Maison des élèves de la Patrie* [Home for children of the nation]. In 1809 the residents were transferred to a Hospice for Abandoned Children and la Pitié became a hospital for the ill.

---

[2] Description by M. Mourier, honorary director of the Assistance publique, in P. Vallery-Radot, "L'ancien hôpital d'Aubervilliers" [The old Aubervilliers hospital], *La Presse Médicale* 1949 (72): 1062–1063; M. Villaret, "Les grandes étapes en hydro-climatologie. Leçon inaugurale de la chaire d'Hydro-climatologie" [Important steps in hydro-climatology. Opening speech for the Chair of Hydrology and therapeutic climatology], *La Presse Médicale* 1928 (95): 1513–1518.
[3] Vallery-Radot, "L'ancien hôpital d'Aubervilliers."

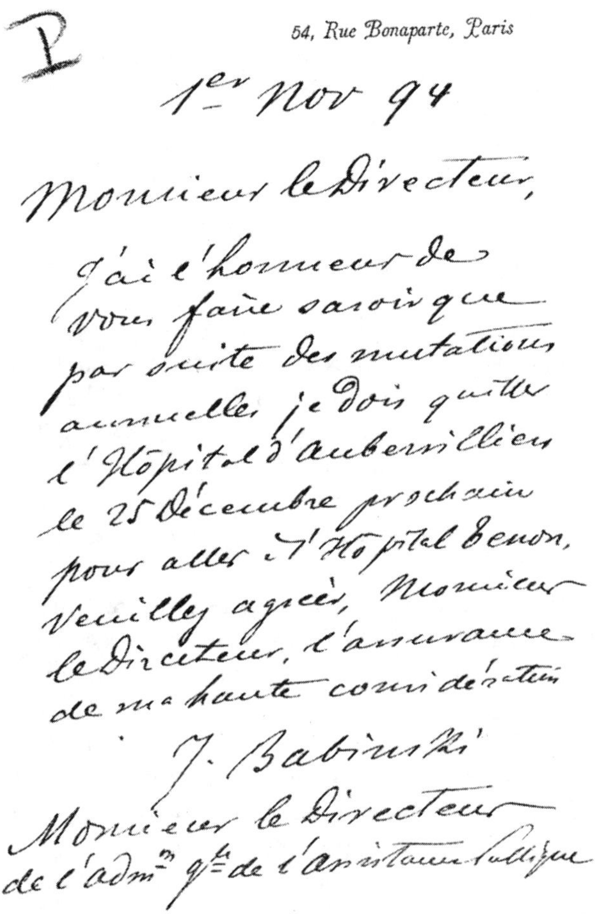

P

54, Rue Bonaparte, Paris

1er Nov 94

Monsieur le Directeur,

J'ai l'honneur de vous faire savoir que par suite des mutations annuelles, je dois quitter l'Hôpital d'Aubervilliers le 25 Décembre prochain pour aller à l'Hôpital Tenon. Veuillez agréer, Monsieur le Directeur, l'assurance de ma haute considération

J. Babinski

Monsieur le Directeur de l'admon gle de l'Assistance publique

Figure 8-1 Letter by Joseph Babinski to the director of the Assistance publique, 1894. (*Source*: Archives of the Assistance publique, Hôpitaux de Paris.)

When Babinski arrived as head of the department of internal medicine on January 1, 1895, La Pitié had both medical and surgical services.[4] He would remain in this position for twenty-seven years, until his retirement in 1922 at the age of sixty-five. This stability was rare among physicians in chief, comparable to the thirty-one years Charcot spent at the Salpêtrière

[4] Decree of the general director of the Assistance publique, dated January 8, 1895, effective January 1, 1895; Nominations of physicians, notice of nominations, Correspondence 1890–1895, Archives de l'Assistance publique, Hôpitaux de Paris, FOSS 791 38/3.

beginning on January 1, 1862. At his death in 1893, Charcot was still active, although he had formally retired as professor at the age of seventy.[5]

The old Pitié was located in a large block of houses in the Fifth Arrondissement of Paris, behind the Jardin des Plantes.[6] It was in a miserable state.[7] André Billy in 1909 painted a bleak picture: "this hospital in decomposition, this cadaverous hospital, like a worm-eaten tomb. The walls ooze misery and death."[8] His description was reinforced by the numerous complaints from people living around the hospital, particularly concerning the smells coming from the morgue.

It was therefore decided to destroy the old Pitié and to build a new one on land belonging to the Salpêtrière. Not everyone was in favor of this project. The reasons offered were numerous: (1) beds for the insane would be significantly reduced at the Salpêtrière; (2) the new hospital would pose a danger for children in the neighboring school, (3) there would be a risk of contagion, (4) the patients' sleep would be disturbed by the noise of the Paris metro, and (5) even the fear that "workers in the builder's yard may get infectious diseases."[9]

The old Pitié was finally torn down in 1912. More than a decade later, between 1922 and 1926, the Great Mosque of Paris, the Clinique Geoffroy Saint-Hilaire, and several residential buildings were constructed on the site (Fig. 8-2).

In March 1895, by decision of the director-general of the Assistance Publique, Paris was divided into different hospital districts; the *Bureau central* was abolished, and for all hospitals the outpatient practice was separated from the wards. The daily consultation was managed by an internist

---

[5] In 1896, besides Babinski, the five physicians who were heads of department at La Pitié were Drs. Jaccoud, Robin, Faisans, Thibierge, and Petit. Nine years later, in 1905, Babinski was still present, but the others had been replaced by Drs. Dalché, Lion, Rénon, Claisse, and Thiroloix. *Almanach National 1896* and *Almanach National 1905*.

[6] *L'Assistance publique en 1900*, 379; *Plans des hôpitaux et hospices civils de la ville de Paris. Levés par ordre du Conseil général d'Administration de ces établissements* [Plans for hospitals and hospices or poor houses of the city of Paris] (Paris, 1820); E. de Labédollière, *Le nouveau Paris* [The new Paris] (Paris: Gustave Barba, 1860); J. Hillairey, *Dictionnaire historique des rues de Paris* [Historical dictionary of the streets of Paris] (Paris: Éditions de Minuit, 1963).

[7] P. Vallery-Radot, *Deux siècles d'histoire hospitalière, de Henri IV à Louis-Philippe (1602–1836)* [Two centuries of hospital history, from Henri IV to Louis Philippe (1602–1836)] (Paris: Éditions Paul Dupont, 1947), 79.

[8] C. Huard and A. Billy, *Paris vieux et neuf. La rive gauche* [Paris, old and new. The left bank] (Paris: Eugène Rey, 1909).

[9] "Le nouvel hôpital de la Salpêtrière" [The new Salpêtrière hospital], *Le Progrès Médical* 1904 (26): 429.

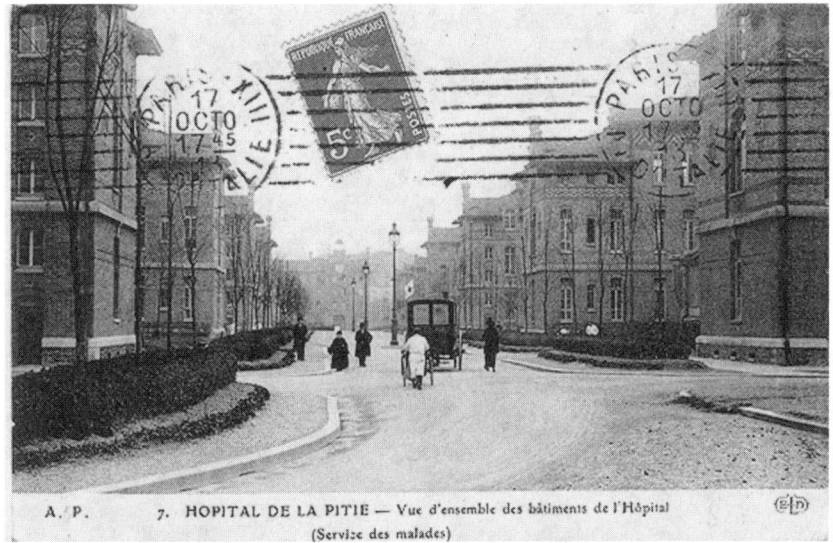

Figure 8-2 Postcard showing the central passage of the new Pitié in 1913. (*Source*: Personal collection, J. Poirier.)

or surgeon, sometimes aided by an associate.[10] Although as a general rule, management of the outpatients was completely detached from that of the wards, there were some exceptions for special pathologies that could be automatically assigned to clinical wards. For example, at La Pitié, Babinski was authorized by the administration to hold a weekly consultation for nervous diseases.[11]

The daily hospital routine of the time gives some insight into Babinski's professional environment. An anecdote shows how seriously the administration took the moral conduct of its staff: in 1895, it levied a deduction of two weeks' wages for any resident who "had received the previous day in his room a woman who spent there the night."[12]

Except for the first Thursday of the month, when the Société de neurologie met, during his first years Babinski arrived every day at the hospital in

---

[10] *L'Assistance publique en 1900*, 155; *Cent ans d'Assistance publique à Paris (1849–1949)* [One hundred years of the Assistance publique in Paris (1849–1949)] (Paris: 3, av. Victoria, 1949).

[11] Conseil de surveillance de l'Assistance publique, meetings of October 31, 1895, and November 14, 1895, 31–32; Archival source.

[12] Conseil de surveillance de l'Assistance publique, meeting of March 7, 1895, 481–482; Archival source.

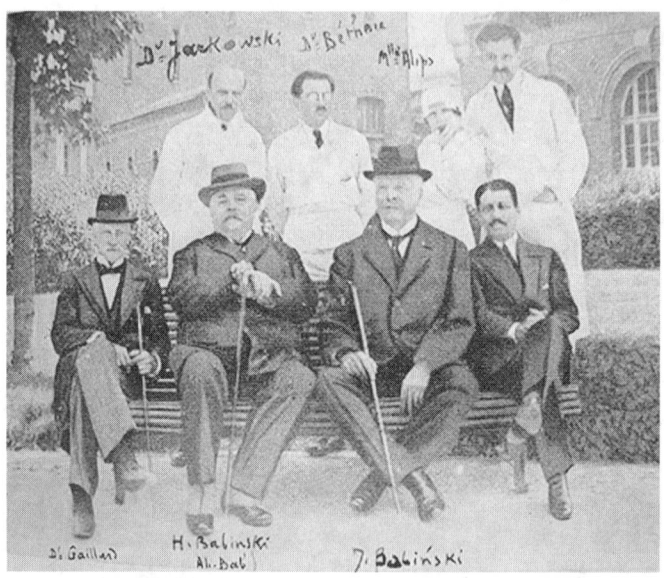

Figure 8-3 Babinski's department at La Pitié. On Babinski's right is his brother, Henri; at far left in the second row (in the white coat) is Jean Jarkowski, and next to him is the head nurse, Ms. Allips. (*Source*: From Albert Charpentier, *Un grand médecin, J. Babinski* [Paris: Typographie François Bernouard, 1934].)

a hackney cab (open during the summer months); later, he arrived in a car driven by a chauffeur who shared his love of silence.[13]

In the old Pitié, Babinski's department was located on the first floor of a building that separated the hospital's two courtyards. It was made up of two long rectangular rooms separated by a landing. A laboratory occupied a small room leading into the men's ward. The consultation room was set up at the end of the women's ward, from which it was separated by a dividing wall, opening through a large door.[14] The men's ward was named after Jenner and the one for women after Laënnec (Fig. 8-3).[15]

In 1900, the mean stay of patients at La Pitié was between twenty-nine and forty-six days.[16] Because Babinski's department was officially one of internal medicine, it is not surprising that patients did not necessarily present

---

[13] A. Tournay, "Babinski dans la vie" [Babinski in everyday life], *La Presse Médicale* 1958 (66): 1485–1489.
[14] Ibid.
[15] *Le Progrès Médical* 1908 (46): 613.
[16] *Annuaire statistique de la ville de Paris*, XXI, 1900 (Paris: Masson, 1902).

neurological pathologies. The admissions register for 1895 shows that bronchial and lung pathologies (tuberculosis, chronic bronchitis emphysemas, pneumonias, pleuresies, congestion of the lungs, flu) accounted for the greatest number of admissions, followed by cardiac diseases (narrowing or insufficiency of the heart orifices, asystoly) and then by a multitude of various diseases and symptoms (kidney insufficiency, diabetes, cirrhosis, anemia, chlorosis, extreme poverty, upset stomach, cachexia, senility, pain, varicose veins, etc.).[17] Neurological pathologies were less common but reflected a wide spectrum of complaints: neuralgias, neurasthenia, syphilitic myelitis, hemiplegias, spasmodic paraplegia, locomotor ataxia, tabes, sciatic, hysteria, facial palsy, lead poisoning, brain softening, tremor, and so on.

Head of a department without any university affiliation (which explained the absence of a chief resident), Babinski was assisted only by hospital staff: a resident (later supplemented by a temporary resident) and four or five non-resident students (see chapter 4). His chief nurse and essential team member for many years was Miss Allips. In addition, former pupils made up a small group of voluntary unpaid associates. Among the most faithful were Albert Charpentier, Auguste Tournay, Jean Jarkowski, and Clovis Vincent, all neurologists (see chapters 3 and 13).

The ophthalmologist was Joseph Chaillous (1872–1934), a former resident who had spent three years in general surgery and then specialized in ophthalmology under Henri Parinaud (1844–1905), Auguste Chevallereau, and Victor Morax (1866–1935).[18] He was successively laboratory assistant and then physician in chief at the Quinze-Vingts Hospital in 1911. Babinski, who appreciated the accuracy of his diagnosis and his professional integrity, entrusted to him the study of eye disorders among his patients.

His electroradiologist was Louis Delherm (1876–1953).[19] After having been resident under Babinski in 1901–1902, he defended his thesis, in 1903, on electrical treatment of common constipation and of muco-membranous colitis.[20] In 1904, Babinski set up a radiological laboratory for Delherm.[21]

[17] Hôpital de la Pitié, Registre des entrées [Register of admissions], 1895, Archives de l'Asistance publique, Hôpitaux de Paris. The total number of patient admissions to the Pitié hospital from January 1 to June 30, 1895, was 4,503.
[18] M.G, V.D. "Joseph Chaillous," *La Presse Médicale* 1934 (35): 717.
[19] *Le Progrès Médical* 1903 (XVIII): 465; G. Pallardy, M. J. Pallardy, and A. Wackenheim, *Histoire illustrée de la radiologie* [Illustrated history of radiology] (Paris: Éditions Roger Dacosta, 1989).
[20] L. Delherm, *Le traitement par l'électricité de la constipation habituelle et de la colite muco-membraneuse* [Electrical treatment of common constipation and muco-membranous constipation] (Paris: Henri Jouve, 1903).
[21] Procès-verbal de la réunion des chefs de service du 5 février 1906 [Minutes of the meeting of department heads on February 5, 1906], Archives de l'Assistance publique,

It was given official status in 1908 with the appointment after competitive examination of the first eleven *radiologues des hôpitaux* (physician in chief for radiology laboratories), including Delherm. After a difficult start, with poor facilities due to lack of financial support and continuous conflicts with the clinicians, Delherm would have an outstanding career in radiology, organizing a modern unit for the whole of the new Pitié.[22] His work dealt with radiology, electrodiagnostics, electrotherapy, and radiotherapy.

The otolaryngologist was G. A. Weill and the histologists Jean Nageotte and Joseph Jumentié (1881–1928).[23] A resident under Babinski in 1910–1911, Jumentié worked in Dejerine's laboratory, defending his thesis in 1911 on the pathological anatomy and clinical aspects of cerebellopontine angle tumors.[24] During World War I, he was an associate of Grasset at a neurological center in Montpellier, then of André Thomas at the Saint-Joseph hospital. In 1925, he carried out a pathological study of the brain of Babinski's famous patient Mouninou; his description of certain major characteristics of the cerebellar lesions confirmed Babinski's clinical observations.[25]

Beginning on June 1, 1911, in anticipation of the imminent opening of the new Pitié, no more patients were admitted to the old Pitié. Outpatients began to be examined at the new hospital at the beginning of July, and the first admissions occurred in August 1911.[26]

At the new hospital, Babinski's department was located on the ground floor of the Benjamin-Delessert ward; two rooms were named after Charcot and Vulpian.[27] Raymond Poincaré (1860–1934), President of France, inaugurated the new Pitié on March 19, 1913, and on that occasion visited Babinski's department.[28]

Hôpitaux de Paris, carton 9 L 128, Hôpital de la Pitié, Activité et fonctionnement de l'établissement.

[22] The radiological department at La Pitié (whose head was Dr. Delherm) was inaugurated in 1934. *L'Informateur Médical*, no. 519, July 22, 1934, in Archives de l'Assistance publique, Hôpitaux de Paris, carton 9 L 128, Hôpital de la Pitié, Activité et fonctionnement de l'établissement. See also M. Hulmann, "Jubilé des vingt-cinq années de services hospitaliers du Dr. Delherm" [Jubilee for the twenty-five-year hospital career of Dr. Delherm], *La Presse Médicale* 1933 (83): 1624.

[23] On Nageotte, see chapter 7. On Jumentié, see M. Laignel-Lavastine, "Joseph Jumentié, nécrologie" [Joseph Jumentié, obituary], *Rev Neurol (Paris)* 1928 (II): 146–147.

[24] *Le Progrès Médical* 1912 (44): 553.

[25] J. Babinski, "Syndrome cérébelleux" [Cerebellar syndrome], *Bulletin de l'Académie de Médecine*, April 23, 1925.

[26] Archives de l'Assistance publique, Hôpitaux de Paris, carton 9L129, La Pitié, Services hospitaliers.

[27] Archives de l'Assistance publique, Hôpitaux de Paris, carton 9 L 128, Hôpital de la Pitié, Activité et fonctionnement de l'établissement.

[28] Ibid.

The Weekly Consultation

Every week, except during the Easter holidays, August, and September, Babinski saw outpatients on Wednesday mornings from 10:00 to 12:00 before an audience of visiting physicians, both French and foreign, and the nonresident medical students, giving lessons emphasizing semiology and examination techniques.[29] He rarely went into the wards, preferring the outpatient room. The visitors sat behind Babinski's chair; the students sat in back of a long table that held various instruments used in neurological examination, a faradic apparatus, and mercury sulfate batteries for the production of galvanic current.[30]

As recalled by all of his pupils, Babinski (like Charcot before him) required his patients, male or female, to disrobe completely before the examination. They undressed and put their clothes back on behind a screen placed at the back of the room. This requirement, which today would be seen as demonstrating a lack of respect for the patient, could be a good subject for further study. Was it common in France prior to Charcot, or did he start it, particularly in reference to female hysteria? Was it common in all medical specialities, or was it particular to neurology and dermatology, which maintained this practice until the 1970s? A. F. Hurst thought that Babinski's semiological discoveries were partly related to this practice, which enabled the doctor to have a full view of the entire body and not just a specific area related to the complaint as expressed by the patient. He recalled that "in English outpatient departments at that time the voluminous clothes, particularly of female patients, made an adequate examination often very difficult."[31] In England the Victorian influence meant that even at the beginning of the twentieth century, doctors tended to examine females in the presence of a third person, which was not systematically the case in France.

Facing his naked patients, Babinski did not speak to them any more than he did to his pupils. Taking the case history was a rapid exercise. In the traditional style of the Paris Medical School at that time, only objective signs as determined by the physician were unquestionable, whereas the symptoms as related by the patient had to be treated with caution. "He was a silent man, as was Charcot, but his students educated themselves by observing his

---

[29] Particularly in *Le Progrès Médical* 1902 (XV): 111; 1902 (XVI): 316; 1903 (XVIII): 325; 1904 (XX): 315; 1911 (XXXI): 139; 1913 (suppl.), 268.

[30] A. Charpentier, "Babinski (Joseph) (1857-1932)," in M. Genty, ed., *Les biographies médicales* [Medical biographies], (Paris: Librairie J. B. Baillière et fils, 1937-39), VI: 17-32.

[31] A. F. Hurst, "Dr. Babinski," *British Medical Journal* 1932 (26): 988.

examination technique. When he had finished with a patient, he dictated in short sentences his main findings. In the following days, he confirmed his initial observations by a new examination of the same patient and tried to detect similarities with other cases."[32]

Given the relatively few laboratory tests in use, the detailed clinical examination remained the primary means of diagnosis. Those tests that were available were quite basic. In 1920,[33] in Babinski's department, 139 measurements of blood urea and 164 sugar and albumin urine tests were carried out. The test for syphilis was in fact the most frequently done (629 Bordet-Wassermann tests were conducted on blood, and 2345 on cerebrospinal fluid), with that for tuberculosis also performed often (195 tests for the Koch bacillus). Histological examinations were very rare. The Benjoin colloïdal reaction described in 1920 by Guillain, Guy Laroche, and Léchelle had not yet found its place in Babinski's laboratory routine.[34] (Table 8-1).

Saturday Clinical Lectures

From May through July, every Saturday at half past ten, Babinski gave a clinical lesson in the lecture hall of La Pitié, attracting a large audience that often included several foreign physicians, who sat in the front row.[35] Babinski was not an orator: he spoke with a certain slowness, and his delivery was sometimes a little jerky.[36] These Saturday lessons were not really theoretical lectures but rather case studies. *Le Journal des Praticiens* frequently published the minutes, recording in detail the clinical notes for each patient.[37] Various

---

[32] L. Rivet, "Joseph Babinski (1857–1932)," *Bulletins et Mémoires de la Société Médicale des Hôpitaux de Paris* 1932 (34): 1722–1733.

[33] Analyses et travaux réalisés dans le laboratoire du Dr Babinski, année 1920 [Laboratory tests and examinations performed in Dr. Babinski's department in 1920], Archives de l'Assistance publique, Hôpitaux de Paris, carton 9L129, La Pitié, Services hospitaliers.

[34] "The Benjoin colloidal reaction, the techniques and results of which the authors reported as early as 1920, offers such clarity and guarantees that at the present time there are few laboratories in France where it is not carried out on a regular basis in examination following spinal tap, in the same way as a blood count or albumin test. This reaction appears more precise than the preceding ones for the diagnosis of nervous syphilis; in one word, it is really specific and represents the best diagnostic test for progressive nervous syphilis." *Le Progrès médical* 1922 (28): 331.

[35] L. Le Sourd, "Le docteur Joseph-François-Félix Babinski (1857–1932)," *Gazette des hôpitaux* 1932 (92): 1681.

[36] M. Loeper, "Babinski," *Le Progrès médical* 1932 (45): 1885.

[37] *Journal des Praticiens*, 1914 (28): 487; 1915 (29): 55, (29): 117; (29): 134; (29): 165; (29): 215; (29): 261; (29): 390; (29): 407; (29): 517; 1916 (30): 103; 1917 (31) (suppl.): 330.

Table 8-1: Laboratory and tests examinations performed in Dr Babinski's department in 1920

BLOOD

Urea assays	139
Differential blood count	96
Haemocultures	33
Wasserman reaction	629
Serodiagnosis	28

CEREBROSPINAL FLUID

Urea assays	19
Cytology examinations	235
Wasserman reaction	235
Sugar assays (encephalitis)	19

KOCH BACILLUS SEARCH

In sputum	
Direct Examination	152
After homogenization	24
In CSF	8
In urine	11

URINE

Albumin and sugar	164
Urea	34
Chlorides and phosphates	25

MISCELLANEOUS SEARCHES

Gonococci	97
Pneumococci	
Staphylococci	
Weber reaction....	

ANIMALS EXPERIMENTAL OPERATIONS

Rabbits	2
Mice	20
Guinea pigs	14
Guinea pigs used for Wasserman test	35

HISTOLOGY

Spinal cord	2
Brain and cerebellar fragments	9
Whole brain (inclusion)	1
Viscera (inclusion, section, analysis)	39

neurological pathologies were presented. For instance, during World War I clinical cases largely concerned hematomyelia with a Brown-Séquard syndrome, post-traumatic half-cutting of the spinal cord, postspasmodic hemiplegia (or posthemiplegia hemichorea), facial palsy from auricular origin, muscular dystrophies, hysteria, myasthenia, and organo-hysteria.

Le Progrès Médical spoke highly and on a regular basis of the merits of these lectures, emphasizing the importance of the meticulous examination of patients that Babinski, with his "incomparable clinical sense," carried out in front of the audience.[38] The journal commented that books were not sufficient to produce a good neurologist, that patient examination should be complete and meticulous, that M. Babinski was the deserving heir of Charcot, and that with him La Pitié had become a well-known center for the teaching of neurological diseases (Fig. 8-4).[39]

> These lectures are far from an artificial series of lessons as they are taught in an annoying way at medical school...The technique for finding signs is performed by the master himself....In summary, M. Babinski offers—and will continue to do so—excellent practical lessons truly useful to the future practitioner. This is what we need and not teaching as it is carried out at the medical school.[40]

Babinski's interest in teaching was also obvious when in 1907 he participated in the founding of the Association d'enseignement médical des hôpitaux de Paris (Association for medical education of the Hôpitaux de Paris) with about forty other physicians, surgeons, and obstetricians, including Lucas-Championnière, Variot, Hirtz, Béclère, Darier, Bazy, Sergent, Souques, and others. This teaching aimed at supplementing the official curriculum of the medical school.[41] On the other hand, it seems that Babinski did not welcome students who had no official affiliation with the hospital.[42]

Private Practice

The salary of a *médecin des hôpitaux* was at that time 1,200 French francs per year (100 francs per month, equivalent today to roughly €15 a month).[43]

---

[38] For instance, Le Progrès Médical 1897 (V): 135; 1902 (XIV): 231; 1903 (XVI): 193; 1905: 356.
[39] Le Progrès Médical 1901: 279.
[40] Le Progrès Médical 1907 (XXIII): 311.
[41] Ibid., 216.
[42] Le Progrès Médical 1894 (XX): 313; 1894 (XX): 395; 1914 (I): 3.
[43] The value of one French franc varied. Equivalents for 1 franc are given here first in 2005 francs and then in 2005 euros (in parentheses). In 1860: F13,62 (€2,04 €); in 1900,

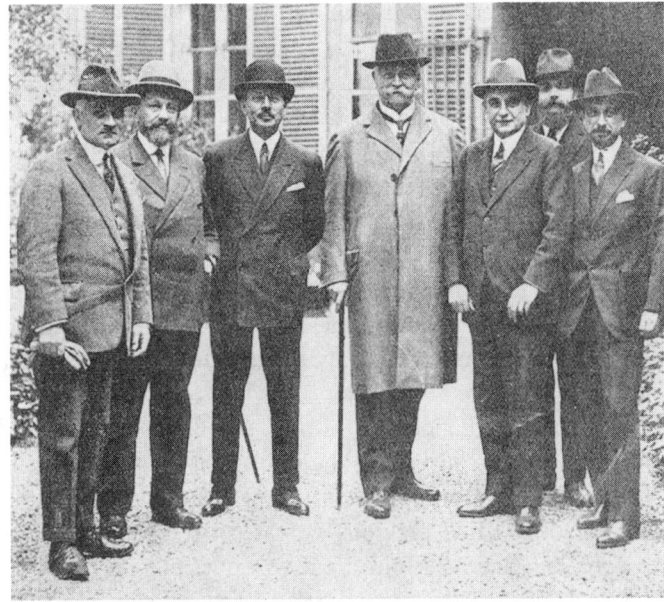

Figure 8-4 Babinski after a meeting of the Société de neurologie, 1927. Next to him, from left to right, are Guillain, Léry, Charpentier, Crouzon, Péhague, and Roussy. (*Source*: Archives of the Académie nationale de médecine, Paris.)

During holiday periods, this salary went to their replacements. Although hospital physicians were poorly paid, in compensation their title carried with it advantages and "gave them the possibility of a private practice and especially of a wealthy one."[44] For that reason, they would work in their private practice in the afternoon, after having spent the morning in the department. Their offices were generally located on the Right Bank, often in the Monceau area. That was the case for Babinski, one of the most sought-after consultants in Paris, with patients coming from all over the world.[45] His fees seemed to have been quite high, sometimes reaching 500 francs for a consultation.[46]

On the walls of his large seven-room apartment located on boulevard Haussmann hung a photograph of his mother, some paintings, one by the Polish painter Olga Boznanska (1865–1940), and portraits of some great

F16,15 (€2,42); in 1910, F17,84 (€2,74); in 1914, F15,03 (€2,25); in 1915, F12,88 (€1,93). In 1920 it decreased to F4,37 (€0,65), and in 1930 it decreased to F2,75 (€0,41).
[44] M. Brueyre, *Conseil supérieur de l'assistance publique* (1898–1899) (IX), no. 68: 55.
[45] Rivet, "Joseph Babinski."
[46] L. Babinski, "Sylwetka Jozefa Babinskiego na tle jego zycia codziennego" [Babinski day by day], *Neurol Neurochir Pol* 1969 (III): 543–546.

figures who had consulted him: the king of Spain, Alfonso XIII (1886–1941, r. 1886–1931), and the victor of Verdun, Philippe Pétain (1856–1951) (Fig. 8-5).[47]

In his private practice he treated on several occasions Marcel Proust (1871–1922), whose correspondence offers some interesting details.[48] For his asthma, Proust was followed by Vaquez, "a nice man, intelligent and serious," who prescribed "one gram of trional two days out of three." In order to regulate his sleep (which occurred mainly during the day), he consulted Dejerine, then Brissaud, "our dear would-be doctor," "the man you have quite to beat to talk about medicine, Brissaud, more handsome and charming than ever," "Brissaud, an admirable individual with a vast intelligence but a bad doctor, who thought (I hardly exaggerate) that you should live on trional."

In 1918, speech disturbances led him to see Babinski, "a famous consultant, whose diagnosis concerning the point that tormented me has been relatively favorable. What remains is to know if he is sincere! I am ready to believe so." Babinski had previously treated Proust's mother for hemiplegia with aphasia. "Babinski told me it was not *éphanie*.[49] But you never know if doctors want to mislead you or mislead themselves." In 1921, Proust again consulted Babinski: "when the most skillful professor tells you 'to pronounce *constantinopolitain* and *artilleur de l'artillerie*,' you do not know what the significance of it may be and he himself believes that you do not know." Babinski advised him to get out of his room and to stop taking sleeping pills. When Proust was at death's door, Babinski, called in by the writer's brother, could only confirm that there was nothing left to do.

The composer Emmanuel Chabrier (1841–1894) was also treated by Babinski, who considered that his condition was related to nervous syphilis contracted in Bordeaux in 1871.[50]

Despite the advantages of an upper-class practice, the great private practitioners did not reap only rewards, especially with patients afflicted by mental illness. The June 28, 1903, issue of the newspaper *Le Temps* reported that a patient of Babinski, left alone for a few moments in a room of the doctor's apartment while the physician was talking with her husband, jumped out of the third-floor window and landed on the pavement below.[51] It is easy to

---

[47] Ibid.
[48] The following quotations from different letters by Marcel Proust are extracted from the well-documented article by D. Mabin, "Proust ou la parole d'un insomniaque" [Proust or the words of an insomniac], *La Presse Médicale* 1993 (22): 1663–1665.
[49] This is possibly a printer's error in the edition of the correspondence: "éphanie" instead of "aphémie" (aphemia). D. Mabin, "Proust ou la parole d'un insomniaque," note 19.
[50] R. Delage, *Emmanuel Chabrier* (Paris: Fayard, 1999).
[51] Reported in *Les Annales Médico-psychologiques*, 1903, 346–347.

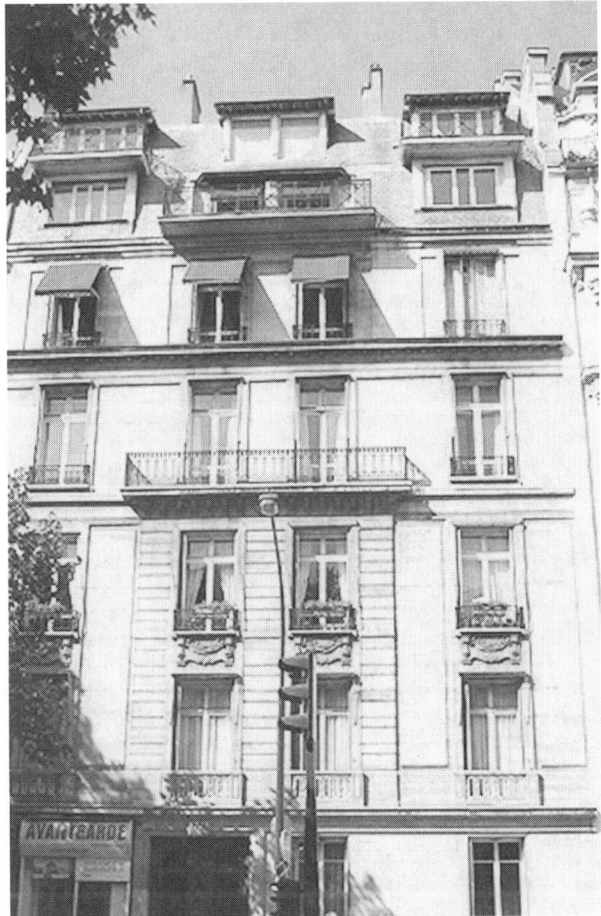

Figure 8-5 Home and office of Joseph Babinski, 170 bis, boulevard Haussmann in Paris. (*Source*: Personal collection, J. Poirier.)

imagine the mental suffering that such an accident may have caused in a man as scrupulous and obsessive as Babinski.

When Babinski had to retire at the end of 1922, his department was taken over by his friend Vaquez, who offered him the opportunity to continue an outpatient practice once a week, assisted by a temporary resident. He benefited also from the presence of two of his faithful associates, Albert Charpentier and Jean Jarkowski, and continued to see patients and publish his findings until 1929.

··· *nine* ···

The Affectionate Admiration of His Students

As Rivet said in his obituary of Babinski, "A man of his caliber had to have had a wide following."[1] This is despite the fact that his nonacademic position carried with it several handicaps. Not being a professor, he could have neither chief residents nor laboratory directors in his department; he could not preside over a thesis nor be on the examining board for the *agrégation*. He had no official assistants, only residents (one or, more rarely two, a year, plus one provisional resident); his team was therefore largely composed of unpaid staff. He had no direct successor because his department was officially considered a department of internal medicine; the neurologists among his pupils could not take over from him when he retired. It was thus his former residents, nonresident students, and auditors of his classes, both French and foreign, who made up the core of his followers.

This having been said, his students demonstrated a level of both admiration and affection far beyond that received by his colleagues, who indeed may have been jealous of these close relationships.[2]

---

[1] L. Rivet, "Joseph Babinski (1857–1932)," *Bulletins et Mémoires de la Société Médicale des Hôpitaux de Paris* 1932 (34): 1722–1733.
[2] "All of his former students are indebted to those, whom we can name—Tournay, Monier-Vinard, Albert Charrin—who until the end supported our mentor and piously closed his eyes." L. Le Sourd, "Le docteur Joseph-François-Félix Babinski (1857–1932)," *Gazette des hôpitaux* 1932 (92): 1681.

In his twenty-nine-year career as head of a department, Babinski was mentor to more than 40 residents and about 150 nonresident students. He supervised the theses of several, notably those of Charles Bourdillon on decompressive craniotomy, André Gendron on spinal cord tumors, Albert Charpentier on the relationship between syphilis and pupillary reflex, Sophie Rosenblum on reflexes of infants during the first year, and Francis Trocmé on decompression methods for brain tumors.[3] He also helped Albert Déchy with his thesis on the significance of the Argyll Robertson sign and the cytology of cerebrospinal fluid.[4] But, as we have already seen, without having professorial status, Babinski could not preside over or be a member of any of the juries for these theses.

Several of Babinski's students would later hold eminent posts in neurology, such as Octave Crouzon (Paris) and Alexandre Barré (Strasburg); in psychiatry, including Georges Heuyer, Jean Nageotte, and Raymond Cestan (Toulouse) (see chapter 7); and even in neurosurgery, with Clovis Vincent and Egas Moniz (Lisbon) (see chapter 13). Others were also in the top ranks of their profession but in areas less directly associated with neurology, such as Louis Delherm, Marcel Labbé, Maxime Laignel-Lavastine, René Moreau, Edouard Rist, Fernand Trémolières, and Maurice Villaret. Certain ones, while not academics, are worthy of note, including Jules Boisseau, Albert Charpentier, André Léri, André Gendron, Raymond Monier-Vinard, and Auguste Tournay (Fig. 9-1).[5]

---

[3] Charles Bourdillon (1891–1963) was a resident in Babinski's department; he became a physician in 1927 as a general practitioner, keeping, however, a double specialty in neurology and dermatology. He played an important role in the French Resistance as early as June 1940; http://perso.wanadoo.fr/fbourdillon/charles.htm. André Gendron, resident under Babinski in 1911–12, defended his thesis on spinal tumors, done by studying twenty-two cases, mostly original, from Babinski's department; Fernand Widal chaired the jury. A. Gendron, *Étude clinique des tumeurs de la moelle et des méninges spinales. Contribution à l'étude des localisations médullaires en hauteur* [Clinical study of spinal cord tumors. About the level of their localisation] (Paris: A. Maloine, 1913), analyzed in *Le Progrès Médical* (1914) (supp., 7). See also chapter 13. A. Charpentier, "Relations entre les troubles des réflexes pupillaires et la syphilis" [Relationships between pupillary reflex disturbances and syphilis], medical thesis, Paris, 1899. Sophie Rosenblum, born in Lodz, Poland, was a nonresident student with Babinski in 1912. Her thesis was *Du développement du système nerveux au cours de la première enfance. Contribution à l'étude des syncinésies, des réflexes tendineux et cutanés et des réflexes de défense* [On the development of the nervous system in early childhood: contribution to the study of synkinesia, tendinous and skin reflexes, and defense reflexes] (Paris: Le François, 1915), analyzed in *Le Progrès Médical* 1914 (supp., 630). F. Trocmé, *De la thérapeutique palliative dans les tumeurs de l'encéphale. Méthodes décompressives (ponction lombaire et trépanation palliative)* [On palliative methods in brain tumors. Decompressive craniotomy and lumbar puncture] (Paris: Henri Jouve, 1909).

[4] A. Déchy, *Le signe d'Argyll-Robertson et la cytologie du liquide céphalo-rachidien* [The Argyll Robertson sign and cerebrospinal fluid cytology], medical thesis, Paris, 1902–3.

[5] Rivet, "Joseph Babinski (1857–1932)."

9. THE AFFECTIONATE ADMIRATION OF HIS STUDENTS

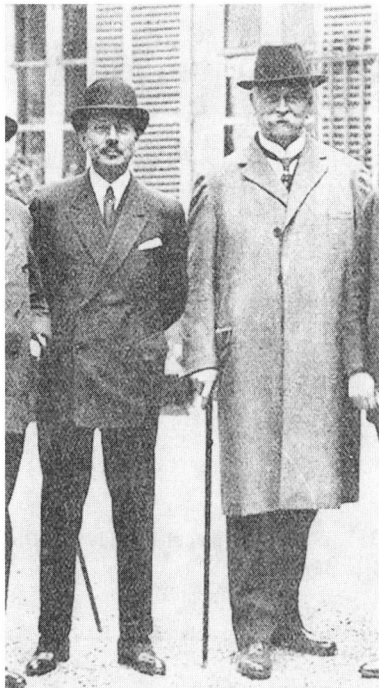

Figure 9-1 Babinski and his pupil Albert Charpentier after a meeting of the Société de neurologie, 1927. (*Source*: Archives of the Académie nationale de médecine, Paris.)

Babinski's *L'œuvre scientifique*, a compendium of his major research papers, was published in 1934 by his closest students: Barré, Chaillous, Charpentier, Crouzon, Delherm, Froment, Gautier, Hartmann, Krebs, Monier-Vinard, Moreau, Plichet, Tournay, Vincent, and Weill.[6]

Students Who Became Close Friends (Table 9-1)

A resident under Babinski in 1909–1910, Alexandre Barré (1880–1967) defended his thesis in 1912 on tabes arthropathies.[7] He formed a friendship with Georges Guillain in the Sixth Army neurological unit during World

---

[6] J. Babinski, *Oeuvre scientifique: recueil des principaux travaux* [Scientific work: Selection of main papers], ed. J. A. Barré, J. Chaillous, A. Charpentier, et al. (Paris: Masson et Cie, 1934).
[7] http://www.whonamedit.com/doctor.cfm/882.html. F. Thiébaut, "Nécrologies. J. A. Barré (1880–1967)" [Obituaries: J. A. Barré (1880–1967)], *Journal of the Neurological Sciences* (Amsterdam) 1968 (6): 381–382.

Table 9-1: Residents (internes) and non resident (externes) students of Babinski

Year	Semester	Internes	Externes
Department of Dr Joseph Babinski (Hôpital de la Porte d'Aubervilliers)			
1894	March 10, 1894–April 30, 1995	Léopold Chauveau Delmond-Bébet (temporary)	Jean-Démétrius Tsakiris Emile Legrand Adrien Girerd
Department of Dr J. Babinski at La Pitié¹			
1895	January 1895–May 1895	Charles Benoit	
	May 1, 1895–January 31, 1896	Marcel Labbé	1/5/1895–31/1/1896 Alexandre Slatinéanu René Lemaître Démêtre Stoïcescu Auguste Dulac
1896	February 2, 1896–January 31, 1897	Léon Levrey	Eugène Pupier Alfred Mirande Roger Brun Pierre Duval
1897	February 1, 1897–February 28, 1898	Edouard Rist	Marcel Hugé, Albert Dufour-Labastide Léon Pauly Maxime Laignel-Lavastine
1898	March 1, 1898–February 28, 1899	Raymond Cestan Louis Le Sourd	François Sémeril Albert Charpentier Charles-Edouard Aubertin Georges Rottenstein
1899	March 1, 1899–February 2, 1900	?	Pierre Vidal René Lemaitre Léon Gibert Albert Barré (died July 14, 1899) replaced by Jules Perrin (1/10/1899–28/2/1900)

(continued)

Table 9-1: Continued

Year	Semester	Internes	Externes
1900	March 1, 1900–September 30, 1900	Léon Bellin	1/3/1900–28/2/1901: Jacques Espitallier André Viteman Edmond Bonamy Maurice Brelet
	October 1, 1900–February 28, 1901	Octave Crouzon	
1901–02	March 1, 1901–September 30, 1901	André Léri	1/3/1901–14/5/1902: Alexandre Pappa Jean Talon Maurice Barbier Paul Podevin (replaced by Bernard Violle)
	October 1, 1901–May 14, 1902	Louis Delherm	
1902–03	May 1, 1902–April 30, 1903	Léopold Braillon	15/5/1902–14/5/1903: Robert Dinet Robert Caruette Florian Budin Serge Rabinovitch
1903–04	May 1, 1903–April 30, 1904	Jules Boisseau	15/5/1903–14/5/1904: André Rousselier Jean Keller Camille De Gandt Raymond Monier-Vinard Vladimir Aïtoff Auguste Tournay
1904–05	May 1, 1904–December 1, 1904	Maurice Villaret	15/5/1904–14/5/1905: Jean Clunet Alfred Offret (exchanged with Edmond Labaude) Henri Flurin Melle Sophie Toufesco Maurice Séjournet
	December 01, 1904–April 30, 1905	Fernand Trémolières	
1905–06	May 01, 1905–April 30, 1906	André Viteman Francisque Lemoine (temporary)	15/5/1905–14/5/1906: Victor Meygret (replaced by Paul Lehucher) Agop Ekmekdjian Gérassimos Rasis

(continued)

Table 9-1: Continued

Year	Semester	Internes	Externes
			(following resignation was replaced by Pierre Astruc) Guy Laroche Paul Crétaux Gendron Wallon
1906–07	May 01, 1906–April 30, 1907	Clovis Vincent Pérol (temporary) as of May 1, then Cadenat from June 11 to July 16	15/5/1906–14/5/1907: Démétri Baisoïu Francis Trocmé Pierre Ménard Alphonse Minaud and Jules Lévy were selected but never reported to duty
1907–08	May 01, 1907–April 30, 1908	Jean Clunet Cesbron (temporary) replaced by Paul Cottenot (ended in October 07)	15/5/1907–14/5/1908: Georges Génil-Perrin Georges Heuyer (replaced by Pierre Hue) André Boutet Robert Marmier Alfred Jacquemin
1908–09	May 01, 1908–April 30, 1909	Auguste Tournay Gustave Clarac (temporary)	15/5/1908–14/5/1909: Robert Dubois Gérald Chevassu-Perigny Pierre Goret (replaced by Francis Bourgeois) Jean Darrieux Jean Audibert (did not report for duty: was replaced by Jean Massé)
1909–10	May 01, 1909–April 30, 1910	Alexandre Barré Adolphe Morancé (temporary)	15/5/1909–14/5/1910: Emile Paley Jacques Durand Ivan Moricand Ernest Pichard (replaced by De Habias) Maurice Delort

(continued)

172

Table 9-1: Continued

Year	Semester	Internes	Externes
1910–11	May 01, 1910–April 30, 1911	Joseph Jumentié Jean Rudelle (temporary)	15/5/1910–14/5/1911: Maxime Leroy Auguste Chardon Paul Blum Georges Imbert (replaced by Elisabeth Kononoff) Henri Ramadier
1911–12	May 01, 1911–April 30, 1912	Paul Cottenot Edouard Krebs (temporary) André Gendron	1/3/1911–29/2/1912 Jacques Fournier Ignace Meyerson André Sorel (replaced by Marguerite Giboulot) René Deron Elizabeth Kononoff
1912–13	May 01, 1912–April 30, 1913	Stephen Chauvet Lépine (temporary 15 February)	1/3/1912–28/2/1913: Gaston Nora Robert Chaperon Sophie Rosenblum Lucien Marx Jean Dagnan-Bouveret Miss Trélat
1913–14		Gauthier Mozer (temporary)	1/3/1913–28/2/1914 Robert Broca Henri Benoist Jacques Wurtz Henri Leroux Jacques Fournier Elisabeth Posuel de Verneaux
1914–15		Jean Dagnan-Bouveret (replaced a resident as of 15 June)	Marcel Dossin Jean Ribeton Jane Mille Jean Moricand Jean Heitz Jean Gallois

(continued)

Table 9-1: Continued

Year	Semester	Internes	Externes
1915–16	?	?	?
1916	?	?	?
1917	?	?	?
1918	October 1, 1918 October 14, 1918	?	Melle Suzanne Maybluh Miss Reverchon
1919	January 2, 1919 January 25, 1919 February 1, 1919 February 15, 1919 September 1, 1919 October 6, 1919 October 12, 1919 November 14, 1919	René Moreau (1/2/1919– 15/4/1920)	2/1/1919–5/10/1919 Dayras (replaced Mrs Masre due to illness) Dussin Ribeton Moricand Fenillé Emile Rousse Mrs Cabonat Besson Desoubry Marcel Ferru
1920	June 18, 1920	Edouard Krebs (16/4/1920– 15/2/1921) Henri Godard	1/3/1920–28/2/1921 Martin Minvielle Marcel Dossin Joseph Gournay Louis Depouilly Philipppe Ginberteau René Jossand Miss Nadine Lachowsky
1921	February 15, 1921– February 14, 1922	André Plichet Louis Bethoux (temporary)	1/3/1921–28/2/1922 Henri Lenfantin Marcel Paillet Jean Christophe Jacques Meyer-May Pierre Bianquis Théodore Fraenkel

(continued)

Table 9-1: Continued			
Year	Semester	Internes	Externes
1922	February 15, 1922	Charles Bourdillon Edouard Hartemann	1/3/1922–28/2/1923 Edmond Charreau Georges Villey Desmeserets Michel Bothézat Melle Lucie Fradiss Nicolle Mayer May Maurice Guyonnaud

¹Beside the Archive documents of the *Assistance Publique* concerning the Pitié Hospital (Registres des appointements, 2 K 15 à 2K 20; Registres d'inscription des employés et gens de service, IK14, IK16, IK18, IK19, IK20, IK22, IK24, IK25, IK26; Etats nominatifs du personnel médical des hôpitaux et hospices—médecins, pharmaciens, internes, externes—1874 à 1910 (449 W 1–24); Externes et internes en médecine dans les hôpitaux de l'Assistance publique: fiches nominatives et suivi et d'évaluation pédagogique, 774 FOSS 1–37), the issues of *Le Progrès Médical*, of *Journal des Praticiens*, of *La Presse Médicale*, and of *Gazette Hebdomadaire de Médecine et de Chirurgie* provide some additional information (however, with numerous mistakes especially in the spelling of the names). During World War I, this analysis was not exhaustive.

War I and engaged in a long-lasting collaboration with him. A subtle and meticulous clinician, professor of neurology in Strasbourg in 1919, he published more than eight hundred scientific papers and founded the *Revue d'Oto-neuro-ophtalmologie*. His name remains associated with the Barré sign (in pyramidal syndrome), Barré-Liéou syndrome, Barré-Masson syndrome, and the most well known, Guillain-Barré or Guillain-Barré-Strohl syndrome. In 1925, he welcomed Babinski with great warmth in Strasbourg and ensured a large audience for his lecture on the importance of questioning in taking case histories and in detecting subjective symptoms.[8]

Jules Boisseau (1878–1961), resident with Darier and Babinski, had a difficult time choosing between dermatology and neurology. His thesis on syphilis was supervised by Professor Gaucher at the Saint-Louis hospital and dedicated to his residency teachers, including Babinski, with whom he worked in

[8] A. Tournay, *La vie de Joseph Babinski* [The life of Joseph Babinski] (Amsterdam: Elsevier, 1967).

1903–4.[9] During World War I, he was in charge of the Neurological Center of Salins and pointed out respectfully to Babinski that the too-frequent diagnosis of physiopathic disorders deprived the front of necessary human resources. Babinski answered that he was convinced by Boisseau's arguments and that, far from being offended by his frankness, he thanked him for it.[10] After the war, Boisseau devoted himself to the fight against venereal disease and to social care, creating in Nice the first outpatient clinic for mothers and children. In 1949, Boisseau published in the *Annales Médico-psychologiques* two extensive papers aiming at demonstrating—contrary to the view of his teacher Babinski—that pithiatism was nothing but malingering.[11]

Raymond Cestan (1872–1934) was a resident with Babinski from March 1, 1898, to February 28, 1899; he defended a thesis in 1899 on Little syndrome and became chief resident under Raymond.[12] Made an associate professor in 1904, he was named to the chair of psychiatry in Toulouse in 1913. His name is associated with two syndromes that he described: Cestan-Chenais brain stem syndrome and Raymond-Cestan syndrome (tumor of the peduncles).

A resident with Babinski in 1907, assistant in the pathological anatomy laboratory directed by Pierre Marie at the Paris University Medical School, associate professor in Nancy, holder of the Legion of Honor, Jean Clunet (1878–1917) died at an early age of typhus fever caught at the Jassy Hospital in Romania, where he was head doctor during World War I.[13] "Quick-witted, with an adventurous disposition, attracted by the unexpectedness of unclear paths," he several times came close to death during the conquest of Morocco and during World War I.[14]

Octave Crouzon (1874–1938) was very impressed and influenced by Pierre Janet; by Georges Dieulafoy (1839–1911), who presided the jury for

---

[9] J. Boisseau, *Traitement local des gommes syphilitiques par les injections d'iodure de potassium* [Local treatment of syphilitic gummas by potassium iodide] (Paris: G. Steinheil, 1906).

[10] P. Cossa, "Jules Boisseau," *La Presse Médicale*, March 18, 1961.

[11] J. Boisseau, "Hystérie et simulation. L'accident pithiatique n'est autre chose qu'un accident simulé" [Hysteria and simulation. A "pithiatic" attack is nothing but a simulated attack], *Annales médico-psychologiques*, July 2 and October 3, 1949. See chapter 15.

[12] http://www.whonamedit.com/doctor.cfm/669.html. Babinski wrote at the end of his residency period: "I was very satisfied with M. Cestan, who during one year worked zealously and with intelligence."

[13] M. Hallion, "Discours du president Hallion, à l'occasion de la mort de M. Clunet, membre de la Société" [Speech of M. Hallion, president, after the death of M. Clunet, member of the Society], *Rev Neurol (Paris)* 1917 (I): 244–246; *Aux médecins morts pour la patrie (1914–18)* [To the physicians who died for their country (1914–18)] (Paris: Baillière/Doin/Masson, 1922), 217; A. R. Brouilhet, *Les héros sans gloire* [Unsung heros] (Paris: Charles Lavauzelle, 1927), 233.

[14] Brouilhet, *Les héros sans gloire.*

his thesis; by Babinski, with whom he was resident in 1900-1; and above all by Pierre Marie.[15] After a training period as resident in his department from May 1902 to May 1903, Pierre Marie considered him "one of the best residents I have ever had." He was responsible for a neurological unit during World War I, then chief of a department at the Salpêtrière from 1919 until his retirement. President of the Société de neurologie de Paris[16] and general secretary of the *Revue Neurologique*, he was named to a chair on medical and social welfare affairs especially established for him. In 1912 he described the cranial and facial malformations, including craniosynostosis and hypoplasia of the facial structures, that are known as Crouzon's disease or hereditary craniofacial dysostosis.[17] Crouzon was honored with the Military Cross and the rank of commander in the Legion of Honor.

Edouard Krebs was a resident under Babinski in 1920. With André Plichet, he was the joint recipient of the Babinski Foundation Prize of the Société de neurologie in 1938.[18]

Marcel Labbé (1870-1939) was a resident under Babinski in 1895-96 and was given a good evaluation at the end of his training period ("I have been satisfied with M. Labbé in all respects"), even if the hospital director had some reservations: "Bright student but a little difficult to deal with."[19]

André Léri (1875-1930), resident in 1901, wrote his thesis on blindness and tabes under the direction of Pierre Marie at Bicêtre (1904).[20] An associate professor, he distinguished himself in neurology (presiding over the Société de neurologie de Paris in 1926), in ophthalmology (he was also president of the Société française d'ophtalmologie), and in bone pathology.[21] He is well known for his description of melorheostosis, or Léri's disease.

---

[15] http://www.whonamedit.com/doctor.cfm/1363.html; O. Crouzon, "Allocution de M. Crouzon, président" [Speech by M. Crouzon, president], *Rev Neurol (Paris)* 1924 (1): 81-82; O. Crouzon, *Des scléroses combinées de la moelle* [Subacute combined degeneration of the spinal cord] (Paris: G. Steinheil, 1904).

[16] Crouzon, "Allocution de M. Crouzon."

[17] *Le Progrès Médical* 1912 (20): 255.

[18] E. Krebs, "Du diagnostic et des indications opératoires dans les complications récentes et tardives des traumatismes cérébraux fermés" [On diagnosis and operative indications in early and late complications of closed head injuries], *Rev Neurol (Paris)* 1939 (71): 369-388.

[19] Archives de l'Assistance publique, Hôpitaux de Paris, 774 FOSS. On Labbé, see F. Huguet, *Les professeurs de la faculté de médecine de Paris. Dictionnaire biographique 1794-1939* [Professors at the Paris Medical School. A biographical dictionary 1794-1939] (Paris: CNRS, INRP, 1991).

[20] http://www.whonamedit.com/doctor.cfm/1599.html; A. Leri, *Cécité et tabès (étude clinique)* [Blindness and tabes (clinical study)] (Paris: J. Rueff, 1904).

[21] *Rev Neurol (Paris)* 1925 (II): 787.

Beginning his medical studies in his hometown of Rouen, André Plichet (1888–1965) was a moving force behind literary and political meetings and took part in drawing up the first socialist student manifesto.[22] Once in Paris, he continued a close association with the socialist student movement and met with Lenin and Jean Jaurès, both of whom he greatly admired. During his studies, he canceled his deferment and began the standard two years of military duty, but just at the end of his service, World War I broke out. He fought in several battles, received positive mention, and was decorated with the Legion of Honor. After the war, he became a resident, under Joseph Babinski and Henri Vaquez, among others. Babinski held Plichet in high esteem and had a great influence on him. From 1923 to 1930, Plichet was a volunteer associate of Babinski, examining patients three times a week at the outpatient practice Babinski had kept in Vaquez's department before presenting the cases to his master. Apart from his medical activities, Plichet had an active interest in artistic and literary life, founding *Tryptique*, a journal devoted to art, literature, and science. At the age of fifty-two, he entered the Resistance movement in immediate response to Charles de Gaulle's call to arms on June 18, 1940. He formed the Libération-Nord unit and edited a weekly underground journal that continued to appear throughout the occupation until liberation. In 1945, he became the editorial secretary of *La Presse Médicale*, a position he held for twenty years, until his death.

Auguste Tournay (1878–1969) was a resident with Babinski in 1908.[23] Member of the Société de neurologie de Paris in 1919, he became its president in 1940. Around 1920, he began at the Collège de France laboratory experiments on nerve section and grafts with rabbits and dogs.[24] For several years he taught psychophysiology at the École des hautes études.[25] He published in 1926 a practical textbook on neurology and in 1934 *Sémiologie*

---

[22] A. Ravina, "Plichet André (1888–1965)," *La Presse Médicale* 1965 (17): 993–995.

[23] P. Nayrac, "In memoriam Auguste Tournay (1878–1969)," *Rev Neurol (Paris)* 1969 (120): 196–197; L. Van Bogaert, "Auguste Tournay (1878–1969)," *Journal of Neurological Sciences* 1970 (10): 197–198; C. Koupernik, "In memoriam: Auguste Tournay (1878–1969)." *Revue de Neuropsychiatrie Infantile* 1969 (17): 331–332; L. Lareng, "Auguste Tournay," *Anesthésie Analgésie (Paris)* 1969 (26): 5–10; P. Passouant, "Personality: Dr. Auguste Tournay," *International Journal of Neurology* 1965 (5): 217–221.

[24] Archives du Collège de France, CDF 22, Art 14, liasse 41.

[25] A. Tournay, P. Chauchard, and M. Sorre, *Conditions et règles de vie* [Life's conditions and rules], vol. VI of H. Piéron, ed., *Traité de psychologie appliquée* [Treatise on applied psychology] (Paris: Presses Universitaires de France, 1958); A. Tournay, "Les régulations organiques de l'affectivité" [Organic control of affectivity], *Bulletin de psychologie, édité par le Groupe d'Etudes de Psychologie de l'Université de Paris*, January 12, 1966, 1–51.

du sommeil [Sleep semiology].[26] He wrote the foreword to *Neurochirurgie du praticien* [Neurosurgery for the general practioner] by Wolinetz.[27] He remained very close to Monier-Vinard, with whom he was a nonresident student under Babinski in 1903–4.[28] Along with Charpentier, he is, without any doubt, the most prolific of those pupils who kept alive the memory of their master.[29]

Nonresident Students Who Remained Exceptionally Faithful

Appointed as a nonresident student in 1895 at the relatively early age of twenty-three, Albert Charpentier held this position for three years, in particular with Babinski (from March 1998 to February 1899), who gave him the evaluation "Very reliable; hard worker, for whom I have nothing but praise," to go along with this comment from the hospital director: "Good student."[30] Charpentier defended his medical thesis in 1899.[31] Becoming a member of the Société de neurologie in 1910, he became its treasurer and substantially contributed to the coffers in 1927 with a personal donation of 2,000

---

[26] A. Tournay, *Neurologie* [Neurology] (Paris: Gaston Doin, 1926). In this book, Tournay made frequent references to Babinski, insisting on the importance of objective signs, quoting the words of Babinski: objective signs are "those that the physician is able to detect by himself, and in the appreciation of which he does not rely on the patient. These objective phenomena cannot be reproduced by will." In the same Babinski tradition, Tournay attached great importance to treatment. A. Tournay, *Sémiologie du sommeil. Essai de neurologie expliquée* [Sleep semiology. Essay on explanative neurology] (Paris: Gaston Doin, 1934).

[27] E. Wolinetz, *Neurochirurgie du praticien* [Neurosurgery for the practitioner], foreword by A. Tournay (Paris: Masson, 1953).

[28] "Whenever with Monier-Vinard, so alive and vibrant, I found once again the companion of our youth which began in that unforgettable year when we first became Babinski's spiritual children. From that point on began our lifelong friendship." A. Tournay, "Discours de l'ancien Président, M. Auguste Tournay" [Speech of the former president, M. Auguste Tournay], *Rev Neurol (Paris)* 1941 (73): 24–26.

[29] A. Tournay, "Joseph Babinski (1857–1932)," *Médecine de France* 1953 (43): 3–10; A. Tournay, "Babinski dans la vie" [Babinski in everyday life], *La Presse Médicale* 1958 (66): 1485–1489; Tournay, *La vie de Joseph Babinski*.

[30] Archives de l'Assistance publique, Hôpitaux de Paris, 774 FOSS.

[31] A. Charpentier, "Relations entre les troubles des réflexes pupillaires et la syphilis" [Relationships between pupillary reflex disturbances and syphilis], medical thesis, Paris, 1899.

francs.[32] Throughout his life, he remained a devoted volunteer associate of Babinski; with Tournay, one of Babinski's most prolific hagiographers; and coeditor of the *Oeuvre scientifique* in 1934 (Figs. 9-2 and 9-3).[33]

Raymond Monier-Vinard (1878–1944), a former nonresident student under Babinski, was at the top of the residency program in 1905, in the same group as Clovis Vincent and Auguste Tournay.[34] After a glorious war record, he was appointed to the Ambroise Paré hospital in 1920 and was characterized as "a person of exceptional distinction, very independent-minded, and with an uncompromising moral rectitude."[35] He was much impressed by Babinski and remained very close to him, publishing in 1935 a short book on neurological semiology dedicated to the memory of his mentor.[36]

In the foreword *to La prothèse fonctionnelle des paralysies et des contractures* (Functional prosthesis in paralyses and contractures) by Maurice Chiray and Jean Dagnan-Bouveret, Babinski wrote a posthumous appreciation of Dagnan-Bouveret, who had been his nonresident student from March 1912 to February 1913 and who had had the opportunity to replace a resident in June 1914 but instead responded to the call to arms. Babinski wrote "I was fortunate to have him as a student; he became my friend, and I appreciated his uncommon moral and intellectual qualities; he had a marked personality and a bright future.... He died on the battlefield felled by an infectious disease caught during duty, in an ambulance on the front."[37] The son of the well-known painter Pascal Dagnan-Bouveret (1852–1929), Jean Dagnan-Bouveret was "intelligent, cultivated, but slightly amateurish."[38] He became

---

[32] *Rev Neurol* 1927 (I): 42; *Rev Neurol (Paris)* 1927 (II): 719–720. When he made the donation, he was living at 3, avenue Hoche, Paris (Seventeenth Arrondissement).

[33] A. Charpentier, *Le Figaro*, October 30, 1932, 2; A. Charpentier, "Un grand médecin, Joseph Babinski (1857–1932)" [A great physician, Joseph Babinski (1857–1932)], *Bulletin Médical*, February 17, 1934; A. Charpentier, *Un grand médecin, Joseph Babinski (1857–1932)* [A great physician, Joseph Babinski (1857–1932)] (Paris: Typographie François Bernouard, 1934); A. Charpentier, "Babinski (Joseph) (1857–1932)," in M. Genty, ed., *Les biographies médicales* [Medical biographies] (Paris: J. B. Baillière, 1937–39), VI:17–32.

[34] A. Sezary, "Raymond Monier-Vinard (1878–1944)," *La Presse Médicale* 1944 (17): 274–275.

[35] Ibid.

[36] R. Monier-Vinard, *Neurologie* (Paris: Masson, 1935); also 2nd ed., 1943.

[37] See Babinski's foreword to M. Chiray and J. Dagnan-Bouveret, *La prothèse fonctionnelle des paralysies et des contractures* [Functional prosthesis in paralysis and contractures] (Paris: Maloine, 1919).

[38] The characterization of Jean Dagnan-Bouveret is from the evaluation by Dr. Roger, under whom Dagnan-Bouveret was a nonresident student at the Hôtel-Dieu; Archives de l'Assistance publique, Hôpitaux de Paris, 774 FOSS. Pascal Dagnan-Bouveret was an "interpreter of mythological and religious subjects as a portraitist, graphic artist and

> ### In memoriam
>
> Géant blond à l'œil bleu, Maître, je vous ai vu
> Poursuivre, obstinément muet, le fil ténu
> Des arcanes profondes
> Jusqu'au jour où, sans morgue, observateur insigne,
> Certain d'avoir trouvé des faits nouveaux, des signes,
> Vous en dotiez le monde.
>
> Souci du pur savant qui n'a rien affirmé
> Qui ne soit démontrable et par lui démontré,
> Impeccable attitude!
> Comme resplendira aux lointains de l'histoire
> L'œuvre de Vérité qui tissait votre gloire
> Et votre inquiétude.
>
> Albert Charpentier

Figure 9-2 Poem in memory of Babinski, by Albert Charpentier. (*Source*: From Albert Charpentier, *Un grand médecin, J. Babinski* [Paris: Typographie François Bernouard, 1934].)

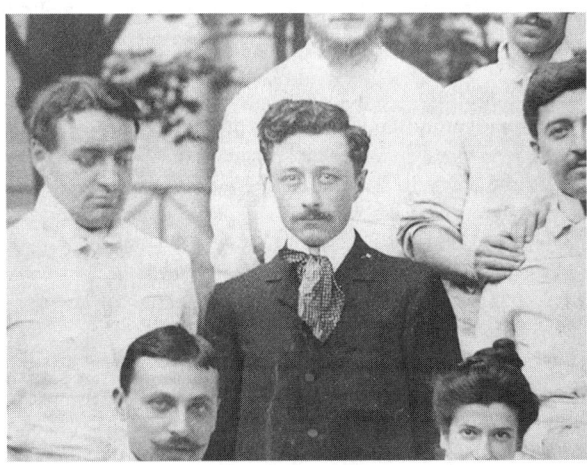

Figure 9-3 Auguste Tournay, resident at the St. Antoine hospital (1906–1907). (*Source*: Personal collection, J. Poirier.)

a professor of philosophy, a resident in psychiatry, and a student of Georges Dumas (1866–1946).[39]

In 1897–98, Maxime Laignel-Lavastine (1875–1953) was a nonresident student with Babinski, then resident and chief resident with Landouzy.[40] His thesis on the solar plexus was chaired by Raymond.[41] He never missed an opportunity to express his everlasting attachment and admiration for Babinski. In his presidential address to the Société de neurologie de Paris in 1928, he recognized that Babinski and Landouzy were the two men who had done the most for his medical education; "he gave me the methodology of thinking correctly and finding the truth in neurology."[42] Becoming a member of the Académie nationale de médecine in 1939, he succeeded Henri Claude in the position of chair at the Clinic for mental diseases at Sainte-Anne hospital. His *Histoire de la médecine* (History of medicine) is a monument to which one may still refer.[43]

Several students of Babinski had brilliant academic careers, as, for example, Maurice Villaret (1877–1946), Babinski's resident in 1904 and also a student of Henri Claude, Pierre Marie, and Bouchard.[44] He became in 1928 the first holder of the chair in therapeutic hydrology and climatology. Georges Heuyer (1884–1977), who founded the field of child psychiatry in France, was a nonresident student with Babinski in 1907.[45]

---

illustrator." He had been a student of Gérome at the School of Fine Arts and also of Corot, receiving the Second Prix de Rome in 1876; E. Bénézit, *Dictionnaire des peintres, sculpteurs, dessinateurs et graveurs* [Dictionnary of painters, sculptors, drawers and engravers], new ed. (Paris: Gründ, 1999).

[39] G. Dumas, *Le surnaturel et les dieux d'après les maladies mentales (essai de théogénie pathologique)* [The supernatural and gods in mental illnesses: an essay in pathological theogony) (Paris : Presses Universitaires de France, 1946).

[40] R. Moreau, "Maxime Laignel-Lavastine," *Rev Neurol (Paris)* 1953 (89): 274–276.

[41] M. Laignel-Lavastine, *Recherches sur le plexus solaire* [Research on the solar plexus] (Paris: Georges Steinheil, 1903).

[42] M. Laignel-Lavastine, "Discours à la Société de Neurologie, réunion du 12 Janvier 1928" [Speech at the Société de neurologie de Paris, meeting of January 12, 1928], *Rev Neurol (Paris)* 1928 (I): 95.

[43] M. Laignel-Lavastine, gen. ed., *Histoire générale de la médecine, de la pharmacie, de l'art dentaire et de l'art vétérinaire* [General history of medicine, pharmaceutics, dentistry and veterinary medicine] (Paris: A. Michel, 1936–49).

[44] M. Villaret, "Les grandes étapes de l'hydro-climatologie" [Important steps in hydro-climatology], *La Presse Médicale* 1928 (95): 1513–1518.

[45] L. Michaux, "Georges Heuyer (1884–1977)," *Nouv Presse Méd* 1978 (7): 383–384; J. L. Lang, *Georges Heuyer, fondateur de la pédopsychiatrie. Un humaniste du XXè siècle* [Georges Heuyer, founder of child psychiatry. A twentieth-century humanist] (Paris: Expansion Scientifique Publications, 1997).

Foreign Physicians Trained by Babinski

Several Polish doctors were part of the larger Babinski circle. Among them, Jean Jarkowski (1880–1929) had a special place, as he was both a volunteer assistant and a friend (see chapter 3). Jerzy Chorobski, one of the founders of Polish neurosurgery, attended Babinski's consultations over a period of several months in 1927 and 1928, and many years later he gave a speech in celebration of the hundredth anniversary of Babinski's birthday.[46] On the same occasion, he quoted a letter in Polish addressed by Henri Babinski to Professeur Orzechowski in which reference is made to the fact that Léon Babinski's father had sent two of his residents from the Evangélique Hospital of Warsaw (Félix Podkolinski and Wladyslaw Filipowicz)[47] for training in Paris under Babinski. Ignace Meyerson was also one of his nonresident students (see chapter 3).

Egas Moniz is probably the most famous among the foreign students of Babinski.[48] The first Portuguese scientist to win a Nobel Prize, he never used his legal name (Antonio Caetano de Abreu Freire), preferring that of Moniz, given to him by his godfather in honor of a hero who resisted the Moors in the twelfth century. Holder of the Neurological Chair in Lisbon (from 1911 to his retirement in 1945), he had studied neurology and psychiatry in Paris with Dejerine, Pierre Marie, Sicard, and Babinski, whom he very much admired. He was very close to the two Babinski brothers, as shown by the paper he published when Babinski died.[49] When he was young, Egas Moniz was intensively involved in politics. Elected to the Portuguese Parliament, he later became ambassador to Spain and then foreign secretary; at the end of World War I, he signed the Treaty of Versailles on behalf of Portugal (June 28, 1919) and held the rank of commander in the Legion of Honor. From 1927 to 1937, Egas Moniz developed the technique of injecting radio-opaque substances into the cerebral arteries, thereby allowing the use of X-rays to localize brain tumors and determine their volume by studying

---

[46] A. Gasecki, "Jozef Babinski wspoltworca wspolcaesnej neurologii i neurochirurgii" [Joseph Babinski, co-founder of the contemporary neurology and neurosurgery], *Neurol Neurochir Pol* 1997 (31), 3: 641–656; J. Chorobski, "Allocution de M. Jerzy Chorobski (Varsovie)" [Speech by M. Jerzy Chorobski (Warsaw)], *Rev Neurol (Paris)* 1958: 637–639.

[47] L. Babinski, "Sylwetka Jozefa Babinskiego na tle jego zycia codziennego" [Joseph Babinski day by day], *Neurol Neurochir Pol* 1969 (III): 543–548.

[48] http://www.upsy.net/upsychologie/ancetres/babinski.html; http://www.upsy.net/upsychologie/ancetres/moniz.htm.

[49] E. Moniz, "Dr. Joseph Babinski," *Lisboa Médica*, November 1932 (IX): 1065.

their displacement.[50] In 1931, Babinski wrote a foreword of praise for the first monograph on angiography.[51] On November 2, 1935, in Lisbon, Egas Moniz and his surgical assistant Almeida Lima performed their first prefrontal leucotomy, sectioning with a surgical knife (leucotome) the fibers connecting the frontal lobe to the thalamus in order to carry out a deafferentation of the frontal lobe. This technique would later be renamed lobotomy by Walter Freeman (1895–1972) when he operated on a schizophrenic patient and inmate in a mental hospital. Publication of favorable results with other patients led to the spread of the method in Portugal and some other countries, in particular Italy, Norway, and the United States.[52] From 1948 to 1957, Freeman, a neurologist, and James Winston Watts (1904–1994), a surgeon at George Washington University, performed the operation on 2,400 patients. In 1949 the Nobel Prize in Physiology or Medicine was given to Egas Moniz for the creation of psychosurgery, an award shared with Walter Rudolph Hess (1881–1973), a Swiss scientist who had worked on diencephalon. After initial enthusiasm for this aggressive surgery, however, its negative effects were emphasized in the following years, and its indications decreased before disappearing to the point that Moniz's Nobel Prize itself became highly questioned. At the age of sixty-five he became paraplegic after being shot by one of his schizophrenic patients, but survived for another seventeen years.

V. Néri, from Italy, Noïca, from Romania, and Grégorie Maranon, from Uruguay, were all neurologists who studied with Babinski. Robert Wartenberg (1887–1956), an American neurologist and graduate of the University of Rostock, worked with Babinski in 1926.[53] In 1933, he became medical director of the Neurological Clinic in Freiburg; persecuted by the Nazis, he left Germany in 1935 and settled in San Francisco, where he became professor of neurology at the University of California there.

---

[50] E. Moniz, "L'encéphalographie artérielle, son importance dans la localisation des tumeurs cérébrales" [Arterial encephalography, its importance in brain tumor localization], *Rev Neurol (Paris)* 1927 (II): 72–90; E. Moniz, "Injections intracarotidiennes et substances injectables opaques aux rayons X" [Injection into the carotid artery of substances impervious to X-rays], *Presse médicale* 1927 (35): 969–971; E. Moniz, *Diagnostic des tumeurs cérébrales et épreuve de l'encéphalographie artérielle* [Diagnosis of brain tumors by arterial encephalography] (Paris: Masson, 1931); E. Moniz, *L'angiographie cérébrale* [Cerebral angiography] (Paris: Masson, 1934).

[51] E. Moniz, *Diagnostic des tumeurs cérébrales et épreuve de l'encéphalographie artérielle* [Diagnosis of brain tumors by arterial encephalography] (Paris: Masson, 1931).

[52] E. Moniz, *La leucotomie préfrontale. Traitement chirurgical de certaines psychoses* [Prefrontal leucotomy. Surgical treatment of some psychiatric disorders] (Torino, 1937).

[53] http://www.whonamedit.com/doctor.cfm/484.html; A. Gasecki and V. Hachinski, "On the names of Babinski," *Canadian Journal of Neurological Science* 1996 (23): 76–79.

U.S.-born Samuel Kinnier-Wilson (1878–1937) graduated from Edinburgh University, worked at the National Hospital for Nervous Diseases in Queen Square, and became professor of neurology at King's College Hospital. He described in 1912 progressive lenticular degeneration, or Wilson disease, which he preferred to be called Kinnier-Wilson disease.[54] He was associated with all the great British names in neurology of that time, in particular Sir William Richard Gowers (1845–1915), Hughlings Jackson, and Sir Victor Horsley (1857–1916). In Paris, he worked first with Pierre Marie, then with Babinski for a year.

From 1897 to 1899, Charles Gilbert Chaddock (1861–1936) stayed with Babinski at La Pitié, and between 1902 and 1921 Chaddock paid him frequent visits. He translated into English some of Babinski's papers and published them in the *Interstate Medical Journal* in 1914. Chaddock remained close to the two Babinski brothers.[55]

Ludo Van Bogaert (1897–1989), of Belgian nationality, assistant to Pierre Marie at the Salpêtrière and to Marcel Labbé at the Charité hospital, also attended the teaching of Charles Foix and Babinski; after returning to Antwerp, he had a prestigious career as a neurologist and a neuropathologist.[56] Otfrid Foerster (1873–1941), a German neurologist and neurosurgeon, professor at the University of Breslau, attended Babinski's lessons, but above all became the disciple of Dejerine during the years 1897–99, showing the greatest admiration for him.[57] Miguel Jimenez Lopez, Erb, Horsley, Flatau, and Baranyi also attended Babinski's consultations and lessons.[58]

Apart from the foreigners, some French nonprofessionals such as Roger Martin du Gard (1881–1958) were regularly present at Babinski's clinical lessons, as well as those of Gilbert Ballet, Fulgence Raymond and Georges Dumas.[59]

---

[54] http://www.whonamedit.com/doctor.cfm/1711.html; "Progressive lenticular degeneration. A familial nervous disease associated with cirrhosis of the liver, doctoral dissertation," *Brain* 1912 (34): 295–507.
[55] P. Bailey, "Joseph Babinski (1857–1932), the man and his works," *World Neurology* 1961: 134–140.
[56] http://georges.dolis.free.fr/Biographies/Biographies_textes_v.htm.
[57] P. Vallery-Radot, "Otfrid Foerster (1873–1941)," *Rev Neurol (Paris)* 1942 (74): 72–74.
[58] http://www.afidro.com/arte_curar/p237/m_tex.htm; Rivet, "Joseph Babinski."
[59] R. Martin du Gard, J. Tardieu, *Lettres croisées (1923–1958)* [Crossed letters (1923–1958)] (Paris: NRF Gallimard, 2003), 240 n. 5.

··· *ten* ···

The Babinski Papers

Despite the encouragement of his friends and colleagues (and perhaps due to an innate shyness), Babinski never found the time to edit an exhaustive compilation of his work. No trace has been found of any personal archive that he may have kept. Reconstructing a complete list of Babinski's medical papers thus has been an interesting but difficult exercise. The major sources are found in two of his own reports and in the 1934 textbook, the *Oeuvre scientifique*, edited by his pupils. In addition, the authors have made an in-depth study of the scientific journals and the minutes of professional organizations in which he published or where his commentaries are recorded.

The 1892 note on his scientific work was intended for his candidacy for the *agrégation*; it contained thirty-one references, mainly on histological and pathological anatomy subjects and a few related to hysteria.[1] The note of 1913, when he was a candidate for the Académie de médecine, was quite naturally more extensive.[2]

The *Oeuvre scientifique*, a volume of 638 pages, published two years after his death, contained 288 publications selected by his pupils.[3] In their introduction, the nature, objectives, intentions, and limits of this publication are

---

[1] J. Babinski, *Notice sur les travaux scientifiques du Dr. J. Babinski* [Note on the scientific papers of Dr. J. Babinski] (Paris: Masson, 1892).

[2] J. Babinski, *Exposé des travaux scientifiques* [Presentation of scientific papers] (Paris: Masson, 1913).

[3] J. Babinski, *Oeuvre scientifique: recueil des principaux travaux* [Scientific work: selection of main papers], ed. J. A. Barré, J. Chaillous, A. Charpentier, et al. (Paris: Masson, 1934).

clearly set forth.[4] They postulated that given the impossibility of reediting all the texts, they were obliged to make choices and deletions, but had not changed any of Babinski's original wordings. A large part of the volume was devoted to the semiological contributions of their mentor.

We have completed the information found in these three sources by the systematic analysis of *Le Progrès Médical* (from 1878 to 1922), the *Bulletins de la Société Anatomique de Paris* (from 1882 to 1889), the *Comptes-rendus Hebdomadaires des Séances et Mémoires de la Société de Biologie* (from 1886 to 1913), the *Archives de Neurologie* (from 1886 to 1895), the *Bulletins et Mémoires de la Société Médicale des Hôpitaux de Paris* (from 1890 to 1932), and the *Rev Neurol* (from 1893 to 1932). From these different sources, we have established a list that we consider as representing quasi-exhaustively the publications and interventions of Babinski (see bibliography).

It is easy to identify two different periods in Babinski's work. During his residency, he was mainly interested in histological and pathological anatomy, as analyzed in chapter 7. Beginning with his association with Charcot in 1885, for whom he was chief resident until 1887, Babinski definitively abandoned his previous interests and became increasingly involved with hysteria, a subject that he would return to from various perspectives throughout his career. He began to study it in the Salpêtrière school manner as taught by Charcot before breaking away from that concept, first by proposing pithiatism, and then later, during World War I circumscribing what he called physiopathic disturbances (see chapter 15).

His first doubts in regard to Charcot's assumptions reflected his conviction that all medical diagnosis must be based upon demonstrable and verifiable facts. To reach this difficult goal in dealing with emotional illness, he would first become a semiologist, eager to detect objective neurological signs that would allow the clinician to distinguish between organic (due to a lesion) and functional (hysterical) illnesses.

The most famous example was certainly the toe phenomenon, characterized by the extension of the big toe during cutaneous plantar excitation, an inversion of normal plantar response known as the Babinski sign (see chapter 11). But the list does not end there: to give just a few examples, Babinski also enriched the semiology of the reflexes, the one of the pupil by a further development of the Argyll-Robertson sign (see below in this chapter), those of the spinal cord compressions, and those of the cerebellum (see chapters 11, 13, and 12, respectively).

[4] Sir Francis Walshe noted that "the works which have been selected are skillfully presented in order to demonstrate the quality of his method and thoughtful way of thinking." F. Walshe, "What place for Babinski in modern neurology," *Rev Neurol (Paris)* 1958 (98): 632–636.

Above and beyond semiology, Babinski remained passionately devoted to therapeutics, becoming increasingly involved in the possibilities offered by surgery for the treatment of central nervous system tumors (see chapters 14 and 13, respectively). Babinski also published several papers on other subjects, particularly on the neurological aspects of syphilis (see below in this chapter).

With the exception of anosognosia, he never showed any deep interest in the semiology of brain functions (see chapter 12). Not very inclined to intellectual speculation, he did not participate in discussions on brain localizations and was not involved in the great dispute on aphasia, when the most famous neurologists of that time, especially Dejerine and Pierre Marie, confronted each other.[5] It is worthy of note that during the three exceptional sessions of the Société de neurologie de Paris devoted to argumentation on aphasia, aside from the two main protagonists, Jutes Dejerine and Pierre Marie, many speakers (Mme Augusta Dejerine, Achille Souques, Edouard Brissaud, André Thomas, Gilbert Ballet, Ernest Dupré, François Moutier, Henri Claude, M. Dufour, Georges Guillain) took the floor, while Babinski, present at all the sessions, remained silent.[6]

Moreover, in contrast to Jules Dejerine and Pierre Marie, Babinski neither wrote nor supervised publication of a neurological treatise drawn from his personal experience or from his works.[7]

Affiliation with Scientific Associations

The majority of Babinski's articles and scientific interventions were presented to professional societies. At the begining of his career, from 1882 to 1889, his voice was heard mainly at the Société anatomique, then from 1886 to 1905 at the Société de biologie (see chapter 7). By the end of his residency, Babinski was attending almost exclusively the Société de biologie, which had been founded in 1848 by Pierre Rayer, Claude Bernard, Charles Robin, Brown-Séquard, and Second, and was less oriented towards pathological anatomy.

---

[5] T. Ott, *Rev Neurol (Paris)* 1958 (98): 660.
[6] Société de neurologie de Paris, meetings of June 11 (*Rev Neurol [Paris]* 1908 (XVI): 611–636), July 9 (*Rev Neurol [Paris]* 1908 (XVI): 974–1023), and July 23, 1908 (*Rev Neurol [Paris]* 1908 (XVI): 1025–1047).
[7] J. Dejerine, *Sémiologie des affections du système nerveux* [Semiology of diseases of the nervous system] (Paris: Masson, 1914); P. Marie, ed., *La pratique neurologique* [Neurological practice] (Paris: Masson, 1911); M. Loeper, "Babinski," *Le Progrès Médical*, 1932 (45): 1885.

He was elected as a full member on July 9, 1887, by thirty-three votes out of thirty-six.[8] From 1886 to 1905, Babinski presented eighteen papers alone or in association with a second author; after an interruption of several years, he published three articles in 1913.[9] With the exception of two in 1886 that still concerned pathological anatomy and histology, all the other articles appearing in the minutes of the Société de biologie concern neurological diseases or hysteria.[10] It was during this period that he focused on the signs marking a distinction between hysteric symptoms and organic signs.[11] His most famous paper concerning the toe phenomenon was delivered in 1896 and

---

[8] *Comptes-rendus Hebdomadaires des Séances et Mémoires de la Société de Biologie* 1887 (IV): 460.

[9] J. Babinski and G. A. Weill, "Désorientation et déséquilibration spontanées et provoquées. La déviation angulaire" [Spontaneous and provoked disorientation and disequilibrium. Angular deviation], *Société de Biologie*, April 26, 1913; J. Babinski, Stephen Chauvet, Jean Jarkowski, "Sur un syndrome de Brown-Séquard par coup de couteau" [Brown-Sequard syndrome by a knife stab], *Société de Biologie*, May 8, 1913; J. Babinski and G. A. Weill, "Mouvements réactionnels d'origine vestibulaire et mouvements contre-réactionnels" [Reactive and counter-reactive movements of vestibular origin], *Société de Biologie*, July 19, 1913.

[10] The two 1886 papers are J. Babinski, "Atrophie musculaire d'origine cérébrale, avec intégrité des cornes antérieures de la moelle et des nerfs moteurs" [Muscular atrophy of brain origin, with no abnormalities in the spinal cord's anterior horns nor of motor nerves], *Comptes-rendus Hebdomadaires des Séances et Mémoires de la Société de Biologie* 1886 (III): 76–78, and J. Babinski, "Sur la présence dans les muscles striés de l'homme d'un système spécial constitué par des groupes de petites fibres musculaires entourées d'une gaine lamelleuse" [On the presence in human striated muscles of a special structure constituted by small neuromuscular spindles], *Comptes-rendus Hebdomadaires des Séances et Mémoires de la Société de Biologie* 1886 (III): 629–631. For the other group, see, for example, J. Babinski, "Recherches servant à établir que certains phénomènes nerveux peuvent être transmis d'un sujet à un autre sous l'influence de l'aimant" [Research in order to demonstrate that some nervous phenomenon may be transmitted from one patient to another under the influence of a magnet], *Comptes-rendus Hebdomadaires des Séances et Mémoires de la Société de Biologie* 1886 (III): 475–477, abstract in *Le Progrès Médical* 1886 (IV): 996; J. Babinski, "Migraine ophtalmique hystérique" [Hysterical ophtalmic migraine], *Comptes-rendus Hebdomadaires des Séances et Mémoires de la Société de Biologie* 1889 (I): 547–549, abstract in *Le Progrès Médical* 1889 (X), 2ème série, No. 35: 223–224.

[11] J. Babinski, "Sur le réflexe cutané plantaire dans certains affections organiques du système nerveux central" [On the cutaneous plantar reflex in some organic diseases of the central nervous system], *Comptes-rendus Hebdomadaires des Séances et Mémoires de la Société de Biologie* 1896 (III): 207–208, abstract in *Le Progrès Médical* 1896 (III): 137 and in *Rev Neurol (Paris)* 1896 (IV): 415; J. Babinski, "Relâchement des muscles dans l'hémiplégie organique" [Muscle loosening in organic hemiplegia], *Comptes-rendus Hebdomadaires des Séances et Mémoires de la Société de Biologie*, 1896 (III): 471–472, abstract in *Rev Neurol (Paris)* 1896 (IV): 467 and in *Le Progrès Médical* 1896 (III): 310–311; J. Babinski, "Des phénomènes des orteils" [On the toes phenomenon], *Comptes-rendus Hebdomadaires des Séances et Mémoires de la Société de Biologie* 1898 (V): 669–700, abstract in *Rev Neurol (Paris)* 1898 (VI): 781–782.

was completed later.[12] The 1886 description of the neuromuscular spindles, not as well known, was nevertheless quite remarkable.[13] Other papers cover a wide range of fields, touching notably on tabes,[14] myopathies,[15] peripheral neuritis,[16] the action of morphine in tetanus,[17] hysteric migraine,[18] voltaïc vertigo,[19] work accomplished with Charrin on pycocyanic infection in rabbits,[20] relaxation of muscles in organic hemiplegia,[21] the contractility

---

[12] Babinski, "Sur le réflexe cutané plantaire." See chapter 11.

[13] Babinski, "Sur la présence dans les muscles striés." See chapter 7.

[14] J. Babinski, "Tabès bénins" [Mild form of tabes], *Comptes-rendus Hebdomadaires des Séances et Mémoires de la Société de Biologie* 1887 (IV): 336–340; J. Babinski and J. Nageotte, "Note sur un cas de tabes à systématisation exceptionnelle" [On a case of tabes with an exceptional systematization], *Comptes-rendus Hebdomadaires des Séances et Mémoires de la Société de Biologie* 1905 (57): 280–283, abstract in *Le Progrès Médical* 1905 (XXI), 3ème série, No. 43: 704.

[15] J. Babinski and I.N. Onanoff, "Myopathie progressive primitive. Sur la corrélation qui existe entre la prédisposition de certains muscles à la myopathie et la rapidité de leur développement (Travail du laboratoire de M. le Prof. Charcot à la Salpêtrière)" [Primitive progressive myopathy. On the correlation between the predisposition of some muscles to myopathy and their rapid development. Work of Pr Charcot's laboratory], *Comptes-rendus Hebdomadaires des Séances et Mémoires de la Société de Biologie* 1888 (V): 145–151.

[16] J. Babinski and M. Zachariade, "Paraplégie crurale par mal de Pott dorsal. Névrites périphériques des membres inférieurs" [Crural paraplegia by a thoracic Pott disease. Peripheral neuritis of the inferior limbs], *Comptes-rendus Hebdomadaires des Séances et Mémoires de la Société de Biologie* 1895 (II): 722–725, abstract in *Le Progrès Médical* 1895 (II): 378 and in *Rev Neurol (Paris)* 1896 (IV): 87–88.

[17] J. Babinski, "De l'action du chlorhydrate de morphine sur le tétanos" [On the action of morphine hydrochlorate on tetanus], abstract in *Le Progrès Médical* 1897 (V): 407–408 and in *Rev Neurol (Paris)* 1897 (V): 656.

[18] Babinski, "Migraine ophtalmique hystérique."

[19] J. Babinski, "De l'influence des lésions de l'appareil auditif sur le vertige voltaïque" [On the influence of lesions of the auditory system on voltaic vertigo], *Comptes-rendus Hebdomadaires des Séances et Mémoires de la Société de Biologie* 1901 (52): 77–80, analyzed in *Rev Neurol (Paris)* 1901 (IX): 1170–117; J. Babinski, "Sur le mécanisme du vertige voltaïque" [On the voltaic vertigo mechanism], *Comptes-rendus Hebdomadaires des Séances et Mémoires de la Société de Biologie* 1903 (LV): 350–353; J. Babinski, "Sur le mouvement d'inclination et de rotation de la tête dans le vertige voltaïque" [On head tilting and rotation in voltaic vertigo], *Comptes-rendus Hebdomadaires des Séances et Mémoires de la Société de Biologie* 1903 (LV): 513–515.

[20] J. Babinski and J.E. Charrin, "De la paralysie pyocyanique. Étude clinique et anatomique" [On paralysis of pseudomonas origin. Clinical and anatomical study], *Comptes-rendus Hebdomadaires des Séances et Mémoires de la Société de Biologie* 1888 (V): 257–259; J. Babinski and J.E. Charrin, "Arthropathies expérimentales. Paralysie pyocyanique" [Experimental arthropathies. Paralysis of pseudomonas origin], *Comptes-rendus Hebdomadaires des Séances et Mémoires de la Société de Biologie* 1889 (I): 545–547, abstract in *Le Progrès Médical* 1889 (X): 223–224.

[21] This trouble, which "is marked by the possibility of the paralyzed members executing some passive movements in greater amplitude than on the normal side…is

of the striate muscles after death,[22] and the transmission of certain nervous phenomena from a patient to another under the influence of a magnet.[23]

In 1890, as soon as he was named *médecin des hôpitaux*, Babinski became a de facto member of the Société Médicale des Hôpitaux de Paris, to which he presented numerous papers, published afterward in the *Bulletin* of the society. The subjects he dealt with between 1890 and 1928 covered a vast spectrum of interests, for example, muscular cramps in cholera,[24] syringomyelia,[25] and quite often hysteria.[26] With Enriquez and Gaston-Durand, Babinski published the case of a young patient presenting signs of coxalgia, which were in fact caused by a reflex muscular spasm related to a latent chronic appendicitis; the appendix resection followed by psychotherapic treatment resulted in a complete cure.[27]

A few months before Charcot's death in 1893, Edouard Brissaud and Pierre Marie founded the *Revue Neurologique*. Babinski was not involved in this task and his name did not appear among the collaborators for the

---

absent in hysterical hemiplegia." Babinski, "Relâchement des muscles dans l'hémiplégie organique."

[22] J. Babinski, "De la contractilité électrique des muscles striés après la mort" [On the electrical contractility of the striate muscles after death], *Comptes-rendus Hebdomadaires des Séances et Mémoires de la Société de Biologie* 1899 (I): 343–346, abstract in *Le Progrès Médical* 1899 (IX), 3ème série, No. 20: 319.

[23] See chapter 3. Babinski, "Recherches servant à établir que certains phénomènes nerveux."

[24] J. Babinski, "Des crampes musculaires dans le choléra et dans d'autres états pathologiques" [On muscular cramps in cholera and other pathological conditions], *Bull. Mém. Soc. Méd Hôp. Paris* 1892 (IX): 845–848, abstract in *Le Progrès Médical* 1892 (XVI), 2ème série, No. 50: 488.

[25] E. Desnos and J. Babinski, "Sur un fait de syringomyélie (présentation de malade)" [On a case of syringomyelia (patient presentation)], *Bull. Mém. Soc. Méd. Hôp. Paris* 1891 (VIII): 652–656.

[26] J. Babinski, "Polyurie hystérique. Influence de la suggestion sur l'évolution de ce syndrome" [Hysterical polyuria. Modification of the syndrome by suggestion], *Bull. Mém. Soc. Méd. Hôp. Paris* 1891 (VIII): 568–574; J. Babinski, "Paralysie hystérique systématique (paralysie partielle ou systématique des fonctions motrices du membre inférieur droit)" [Systematic hysterical paralysis (partial or systematic paralysis of the functions of the right inferior limb)], *Bull. Mém. Soc. Méd. Hôp. Paris* 1892 (IX): 533; J. Babinski, "Paralysies hystériques systématiques. Paralysie faciale hystérique" [Systematic hysterical paralysis. Hysterical facial palsy], *Bull. Mém. Soc. Med. Hôp. Paris* 1892 (IX): 706, abstract in *Le Progrès Médical* 1892 (XVI): 409; J. Babinski, "Paralysie faciale hystérique" [Hysterical facial palsy], *Bull. Mem. Soc. Méd. Hôp. Paris* 1892 (IX): 738, abstract in *Le Progrès Médical* 1892 (XVI):414–415.

[27] J. Babinski, "Pseudo-coxalgie et appendicite" [Pseudo-coxalgia and appendicitis], *Bull. Mém. Soc. Méd. Hôp. Paris* 1913 (XXXV): 191–199.

first issue.[28] Several years later, as of 1899, when the *Rev Neurol* became the official journal of the Société de neurologie de Paris, and published every month the minutes of its sessions, Babinski's works appeared regularly in the journal after their oral presentation at the assembly. Following Brissaud's death in 1909, the *Rev Neurol* was run by a Directory Committee composed of Joseph Babinski, Pierre Marie, and Achille Souques, which remained unchanged until 1923; Babinski continued as a member until his death.[29]

Founded in Paris on June 8, 1899, six years after the *Revue Neurologique*, the Société de neurologie de Paris was intended to bring together periodically physicians concerned with nervous diseases. It was composed of full and associate members from France and foreign countries. Every month, except in August, September, and October, the members had the opportunity to give oral presentations (maximum fifteen minutes) or could show a patient or anatomical specimen. The Advisory Committee consisted of Alix Joffroy (president), Fulgence Raymond (vice president), Pierre Marie (general secretary), Henry Meige (secretary for the sessions), and Achille Souques (treasurer); the founding members were Achard, Babinski, Ballet, Brissaud, Dejerine, Dupré, Gilles de la Tourrette, Gombault, Klippel, Parinaud, Parmentier, and Richer. The first open session took place on July 6, 1899 at which Babinski read a paper, "Du 'phénomène des orteils' dans l'épilepsie" [On the toes phenomenon in epilepsy].[30]

As behooved the founding members of the society, Babinski regularly attended the meetings and the general assembly. By seniority, he was elected president in 1907.[31] He showed on the occasion of his short presidential speech that he could be humorous by underlying "the cordiality of

[28] List of the collaborators of the *Revue Neurologique*: Blin, Blocq, Boix, Bresson, Charcot (Jean), Chrétien, Feindel, Guinon, Habel, Hallion, Huet, Landowski, Marinesco, Souques, Zuber; special collaborators: Boulloche (child neurology), Chipault (surgery), Janet (psychology), Rochon-Duvigneaud (ophthalmology), Ruault (ear, nose, and throat), Thibierge (dermatology). *Rev Neurol (Paris)* 1893 (I): 4.

[29] "The new directors will be faithful to the program of the founding members. The same community of origin—Charcot's school—gather them together, as well as their editorial interests. It is the safest guarantee that the individual efforts will move forward in the same direction as that of the past eighteen years." Foreword, *Rev Neurol (Paris)* 1911 (XXI): 1–2.

[30] J. Babinski, "Du phénomène des orteils dans l'épilepsie" [On the toes phenomenon in epilepsy], *Rev Neurol (Paris)* 1899 (VII): 512–513.

[31] Beginning at its foundation, "the oldest full member was designated for a year as president." In 1919, age was no longer taken into account, but rather the length of full membership. *Rev Neurol (Paris)* 1919 (V): 425. For 1907, the committee was composed of J. Babinski, president; M. Klippel, vice president; Pierre Marie, general secretary; Henry Meige, secretary for the sessions; and A. Souques, treasurer.

our relationship," the meetings "never disturbed, as in other assemblies, by stormy debates," "the perfect serenity in our discussions" (see appendixes to this chapter). As we can see from reading the minutes of the sessions, this was far from being the case; the minutes, to say the least, reflect the heat and even the aggressiveness of the verbal exchanges, which would find their apogee a year later in the famous 1908 debate on aphasia.

Babinski was also on the boards of different bodies of the society and was unanimously elected in 1919 to be a member of the *Commission du fonds J. Dejerine*, which evaluated the research grant purposes and selected the recipients (with his mandate renewed in 1921 and again in 1924), and a member of the Commission des réunions neurologiques annuelles, concerned with the annual neurological meetings.[32] He proposed that Parkinsonian syndromes should be the theme of the annual meeting in 1921; recall that Babinski did not like to examine patients with Parkinson disease, as his father had suffered from it and he feared that he himself would one day be affected, which was indeed, unfortunately the case.[33] In 1923, he was appointed as president of the Comité d'organisation du centenaire de Charcot, to handle the events celebrating Charcot's centenary, with Pierre Marie, Albert Pitres, Paul Richer as honorary president, and Achille Souques as general secretary.[34] He was also a member of the Commission pour le Prix Charcot, introduced in 1925 by the Société de neurologie.[35] For the commemoration of the Vulpian centennial, Babinski was named to the honorary committee and was one of the vice presidents of the organizational committee.

After his official retirement in 1922, Babinski continued to attend the meetings of the Société de neurologie and to publish for several years. On January 11, 1925, he presided over the international meeting of the Société de neurologie in Strasbourg, where he met again his associate Alexandre Barré, who had become professor of neurology in that city. His last intervention at the Société de neurologie took place in 1930.[36]

---

[32] The commission du fonds J. Dejerine was composed of J de Massary (president of the society), Henry Meige (general secretary), Mme Dejerine, Babinski, and André Thomas. See *Rev Neurol (Paris)* 1919 (V): 446–447; *Rev Neurol (Paris)* 1924 (II): 660. In 1921, the commission on annual meetings was composed of Pierre Marie, Babinski, Souques, H. Claude, and H. Meige. See *Rev Neurol (Paris)* 1921 (VI): 715.

[33] The minutes of this annual meeting are in *Rev Neurol (Paris)* 1920 (7): 748. M. Souques was named rapporteur. L. Rivet, "Joseph Babinski (1857–1932)." *Bull. Mém. Soc. Méd. Hôp. Paris* 1932 (34): 1722–1733.

[34] *Rev Neurol (Paris)* 1924 (I):72–73.

[35] *Rev Neurol (Paris)* 1925 (II): 789–791. The commision was presided over by Guillain.

[36] J. Babinski, intervention of 66 lines (pp. 1171–1173) about the communication of A. Radovici, "L'hystérie et les états hystéroïdes organiques" [Hysteria and hysteria-like organic conditions], *Rev Neurol (Paris)* 1930 (I): 1164–1173.

To show his attachment to the Société de neurologie de Paris, in a codicil to his will he bequeathed the society 50,000 francs "in order to create with the income of this sum a prize similar to the Dejerine prize, awarded every third year to a work on neurology."[37] In 1933, the society created a commission of five members, all former students and friends of Babinski: Clovis Vincent, Octave Crouzon, Alexandre Barré, Albert Charpentier, and Auguste Tournay. This commission was in charge of selecting the first recipients of the Babinski Fund.[38] Edouard Krebs and André Plichet, both of them former residents under Babinski, received the prize from the Société de neurologie in 1938.[39]

Aside from the four main scientific societies that published the greater part of his works, a small number of the papers appeared in other journals such as the *Bulletin de l'Académie de Médecine, La Presse Médicale, Revue de Médecine, Annales de Médecine, Journal du Praticien, Bulletin Médical, Le Progrès médical, Gazette Hebdomadaire de Médecine et de Chirurgie, Semaine médicale, Encéphale,* and *Comptes-rendus de l'Académie des Sciences.* Often these were reissues of previous publications.

Babinski, Above All a Semiologist

Babinski often and at great length expressed himself on the importance of semiology. Whether at a lesson given in 1904 at the Pitié or a conference held in 1925 on the occasion of the neurological meeting in Strasbourg, he insisted that certain methods must to be followed to lead to an exact diagnosis.[40] His conception of semiology was founded on the importance of objective signs, those that do not depend on the patient's will. He emphasized as well the errors in diagnosis that may arise when the patient is prone to conscious or unconscious simulation or open to involuntary suggestion, particularly by the physician. He explained how to avoid such traps when

---

[37] Letter of M. Dufour, notary in Paris, to the general secretary of the Société de neurologie, November 17, 1932, *Rev Neurol (Paris)* 1932 (II): 714.
[38] *Rev Neurol (Paris)* 1933 (II): 886.
[39] E. Krebs, "Du diagnostic et des indications opératoires dans les complications récentes et tardives des traumatismes cérébraux fermés" [On diagnosis and operative indications in early and late complications of closed head injuries], *Rev Neurol (Paris)* 1939 (71): 369–388.
[40] J. Babinski, "Quelques considérations sur l'interrogatoire en clinique et les symptômes subjectifs" [Some considerations on clinical interrogation and subjective symptoms], *Rev Neurol (Paris)* 1925 (I): 297–310 (no. 281 in Babinski, *Oeuvre scientifique*).

questioning the patient. In particular, Babinski championed the importance of a complete and systematic neurological exam:

> I estimate that diagnostic errors are usually less often related to a false interpretation than to a defective observation of symptoms, that is more to errors in semiology.... Before concluding, I want to give you some final practical advice. You have to look for all or at least the majority of these objective signs in each patient you are examining or treating; once the habit has been acquired, you will do it rapidly and to a certain extent unconsciously. You will often find, for the benefit of your patients, disorders that otherwise could have been overlooked. You will be able to make a correct diagnosis, and in any case, by acting in this way, you will not make glaring mistakes, harmful to your reputation, and what is more serious, likely to harm those who have placed their confidence in you.[41]

In chapters 11 through 15, we shall discuss the fundamental contributions of Babinski to neurological semiology, especially the toe phenomenon or Babinski sign, the tendinous and defense reflexes, pupillary semiology, cerebellar symptomatology, localization of spinal cord tumors, the distinction between organic and hysterical, anosognosia, and physiopathic disturbances.

Syphilis of the Nervous System

In the nineteenth century and the first half of the twentieth, together with tuberculosis and alcoholism, syphilis was a major public health problem in France.[42] The turning point in the understanding of the disease began with the discovery in 1905, by Fritz Schaudinn (1871–1906) and Paul Hoffmann (1868–1959), of *Treponema palllidum*, the germ responsible for the infection,

---

[41] J. Babinski, "Introduction à la sémiologie des maladies du système nerveux. Des symptômes objectifs que la volonté est incapable de reproduire. De leur importance en médecine légale" [Introduction to nervous disease semiology. On the objective signs which cannot be voluntarily reproduced. Their importance in forensic medicine], *Gazette des Hôpitaux*, October 11, 1904 (no. 108 in Babinski, *Oeuvre scientifique*).

[42] "At the beginning of the nineteenth century, the files of the insurance companies disclosed that between 14 and 15 percent of deaths was due to syphilis. Another analysis gives a figure of 17 percent. A third one carried out between the two wars suggested that a tenth of the population was probably affected, this meaning that 140,000 persons died yearly, and there were 40,000 births followed by death every year [due to maternal infection]. It was one of the great causes of madness." T. Zeldin, *Histoire des passions françaises, I, Ambition et Amour* [History of French passions, I: ambition and love] (Paris: Seuil, 2002), 357.

and the development in 1906 by August Paul von Wassermann (1866–1925) of the chemical reaction named after him. Carried out on blood serum or cerebrospinal fluid, this reaction is a diagnostic test for syphilis, derived from the reaction of the deviation of the complement, discovered in 1901 by two Belgian biologists, Jules Bordet (1870–1961) and Octave Gengou (1875–1957). Generally known in France as the *réaction de Bordet-Wassermann* or *BW* (pronounced *Bé-Vé*), for a long time it was systematically practiced on all patients entering the hospital.

As were most of the physicians of his time, Babinski was preoccupied by syphilis, especially its neurological aspects. This marked interest appeared throughout his career, as seen in about twenty papers published on the subject, mainly in the *Bulletin de la Société Médicale des Hôpitaux de Paris* and the *Revue Neurologique*, as well as about twenty interventions (see bibliography) during discussion of articles presented by speakers at the Société de neurologie de Paris, notably during the special session devoted to tabes in 1911 and during the annual meeting of the *Société* in 1920 dealing with the clinical aspects of nervous syphilis and its treatment.[43]

As early as 1887, he had published in the bulletin of the Société anatomique two papers on tabetic arthropathies and one in that of the *Société de Biologie* on the mild forms of tabes.[44] After having drawn attention to the weakening or absence of the Achilles reflex in sciatica, Babinski noted two years later that the same modifications may be observed in tabes.[45] He defended the idea that the modifications of this reflex in tabes was as important as the Westphal sign, particularly since, not exceptionally, the knee reflex may

---

[43] At the 1911 session Babinski offered seven interventions—10 lines (p. 762), 7 lines (765), 15 lines (766), 18 lines (769–770), 26 lines (770–771), 6 lines (776), 58 lines (778–779)—in the special session (December 14, 1911) of the Société de neurologie de Paris, "Sur la délimitation du tabes" [On the delimitation of tabes], *Rev Neurol (Paris)* 1911 (XXII): 721–812. For his contributions to the 1920 annual meeting, see his intervention of 3 lines (p. 626), "Sur l'influence des races dans le tabes" [On racial influence in tabes], concerning the report of J. A. Sicard, "Syphilis nerveuse et son traitement" [Nervous syphilis and its treatment], *Rev Neurol (Paris)* 1920 (XXXVI): 609–748.

[44] J. Babinski, "Arthropathies des ataxiques" [Arthropathies in ataxic patients], *Bulletins de la Société Anatomique de Paris*, 1887 (I): 624–626; J. Babinski, "Ataxie locomotrice—Arthropathie tabétique—Rhumatisme chronique" [Locomotor ataxia—Tabes arthropathies—Chronic rheumatism], *Bulletins de la Société Anatomique de Paris* 1887 (I): 669–672; Babinski, "Tabes bénins."

[45] J. Babinski, "Abolition du réflexe de tendon d'Achille dans la sciatique" [Achilles reflex abolition in sciatica], *Bull. Mém. Soc. Méd. Hôp. Paris* 1896 (XIII): 887–889; J. Babinski, "Sur le réflexe du tendon d'Achille dans le tabes" [On the Achilles reflex in tabes], *Bull. Mém. Soc. Méd. Hôp. Paris* 1898 (XV): 679–684, abstract in *Le Progrès Médical* 1898 (VIII), 3ème série, No. 44: 301.

be present whereas the Achilles reflex has disappeared.[46] On this occasion, he insisted on the importance in any neurological exam of routinely studying this reflex with the appropriate technique (the patient kneeling on a seat).

He also drew attention to the frequency of marital tabes, and considered that tabes caused by hereditary syphilis was more frequent than generally thought.[47] Often appearing in a mild form, it calls for a systematic examination, especially since its evolution may be favorably influenced by an intensive and prolonged mercury treatment.[48] With Barré, he showed that transmission of syphilis between family members was also frequent, often latent, calling for systematic screening of husband, wife, and children by the Wassermann test.[49] He also pointed out that stomach pain caused by a small ulcer near the pylorus may mimic tabetic gastric pain, and underlined the serious therapeutic consequences.[50] He reported with Nageotte an exceptional case of tabes with a normal knee reflex.[51] In collaboration with Chaillous, he studied the visual field and central vision during tabetic atrophy of the optic nerve and showed that there was no specific modification of the field in this pathology.[52] He also drew attention to the rarity of central scotoma in optic atrophy of the tabes; if one was present, he recommended looking for another lesion, particularly a retrobulbar neuritis of alcoholic, nicotinic, or more rarely infectious origin.[53] Babinski became interested as well in the different forms of pseudo-tabes and with Jumentié reported two cases of meningeal hemorrhage that he connected to syphilitic lesions of the meninges or arteries.[54]

[46] The Westphal sign is the abolition of the knee reflex in tabes.

[47] J. Babinski, intervention of 33 lines (pp. 340–341) concerning the communication of Souques, "Tabes conjugal" [Marital tabes], *Rev Neurol (Paris)* 1900 (VIII): 338–341.

[48] J. Babinski, "Tabes hérédo-syphilitique (tabes héréditaire)" [Hereditary syphilitic tabes], *Bull. Mém. Soc. Méd. Hôp. Paris* 1902 (XIX): 884–889, abstract in *Le Progrès Médical* 1902 (XVI), 3ème série, No. 44: 284. See chapter 14.

[49] J. Babinski and J.A. Barré, "Contribution à l'étude de la syphilis familiale (recherches à l'aide de la méthode de Wassermann" [Contribution to the study of family syphilis (using the Wasserman method)], *Bull. Mém. Soc. Médicale des Hôpitaux de Paris* 1906 (XXIX): 595–598, abstract in *Le Progrès Médical* 1910 (XXIII): 328.

[50] J. Babinski, S. Chauvet, and G. Durand, "Un cas de crises gastriques tabétiformes liées à l'existence d'un petit ulcus juxta-pylorique" [About a case of gastric tabes-like pain due to a small ulcer near the pylorus], *Rev Neurol (Paris)* 1913 (XXV): 436–438.

[51] Babinski and Nageotte, "Note sur un cas de tabes à systématisation exceptionnelle."

[52] J. Babinski and J. Chaillous, "Du champ visuel et de la vision centrale dans l'atrophie tabétique des nerfs optiques" [On visual field and central vision in tabetic optic nerve atrophy], *Comptes-rendus de la Société d'Ophtalmologie de Paris*, February 7, 1907.

[53] J. Babinski, "Sur une forme de pseudo-tabes (névrite rétrobulbaire infectieuse et troubles dans les réflexes tendineux)" [On a case of pseudo-tabes (infectious neuritis and pertubation in tendinous reflexes)], *Rev Neurol (Paris)* 1900 (VIII): 622–625.

[54] J. Babinski, intervention of 13 lines (p. 272) concerning the presentation of P. Marie et G. Guillain, "Vitiligo et symptômes tabétiformes" [Vitiligo and pseudo-tabes symptoms],

Going against the general opinion of most physicians of his time, Alfred Fournier (1832–1914), first professor of the Clinic of Cutaneous and Syphilitic Diseases at the Saint-Louis hospital, had demonstrated, in 1876, the syphilitic origin of tabes and general paralysis.[55] Babinski shared that view, as did Raymond.[56]

Babinski, most often in collaboration with Albert Charpentier, published several articles on pupillar semiology, particularly in relation to the pupillar reflex and the Argyll-Robertson sign.[57] For him, the disappearance of the pupil reflex to light, if permanent and not related to an eyeball lesion or paralysis of the third nerve, "is the sign of a disturbance of the central nervous system, quite surely of syphilitic origin: the...patient who presents such signs is a candidate for diagnosis of tabes or general paralysis."[58]

Babinski thought that patients with syphilis, even without any visible sign of tabes, general paralysis, or another neurological sign, might nevertheless show an Argyll-Robertson sign. It was therefore for him a sign of "acquired or hereditary syphilis quite or completely pathognomonic."[59] During the discussions following presentation of papers at the Société médicale des hôpitaux de Paris or at the Société de neurologie, Babinski intervened several times to

---

Rev Neurol (Paris) 1902 (X): 273–274; J. Babinski, "Pseudo-tabes spondylosique" [Spondylotic pseudo-tabes], *Rev Neurol (Paris)* 1903 (XI): 645; J. Babinski and C. Gautier, "Pseudo-tabes et filariose sanguine" [Pseudo-tabes and filariasis], *Rev Neurol (Paris)* 1914 (XXVII): 856–857; J. Babinski and J. Jumentié, "Contribution à l'étude de l'hémorragie méningée" [Contribution to the study of meningeal hemorrhage], *Bull. Mém. Soc. Méd. Hôp. Paris* 1912 (XXXIII): 744–749, abstract in *Le Progrès Médical* 1912 (23): 290.

[55] A. Fournier, *De l'ataxie locomotrice d'origine syphilitique* [On locomotor ataxia of syphilitic origin] (Paris: Masson, 1876).

[56] J. Babinski, "Association de tabes et de lésions syphilitiques" [Association between tabes and syphilitic lesions], *Rev Neurol (Paris)* 1900 (VIII): 625–626; F. Raymond, *Etiologie du tabes dorsal* [Tabes dorsalis etiology] (Paris: Aux bureaux du Progrès Médical, Veuve Babé et Cie, 1892).

[57] The sign was first described in 1869 by the Scottish ophthalmologist Argyll Robertson. See A. Robertson, "On an interesting series of eye symptoms in a case of spinal disease, with remarks on the action of belladonna on the iris," *Edinburgh Medical Journal* 1869 (14): 696–708; A. Robertson, "Four cases of spinal myosis: with remarks on the action of light on the pupil, iris," *Edinburgh Medical Journal* 1869 (15): 487–193. (These two references are cited by J. M. S. Pearce, "The Argyll Robertson pupil," *Journal of Neurology, Neurosurgery and Psychiatry* 2004 [75]: 1345.) For Babinski's and Charpentier's research on the sign, see A. Charpentier, "Relations entre les troubles des réflexes pupillaires et la syphilis" [Relationships between pupillary reflex disturbances and syphilis], medical thesis, Paris, 1899.

[58] J. Babinski, "Des troubles pupillaires dans les anévrismes de l'aorte" [On pupillary perturbations in aortic aneurysms], *Bull. Mém. Soc. Hôp.Paris* 1901 (XVIII): 1121–1124, abstract in *Le Progrès Médical* 1901 (XIV): 391 and in *Rev Neurol (Paris)* 1902 (X): 459.

[59] Babinski, "Des troubles pupillaires dans les anévrismes de l'aorte."

reaffirm this opinion.[60] He was more precise in 1907, when he stated, "If you cannot absolutely affirm that this sign is characteristic of syphilis, neither can you demonstrate that it is related to another cause."[61] There was consensus on this point. For instance, Dufour noted that pupil irregularity has a considerable value in the diagnosis of syphilis, and that the Argyll-Robertson sign had been observed only in patients with syphilis, general paralysis, or tabes.[62] Others were more reserved: "From a practical point of view, the presence of an Argyll-Robertson sign leads to suspicion of syphilis, according to the rule established by M. Babinski. According to the authors, however, until the evidence has been demonstrated by pathological anatomy, it should be admitted that this sign indicates an initial tabes or general paralysis, either isolated, or associated with other nervous diseases of syphilis."[63]

[60] J. Babinski, intervention of 4 lines (p. 622), concerning the presentation of J. Piltz (from Warsaw), "Sur quelques nouveaux symptômes pupillaires dans le tabes dorsal" [On some new pupillary symptoms in tabes dorsalis], *Rev Neurol (Paris)* 1900 (VIII): 593–597; J. Babinski, concerning the minutes, "De l'inégalité pupillaire dans les anévrismes" [Pupillar asymmetry in aneurysms], *Bull. Mém Soc. Méd. Hôp. Paris* 1901 (XVIII): 1155–1156 and abstract in *Rev Neurol (Paris)* 1902 (X): 459–460; J. Babinski, concerning the minutes, "Signe d'Argyll-Robertson et syphilis" [The Argyll-Robertson sign and syphilis], *Bull. Mém. Soc. Méd. Hôp. Paris* 1902 (XIX): 149–150; J. Babinski, intervention of 30 lines (pp. 277–278), concerning the presentation of Joffroy and Schrameck, "Des rapports de l'irrégularité pupillaire et du signe d'Argyll-Robertson" [On the relationship between pupillary asymmetry and the Argyll-Robertson sign], *Rev Neurol (Paris)* 1902 (X): 275–279; J. Babinski, intervention of 2 lines (p. 1516) concerning the presentation of F. de Lapersonne and A. Cantonnet, "Signe d'Argyll-Robertson unilatéral avec coexistence, du même côté, d'un syndrome oculo-sympathique incomplet" [A unilateral Argyll-Robertson sign coexisting with a partial oculo-sympathetic syndrome], *Rev Neurol (Paris)* 1909 (XVIII): 1515–1517.

[61] J. Babinski, intervention of 14 lines (p. 1304) concerning the presentation of Félix Rose and F. Lemaître, "Deux cas de syringomyélie avec signe d'Argyll Robertson" [Two cases of syringomyelia with an Argyll-Robertson sign], *Rev Neurol (Paris)* 1907 (XV): 1300–1304. Babinski was not therefore convinced by the cases reported particularly by Dejerine of Argyll-Robertson sign observed in interstitial hypertrophic neuritis. J. Babinski, intervention of 13 lines (pp. 536–537) concerning the presentation of J. Dejerine and A. Thomas, "Examen histolologique d'un cas de névrite interstitielle hypertrophique et progressive de l'enfance, suivi d'autopsie" [Histological examination of a case of progressive interstitial hypertrophic neuritis in a child, followed by autopsy], *Rev Neurol (Paris)* 1902 (X): 534–537; J. Babinski, intervention of 6 lines (pp. 559–560) concerning the presentation of P. Marie, "Forme spéciale de névrite interstitielle hypertrophique progressive de l'enfance" [A special form of progressive interstitial hypertrophic neuritis in a child], *Rev Neurol (Paris)* 1906 (XIV): 557–560.

[62] H. Dufour, "Relations existant entre les troubles pupillaires, la syphilis, le tabes et la paralysie générale" [Relationships between pupillary pertubations, syphilis, tabes, and paralysis of the insane], abstract in *Le Progrès Médical* 1902 (XV): 411.

[63] R. Cestan and M. Dupuy-Dutemps, "Sur le signe pupillaire d'Argyll-Robertson" [On the pupillary sign of Argyll-Robertson], abstract in *Le Progrès Médical* 1902 (XVI): 106.

Based on the work of Widal, Sicard, and Ravaut, Babinski became interested in the results of cytodiagnosis of the cerebrospinal fluid in neurological diseases, particularly in terms of its relation with syphilis and the Argyll-Robertson sign.[64] In his thesis in 1903, Albert Déchy made a general review of the problem.[65] After having studied twenty-three cases in the departments of Widal and Babinski, he observed that in patients presenting an Argyll-Robertson sign, one consistently finds a lymphocytosis reaction into the cerebrospinal fluid.[66] The author concluded that this was proof that the Argyll-Robertson sign expresses an organic lesion of the nervous system with meningeal irritation. He considered that lymphocytosis, an objective biological sign, was "pathognomonic of nervous system syphilis" if coexisting with an Argyll-Robertson sign.

Today, there is a widespread agreement that the Argyll-Robertson sign, even if very typical of tertiary nervous syphilis (tabes and general paralysis), may be observed more rarely in diabetes, hereditary hypertrophic neuropathies such as Dejerine-Sottas disease or Thévenard diseases, multiple sclerosis, and sarcoidosis or tumoral vascular lesions of the pons in the vicinity of the periaqueductal area.

In an article typical of his rigorous method, caution, semiological finesse, and profound desire to arrive at an exact diagnosis, Babinski reported in detail certain cases of pseudo-abolition of pupillar reflex to light that were difficult to understand, and he recommended looking for the Argyll-Robertson in a dark room.[67] With his talented observations, Babinski anticipated the

[64] F.Widal, J.A. Sicard. Valeur diagnostic de la ponction lombaire dans les affections nerveuses [Diagnostic value of lumbar puncture in nervous diseases] In Bouchard, "Traité de pathologie générale," T. VI, p. 621e; J. Babinski and J. Nageotte, "Contribution à l'étude du cytodiagnostic du liquide céphalo-rachidien dans les affections nerveuses" [Contribution to the cytodiagnosis study of cerebrospinal fluid in nervous diseases], *Bull. Mém. Soc. Méd. Hôp. Paris* 1901 (XVIII): 537–548, abstract in *Le Progrès Médical* 1901 (XI), 3ème série, No. 23: 358; J. Babinski, "Lymphocytose dans le tabes et la paralysie générale" [Lymphocytosis in tabes and paralysis of the insane], *Rev Neurol (Paris)* 1903 (XI): 341.

[65] A. Déchy, "Le signe d'Argyll Robertson et la cytologie du liquide céphalo-rachidien" [The Argyll-Robertson sign and cerebrospinal fluid cytology], medical thesis, Paris, 1902–3.

[66] In his thesis, presided by Professor Gilbert but inspired by Fernand Widal, Déchy thanks "MM. Babinski, physician at la Pitié, and Nageotte, associate at Bicêtre, for the kindness with which they have received us in their departments and have given advice."

[67] J. Babinski, "De l'influence de l'obscuration sur le réflexe des pupilles à la lumière et de la pseudo-abolition de ce réflexe" [On the influence of forced obscurity on the pupillary reflex to light and the pseudo-abolition of this reflex], *Rev Neurol (Paris)* 1905 (XIII): 1214–1218. Several excerpts from this brilliant paper are given in the appendix at the end of this chapter.

work of William John Adie (1886–1935) when in 1931 the latter described the tonic pupil, attached to a special nonsyphilitic disease, and which corresponds to a benign, idiopathic disturbance of sympathetic origin.

The Babinski Syndromes

In the next set of syndromes, Babinski's name is associated with that of another author, either because of a true collaboration (Babinski-Vaquez, Babinski-Nageotte, Babinski-Froment) or corresponding to the independent description of the same syndrome by two different authors, where it is sometimes difficult to determine who had been the first (Anton-Babinski, Babinski-Frölich).

In the June 1900 issue of the *Revue Neurologique*, Babinski reported the case of a young girl, seventeen years old, who had suffered for years from headaches and seizures.[68] When examining her, he observed a bilateral papilledema, obesity, the infantile aspect of the genital organs, and amenorrhea. There was neither acromegaly nor gigantism. At the postmortem examination, a tumor lying in the sella turcica was found. The histological exam done by Onanoff (who would use it as thesis material) showed "an epithelioma developed from the pituitary gland epithelium of malpighian type...with a myxomatous degeneration of the conjunctive stroma."[69] A year later, in 1901, Alfred Frölich (1871–1953) described a similar case, leading to the name Babinski-Frölich syndrome (Figs. 10-1 and 10-2).[70]

Contrary to the general opinion that associated pupillary troubles in patients presenting an aortic aneurysm of the aorta were related to a

---

[68] J. Babinski, "Tumeur du corps pituitaire sans acromégalie et avec arrêt de développement des organes génitaux" [Tumor of the pituitary gland without acromegaly and absence of development of the genital organs], *Rev Neurol (Paris)* 1900 (VIII): 531–533.

[69] This histological description corresponds to what is known today as craniopharyngioma.

[70] Frölich, a pioneer in neuroendocrinology, was a professor of pharmacology and toxicology at the University of Vienna until 1939, when Nazism obliged him to flee to the United States, where he pursued his work at the Jewish Hospital of Cincinnati. On the syndrome, see A. Frölich, "Ein Fall von Tumor der Hypophysis cerebri ohne Akromegalie" [One case of hypophyseal tumor without acromegaly], *Wiener klinische Rundschau* 1901 (15): 833–836, 906–908. However, Professor E. Herman claimed that the syndrome should be named Pechkranc-Babinski-Frölich syndrome, as Dr. Pechkranc, from the Na Czystem hospital in Warsaw, had described it in German before the other two authors; E. Herman, *Josef Babinski*, Warszawa, 1965 (Panstwowy: Zaklad Wydawnictw Lekarskich), cited in A. Gasecki, "Jozef Babinski wspoltworca wspolcaesnej neurologii i neurochirurgii" [J. Babinski, co-founder of neurology and neurosurgery], *Neuro Neurochi Pol* 1997 (XXXI): 641–656.

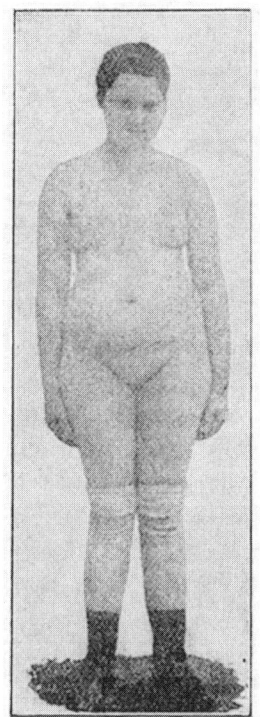 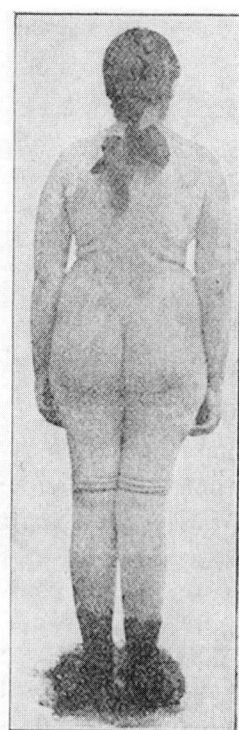

Figure 10-1 Adiposo-genital syndrome, front and back view of the patient. (*Source*: From J. Babinski, "Tumeur du corps pituitaire sans acromégalie et avec arrêt de développement des organes génitaux," [Tumor of the pituitary gland without acromegaly and absence of development of the genital organs] *Rev Neurol [Paris]* 1900 [VIII]: 531–533.)

compression of the sympathetic ganglion or of the small nerves leaving it, Babinski attributed the aortic lesions and the pupillary modifications to the same cause, syphilis.[71] Vaquez proposed naming this association of pupillary abnormalities and aortic lesions Babinski syndrome, but posterity usually refers to it as Babinski-Vaquez syndrome.[72]

---

[71] J. Babinski and A. Charpentier, "De l'abolition des réflexes pupillaires dans ses relations avec la syphilis" [On the relationships between pupillary reflex abolition and syphilis], *Bull. Mém. Soc. Méd. Hôp. Paris* 1901 (XVIII): 502–506, abstract in *Le Progrès Médical* 1901 (XIII): 345; Babinski, "Des troubles pupillaires dans les anévrismes de l'aorte."

[72] H. Vaquez, "Les troubles pupillaires dans les lésions aortiques" [On pupillary perturbations in aortic lesions], *Le Progrès Médical* 1902 (XV): 103. See also *Le Progrès Médical* 1905 (XXI): 7. On Vaquez, see chapter 4.

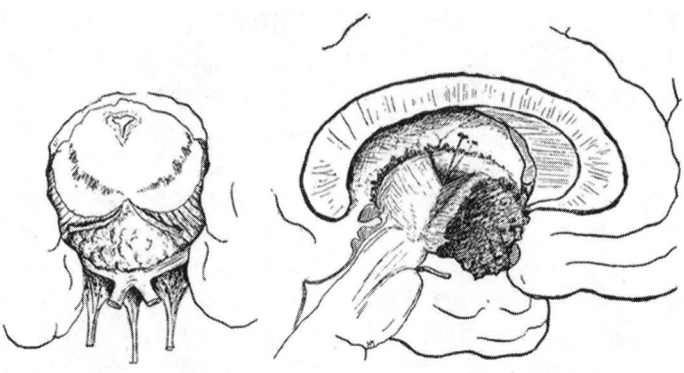

Figure 10-2 Adiposo-genital syndrome, drawing of the macroscopic aspect of the hypophyseal tumor. (*Source*: From J. Babinski, "Tumeur du corps pituitaire sans acromégalie et avec arrêt de développement des organes génitaux," *Rev Neurol [Paris]* 1900 [VIII]: 531–533.)

Observed by the researchers in three cases, Babinski-Nageotte syndrome is caused by unilateral ischaemic lesions of the medulla oblongata from syphilitic origin; it is clinically marked by vertigo, hemiplegia with hemianesthesia on the opposite side of the lesion, and hemiasynergy with lateropulsion and myosis on the homolateral side.[73]

Babinski-Froment syndrome associates trophic and vasomotor disturbances, a diffuse amyotrophy, an exaggeration of the tendinous reflexes, and muscular contraction.[74]

---

[73] J. Babinski and J. Nageotte, "Hémiasynergie, latéropulsion et myosis bulbaires avec hémianesthésie et hémiplégie croisées" [Lesions of the medulla oblongata with hemiasynergy, lateropulsion and myosis with hemianesthesia and hemiplegia on the opposite side], *Rev Neurol (Paris)* 1902 (X): 358–365; J. Babinski and J. Nageotte, "Lésions syphilitiques des centres nerveux. Foyers de ramollissement dans le bulbe. Hémiasynergie, latéropulsion et myosis bulbaires avec hémianesthésie et hémiplégie croisées" [Syphilitic lesions in the central nervous system: ischemic lesions of the medulla oblongata; hemiasynergy, lateropulsion, and myosis with hemianesthesia and hemiplegia on the opposite side], *Nouvelle iconographie de la Salpêtrière* 1902 (XV): 492–512.

[74] http://www.whonamedit.com/synd.cfm/1972.html. Jules Froment (1878–1946) was a neurologist from Lyon. He described a sign of ulnar paralysis: if a patient holds a sheet of paper between his thumb and index finger, the thumb flexes in the case of ulnar paralysis. This sign, named the Froment sign, had in fact been described before in 1904, by Breeman. Froment also identified a hereditary syndrome corresponding to an autosomic dominant olivo-ponto-cerebellar atrophy; J. Froment, P. Bonnet, and A. Colrat, "Hérédodégénérations rétinienne et spino-cérébelleuse; variantes ophtalmoscopiques et neurologique présentées par trois générations successives" [Hereditary degenerative

One of the most quoted of Babinki's papers is a brief communication presented at the Neurological Society of Paris on June 11, 1914.[75] Babinski succinctly described two patients with a left severe hemiplegia, without intellectual or affective disturbances, who "ignored or appeared to ignore" their paralysis. He coined the term *anosognosia* (from the Greek *agnosia*, lack of knowledge; *nosos*, disease) to describe this special "mental disorder," which is a disturbance of cognition. However, Babinski pointed out that some other patients, although aware of their motor deficit, did not seem to be affected by it. He proposed the term *anosodiaphoria* for this disorder (from the Greek *adiaphoria*, indifference, lack of concern), which is more a disturbance of affect. Babinski briefly discussed the possible mechanism of anosognosia. He rejected the possibility that it was an attempt by the patient to maintain self-esteem, and suggested that anosognosia is probably real, linked to sensory deficits. Moreover, in the conclusion of his report, he wrote with remarkable intuition: "it should be pointed out that these patients presented a left hemiplegia. Could anosognosia be linked to lesions of the right hemisphere?"

Unawareness of left hemiplegia is frequently termed, in France, Anton-Babinski syndrome. Gabriel Anton (1858–1933) was an Austrian neurologist and psychiatrist, pupil of Theodor Hermann Meynert (1833–1892), who succeeded Karl Wernicke (1848–1905) in Halle. He described patients with cortical blindness or deafness who were unaware of their deficits.[76] However, in the English-language literature, Anton syndrome usually refers only to visual anosognosia. In the discussion following Babinski's initial report, Gilbert Ballet (1853–1916) said, without quoting Anton's paper: "Unawareness of the deficit, similar to that reported by M. Babinski in hemiplegic patients, is sometimes observed in patients with brain tumors who deny any visual trouble although they present with a total blindness."[77]

Babinski, in 1918, reasserted his view on anosognosia and suggested the role of a cortical lesion resulting in a disorder of attention or memory

---

retinal and spino-cerebellar lesions: opthalmoscopic and neurological variations observed through three successive generations], *J Méd Lyon* 1937: 153–163.

[75] J. Babinski, "Contribution à l'étude des troubles mentaux dans l'hémiplégie organique cérébrale (anosognosie)" [Contribution to the study of mental disorders in organic cerebral hemiplegia (anosognosia)], *Rev Neurol (Paris)* 1914 (XXVII): 845–848.

[76] G. Anton, "Über die Selbstwahrnehmung der Herderkrankungen des Gehirns durch den Kranken bei Rindenblindheit und Rindentaubheit" [On the self-perception of focal brain lesions in patients with cortical blindness or cortical deafness], *Archiv für Psychiatrie und Nervenkrankheiten (Berlin)* 1899 (32): 86–127.

[77] J. Babinski, "Contribution à l'étude des troubles mentaux dans l'hémiplégie organique cérébrale (anosognosie)" [Contribution to the study of mental disorders in organic cerebral hemiplegia (anosognosia)], *Rev Neurol (Paris)* 1914 (XXVII): 845–848.

regarding the limb paralysis. At this session, Pierre Marie pointed out that "such psychic disorder that is reported by M. Babinski" is not restricted to left hemiplegia, but can be observed in other neurological deficits due to a cortical or subcortical lesion large enough to produce sensory deficits. The name Anton-Babinski syndrome should therefore only be applied to a general sense of unawareness of neurological deficits. In a third short presentation, in 1923, Babinski reported the case of a patient from Dr. Lutenbacher who had a reversible left hemiplegia associated with anosognosia.

The term *anosognosia* has been widely accepted by the neurological community to describe unawareness of neurological deficits such as hemianopsia, cortical blindness, linguistic, or memory deficits; the term *anosodiaphoria* is no longer in use.[78] However, the cause of unawareness of neurological deficits remains controversial, involving neurological as well as psychological mechanisms.[79] Psychological mechanisms are usually described under the term *denial*, a translation of the term first used by Freud (*Verleugnung*) to describe the negation of reality that he considered as the main mechanism of psychosis.[80] The term *denial* was later applied by Weinstein and Kahn to a psychological defense mechanism that emerges when subjects undergo major stressful events.[81] Neurological mechanisms stress the major role of the right hemisphere and frontal lobe dysfunction. In the past two decades, several neuropsychological mechanisms have been proposed, based on disturbances of attention, consciousness, self-perception or memory.[82]

Miscellaneous

Babinski published numerous papers covering various fields of neurology, as seen in the contents of the *Oeuvre scientifique* (see appendixes at the end of this chapter). We do not intend to analyze all of them, but will mention some examples showing the extent and diversity of Babinski's medical interests.

[78] G. P. Prigratano and D. J. Schacter, *Awareness of Deficit after Brain Injury: Clinical and Theoretical Issues* (New York: Oxford University Press, 1991).
[79] R. Trouillet, M. C. Gely-Nargeot, and C. Derouesné, "Méconnaissance des deficits dans la maladie d'Alzheimer: une approche multimodale" [Unawareness of deficits in Alzheimer's disease: a multidimensional approach], *Psychologie et Neuropsychiatrie du Vieillissement* 2003 (1): 99–110.
[80] S. Freud, *Abriss der Psychanalysis* [An outline of Psychoanalysis] *Gesamte Werke* 1938 (XVII): 134.
[81] E. A. Weinstein and R. L. Kahn, *Denial of Illness: Symbolic and Physiological Aspects* (Springfield, Ill.: Thomas, 1955).
[82] P. Vuilleumier, "Anosognosia: The Neurology of Beliefs and Uncertainties," *Cortex* 2004 (XL): 9–17.

At the August 1895 meeting in Bordeaux, the Congrès des aliénistes et neurologistes devoted a session to the thyroid gland and Basedow disease. Babinski intervened to report that he had observed in his personal practice two cases associating Basedow disease and myxedema, but that they were rather contradictory to the hypothesis of toxins or antitoxins either in excess or deficiency, according to the pathology. "It is difficult to understand that the same production can be both excessive and deficient."[83]

In a patient showing a left-sided tongue palsy following a traumatic lesion of the hypoglossal nerve, Babinski noted a hemiatrophy of the tongue; he reported that when he "pulled out the tongue, it is deviated toward the paralyzed side. In the resting position the tongue is quite normal; but if the patient opens his mouth with force, the tongue is deviated toward the normal side. The same phenomenon has been observed in the rabbit when the hypoglossal nerve has been cut."[84]

In spasmodic torticollis, Babinski raised argumentation in favor of its organic origin, as opposed to the idea of a psychological etiology (mental torticollis).[85] In his first report, in 1900, after having observed a cutaneous plantar response in extension in his patient, Babinski wondered whether there could be "some irritation of the pyramidal system, the nature of which I cannot specify."[86] It is the same discussion with the patient reported in 1901.[87] The case presented at the Société de neurologie in 1922 was slightly different, as there was an association of spasmodic torticollis, pyramidal signs, and athetosic movements of the lower left limb. On the basis of these cases, Babinski concluded that the organic origin of the torticollis previously

[83] J. Babinski, "Coincidence entre le syndrome de Basedow et certains symptômes du myxoedème" [coincidence between Basedow syndrome and some signs of myxoedema], *Rev. Neurol (Paris)* 1895 (3), No. 16: 484, summary in *Le Progrès Médical* 1895 (II) :88.
[84] J. Babinski, "Hémiatrophie de la langue" [Tongue hemiatrophy], *Bull. Mém. Soc. Méd. Hop. Paris* 1896 (XIII): 671–675, abstract in *Le Progrès Médical* 1896 (IV): 133.
[85] J. Babinski, "Sur un cas d'hémispasme (contribution à l'étude de la pathogénie du torticolis spasmodique) [On a case of hemispasm (contribution to the study of spasmodic torticollis)], *Rev Neurol (Paris)* 1900 (VIII): 142–147; J. Babinski, "Sur le spasme du peaucier du cou" [On the platysma muscle spasm], *Rev Neurol (Paris)* 1901 (IX): 693–696; J. Babinski, "Torticollis mental ou torticolis spasmodique" [Mental or spasmodic torticollis], *Rev Neurol (Paris)* 1904 (XII): 1206; J. Babinski, "Torticolis spasmodique" [Spasmodic torticollis], *Rev Neurol (Paris)* 1921 (37): 367–371; J. Babinski, E. Krebs, and A. Plichet, "Torticollis spasmodique avec lésion du système nerveux central. Exostoses ostéogéniques multiples" [Spasmodic torticollis with lesions in the central nervous system. Multiple osteogenic exostosis], *Rev Neurol (Paris)* 1922 (38): 587–593, abstract in *La Presse Médicale* 1922 (23): 251–252; J. Babinski, "De la section du spinal externe dans le torticolis spasmodique" [On the section of the peripheral spinal accessory nerve in spasmodic torticollis], *Rev Neurol (Paris)* 1924 (I): 452–457.
[86] Babinski, "Sur un cas d'hémispasme."
[87] Babinski, "Sur le spasme du peaucier du cou."

labeled "mental" was indeed confirmed; taking into account the athetosic movements, "one may admit that the causal lesion is situated near the central grey nuclei."[88]

Babinski drew attention in several publications to the value of a cytological exam of cerebrospinal fluid in some forms of meningitis but also in different diseases of the spinal cord and brain.[89] He pointed out that a lesion in the medulla oblongata, without impeding the voluntary motor function, may create vasomotor and thermic disturbances: vasodilatation and hyperthermy on one side of the body or vasoconstriction and hypothermy on the other side. He gave to his observation the name of bulbar thermoasymmetry.[90] Concerning the paper of Huchard and Bergouignan on the "Influence of the aneurysms of the aorta on lung diseases," Babinski "recalled the harmful effect of the section of the vagus nerve on lung condition on the same side in the tubercular rabbit."[91] Observing the case of a patient presenting a persisting tremor of the right upper limb after a concussion secondary to a shell explosion, he discussed the various interpretations that could be given (organic, physiopathic, or neuropathic origin).[92] During World War I, in collaboration with Heitz, he studied arterial obstruction, especially traumatic, and the vasomotor disturbances of reflex or central origin.[93] Later

---

[88] Babinski, Krebs, and Plichet, "Torticolis spasmodique avec lésion du système nerveux central."

[89] See *Le Progrès Médical* 1901 (XXI), 3ème série, No. 23: 358.

[90] J. Babinski, "Thermo-asymétrie d'origine bulbaire" [Thermal sensory disturbance originating in the medulla oblongata], *Rev Neurol (Paris)* 1905 (XIII): 452; *Rev Neurol (Paris)* 1905 (XIII): 568–572; J. Babinski, "Lésion bulbaire unilatérale: thermo-asymétrie et vaso-asymétrie; hémianesthésie alterne à forme syringomyélique" [Unilateral bulbar lesion: thermal sensory and vasomotor disturbances; alternate hemianesthesia, syringomyelia-like], *Rev Neurol (Paris)* 1906 (XIV): 1177–1182.

[91] J. Babinski, Discussion on the presentation of M. Huchard and M. Bergouignan, "Anévrisme latent de la crosse de l'aorte avec pneumonie massive et nécrosante gauche par compression du nerf pneumogastrique gauche" [Latent aortic aneurysm with massive necrosing pneumonia by compression of the left vagus nerve], *Bull. Mém. Soc. Méd. Hôp. Paris* 1901 (XVIII): 1183, abstract in *Le Progrès Médical* 1901 (XIV): 410.

[92] J. Babinski and R. Dubois, "Tremblement du membre supérieur droit consécutif à une commotion par éclatement d'obus" [Tremor of the right superior limb following a commotion by shell explosion], *Journal du Praticien* 1917: CCCXXX.

[93] J. Babinski and J. Heitz, "À propos d'un cas de claudication intermittente par endartérite oblitérante" [On a case of intermittent claudication by obstructive endarteritis], *Rev Neurol (Paris)* 1917 (IV–V): 257–258; J. Babinski and J. Heitz, "Paraplégie organique. Troubles vaso-moteurs au membre supérieur droit, avec méiopragie et sans modification locale des réflexes ostéo-tendineux" [Organic paraplegia. Vasomotor pertubations of the right superior limb without modification of the tendinous reflexes], *Rev Neurol (Paris)* 1917 (IV–V): 258–259; J. Babinski and J. Heitz, "De la claudication intermittente après ligature de l'artère principale du membre inférieur" [On intermittent claudication

in his life, Babinski, who had some reluctance to examine patients with Parkinson disease, wrote a few articles on this disease.[94]

APPENDIXES

J. Babinski, Oeuvre scientifique *(Paris: Masson, 1934)*

Introduction   Babinski is dead; his work is now part of the history of neurology.

Much of this work has already been integrated into the daily life of neurologists, and lives on in their routine examination of patients.

But the other part, written from 1882 to 1932 in notes and sparse papers in journals, corresponding to 288 bibliographical references, was subject to the disadvantages of such dispersion.

That is why Babinski's pupils have collected the essential components of this *Oeuvre scientifique,* not so much to preserve it from being forgotten (an improbable hypothesis) but rather to help all present and future neurologists, for whom otherwise it would become less and less accessible.

In view of the impossibility of issuing a simple reprint of all the original texts, in a chronological order, they have taken the responsibility of making choices and some cuts, with, however, the rule never to add a line to the original Babinski's texts.

Taking the best inspiration they could from the spirit of their mentor, they have largely drawn examples from those he had personally overseen in the *Exposé des travaux scientifiques du Dr Babinsk*i, published in 1913 (Paris, Masson et Cie) and which had yet to be completed.

---

following ligature of the main artery of the inferior limb], *Rev Neurol (Paris)* 1918 (34): 175–178; J. Babinski and J. Heitz, "Les oblitérations artérielles traumatiques. Du rétablissement de la circulation après oblitération de l'artère principale d'un membre" [Traumatic arterial obstructions. Circulatory restoration after obstruction of the main artery of a limb], *Archives des maladies du coeur, des vaisseaux et du sang* 1918 (11): 481; J. Babinski and J. Heitz, "Les altérations artérielles traumatiques. Des troubles que détermine la lésion de l'artère dans les fonctions du membre blessé" [Traumatic arterial lesions and their consequences on the functions of the injured nerve], *Archives des maladies du coeur, des vaisseaux et du sang,* December 1919.

[94] J. Babinski, J. Jarkowski, and A. Plichet, "Kinésie paradoxale. Mutisme parkinsonien" [Paradoxical kinesthesis. Parkinonian mutism], *Rev Neurol (Paris)* 1921 (37): 1266–1270; J. Babinski and A. Charpentier, "Syndrome parkinsonien fruste post-encéphalitique. Troubles respiratoires" [Mild parkinsonian syndrome after encephalitis. Respiratory disturbances], *Rev Neurol (Paris)* 1922 (38): 1369–1377.

However, they thought that they were not obliged to follow too strictly the plan of this *Exposé*; thus, they have placed at the beginning of this book the texts where Babinski has insisted on his method and they have underlined, by according to it a large place, everything by which the neurologist has so decisively contributed to neurological semiology.

The book is divided into several parts, which can themselves be subdivided in function of their importance.

The texts in each section are placed in chronological order and reproduced either in full or by abstracts, beginning with date and reference.

Exceptionally, when too many deletions risks to create gaps or on the contrary when the full text would have been at the origin of prolonged developments, a more condensed version has been inserted, retaining the notice that Babinski himself has used in his *Exposé*, the reference always being mentioned.

Babinski said also in the foreword to the *Exposé*: "Some phenomena that I have described could be placed in different subdivisions; I always tried to put them in the chapter that seemed the most appropriate, to avoid repetition."

We have applied the same principle to distribute the texts in the present volume, the general outline being as follows: the method in semiology; the semiology, brain tumors, non pyramidal diseases, cerebellar, medulla oblongata and labyrinthic pathology; paraplegies and spinal cord affections, peripheral nerves and muscular diseases, hysteria and pithiatism, physiopathic disturbances, therapeutics."

Table of contents

First part: The semiological method

Introduction to the semiology of the nervous system

About objective symptoms which cannot be produced voluntarily and their importance in forensic medicine

Some considerations on clinical questioning and subjective symptoms

Second part: Semiology

Fundamentals in organic semiology

About the cutaneous plantar reflex in some organic central nervous system diseases

The toe phenomenon and its semiological significance

About the toes abduction

Tendinous and bone reflexes

Organic brachial monoplegia

Active and passive movements

Differential diagnosis between organic and hysterical hemiplegias

Contribution to the study of mental disorders in cerebral organic hemiplegia (Anosognosia)

Defense reflexes. Clinical study

Defense reflexes

About the conjugate movements

Modifications of the cutaneous reflexes under the influence of compression by Esmarch bandage

About hyperreflectivity in hyperalgesia

Reappearance, provoked and transitory, of voluntary motion in paraplegia

Ocular semiology

About the influence of forced obscurity on the pupillary light reflex and of the pseudo-abolition of this reflex

Pupillary modifications in aortic aneurysm of this reflex

Cerebellar semiology

Cerebellar asynergy

Symptoms of cerebellar diseases and their significance

Vestibular semiology

Electrology

About striate muscle contractility after death

Slowness of the faradic shock

Slowness of the tendinous-reflex shock

Advanced fusion of the faradic shocks

Third part: Brain compression and tumors

Pituitary gland tumors without acromegaly and absence of genital organs development

Papilledema cured by cranial trepanation

Two cases of temporal lobe tumors

About decompressive craniectomy

Fourth part: Nonpyramidal diseases

On a case of hemispasm

On neck spasm

Spasmodic torticollis associated with a central nervous lesion

On degeneration and regeneration of the sternocleidomastoid muscle after section of the spinal accessory nerve

On section of the spinal accessory nerve in spasmodic torticollis

On the combined flexion of thigh and trunk in Sydenham chorea

Paradoxical kinesia. Parkinsonian mutism

Mild parkinsonian syndrome, post-encephalitis. Respiratory disorders

Fifth part: Cerebellar, bulbar, and labyrinthic disorders

Cerebellar disorders

First case

Cerebellar syndrome

Hemiasynergy

Lateropulsion and myosis with crossed hemianesthesia and hemiplegia from bulbar origin

Bulbar disorder

Asymetric thermoanesthesia from bulbar origin

Labyrinthic disorders

Sixth part: Paraplegias—Spinal cord disorders

Multiple sclerosis—Paraplegia

Multiple sclerosis

A case of paraplegia secondary to an organic lesion without degeneration of the pyramidal system

On the paralysis by compression of the pyramidal system without secondary degeneration

Organic spasmodic paraplegia with flexion spasm and involuntary muscular contractions

Sympathetic and spinal hemisyndrome of the irritative type, with an intermittent and rhythmic evolution

Tabes and pseudo-tabes

On the Achilles reflex in tabes

On a form of pseudo-tabes

On visual field and central vision in tabetic atrophy of the optic nerves

Spinal cord compressions

Brown-Séquard syndrome from knife stabbing

Remarks on the persistence of radicular sensitive areas in spinal paraplegias with anaesthesia

On the localization of spinal cord compressions. How to be precise in their topography and determine their inferior level by the study of defense reflexes

Tumor of the meninges. Crural paraplegia by compression of the cord; ablation of the tumor; recovery

Hypertrophic cervical meningitis Contribution on the study of anesthesia in thoracic cord compressions

Some documents in relation to spinal cord compression

Crural paraplegia by an epidural tumor. Operation and recovery

Hypertonic crural monoplegia with anaesthesia on the same side but without pyramidal signs: Sacro-lumbar intramedullary tumor

About the diagnosis of spinal cord compression

Fibrinous meningitis with hemorrhage. Spasmodic paraplegia. Lumbar punctures. Mercury treatment. Recovery

Spinal dorsal compression

Seventh part: Nerve disorders

On neuritis

Peripheric facial hemispasm

Eighth part: Muscular disorders

Progressive myopathy: about the correlation of the predisposition of some muscles to myopathy and the rapidity of growth

On idiomuscular excitability and the tendinous reflexes in progressive primitive myopathy

Ninth part: Hysteria—Pithiatism

Definition of hysteria

My conception of hysteria and hypnotism

Pulling apart traditional hysteria

Pithiatism

On hypnotism in therapeutic and forensic medicine

Hysteria and pithiatism

Hysteria during the war

Hysteria—pithiatism in war neurology

Tenth part: Physiopathic disorders

Nervous disturbances of reflex origin

Eleventh part: Therapeutics

About mercury treatment in the tabetic sclerosis of the optic nerves

Therapeutic results of lumbar puncture in optic neuritis of intracranial origin

Treatment of ear disorders especially of auricular vertigo by lumbar puncture

On the treatment of extramedullary tumors

On the treatment of facial neuralgia by high intensity voltaic currents

Generalized spasm by compression of the cervical cord, greatly improved by X-ray therapy

About X-ray therapy in spasmodic spinal paralysis

Radiotherapy in sciatica intensity voltaic currents

An example of Babinski's rigor, prudence, and method

J. Babinski, "De l'influence de l'obscuration sur le réflexe des pupilles à la lumière et de la pseudo-abolition de ce réflexe" [On the influence of forced obscurity on the pupillary reflex to light and on the pseudo-abolition of this reflex], *Rev Neurol (Paris)*, 1905 (XIII): 1214–1218. [Extracts from *Œuvre scientifique*]

> Because the study of papillary disorders is of fundamental importance, I think that one cannot be too precise in determining the conditions which may interfere with the state of the pupil...
> Examining a young lady with epilepsy,... I was struck by the fact that her pupils, immediately explored, as I usually do, after her entrance to a dark room, were dilated without any reaction to light. But by doing a new examination a few minutes after the first, the patient during this time having remained in the dark, I noticed that the light excitation then provoked a weak but clear pupillary contraction.
> These two successive exams were giving apparently contradictory results, and I thought it would be interesting to know the reason for this difference. To that end, during about ten consecutive days I made observations and experiments that provided information, at least partially. I must say firstly that in this patient, the pupillar contractility presented daily fluctuations, the causes of which I don't really know, but I am quite sure to have determined at least one of them. I can thus state that light has a tendency to exhaust the reflex, and on the contrary that darkness reinforces it. For this reason, when the exam is performed in a dark room, the reflex, weak or absent when the patient penetrates the room, becomes stronger when the patient has stayed in

the dark for some time. I shall also call attention to the fact that the complete exhaustion of the reflex appears sometimes after two or three excitations followed again by a pupillary reaction; this is why the reflex is generally weaker on clear days than on dark ones....

So we have here a patient whose reflex to light is weak, eventually absent, when it is observed in the conditions which have been specified.... Whatever it is, we are in the presence of an abnormal state, a perturbation which may be named (only to set the ideas) a *pseudo-abolition of the light reflex.* I shall say to complete the description of this problem that the patient's pupils react to convergence and accommodation.... If you are not aware of the possibility of confusing pseudo-abolition with the true abolition of the light reflex, there is a risk of making a serious practical error. I am persuaded that sometimes one may be confused; this could be an explanation for the so-called successive disappearance and reappearance of the Argyll-Robertson sign noted by some observers; I always cast doubt on it, without however categorically denying them. But if attention is drawn to this cause of error, it is easy to avoid it. In fact, when we are in presence of a true abolition of the pupillary reflex to light, the trouble persists, no matter what the intensity of the light source; it persists despite the use of obscurity, whatever its prolongation, and the consensual reflex is also abolished.

The study of these reported facts led me to wonder if by artificially creating obscurity one would not be able to reinforce the reflex to light, even in the normal state. Experiments conducted on about twenty persons without any ocular disturbance nor organic disease of the central nervous system gave me a clearly positive result in the majority of cases; therefore, this is a physiological phenomenon easy to verify. In order to avoid any confusion, even if I repeat what I have said before, I am going to indicate precisely the conditions which allow to objective this fact. The patient, after having had an eye completely closed, must stay, during half an hour, in a well-lit room, in daylight; then he has to go to a dark room, and by a lateral lighting with a candle of the eye that has remained open, one may determine firstly the degree of pupil dilatation as the intensity of his reflex to light; when this has been accomplished, this eye is closed while the covering of the other one is removed; the pupil is immediately examined with the same technique as before. This comparison leads to the conclusion that, if we do not take into account the dilatation created by obscurity and observed only temporarily when the eye is uncovered, the pupil of the covered eye is smaller than the other, due obviously to the fact that light is more active on the reflex center. Furthermore, the pupillary reflex movements observed by the usual technique are generally quicker on that side; a pupillary asymmetry is thus artificially created, more or less pronounced according to the brightness of the day of the experiment and which persists over a variable time; generally, when the two eyes are opened, equilibrium is rapidly established.

It is necessary to recall that the fact of creating obscurity which reinforces the light reflex leads also to regeneration of purple in the retina (see on that subject the work of Parinaud, *La Vision*). Given that, one may ask if there is not between these two phenomena a relationship of cause and effect. It may be because the retina, subjected to obscurity has acquired fluorescent properties that the reflex to light becomes stronger. If such were the case, we should admit that erythropsin plays an important role in the production of this reflex. In defense of this still hypothetical theory, I shall mention the following facts: I have noticed that, in the wood owl, the retina of which contains a lot of purple, the reflex to light is especially vivid, but on the contrary in the hen whose retina is deprived of erythropsin, this reflex is weak; to support this concept, one may also put forward the pupil status in hemeralopia, a disease related to a purple alteration (Parinaud) and where the reflex to light is weak or absent.

From these observations and experiments, I can draw the following conclusions:

1. Creating obscurity reinforces the pupillar reflex to light and allows one to create artificially, in a normal subject, a transitory difference in pupil size.
2. There is a pupillary disturbance, of still undetermined origin, which may be called *pseudo-abolition of the reflex to light*, which can be confusing, but which, by the use of an intensive lightening or with a prior exposition to obscurity, and by the conservation of the consensual reflex, may be distinguished from the true absence of the reflex to light, caused by a chronic syphilitic meningitis.

··· *eleven* ···

The Reflexes and the Sign*

When Babinski prepared his candidacy for the *agrégation* in January 1892, the bibliographical notes on his clinical research did not reflect any particular interest in cutaneous or tendon reflexes. Only a few years later did the subject of reflexes become his predominant focus, a leitmotiv that emerged as a unifying thread of his work: "find objective signs that allow the distinction between organic neurological disorders and those of a functional or hysteric origin, separating with certitude organic and functional problems."[1]

The Babinski Sign

Cutaneous reflexes were known before the discovery of what is now called the Babinski sign.[2] In his 1886 book, the well-known British neurologist Sir William Richard Gowers mentioned two as being the most important: the plantar reflex and the cremasteric and abdominal cutaneous reflex (suppressed on the paralyzed side of an organic hemiplegia).[3] Grigorii Ivanovich

---

* This chapter was written with the collaboration of Philippe Ricou, MD.
[1] G. Schaltenbrand, Société Française de Neurologie, meeting of June 2, 1958, *Rev Neurol (Paris)* 1958 (98): 640–668.
[2] R. Wartemberg, *Les réflexes dans l'examen neurologique* [Reflexes in neurological examinations] (Paris: J. B. Baillière, 1954); C. G. Goetz, "History of the extensor plantar response: Babinski and Chaddock signs," *Seminars in Neurology* 2002 (22): 391–398.
[3] W. R. Gowers, *A Manual of Diseases of the Nervous System*, vol. I: *Diseases of the Spinal Cord and Nerves* (London: J. & A. Churchill, 1886); Anton Julius Friedrich Rosenbach

Rossolimo (1860–1928) described in 1891 the anal reflex.⁴ But the inevitable search for precursors here, as in any retrospective study, is both futile and of no particular interest, because even if the extension of the big toe had already been observed within the context of the plantar reflex, no special significance had been attached to it.⁵ For example, Adolph Strümpell (1853–1925) did not mention this possibility in the chapter of his 1885 internal pathology treatise that dealt with cutaneous and tendon reflexes.⁶

At the February 22, 1896, meeting of the Société de Biologie, Babinski, who was an honorary member of the society, submitted a paper, the text of which was published later and consisted of twenty-eight lines:

> I have observed in a certain number of cases of hemiplegia or crural monoplegia caused by organic lesion of the central nervous system a modification in the plantar reflex, which I can describe in a few words.
>
> On the normal side, a pinprick of the plantar foot causes, as is usual, a flexion of the thigh toward the pelvis, of the leg toward the thigh, of the foot toward the leg, and of the toes toward the metatarsus. On the paralyzed side, the same stimulation causes, as is usual in the normal situation, a flexion of the thigh toward the pelvis, of the leg toward the thigh, and of the foot toward the leg, but the toes, instead of going into flexion, perform a movement of extension on the metatarsus.
>
> I have had the opportunity to observe this disorder in cases of recent hemiplegia, dating back only a few days, as well in spasmodic hemiplegias lasting for several months; I have observed it in patients unable to voluntarily move their toes, but also in those who were able to perform voluntary movements of their toes. I must add, however, that this perturbation is not constant.
>
> I have also observed in several cases of crural paraplegia of organic origin an extension movement of the toes after pinprick of the plantar foot, but

(1842–1923), *Archives fur Psychiatrie. und Nervenkr*, VI, 845—*Centralbl. f. Nerv.* II, p. 193, and Moell (D. Arch. f. klin. Med., XXII, 279.), cited in J. Grasset, *Traité pratique des Maladies du système Nerveux* [Practical treatise of diseases of the nervous system], 2nd ed. (Paris: Adrien Delahaye & Lecrosnier, 1881).

⁴ G. I. Rossolimo, "Der Analreflex, seine Physiologie und Pathologie" [Physiology and pathology of anal reflex], *Neurologisches Centralblatt* 1891 (4): 257–259.

⁵ A. Strümpell, "Symptomenbild der Amyotrophischen Lateral Sclerose, Combinirte Erkrankung der Pyramidenbahnen und gewisser Fasersysteme in den Hintersträngen" [Signs of amyotrophic lateral sclerosis with combined lesions of pyramidal tract and posterior columns], *Archives fur Psychiat* 1880 (11): 32–36, cited in Goetz, "History of the extensor plantar response"; E. Remak, "Zur localisation der spinalen Hautreflexe des Unter extremitäten" [On localization of lower limbs cutaneous reflexes], *Neurologisches Centralblat* 1893 (12): 506–512, analyzed in *Rev Neurol (Paris)* 1893 (I): 690; J. Van Gijn, "Remak and the plantar response," *Lancet* 1996 (348): 338–339.

⁶ Ernst Adolf Gustav Gottfried von Strümpell was a German neurologist, professor at Leipzig, and known in France particularly for his description of family paraplegia or Strumpell-Lorrain disease. See his *Traité de pathologie interne* [Treatise on internal pathology], vol. II, part 1, *Maladies du système nerveux* [Diseases of the nervous system] (Paris: Librairie F. Savy, 1885), 59–65.

because in this case there is no possible comparison between the two sides, the conclusion from the demonstration is less obvious.

In summary, the reflex movement caused by the pinprick of the plantar foot in crural paralysis related to a central nervous disorder shows a modification not only in its intensity, which is known, but also in its characteristics.

This short historical text was the first report on the toe phenomenon. It is a model of style and concision, allowing Sir Francis Walshe to confide: "Ah! If only young people today could do us the favor of stating their observations and their ideas in such clear a language and with such an economy of words (Fig. 11-1)."[7]

Babinski demonstrated in this article that when the plantar foot is pinpricked in a hemiplegic patient, the big toe on the paralyzed side, instead of going into flexion, performs an extension movement toward the metatarsus, indicating an organic lesion of the central nervous system. After a more complete description at the neurological meeting in Brussels in 1897, Babinski published another article on the phenomenon in 1898:

> This sign seems to correspond to a lesion of the pyramidal system and may be found in diffuse meningoencephalitis, partial epilepsy, cerebrospinal meningitis, strychnine poisoning, spasmodic spinal paraplegia, etc. This sign is often associated with a hyperreflectivity and with spinal epilepsy; it may occur before these modifications.[8]

Both Babinski himself and his pupils would come back frequently to his sign and its diagnostic value.[9] He also indicated that in some normal individuals, the big toe may remain immobile when the plantar foot is stimulated, but an extension is never observed.

Babinski insisted, in his usual manner, on the importance of technique in the detection of the sign. To relax the leg and foot muscles, he recommended

---

[7] F. Walshe, "Où situer Babinski dans la neurologie moderne" [What is the place of Babinski in modern neurology], *Rev Neurol (Paris)* 1958 (98): 632–636.

[8] *Le Progrès Médical* 1898 (VIII), No. 27: 7.

[9] Among several references, we may cite J. Babinski, "Du 'phénomène des orteils' dans l'épilepsie" [On the toes phenomenon in epilepsy], *Rev Neurol (Paris)* 1899 (VII): 512–513; J. Babinski, "Sur les scléroses combinées" [On subacute combined degeneration], *Journal de Neurologie* 1900 (V): 417–418; J. Babinski, "Sur la transformation du régime des réflexes cutanés dans les affections du système pyramidal" [On the modifications of cutaneous reflexes in pyramidal system diseases], *Rev Neurol (Paris)* 1904 (XII): 58–62; J. Babinski, interventions of 4 lines (p. 95) and of 20 lines (p. 96), concerning the paper "Sur la transformation du régime des réflexes cutanés dans les affections du système pyramidal," *Rev Neurol (Paris)* 1904 (XII): 94–96; G. Marinesco, "Étude sur le phénomène des orteils (signe de Babinski)" [Study on the toes phenomenon (Babinski sign)], *Rev Neurol (Paris)* 1903 (XI): 489–502.

asking the patient to close his eyes and not informing him of the maneuver before it was done. The leg is supported with one hand after a light flexion on the thigh, while the other hand tickles or pinpricks the plantar foot. He laid out the data that allows a distinction between the normal reflex movement (with a flexion of the big toe), the pathological one (with an extension), and voluntary movement caused by too strong a stimulation, a hysterical phenomenon, or an attempt at malingering. The toe phenomenon is the sign

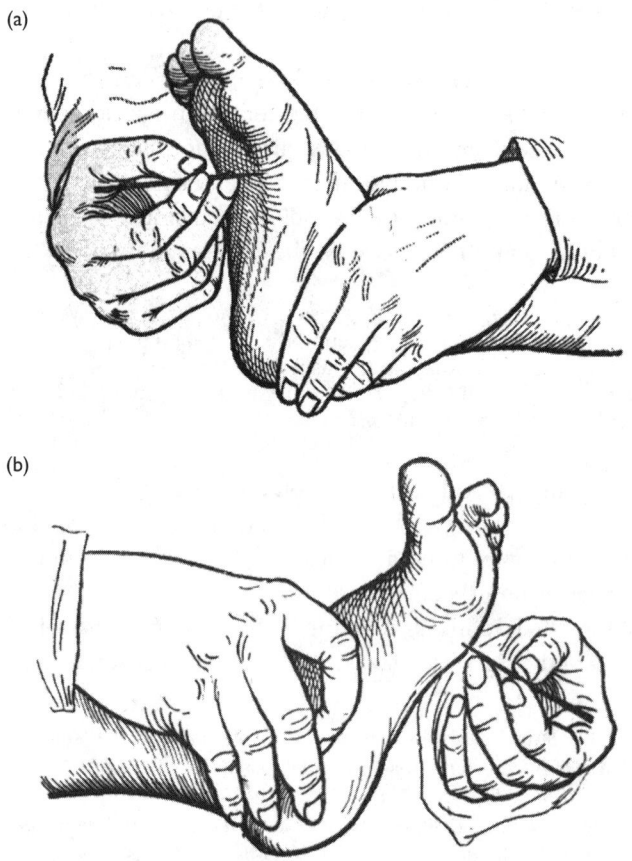

Figure 11-1 Babinski's sign. (a) Normal plantar reflex. (b) Toe phenomenon. (c) "Small Cowper Madonna" (c. 1505, oil on panel) painted by Raphael (1483–1520). Note the extension of the child's big toe while his mother is touching the sole of his foot. (*Sources*: [a and b] From J. Babinski and J. Froment, *Hystérie-pithiatisme et troubles nerveux d'ordre réflexe en neurologie de guerre* [Paris: Masson et Cie, 1917]. [c] Widener Collection, National Gallery of Art, Washington, D.C.)

(c)

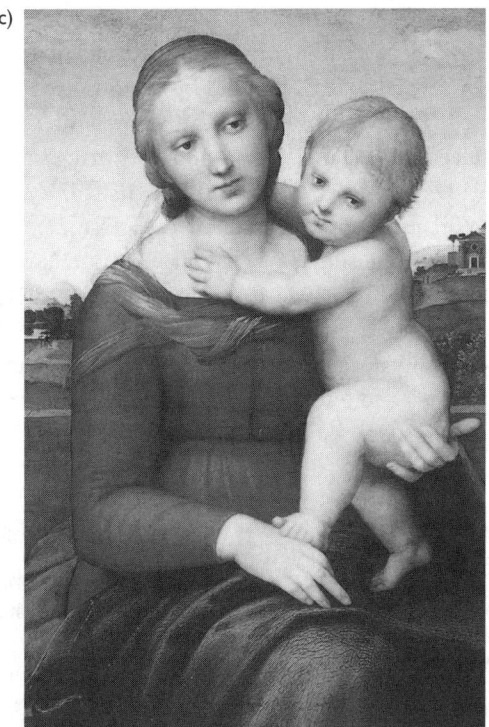

Figure 11-1 Continued.

of a dysfunction in the pyramidal tract, but its intensity is not proportional to that of the paralysis. Its semeiological value is even more important when the tendinous reflexes are normal.

Babinski also drew attention to the fact that before a baby starts to walk, when development of the pyramidal system is not complete, one may observe an extension of the big toe after tickling the plantar foot.[10] As Neelon and Harvey note, this gave rise to many reports by Babinski's associates and later by other authors.[11] The usefulness as a clinical sign of the big toe extension in

---

[10] At birth, extension of the big toe is a rule; it disappears in general around the age of five to six months, and after three years, flexion is the rule. A. Leri, "Le réflexe des orteils chez les enfants (valeur diagnostique et pronostique de l'extension et de la flexion des orteils)" [The toes reflex in childhood (diagnostic and prognostic value of the toes extension and flexion)], *Rev Neurol (Paris)* 1903 (XI): 689–692.

[11] F. A. Neelon and E. N. Harvey, "The Babinski sign," *New England Journal of Medicine* 1999 (340): 196. For a report by one of Babinski's students, see, for example, S. Rosenblum, *Du développement du système nerveux au cours de la première enfance*.

the newborn or young baby remains limited, since such a flexion may be seen in normal subjects.[12] Some authors have pointed out that the big toe extension was visible in several infants painted by famous artists of the past, such as Sandro Botticelli (1445–1510), Raphael (the byname of Raffaello Sanzio, 1483–1520), Leonardo da Vinci (1503–1507), Correggio (the byname of Antonio Allegri, 1494–1534), or Peter Paul Rubens (1577–1640).[13] (Fig. 11-1c)

There are several different accounts of the circumstances surrounding Babinski's discovery of the sign. Robert Wartenberg (1887–1956) quoted the account Babinski provided in 1926 in response to a question: at the time of his first description, neurologists were mainly concerned with the distinction between organic and hysteric hemiplegia, and for this reason Babinski had checked all the reflexes and found that in organic hemiplegia the response to plantar stimulation was an extension and not a flexion.[14]

Barré's version, quoted by Fauconnet, was more poetic:

> Babinski, when passing through the women's ward at La Pitié, was accustomed, in a nice and affectionate gesture, to pat the plantar foot of his patients, who, during the summer months, partially removed their bedclothes. One of them, a hysteric, attracted the attention of the master by the fact that she was not able to produce an extension of her big toe, in contrast to the patient next to her, who had a spinal cord compression.[15]

Despite some immediate but ephemeral reservations, the toe phenomenon was rapidly recognized and adopted by neurologists all over the world.[16] It

---

Contribution à l'étude des syncinésies, des réflexes tendineux et cutanés et des réflexes de défense [Development of the nervous system during early childhood. Contribution to a study of syncinesis, tendon, cutaneous and defense reflexes] (Paris: Le François, 1915). For reports by other authors, see, for instance, C. Juarros, "Le signe de Babinski chez les nouveau-nés" [The Babinski sign in the newborn], *Rev Neurol (Paris)* 1930 (II): 695–70; G. D. Kumhar, T. Dua, and P. Gupta, "Plantar response in infancy," *European Journal of Paediatric Neurology* 2002 (6): 321–325; Y. T. Ng and J. B. Bodensteiner, "The extensor plantar response in neonates is not the same as the Babinski sign," *Pediatric Neurology* 2005 (32): 218–219.

[12] E. D. Ross, J. Velez-Borras, and N. P. Rosman, "The significance of the Babinski sign in the newborn—a reappraisal," *Pediatrics* 1976 (57): 13–15.

[13] T. E. Cone Jr. and S. Khoshbin, "Botticelli demonstrates the Babinski reflex more than 400 years before Babinski; pediatrics in art," *American Journal of Diseases of Children* 1978 (132): 188; E. W. Massey and L. Sanders, "Babinski's sign in medieval, Renaissance, and baroque art," *Archives of Neurology* 1989 (46): 85–88; comment in *Archives of Neurology* 1989 (46): 1046, 1047; 1990 (47): 253.

[14] R. Wartenberg, "The Babinski reflex after fifty years," *JAMA* 1947 (135): 763–767.

[15] E. Fauconnet, "Joseph Babinski et la naissance de la neurochirurgie française" [Joseph Babinski and the birth of French neurosurgery], thèse de doctorat en médecine, Faculté de médecine de Rennes, 1985.

[16] M. Vires and A. Calmettes. "Recherches sur le phénomène des orteils (signe de Babinski)" [Research on the toes phenomenon (Babinski sign)], *Rev Neurol (Paris)* 1900

became usual to call it the "Babinski sign." Pierre Marie noted that "since the day he made it known, the reflex described as the 'toe phenomenon' was quite universally and rightly called the 'Babinski reflex.'"[17] As early as 1898, Van Gehuchten informed the Belgian neurological community of the existence of the sign.[18] In 1899, British physicians were told of the sign, its significance, and its great semiological interest through an article by the London physician James Stansfield Collier (1870–1919), published in *Brain*.[19] In the first edition, dated 1901, of his text on the semiology of the nervous system, Dejerine devoted about ten lines to the toe phenomenon and discussed its presence or absence in hysteric hemiplegias.[20] His conclusion, however, left room for doubt: "The question remains a subject of discussion; the toe phenomenon is, like other clinical signs, a mark of presumption, but not of an absolute certainty, of an alteration of the pyramidal system." In 1903, the great Polish neurologist Samuel Vulfovitsj Goldflam (1852–1932) took up the cause of the Babinski reflex.[21]

In 1913, referring to the toe phenomenon, Babinski wrote, "It has become usual, in France as well as in foreign countries, to call it 'the Babinski sign.'"[22] He also quoted thirty-five references in French and foreign papers that confirmed the diagnostic value of his sign. He ended his listing as of 1903, because "since that date, the value of the toe phenomenon has been unanimously accepted; there are no clinical observations in relation to a

(VIII): 535–553; H. Oppenheim, discussion, p. 612, of W. Koenig, "Über die bei Reizung der Fussohle zu beobachtenden Reflexerscheinungen mit besonderer Berücksichtigung der Zehenreflexe bei den verschiedenen Formen der cerebralen Kinderlähmung" [On reflex signs observed by plantar foot stimulation especially of the toes reflex in different forms of infantile cerebral palsy], *Neurologisches Centralblatt* 1899 (18): 610–613.

[17] P. Marie, discussion in J. Babinski, "Sur le prétendu réflexe antagoniste de Schaefer" [On the so-called antagonist reflex of Schaefer], *Rev Neurol (Paris)* 1900 (VIII): 52–53.

[18] A. Van Gehuchten, "Le phénomène des orteils" [The toes phenomenon], *Journal de Neurologie* 1898 (III): 153–155; A. Van Gehuchten, "À propos du phénomène des orteils" [Concerning the toes phenomenon], *Journal de Neurologie* 1898 (III): 284–286.

[19] J. S. Collier, "An investigation upon the plantar reflex, with reference to the significance of its variations under pathological conditions, including an inquiry into the etiology of acquired pes cavus," *Brain* 1899 (23): 71–99. See also J. Fulton, "Joseph François Félix Babinski 1857–1932," *Archives of Neurology and Psychiatry* 1933 (29): 168–174.

[20] J. Dejerine, "Sémiologie des affections du système nerveux" [Semiology of diseases of the nervous system], in C. Bouchard, ed., *Traité de pathologie générale* (Paris: Masson, 1901), 5:359–1168.

[21] S. Goldflam, "Zur Lehre von den Hautreflexen an den Unterextremitäten (insbesondere des Babinskischen Reflexes)" [Contribution to the study of cutaneous reflexes of the inferior limb (particularly of the Babinski reflex)], *Neurologisches Centralblatt* 1903 (23): 1119 and 1903 (24): 1137.

[22] J. Babinski, *Exposé des travaux scientifiques du Dr J. Babinski* [Presentation of scientific papers of Dr. J. Babinski] (Paris: Masson et Cie, 1913), 38.

neurological pathology where its presence or absence has not been specifically mentioned."[23]

Quite rightly, Fulton recalled that it is because of the sign that Babinski's name is "frequently on the lips of every student of medicine in every corner of the globe."[24] Sir Francis Walshe added: "Each time that I encounter it, I always find the same appeal in the toe phenomenon."[25].

In 1903, seven years after his first publication on the toe phenomenon, Babinski described the toes abduction sign, which he considered "a complement to the big toe sign": it consists of a more or less marked abduction of one or several toes after plantar foot stimulation. Babinski indicated that this phenomenon is frequently observed in disorders of the pyramidal system but rarely found in normal subjects. He also noted that in the infant, where the formation of the pyramidal system is not fully developed, tickling of the plantar foot results in a big toe extension generally associated with toe abduction. His cautious conclusion was that the toe abduction "constituted a sign of probability in favor of the diagnosis of a perturbation of the pyramidal system, a sign that may be valuable in some dubious cases."[26]

In a second note appearing a few months later, Babinski completed the description of the toes abduction reflex by discussing the associated abduction observed, for example, during the flexion-extension movements of the trunk toward the pelvis.[27] He assigned the same importance to these two varieties of toe abduction, considering that they are "quite surely" proof of a pyramidal system disturbance. He thought that the name "fan sign," proposed by Dupré, was "a vivid expression that may be kept in mind"; he did add, though, that it "could be preferable to be satisfied with the term 'toe abduction,' to which, depending upon the circumstances, may be added the words 'reflex-associated' or 'reflex' and 'associated.' "[28]

Today no one questions that the Babinski sign is a reliable indication of a pyramidal disorder. There are, however, some exceptions, as can be seen in the following examples, where the sign may be observed quite apart from any lesion of the cerebrospinal tract or even from any neurological disorder.[29]

---

[23] Ibid., 50–52.

[24] J. F. Fulton, "Science in the clinic as exemplified by the life and work of Joseph Babinski," *Journal of Nervous and Mental Diseases* 1933 (77): 121–133.

[25] Walshe, "Où situer Babinski dans la neurologie moderne."

[26] J. Babinski, "De l'abduction des orteils" [On the toes abduction], *Rev Neurol (Paris)* 1903 (XI): 728–729.

[27] J. Babinski, "De l'abduction des orteils (signe de l'éventail)" [On the toes abduction (fan sign)], *Rev Neurol (Paris)* 1903 (XI): 1205–1206.

[28] Ibid.

[29] Babinski himself pointed out that the Babinski sign is not uncommon during infantile paralysis (poliomyelitis), but that in this disease, lesions may not be limited to the

Typical cases include scopolamine or strychnine poisoning, chloroform narcosis, hypoglycemia, coma, the apnea phase of Cheyne-Stokes respiration, or cardiac insufficiency.[30] Exceptionally, the Babinski sign may be absent in authentic dysfunctions of the pyramidal tract.

It is also recognized that cold may influence the appearance of the sign. Consequently, it is a good rule to warm up the feet before looking for the sign.[31] Ischemia has the same impact as cold: Babinski showed that with the Esmarch compressive bandage, the toe sign disappeared.[32] Boveri remarked that the sign may appear or disappear depending on the patient's position in bed.[33] Finally, in some cases, the act of testing for the plantar reflex on one side may be responsible for a contralateral response of the opposite big toe: this "crossed reflex" is a possibility that Babinski had already pointed out.[34]

Works dedicated to the Babinski sign and particularly to its physiology and physiopathology are so extensive that it is out of the question to mention

---

anterior horns of the spinal cord and could reach the lateral columns, where the pyramidal tracts are located. Babinski, *Exposé des travaux scientifiques*. See also A. Rouquier and D. Couretas, "Le signe de Babinski en dehors des lésions pyramidales, extension de l'orteil chez deux malades atteints de funiculite lombo-sacrée avec amyotrophie globale des fléchisseurs et des extenseurs des orteils et du pied, origine périphérique de ce signe," [Babinski sign apart from the pyramidal lesions: toe extension in two patients presenting a lumbo-sacral funiculitis with a global amyotrophy of the toes flexor and extensor muscles; peripheral origin of the sign], *Rev Neurol (Paris)* 1926 (2): 167–174; S. P. Kumar, "The Babinski sign. A critical review," *Journal of the Association of Physicians of India* 2003 (51): 53–57.

[30] J. Lhermitte and Y. Dupont, "Le signe de Babinski à paroxysmes rythmés par l'insuffisance cardiaque" [Paroxysmal rhythmic Babinski sign with cardiac insufficiency], Société de Biologie, meeting of June 29, 1929, abstract in *Rev Neurol (Paris)* 1929 (II): 357; J. Lhermitte and Y. Dupont, "Le signe de Babinski à évolution rythmée par l'insuffisance cardiaque" [Paroxysmal rhythmic Babinski sign with cardiac insufficiency], *Rev Neurol (Paris)* 1929 (II): 92–96.

[31] D. Noïca and A. Radovici, "Abolition du signe de Babinski par le froid et sa réapparition par la chaleur" [Abolition of the Babinski sign with cold and reappearance by heat], *Rev Neurol (Paris)* 1919 (12): 891–893.

[32] J. Babinski, "Modification des réflexes cutanés sous l'influence de la compression par la bande d'Esmarch" [Modification of the cutaneous reflexes under compression by Esmarch bandage], *Rev Neurol (Paris)* 1911 (XXII): 651–652.

[33] P. Boveri, "Sur la présence ou disparition du phénomène de Babinski suivant la position du malade" [On the presence or absence of the Babinski phenomenon according to the patient's position], *Rev Neurol (Paris)* 1916 (7): 143–144.

[34] J. C. Gautier, E. Pierrot-Desseilligny, C. Morin, et al., "Extension croisée du premier orteil. Étude clinique et neurophysiologique" [Cross-extension of the big toe. Clinical and neurophysiological study], *Rev Neurol (Paris)* 1980 (136): 521–529; J. Babinski, "Du phénomène des orteils et de sa valeur sémiologique" [On the toes phenomenon and its semiological value], *Semaine Médicale* 1898 (18): 321–322.

them all here.[35] The interested reader may refer to Tournay's impressive report,[36] Roger's papers,[37] Fulton's book,[38] and Walshe's article,[39] as well as to Van Gijn's numerous publications, all of which contain exhaustive bibliographies.[40] The pseudo-Babinski sign, which may be observed in

[35] L. Barraquer-Ferre, "Contribution à l'étude du réflexe plantaire pathologique" [Contribution to the study of the pathological plantar reflex], *Rev Neurol (Paris)* 1930 (I): 174–182; B. Estanol Vidal, E. Huerta Diaz, and G. Garcia Ramos, "100 years of the Babinski sign," *Rev Invest Clin* 1997 (49): 141–144; V. Jay, "The sign of Babinski," *Archives of Pathology and Laboratory Medicine* 2000 (124): 806–807; S. P. Kumar and D. Ramasubramanian, "The Babinski sign—a reappraisal," *Neurology India* 2000 (48): 314–318; J. W. Lance, "The Babinski sign," *Journal of Neurology, Neurosurgery and Psychiatry* 2002 (73): 360–362; J. Pearce, *Fragments of Neurological History* (London: Imperial College Press, 2003), 352–354; Kumar, "The Babinski sign. A critical review."

[36] A. Tournay, "Le signe de Babinski. Caractéristiques, mécanisme et signification" [The Babinski sign: its characteristics, mechanism and significance], in *Rapport de neurologie, Congrès des médecins aliénistes et neurologistes de France et des pays de langue française, XXXth session, Genève-Lausanne, August 2–7, 1926* (Paris: Masson et Cie, 1926), abstract in *Rev Neurol (Paris)* 1926 (II): 471–473.

[37] H. Roger, "Signe de Babinski et réflexe cutané plantaire normal: mode de recherche et caractères cliniques" [The Babinski sign and normal plantar cutaneous reflex: research methodology and clinical aspects], *Sud Médical et Chirurgical* 1926: 105–117; H. Roger, "Valeur sémiologique du signe de Babinski" [Semiological significance of the Babinski sign], *Gazette des Hôpitaux* 1926: 597–606; H. Roger, "Physiologie pathologique du signe de Babinski" [Pathological significance of the Babinski sign], *Marseille Médical* 1926: 954–973; H. Roger, "À propos du signe de Babinski" [Concerning the Babinski sign], *XXXè Congrès des Aliénistes et Neurologistes de langue française* (Genève: 1926), 160–164, analyZed in *Rev Neurol (Paris)* 1927 (II): 288–289.

[38] J. F. Fulton and A. D. Keller, *The sign of Babinski. A study of the evolution of cortical dominance in primates* (Springfield, Ill.: Charles C. Thomas, 1932).

[39] F. Walshe, "The Babinski plantar response, its forms and its physiological and pathological significance," *Brain* 1956 (LXXIX): 529–556.

[40] J. Van Gijn, "Equivocal plantar response: a clinical and electromyographic study," *Journal of Neurology, Neurosurgery and Psychiatry* 1976 (39): 275–282; J. Van Gijn, *The plantar reflex. A historical, clinical and electromyographic study* (Meppel: Krips Repro, 1977); J. Van Gijn and B. Bonke, "Interpretation of plantar reflexes: biasing effect of other signs and symptoms," *Journal of Neurology, Neurosurgery and Psychiatry* 1977 (40): 787–789; J. Van Gijn, "The Babinski sign and the pyramidal syndrome," *Journal of Neurology, Neurosurgery and Psychiatry* 1978 (41): 865–873; J. Van Gijn, "Testing the plantar reflex," *Journal of Neurology, Neurosurgery and Psychiatry* 1987 (50): 502–503; J. Van Gijn, "Plagiarism: Babinski, art, and originality," *Archives of Neurology* 1989 (46): 1046; P. G. Raijmakers, M. C. Cabezas, J. A. Smal, et al., "Teaching the plantar reflex," *Clinical Neurology and Neurosurgery* 1991 (93): 201–204; J. Van Gijn, "The Babinski reflex," *Postgrad Medical Journal* 1995 (71): 645–648; J. Van Gijn, "The Babinski sign: the first hundred years," *Journal of Neurology* 1996 (243): 675–68; Van Gijn, "Remak and the plantar response"; J. Van Gijn, *The Babinski Sign, a Centenary* (Utrecht: Universiteit Utrecht, 1996); J. Van Gijn, "The Babinski sign," *Practical Neurology* 2002 (2): 42–44; J. Van Gijn, "Should the Babinski sign be part of the routine neurologic examination?" *Neurology* 2006 (23): 1607–1609.

peripheral neuropathies or in some myopathies, is of no particular diagnostic significance today, as is well known.[41]

Many physicians have made efforts to find variations of the sign, as a means of rendering a doubtful Babinski sign more readable.[42] Shaltenbrand recalled that there have been "numerous descriptions of sites on the leg, the stimulation of which provokes the reflex. The leg therefore would be like an advertising column where each neurologist may post his name. All these signs are only variations on the Babinski sign."[43]

All these maneuvers have a common point with the Babinski sign, which is to underline a pyramidal syndrome and therefore to distinguish an organic hemiplegia from a hysterical one.[44] The Strümpell sign, described in 1899, is related to a big toe extension activated by rubbing the tibial crest.[45] In the Schaefer sign, the big toe extension is linked to a pinching of the Achilles tendon. Schaefer considered this sign as an antagonistic tendon reflex.[46] However, this was strongly refuted by Babinski: "This so-called antagonistic reflex is nothing other than the toe phenomenon, which may be created not only by the tickling of the plantar foot but also by stimulation of the skin in other places."[47] In the Oppenheim sign, the extension of the big toe appears after a downward rubbing of the anteromedial part of the tibia.[48] In

[41] L. Gomez-Fernandez and D. J. Calzada-Sierra, "Pseudobabinski," *Rev Neurol (Spain)* 2001 (32): 799; L. Gomez-Fernandez and D. J. Calzada-Sierra, "Replica: Reflejo de Babinski, si; signo de Babinski, no; pseudobabinski, nunca!" *Rev Neurol (Spain)* 2002 (34): 699–700; F. E. Leon-Sarmiento, L. J. Prada, "Reflejo de Babinski, si; signo de Babinski, no; pseudobabinski, nunca!" *Rev Neurol (Spain)* 2001 (33): 1200; F. E. Leon-Sarmiento and L. J. Prada-Moreno, "Pseudobabinski y pseudorrespuestas," *Rev Neurol (Spain)* 2003 (36): 299–300.
[42] "Many tried to jump onto the bandwagon of Babinski's clinical shibboleth: Chaddock, Gordon, Oppenheimer and Yoshimura each tendered their modifications, but in .this context at least, they were '*deuxième cru*' in comparison to Babinski's discovery of the sign so succinctly described by Remak. For an excellent detailed review, see van Gijn" (Pearce, *Fragments of Neurological History*, 354). See also R. Grant, "The neurological assault on the great toe (1893–1911)," *Scot Med J* 1987 (32): 57–59.
[43] G. Schaltenbrand, *Rev Neurol (Paris)* 1958 (98): 640.
[44] M. S. Okun and P. J. Koehler, "Babinski's clinical differentiation of organic paralysis from hysterical paralysis. Effect on US neurology," *Arch Neurol* 2004 (61): 778–783; P. J. Koehler and M. S. Okun, "Important observations prior to the description of the Hoover sign," *Neurology* 2004 (63): 1693–1697.
[45] A. V. Strümpell, "Über das Verhalten der Haut- und Sehnenreflexe bel Nervenkranken," *Neurologishes Centralblatt* 1899 (18): 617–619.
[46] Schaefer, "Üeber einen antagonistischen reflex" [On the antagonist reflexes], *Neurologisches Centralblatt* 1899 (22): 1016–1018.
[47] J. Babinski, "Sur le prétendu réflexe antagoniste de Schaefer" [On the so-called antagonist reflex of Schaefer], *Rev Neurol (Paris)* 1900 (8): 52–53.
[48] H. Oppenheim, "Zur Pathologie der Hautreflexe an den unteren Extremitäten" [On lower limb cutaneous reflexes pathology], *Monatsschrift für Psychiatrie und Neurologie*

the Gordon sign, the extension corresponds to pressure on the calf muscles (triceps sural).[49] To look for the Rossolimo sign, one flicks the toes on the plantar surface of the second phalanx, which results if there is a disorder of the pyramidal tract, in a toes flexion instead of the normal reflex.[50]

The lateral malleolus sign, or Chaddock reflex, was formally described by the American physician Charles Gilbert Chaddock (1861–1936), professor of neuropsychiatry at Marion Sims-Beaumont College of St. Louis University, in 1911.[51] If there is a pyramidal disturbance, skin stimulation below the

1902 (12): 421–423, 518–530. Hermann Oppenheim (1858–1919) was a famous German neurologist. Babinski signaled (Babinski, *Exposé des travaux scientifiques*) that the Oppenheim sign was nothing other than the Babinski sign, and that has been "anyway a remark made by several authors, and particularly by Yoshimura, from Tokyo (see "Über das Babinski'sche phaenomen," *Aus der medicinischen Facultät der Kaiserlich Japanischen Universität zu Tokio*, Bd. VIII, Heft 2, 1908, S. 220).

[49] Alfred Gordon (1874–1953) was an American neurologist who did his medical studies in Paris. A. Gordon, "Réflexe paradoxal des fléchisseurs. Leurs relations avec le réflexe patellaire et le phénomène de Babinski" [The paradoxic reflex of flexor muscles. Its relationship with patellar reflex and the Babinski phenomenon], *Rev Neurol (Paris)* 1904 (21): 1083–1084; A. Gordon, "A new reflex: paradoxic flexor reflex and its diagnostic value," *Amer Med* 1904 (8): 971, cited in Goetz, "History of the extensor plantar response"; A. Gordon, "A new reflex: paradoxic flexor reflex," *Journal of Nervous and Mental Diseases* 1905 (32): 123–124; A. Gordon, "A further contribution to the study of the 'paradoxic reflex,'" *Journal of Nervous and Mental Diseases* 1906 (33): 415–418; A. Gordon, "Diagnostic significance of the paradoxic reflex. New anatomical evidence of its practical importance," *Journal of the American Medical Association* 1911 (LVI): 805–807; S. Goldflam, "Sur la valeur clinique du signe de Gordon, réflexe paradoxal des fléchisseurs, phénomène paradoxal des orteils et du mollet" [On the clinical value of the Gordon sign, the paradoxic reflex of flexor muscles, paradoxic phenomenon of the toes and calf], *Rev Neurol (Paris)* 1925 (I): 592–603; A. Gordon, "Sur la valeur clinique du réflexe paradoxal" (answer to Goldflam), *Rev Neurol (Paris)* 1926 (I): 11–14.

[50] Grigorii Ivanovich Rossolimo (1860–1928) was a famous Russian neurologist. G. I. Rossolimo, "Pathologie der Spinalreflexe" [Spinal reflexes pathology], *Journal nevropatologii i psichiatrii* 1902 (2): 239; G. Rossolimo, "Le réflexe profond du gros orteil" [Deep reflex of the big toe], *Rev Neurol (Paris)* 1902 (15): 723–724; G. I. Rossolimo, "Der Zehenreflex (ein speziell pathologischer Sehnenreflex)" [The toes reflex (a specific pathological reflex)], *Neurologisches Centralblatt* 1908 (27): 452, cited in M. J. Madonick and N. Savitsky, "Statistical control studies in neurology, V: The Rossolimo sign," *AMA Archives of Neurology and Psychiatry* 1954 (72): 365–374; G. I. Rossolimo, "Mein Zehenreflex" [My toes reflex], *Deutsche Zeitschrift für Nervenheilkunde* 1927 (97): 172. See also R. Satran, "Chekhov and Rossolimo. Careers in medicine and neurology in Russia 100 years ago," *Neurology* 2005 (64): 121–127.

[51] C. G. Chaddock, "A preliminary communication concerning a new diagnostic nervous sign," *Interstate Medical Journal* 1911 (18): 742–746; C. G. Chaddock, "An explanation of the external malleolar sign made with a view to incite study of it to determine its place in semiology," *J Mo State Med Assoc* 1911 (8): 138–144; C. G. Chaddock, "The external malleolar sign," *Interstate Medical Journal* 1911 (18): 1026–1038. See also Okun

lateral malleolus causes an extension of the big toe and eventually a fan sign. Chaddock had worked in Babinski's department from 1897 to 1899; he translated several of Babinski's papers into English and also made the sign known in the United States as early as 1899. In 1906, five years before Chaddock, the Japanese physician Kisaku Yoshimura (1879–1945) had described the same sign, but only in a Japanese journal.[52] Yoshimura was also the first to propose the use of electrical stimulation to activate the toe phenomenon.[53] The lateral malleolus reflex of Balduzzi consists of a dorsal extension of the foot after percussion of the anterior rim of the lateral malleolus in the presence of a pyramidal disorder; it could be related to the extension of the reflexogenic zone of the Piotrowski phenomenon (extension of the foot caused by percussion of the anterior leg muscle).[54]

Writing during World War I, Pierre Marie and Henri Meige noted that soldiers' "plantar sensitivity may have been blunted by long walks, prolonged standing position, wet shoes, etc." They then described an alternative test that could be done with such individuals: a foot adduction can be evoked by stimulation of the skin with a pin or a blunt point along the medial border of the foot, from the base of the big toe toward the heel.[55] In 1916 Egas Moniz described the sign of plantar flexion of the big toe with the leg flexed, noting that he had observed that in some cases "the toe phenomenon was only activated by the plantar flexion of the foot with the leg in flexion," while the Babinski sign and all other substitutes were negative.[56] The Bing sign appears in cases of a pyramidal lesion: after a pinprick of the dorsal part of the toe or the foot, there is an extension of the big toe.[57] Austregesilo and

---

and Koehler, "Babinski's clinical differentiation of organic paralysis from hysterical paralysis"; Goetz, "History of the extensor plantar response."

[52] K. Yoshimura [On Babinski's phenomenon], *Igaku Chuo Zasshi* 1906 (4): 533–549, 824–841, 939–955, cited in K. Tashiro, "Kisaku Yoshimura and the Chaddock reflex," *Archives of Neurology* 1986 (43): 1179–1180.

[53] Tashiro, "Kisaku Yoshimura and the Chaddock reflex."

[54] K. Sagin, "Le réflexe de la malléole externe et le phénomène de Piotrowski" [Lateral malleolus reflex and the Piotyrowski phenomenon], *Rev Neurol (Paris)* 1927 (I): 319–325.

[55] P. Marie and H. Meige, "Le réflexe d'adduction du pied" [Adduction of the foot reflex], *Rev Neurol (Paris)* 1916 (XXIX): 420–422.

[56] E. Moniz, "Le signe de la flexion plantaire du gros orteil avec la jambe en flexion" [The big toe plantar flexion reflex with the leg flexed], *Rev Neurol (Paris)* 1916 (30): 173–176. However, there is every reason to believe that one should read "extension" and not "plantar flexion" of the big toe.

[57] Paul Robert Bing (1878–1956) was a German-Swiss neurologist. P. R. Bing, "Zur diagnostischen Bewertung der Varietäten des Babinski' schen Reflexes," *Schweizer Archiv für Neurologie und Psychiatrie (Zurich)* 1918 (3): 89–94.

Esposel provoked the toe phenomenon by pressure on the thigh;[58] Juster did so by a light rubbing of the lateral side of the dorsal foot face;[59] Roch, from Geneva, rubbed the back of the foot as well but closer to the toes, at the level of the metatarsus.[60] The "sign of the painful toe"consisted of an extension of the big toe activated by strong pressure from the thumb and index finger on the distal phalanx of the four last toes at the same time.[61]

Victor Gonda (1889–1959), an American neurologist of Hungarian origin, described in 1942 at the Chicago Neurological Society a new method to activate extension of the big toe in cases of pyramidal disorder.[62] The technique, which was in fact an application to the foot of the Hoffmann sign previously described for the hand, consisted of grabbing the distal phalanx of the fourth toe between the thumb and index finger for six to eight seconds, forcing a plantar flexion. With a pyramidal tract lesion, one may note an extension of the big toe. This is called both the Gonda sign and the Gonda-Allen sign.[63] To provoke extension of the big toe, it is sometimes sufficient merely to expose the foot by lifting up the bedsheet (a technique sometimes known as "the 'bedsheet' Babinski") or by pulling off the patient's socks; at other times no maneuver at all is necessary to produce the extension of the big toe, which may appear spontaneously and continuously.[64]

---

[58] A. Austregesilo and F. Esposel, "Le phénomène de Babinski provoqué par l'excitation de la cuisse" [The Babinski phenomenon provoked by rubbing of the thigh], *L'Encéphale* 1912 (5): 429–437.

[59] E. Juster (presented by M. Crouzon), "La friction du bord externe de la face dorsale du pied permet d'obtenir, dans certains cas de lésion pyramidale une extension du gros orteil plus manifeste" [Rubbing the lateral part of the dorsal side of the foot allows in some cases to obtain, in the case of a pyramidal lesion, a more obvious extension of the big toe], *Rev Neurol (Paris)* 1927 (II): 472–473.

[60] M. Roch, "Le phénomène des orteils provoqué par friction du dos du pied" [The toes phenomenon provoked by rubbing the dorsal side of the foot], *Rev Neurol (Paris)* 1928 (I): 120.

[61] J. B. Grossman, "Un nouveau réflexe pathologique: l'orteil douloureux" [A new pathological reflex: the painful toe], *Rev Neurol (Paris)* 1927 (II): 370–372.

[62] V. E. Gonda, "A new tendon stretch reflex: its significance in lesions of the pyramidal tract," *Archives of Neurology and Psychiatry* 1942 (48): 531–537; V. E. Gonda, "Ein neuer Sehnen-Streckreflex. Seine Bedeutung bei Erkrankung der Pyramidenbahnen" [A new tendinous stretch reflex: its significance in lesions of pyramidal tract], *Schweiz Arch Neurol Psychiatr* 1953 (71–72): 97–99. On Gonda, see L. Kiss, "Rozsahegytol Chicagoig: Gonda Viktor (1889–1959)—egy meltatlanul elfeledett amerikai magyar orvos" [From Rozsahegy to Chicago: Victor Gonda (1889–1959)—a forgotten Hungarian-American physician], *Orv Hetil* 2005 (146): 853–855.

[63] I. M. Allen, "Application of a stretch reflex for identification of lesions of upper motor neurons," *NZ Med J* 1945 (44): 227–233, cited in Goetz, "History of the extensor plantar response."

[64] J. R. Berger and M. Fannin, "The 'bedsheet' Babinski," *Southern Medical Journal* 2002 (95): 1178–1179; J. A. Sicard, "Extension continue du gros orteil. Signe de réaction

Other less well-known methods have also been reported. For instance, Gordon in 1911 described the finger phenomenon, the equivalent for the hand of the Babinski sign.[65] Compression of the anterior side of the wrist facing the pisiform bone results in an extension of the fingers, which sometimes become fan-shaped. Hindfelt and colleagues, at Lund University in Sweden, described in 1976 the cross upgoing toe sign (CUT sign), which consists of a "slow, tonic dorsiflexion of the great toe when the contralateral elevated leg is firmly depressed in the supine patient."[66] These authors thought that this CUT sign "seems to be a reliable and more sensitive reflex than the Babinski reflex"; however, they concluded that "the CUT reflex does not replace the Babinski reflex, but may be a useful adjunct in clinical diagnostics." In fact, the value of the CUT sign has been challenged by several other authors.[67] In 1992, Vladimir Hachinski, an American neurologist of Polish origin, described the "upgoing thumb sign," which he considered an equivalent of the Babinski sign in the hand.[68] It is characterized by a thumb extension on the side of the pyramidal disturbance when the arms are stretched out and the two palms are placed facing each other. Hachinski's short note gave rise to different opinions, some positive, others very doubtful or even completely hostile.[69] The Szapiro method consisted of putting into plantar flexion the last four toes, a maneuver that was supposed to make the extension of the big toe during stimulation of the plantar foot more obvious.[70] Mieczysalw Krawczyk firmly stated that this technique provoked a false Babinski sign and thus made the interpretation of the sign more difficult; he recommended the opposite, a dorsal extension of the last

pyramidale" [Continuous extension of the big toe. A sign of pyramidal reaction], *Rev Neurol (Paris)* 1911 (22): 405–407.

[65] A. Gordon, "Le phénomène des doigts" [The fingers phenomenon], *Rev Neurol (Paris)* 1912 (20): 421–424.

[66] B. Hindfelt, I. Rosen, and J. Hanko, "The significance of a crossed extensor hallucis response in neurological disorders: a comparison with the Babinski sign," *Acta Neurologica Scandinavica* 1976 (53): 241–250.

[67] S. Andenaes, "Babinski reflex and the CUT reflex—a comparative study," *Acta Neurologica Scandinavica* 1979 (60): 260–263; E. W. Willoughby and R. Eason, "The crossed upgoing toe sign: a clinical study," *Annals of Neurology* 1983 (14): 480–482.

[68] V. Hachinski, "The upgoing thumb sign," *Archives of Neurology* 1992 (49): 346.

[69] For a positive opinion, see H. S. Tamm, "The upgoing thumb: a sign in search of a name," *Archives of Neurology* 1993 (50): 239. As an example of a doubtful opinion, see M. E. Mahler, "Specificity of the upgoing thumb," *Archives of Neurology* 1993 (50): 239. And for a hostile view, see G. N. Fuller, S. B. Blunt, and M. T. Silva, "Babinski yes, Hachinski no," *Archives of Neurology* 1993 (50): 239. See also the answer by Hachinski to the previous comments: V. Hachinski, A. P. Gaesecki, P. Maher, et al., "Reply," *Archives of Neurology* 1993 (50): 239–240.

[70] M. Krawczyk, "Watpliwy odruch Babinskiego—a metoda Szapiro" [Doubtful Babinski reflex—and the Szapiro method], *Neur Neurochir Pol* 1996 (30): 887–888.

four toes.[71] One could quote more examples, such as the Stransky, Mandal Bechtrew, Throckmorton, Allen-Checkley, and Cornell signs.[72]

In summary, one can say that the multiplicity and apparent diversity of these signs of pyramidal disorders only show that the reflexogenic zone at the origin of the extension of the big toe is much more extensive than originally thought. This zone may eventually concern the entire half of the body on the pathological side.[73]

On the occasion of the fiftieth anniversary of the description of the sign, Robert Wartenberg concluded:

> Despite the endless number of "modifications" and the bombastic claims of their discoverers and rediscoverers, it has been my experience that the good old method of Babinski, carefully applied, is by far the best and most reliable. A method which is really superior still remains to be discovered after fifty years.[74]

In the era of CT scans and MRI, one may well ask what the significance is of the Babinski sign in medical practice today. Does the test provide a decisive piece of information or an interesting contribution, or is it just a habit?[75] The discussion is not new: supporters and detractors of the Babinski sign have confronted each other for decades.[76] Most practitioners still find the Babinski sign to be superior to all its rivals.[77] In 1996, Barraquer-Bordas concluded:

> One hundred years after its subtle description—simple and brilliant at the same time—by Joseph François Félix Babinski, and while we are flooded by morphological and functional neuroimagery, which without any doubt is very useful, his sign remains of major diagnostic importance at the patient bedside.[78]

---

[71] Ibid.

[72] The first four are cited in Kumar and Ramasubramanian, "The Babinski sign—a reappraisal." The last is cited in Krawczyk, "Watpliwy odruch Babinskiego."

[73] G. Guillain and J. Dubois, "Le signe de Babinski provoqué par l'excitation des téguments de tout le côté hémiplégié dans un cas d'hémiplégie infantile" [Babinski sign provoked by cutaneous stimulation of the hemiplegic side in a case of infantile hemiplegia], *Rev Neurol (Paris)* 1914 (27): 614–616.

[74] Wartenberg, "The Babinski reflex after fifty years."

[75] D. K. Ziegler, "Is the neurologic examination becoming obsolete?" *Neurology* 1985 (35): 559; T. H. Glick, "Toward a more efficient and effective neurologic examination for the twenty-first century," *European Journal of Neurology* 2005 (12): 994–997.

[76] The main protagonists are quoted in T. M. Miller and S. C. Johnston, "Should the Babinski sign be part of the routine neurological examination?" *Neurology* 2005 (65): 1165–1168.

[77] See J. F. Ditunno and R. Bell, "The Babinski sign: 100 Years on. Still rivals current technology in its precision, reliability, convenience, and cost," *British Medical Bulletin* 1996 (313): 1029–1030.

[78] L. Barraquer-Bordas, "Que nous offre le signe de Babinski cent ans après sa description?" [What is the significance of the Babinski sign 100 years after its description?] *Rev Neurol (Paris)* 1998 (154): 22–27.

Several studies have evaluated how frequently any particular sign was present in control groups.[79] For example, out of 2,500 patients free of any neurological disorder, Madonick found the following frequencies of occurrence: Babinski sign, 4.3 percent; Rossolimo sign, 2.5 percent; Oppenheim sign, 2.2 percent; Hoffman sign, 2.1 percent; Gordon sign, 1.3 percent; absence of cutaneous abdominal reflexes, 16.5 percent.[80] In 2005, Brazilian neurologists demonstrated that out of 100 patients with no pyramidal disorder, 10 percent nevertheless presented an extension of the big toe.[81]

Other authors have compared the sensitivity of the different methods used for the demonstration of the big toe extension in cases of pyramidal system disorder. Some concluded that the Gonda-Allen sign (86 percent sensitivity) and the Babinski sign (76 percent sensitivity; the difference is non-significant) have better accuracy than all other tests, especially those for the signs of Allen-Checkley (63 percent), Chaddock (63 percent), Oppenheim (50 percent), and Gordon (22 percent).[82] Other authors considered that the Gonda-Allen sign (with 90 percent sensitivity) was ahead of the Allen-Checkley (82 percent), Babinski (75 percent), Chaddock (74 percent), and Cornell (54 percent) signs.[83]

Several recent papers, particularly two published in 2005 in the journal *Neurology*, keep the controversy alive.[84] While Landau (of Washington

---

[79] Madonick and Savitsky, "Statistical control studies in neurology, V"; M. J. Madonick, "Statistical control studies in neurology, VII: The Oppenheim sign," *AMA Archives of Neurology and Psychiatry* 1956 (76): 247–251; M. J. Madonick, "Statistical control studies in neurology, IX: The Gordon sign," *Journal of Nervous and Mental Diseases* 1958 (126): 221–224; M. J. Madonick, "Statistical control studies in neurology, X: Relationship between frequencies of reflexes in a group of 2500 non-neurological patients: Babinski, Hoffmann, Rossolimo, Oppenheim, Gordon and absent cutaneous abdominal reflexes," *Journal of Nervous and Mental Diseases* 1960 (131): 547–549; P. Maranhao-Filho, E. Dib, and R. G. Ribeiro, "Sinais de Babinski e Chaddock sem disfunçao piramidal aparente," *Arq Neuropsiquiatr (Brazil)* 2005 (63): 484–487.

[80] Madonick, "Statistical control studies in neurology, X."

[81] Maranhao-Filho, Dib, and Ribeiro, "Sinais de Babinski e Chaddock."

[82] S. H. Cheon, J. C. Kim, and K. S. Lee, "Extensor toe signs elicited by various methods in cerebral palsy children," *J Korean Child Neurol Soc* 2002 (10): 298–304 (article in Korean, abstract in English).

[83] D. Ghosh and S. Pradhan, "Extensor toe sign by various methods in spastic children with cerebral palsy," *Journal of Child Neurology* 1998 (13): 216–220. Comment in *J Child Neurol* 1999 (14): 337 and 337–340.

[84] W. Landau, "Plantar reflex amusement. Misuse, ruse, disuse, and abuse," *Neurology*, 2005 (65): 1150–1151; Miller and Johnston, "Should the Babinski sign be part of the routine neurologic examination?" See also R. Holloway, "The Babinski sign: thumbs up or toes down?" *Neurology* 2005 (65): 1147.

University in St. Louis) defended the Babinski sign, Miller and Johnston (from the University of California at San Francisco) were more skeptical. They compared the reproducibility, sensitivity, and specificity of the Babinski sign to the slowing observed during fast movements (in this case foot tapping), which is also a sign of a pyramidal disorder. They concluded that the slowing in foot tapping was more useful than the Babinski sign for identifying a pyramidal dysfunction. However, the authors recognized that, in contrast to tapping, the Babinski sign may be evaluated with noncooperative or comatose patients and that it may also serve to detect a pyramidal disorder in patients having predominantly a peripheral motor neuron dysfunction.

Finally, it is not without interest to note a patient's reaction to his doctor's search for a Babinski sign:

> The demonstration of the Babinski response is the most excruciating uncomfortable physical examination I know. Students, house physicians, registrars, research fellows, neurologists, and neurosurgeons alike cannot resist the masochistic urge to elicit a response even when they know that it has been strongly positive for years. How many hours of neurological time have been expended on the performance of this ritual? I would estimate that if this test was outlawed we could dispense with about a tenth of consultant neurologists.[85]

The Other Babinski Signs

The Babinski sign is so well known that one tends to forget that Babinski described numerous other signs. In *Dorland's Medical Dictionary*, four others are cited:[86]

1. Suppression or the weakness of the Achilles reflex in sciatica, demonstrating an organic pathology and allowing the distinction between true sciatica and pseudo-sciatica[87]
2. Maneuver of the combined flexion of the thigh and trunk, a part of the cerebellar semiology (see chapter 12), but which at the same

---

[85] P. H. Rayner, "The Babinski sign. Eliciting the sign brings out doctors' masochistic tendencies," *British Medical Journal* 1997 (314): 374.

[86] *Dorland's Illustrated medical dictionary*, 30th ed. (Philadelphia: W. B. Saunders, 2003).

[87] J. Babinski, "Abolition du réflexe de tendon d'Achille dans la sciatique" [Abolition of the Achilles reflex in sciatica], *Bulletins et Mémoires de la Société Médicale des Hôpitaux de Paris* 1896 (XIII): 887–889.

time signals a pyramidal syndrome, helping to distinguish an organic hemiplegia from a hysterical one[88]
3. Babinski plathysma sign, observed when there is an absence or diminution of the contraction of this muscle in hemiplegia or peripheral facial palsy[89]
4. The pronation sign—in organic hemiplegia, the hand of the paralyzed side is generally in pronation; if, by a passive movement it is placed in supination and is left in this position, it will return to pronation, demonstrating the organic character of hemiplegia[90]

Finally, there is yet another sign identified by Babinski: with a facial hemispasm, one may observe a paradoxical raising of the eyebrow (by contraction of the medial part of the frontal muscle) during eye closing (by contraction of the eyelid orbicular).[91]

---

[88] Many equivalents of this maneuver have been described, under different names, particularly the Bychowski sign (Zygmunt Bychowski, Polish physician, 1860–1935), the Hoover sign (Charles Franklin Hoover, American physician, 1865–1927), or the Grasset (Joseph Grasset, French physician, 1849–1918), Grasset-Gaussel (Amans Gaussel, French physician, 1871–1937), Grasset-Bychowski, or Grasset-Gaussel-Hoover sign. P.J. Koehler and M.S. Okun, "Important observations prior to the description of the Hoover sign," *Neurology* 2004 (63): 1693–1697. See also J. Lhermitte, "De la valeur de 'l'opposition complémentaire' comme moyen de diagnostic entre les hémiplégies organiques et les hémiplégies fonctionnelles" [On the diagnostic value of complementary opposition as a means of differentiating between organic and functional hemiplegia], *Semaine Médicale* 1908: 565–567, and J. Lhermitte, "Les petits signes de l'hémiplégie organique et leur valeur sémiologique" [The minor signs of organic hemiplegia and their semeiological value], *Rev Neurol (Paris)* 1911 (19): 407. One may also add the Strümpell phenomenon, which Marie and Crouzon reminded us of: if the flexion of the leg toward the thigh is impeded, this activates, in the case of a pyramidal tract lesion, an involuntary contraction of the anterior leg muscle on the same side, causing a raising of the medial border of the foot and a rotation inside of the plantar foot (P. Marie and O. Crouzon, "Le phénomène du jambier antérieur (phénomène de Strümpell)" [Leg muscle phenomenon (Strumpell phenomenon)], *Rev Neurol (Paris)* 1903 (XI): 729–731.

[89] J. Babinski, "Spasme associé du peaucier du cou du côté sain dans l'hémiplégie organique" [Associated spasm of the platysma muscle on the healthy side in organic hemiplegia], *Bulletins et Mémoires de la Société Médicale des Hopitaux de Paris* 1897 (XIV): 1103–1104; J. Babinski, "Sur le spasme du peaucier du cou" [On the plathysma muscle spasm], *Rev Neurol (Paris)* 1901 (IX): 693–696; Babinski, *Exposé des travaux scientifiques*, 119–120; F. E. Leon-Sarmiento, L. J. Prada, and M. Torres-Hillera, "The first sign of Babinski" *Neurology* 2002 (59): 1067. In fact, the plathysma muscle is innervated by the facial nerve.

[90] J. Babinski, "De la pronation de la main dans l'hémiplégie organique" [On hand pronation in organic hemiplegia], *Rev Neurol (Paris)* 1907 (XV): 755.

[91] J. Babinski, "Hémispasme facial périphérique" [Peripheral facial hemispasm], *Rev Neurol (Paris)* 1905 (XIII): 443–450; J. L. Devoize, "The 'other' Babinski's sign: paradoxical

The Tendon and Bone Reflexes

Wilhelm Heinrich Erb (1840–1921), professor of neurology at Heidelberg, and Carl Friedrich Otto Westphal (1833–1890), professor of psychiatry in Berlin, published separately in the same issue of the *Archiv fur Psychiatrie und Nervenkrankheiten*, January 1895, a paper on the reflex phenomenon.[92] Both recalled that many physicians had already identified the role of tendon reflexes, particularly the patellar reflex (what Westphal called the knee phenomenon and Erb called the patellar tendon reflex), without giving them a precise diagnostic value in nervous pathology.

Within five or ten years of the first publication of those two papers, the reflex percussion had become routine in neurological examinations and the diagnostic interest of the absence of Gowers's knee jerk in tabes (the Westphal sign) was widely known.[93] However, by the end of the century the great French neurological textbooks were still mostly silent concerning reflexes. In Charcot, Bouchard, and Brissaud's 1894 medical textbook, Hallion did not mention tendon reflex perturbations in clinical semiology of peripheral nerve palsies in his chapter on diseases of the muscles and nerves.[94] In this same volume, Babinski wrote the chapter on neuritis.[95] Only one page was dedicated to cutaneous and tendon reflexes; he concluded that "in neuritis, the diminution or absence of tendon reflexes is a rule, their increase a rarity, and the clonus may be considered, until new data appear, as absent in the semiology of this affection."

The same applies to Debove and Achard's *Manuel de Médecine* (1896), where in the chapter written by Pierre Boulloche, there was, for example, no

---

rising of the eyebrow in hemifacial spasm," *Journal of Neurology, Neurosurgery and Psychiatry* 2001 (70): 516.

[92] W. H. Erb, "Über Sehnenreflexe bei Gesunden und bei Rückenmarkskranken" [On tendinous reflexes in healthy patients and those with spinal cord lesions], *Archives für Psychiatrie und Nervenkrankheiten* 1875 (5): 792–802; C. Westphal, "Über einige Bewegungs-Erscheinungen an gelähmten Gliedern," *Archives für Psychiatrie und Nervenkrankheiten* 1875 (5): 803–834. See also M. Bonduelle, "Découverte des réflexes tendineux, Erb-Westphal-1875" [The discovery of tendinous reflexes, Erb-Westphal 1875], *Rev Neurol (Paris)* 2000 (156): 427–429 and E. D. Louis, "Erb and Westphal: simultaneous discovery of the deep tendon reflexes," *Seminars in Neurology* 2002 (22): 385–390.

[93] Gowers, *A Manual of Diseases of the Nervous System*, vol. 1: *Diseases of the spinal cord and nerves*.

[94] J.M.Charcot, Ch. Bouchard, and E. Brissaud, *Traité de médecine* [Treatise on medicine] (Paris: Masson, 1894), V: 835–936.

[95] J. Babinski, "Des névrites" [On neuritis], in Charcot, Bouchard, and Brissaud, *Traité de médecine*, VI: 649–834 (cutaneous and tendinous reflexes in neuritis are covered in pp. 737–739).

reference to the knee reflex in crural nerve palsy; he was more interested in the electrical reactions (muscular faradic contractility).[96]

In the first edition, published in 1901, of his *Sémiologie des affections du système nerveux* (Semiology of diseases of the nervous system), Dejerine briefly mentioned Babinski's discovery of the early disappearance of the Achilles reflex in tabes, underlining, however, "that it is not proven that it usually occurs before that of the knee reflex."[97]

The four lessons on tendon and bone reflexes published by Babinski in 1912 in the *Bulletin Médical* represented a particularly complete survey of the knowledge at that time and of Babinski's personal contribution to neurological semiology.[98] A review of that paper in *Le Progrès Médical* was very positive: "We cannot say too much in favor of this paper.... One will find the main qualities of the physician of La Pitié: clarity and clinical sense."[99]

In the first lesson, after some historical background and discussion of physiology, Babinski set out techniques for testing tendon reflexes (accompanied by photographs) that he recommended be carried out during every neurological exam:

> The hand, helped by the hammer, asks questions of the nervous system, which through these reflexes gives a clear response to these questions. The disclosures obtained in this way are very valuable: one may find the damage to its structure; sometimes, like in geometry, the location and the extent of the lesion can be precisely determined, putting the doctor on his guard against the serious dangers that threaten the patient. Such a dialogue, from which lies and errors are excluded for the one who knows this language, is able in a short time to reveal secrets that otherwise would have been unknown.[100]

---

[96] P. Boulloche, "Paralysies des nerfs périphériques" [Peripheral nerve palsies], in G. M. Debove and C. Achard, *Manuel de médecine*, vol. IV: *Maladies du système nerveux* (1896): 30–95.

[97] J. Dejerine, "Sémiologie des affections du système nerveux" [Semiology of diseases of the nervous system], in C. Bouchard, *Traité de pathologie générale* (Paris: Masson, 1901), V: 359–1168. See also chapter IX, "Sémiologie des réflexes" [Reflex semeiology], pp. 990–1017.

[98] J. Babinski, "Réflexes tendineux et réflexes osseux, leçons faites à l'hôpital de la Pitié recueillies par MM. Albert Charpentier et J. Jarkowski et revues par l'auteur" [Bone and tendinous reflexes, lessons delivered at the Pitié Hospital collected by MM. Albert Charpentier et J. Jarkowski and reviewed by the author], *Le Bulletin Médical* 1912 (19): 929–936, 953–958, 985–990, 1053–1059. Reprinted as *Extrait du Bulletin Médical, 19 et 26 octobre, 6 et 23 novembre 1912* (Paris: Imprimerie typographique R. Tancrède, 1912). Analysis in *Le Progrès Médical* 1913 (17): 220.

[99] C. Paul-Boncour, "Réflexes tendineux et réflexes osseux" [Bone and tendinous reflexes], *Le Progrès Médical*, 1913 (XXXIII), No. 17: 220.

[100] Babinski noted "that in purely clinical work it is not possible to find, before 1862, any indications on the subject presently discussed." J. Babinski. *Réflexes tendineux et réflexes osseux, Leçons faites à l'Hôpital de la Pitié, recueillies par MM Albert Charpentier et*

Babinski discussed in detail how the reflexogenic areas should be percussed and the best positions to adopt in order to avoid any error in interpretation. For example, the Achilles reflex should be studied with the patient kneeling on a chair, the feet dangling. The main data on reflexes in the normal subject were then considered.

The second lesson was devoted to the diminution or absence of these reflexes and the corresponding diseases, and the third to their exaggeration. The last lesson dealt with the relation between tendon and cutaneous reflexes. In conclusion, Babinski once more affirmed his certitude that hysteria never modifies tendon reflexes.

Many other papers by Babinski and by his pupils demonstrate the extreme importance that Babinski attached to the reflexes and particularly to the diagnostic method to be followed. Auguste Tournay recounted that thanks to a medical officer of the *Garde républicaine* who had listened to his lectures, Babinski had been able to percuss all the Achilles tendons "available" at the Célestins barracks.[101]

The traditional method of percussing was with the ulnar border of the hand.[102] However, Babinski (as well as some other neurologists) recommended the use of a reflex hammer.[103] In 1892, at the November 18 meeting of the Société Médicale des Hôpitaux, Babinski had previously

> presented in the name of M. Paul Blocq an instrument built by M. Mathieu to be used in the study of the tendon reflexes. Until then the hammers used for thorax percussion were utilized. This new apparatus was in fact composed of two hammers. That for percussion has the advantage of a variable weight (from 60 to 150 grams); it has two unequal surfaces by their area and is covered by a material that does not deteriorate. The other, completing the first one, when applied to different surfaces, allows one to study the jaw, brachial biceps, thigh adductor muscles reflexes, etc. In conclusion, this instrument seems perfectly adapted to the different particularities of this type of clinical exploration.[104]

J Jarkovski et revues par l'auteur [Bone and tendinous reflexes, Lessons delivered at the Pitié hospital, collected by MM. A. Charpentier and J. Jarkovski and reviewed by the author], *Bulletin Médical* 1912, 19, 26 October, 6 and 23 November.

[101] A. Tournay, "Joseph Babinski (1857-1932)," *Médecine de France* 1953 (43): 3-10.

[102] Grasset, *Traité pratique des maladies du système nerveux*.

[103] Previously Charcot recommended using the Skoda hammer. D. J. Lanska, "The history of reflex hammers," *Neurology* 1989 (39): 1542-1549.

[104] J. Babinkski, "Présentation d'instrument" [Presentation of an instrument], *Bulletins et Mémoires de la Société Médicale des Hôpitaux de Paris* 1892 (IX): 820-821; *Le Progrès Médical* 1892 (XVI): 435-436. This "double-sided hammer, with a weight graduation by Paul Blocq" is advertised, beside and among others, as the "hammer of Dr. Dejerine" and the "hammer with an automatic central percussion and graduation of Dr. Maurice

II. THE REFLEXES AND THE SIGN   239

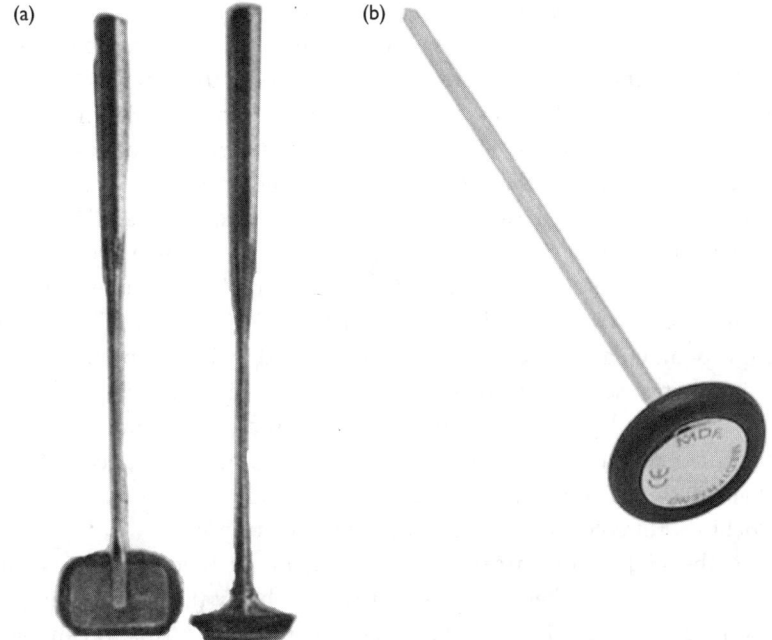

Figure 11-2 Babinski hammer. (*Sources*: (a) From J. Babinski, "Réflexes tendineux et réflexes osseux," *Le Bulletin Médical*, October 26, 1912. (b) From catalogue, MDF Instruments Direct, Inc., Agoura Hills, California.)

In his 1912 paper, Babinski described the two hammers he used (Fig. 11-2):

> I turn to the point of percussion. It should not be practiced with the ulnar border of the hand, as many still do; one of the disadvantages, among others, is related to the fact that the stroke is given to too large an area. It is necessary to use a special hammer, of which different models exist. Here are two that I generally use. One is composed of a handle made of nickel-plated steel, 20 to 25 centimeters long, fixed to the center of a disk of the same material, the circumference of which is gouged with a groove covered by a rubber ring. In the second specimen, the advantage of which is that it can be easily placed in the pocket, the handle is similar to the previous, but the disk is replaced by a rectangular plate, which is on the same plan as the handle; it is also covered by a rubber ring in its peripheral groove. These hammers possess elastic capacity suitable for their intended functions.[105]

Dupont" in the catalogue of Maison Mathieu, "fabrique d'instruments de chirurgie, orthopédie, prothèse, physiologie, anthropologie, coutellerie fine," Paris, n.d. (ca. 1907).
[105] Babinski, "Réflexes tendineux et réflexes osseux."

Nothing in this text presupposes that Babinski was the inventor of these two models of reflex hammers; he only said that they were the two he generally used. However, they were (and are still) known under the name of "Babinski hammers." An Internet search gives as many references to Babinski hammers as to the Babinski sign, and all medical instrument catalogues offer the Babinski reflex hammer, the most frequently used in France. The hammer as described by Babinski was later modified—for example, adding a telescopic handle. The American neurologist Abraham Rabiner (1892–1986) popularized the use of the Babinski hammer in the United States, modifying it by a head screwed to the handle, allowing orientation in two directions (perpendicular or parallel to the handle) and by its sharp tip, allowing it to roughly test sensitivity. This modified hammer is sometimes called the Babinski-Rabiner hammer. In connection with that, some said that during a gala dinner in Vienna in 1920, Babinski and Rabiner quarreled with each other about the hammers and came to blows.[106] In a gesture of reconciliation, Babinski offered Rabiner his own hammer as a gift.

Since the end of the nineteenth century, many reflex hammers have been invented and marketed.[107] The first was probably that devised by John Madison Taylor (1855–1931) in Philadelphia in 1888.[108] This Taylor hammer was nicknamed the "tomahawk reflex hammer" because of its head shape. Many other models have followed, particularly the ones developed by William Christopher Krauss (1863–1909) in Buffalo, New York, in 1894; Bernhardt Berliner in Berlin in 1910; Jules Dejerine in Paris, recommended to physicians as early as 1899;[109] and Ernest L. O. Troemner (1868–1930) in Hamburg in 1910. There are also those of Buck, Stookey, Queen Square, Vernon, and Henri Meige (1866–1940), who modified and standardized the reflex hammer developed by Josef Skoda (1805–1881).[110]

---

[106] Pearce, *Fragments of Neurological History*, 341–346; Lanska, "The history of reflex hammers"; T. Brückner, "Der Reflexhammer. Infos über ein wichtiges Utensil für Medizinstudenten und Ärzte," http://www.thieme.de/viamedici/studienort_hannover/klinik/reflexhammer.html#anker13.
[107] F. Schiller, "The reflex hammer. In memoriam Robert Wartenberg (1887–1956)," *Medical History* 1967 (11, 1): 75–85; F. Pinto, "A short history of the reflex hammer," *Practical Neurology* 2003 (3): 366–371; Lanska, "The history of reflex hammers."
[108] D. J. Lanska and M. J. Lanska, "John Madison Taylor (1855–1931) and the first reflex hammer," *Journal of Child Neurology* 1990 (5): 38–39.
[109] P. Michaut, Pour devenir médecin [To become a physician], *Schleicker frères (Paris)* 1899: 125.
[110] D. J. Lanska, "The Stookey reflex hammer," *Journal of Child Neurology* 1995 (10): 23–24. The Vernon hammer for children is similar to that of Babinski, but smaller; that is the reason why it is sometimes named the Babinski-Vernon hammer.

When looking for reflexes, the muscles of the explored segment should be well loosened, and Babinski recommended, as did many others, the use of Jendrassik's maneuver (Fig. 11-3 and 11-4):

> When, for example, you are searching for the knee reflex, you ask the patient to join his hands and to strongly pull on the entwined fingers; just at the moment when he carries out this order, you percuss the tendon; this is the excellent method devised by Jendrassik.[111]

Obsessed, as always, by the risk of confounding hysterical symptoms with a true neurological disease, Babinski recommended that in difficult cases the reflexes be studied under general anesthesia.[112] This effectively eliminates any activity caused by the patient's will and renders indisputable any exaggeration in the reflex response, a fundamental point for the distinction of organic versus hysteric or malingering affections.

In 1898, the same year as his final description of the toe phenomenon, Babinski demonstrated that the abolition or diminution of the Achilles reflex in tabes was as important as that of the knee reflex (Westphal sign).[113] It may be that only one of these reflexes is abolished; therefore, he recommended looking for modifications in both, not only the knee reflex (see chapter 10).

Babinski also described the inversion of some tendon reflexes. At the October 19, 1910, meeting of the Société médicale des hôpitaux, he reported that percussion of the lower extremity of the radius normally causes a flexion of the forearm toward the arm, possibly with flexion of the fingers in cases of "a strong reflex," but never in a normal state was an isolated finger flexion observed.[114] This phenomenon, which he proposed be named the "inversion of the radial reflex," has only been found in patients presenting a cervical cord lesion (syringomyelia, tumor), particularly at the level of the fifth cervical vertebra. From that, he concluded that "the inversion of

---

[111] Babinski, "Présentation d'instrument"; Gowers, *A Manual of Disease of the Nervous System*, vol. 1: *Diseases of the spinal cord and nerves*. On the Hungarian physician Erno Jendrassik, see E. Pasztor, "Erno Jendrassik (1858–1921)," *Journal of Neurology* 2004 (251): 366–367.

[112] J. Babinski, J. Froment, "Les modifications des réflexes tendineux pendant le sommeil chloroformique et leur valeur en sémiologie" [Modifications of tendinous reflexes during chloroform sleep and their semiological value], *Journal des Praticiens* 1915: 686.

[113] J. Babinski, "Sur le réflexe du tendon d'Achille dans le tabès" [On the Achilles reflex in tabes], *Bull. Mem. Soc. Méd. Hôp. Paris* 1898 (XV): 679–684; J. Babinski, "Sur les scléroses combinées" [Subacute combined degeneration], *Journal de Neurologie* 1900 (V): 417–418.

[114] J. Babinski, "Inversion du réflexe du radius" [The inverted radial reflex], *Bulletins et Mémoires de la Société Médicale des Hôpitaux de Paris* 1910 (XXX): 185–186.

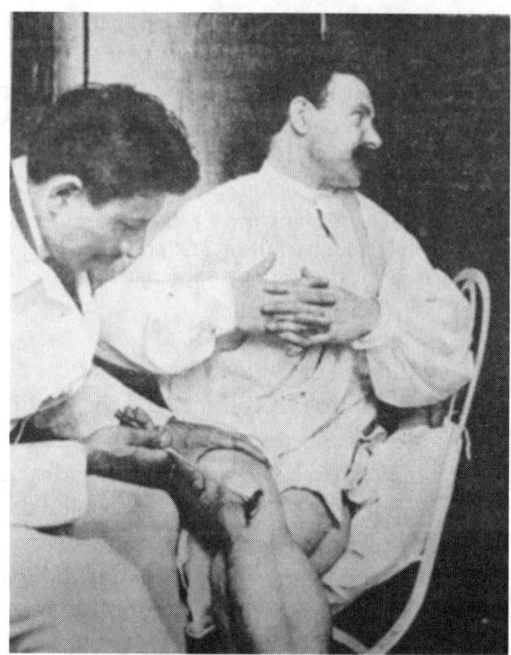

Figure 11-3 Looking for the knee reflex. (*Source*: From J. Babinski, "Réflexes tendineux et réflexes osseux," *Le Bulletin Médical*, October 26, 1912.)

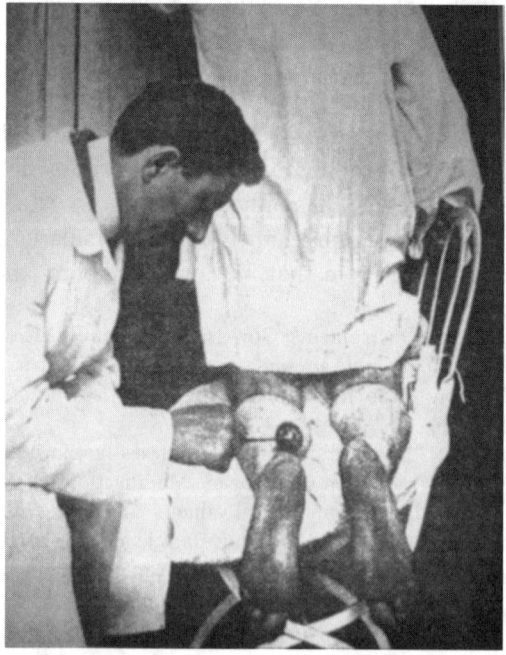

Figure 11-4 Looking for the Achilles reflex. (*Source*: From J. Babinski, "Réflexes tendineux et réflexes osseux," *Le Bulletin Médical*, October 26, 1912.)

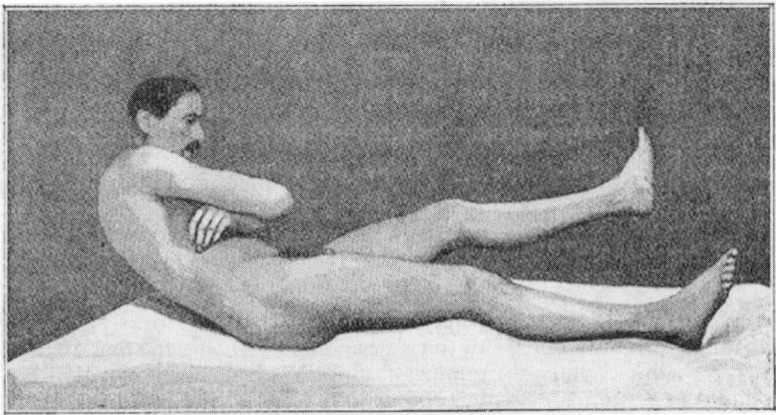

Figure 11-5 Organic left hemiplegia one year after its onset. Combined flexion of the trunk and thigh on the left side. (*Source*: From J. Babinski, *Exposé des travaux scientifiques* [Paris: Masson et Cie, 1913].)

the radial reflex constitutes a sign that, by itself, allows the physician to be quite certain that there is a cervical lesion and may contribute to identifying its precise location." He also described the inversion of the tricipital reflex, which he named "paradoxical reflex of the elbow," and interpreted it thus:

> In a normal state, percussion of the lower extremity of the humerus causes a flexion of the forearm, except when it is performed at the level of the triceps tendon, the effects on the tendon stimulation being stronger than those depending upon the shaking of the underlying bone. In a pathological state, when the extension reflex is abolished or decreased, the reflex movement of flexion appears, even when the triceps tendon is percussed.[115]

Babinski did not fail to mention the reflex inversions noticed by other authors, such as the paradoxical knee reflex of Benedikt and the inversion of the ulnar reflex described by Pierre Marie and Barré. Finally, although its use is quite limited, we may cite the paper of his pupil and friend Jean Jarkowski on the vertebral reflexes, resulting from percussion of the spinal column (Fig. 11-5).[116]

---

[115] Ibid.; also J. Babinski, intervention of 21 lines (pp. 511–512) concerning the paper of A. Souques, "Inversion du réflexe tendineux du triceps brachial dans l'hémiplégie associée au tabès" [Inverted brachial triceps reflex in hemiplegia associated with tabes], *Rev Neurol (Paris)* 1911 (XXI): 510–512.

[116] J. Jarkowski, "Sur les réflexes vertébraux" [On vertebral reflexes], *Rev Neurol* 1929 (I): 628–631.

Spinal Epilepsy or Clonus

Brown-Séquard in 1856 labeled as "spinal epilepsy" the convulsive movements observed in the part of the body below a spinal cord section.[117] In 1862, Vulpian and Charcot noted the same phenomenon in a case of multiple sclerosis, and several papers of the Salpêtrière school mentioned it in the years 1866, 1868, and 1869.[118] With his habitual precision, Babinski meticulously described the art of detecting this condition:

> Holding the leg immobile with the left hand and grabbing the foot extremity with the right hand, the examiner abruptly bends the foot toward the leg, still held in position. There is an epilepsy-like trepidation when this impulse causes a rapid succession of flexions and extensions, giving to the sustaining hand on the foot the feeling of a perfect rhythm.[119]

Babinski maintained that this was not epilepsy; rather, the clonus, which most often is seen at the level of the foot or of the patella, was evidence of an increase in intensity of the tendon reflexes (hyperactivity): "There is hyperactivity when, in a patient who does not voluntarily contract his muscles, tendon stimulation causes in the corresponding group of muscles a series of rhythmic reflex contractions."[120] He described the clinical tests used to distinguish between *complete clonus* (the sign of a pathological hyperactivity, having the same significance as a polycinetic reflex) and partial clonus (commonly found in subjects "whose nervous system should be considered as perfectly normal"). Babinski, always a little suspicious of his colleagues,

---

[117] C.E. Brown-Séquard, "Recherches expérimentales sur la production d'une affection convulsive épileptiforme, à la suite de lésions de la moelle épinière" [Experimental research on the production of an epileptic-like convulsive disease following a spinal cord lesion], *Archives générales de médecine (Paris)* 1856 (7): 143–149; C.E. Brown- Séquard "Note sur les faits nouveaux concernant l'épilepsie consécutive aux lésions de la moelle épinière" [Note on new data concerning epilepsy following spinal cord lesions], *Journal de la Physiologie de l'homme et des animaux* 1858 (I): 472–478.

[118] J. Grasset, *Traité pratique des maladies du système nerveux*.

[119] J. Babinski, "De l'épilepsie spinale (procédés pour la faire apparaître quand elle est latente)" [On spinal epilepsy (how to make it clear when it is latent)], *Rev Neurol (Paris)* 1903 (XI): 111–112.

[120] The relation between clonus and hyperreflectivity was known for several years. See Grasset, *Traité pratique des maladies du système nerveux*; Gowers, *A manual of disease of the nervous system*, vol. 1: *Diseases of the spinal cord and nerves*; Louis, "Erb and Westphal." The word *clonus* comes from Erb and Westphal (Grasset, *Traité pratique des maladies du système nerveux*). Babinski, "De l'épilepsie spinale"; J. Babinski, "Trépidation épileptoïde et hémiparésie chez une hystérique" [Clonus and hemiparesis in a hysterical patient], *Rev Neurol (Paris)* 1903 (XI): 733.

added: "It is just as true that if one does not pay enough attention, as many physicians do with a rapid exam, one may be exposed to the danger of confusing the two types of spinal epilepsy."[121]

Defense Reflexes

Defense reflexes are present when "the reflex movements of foot, leg or thigh flexion are obviously increased, similar to those observed in animals or man after a horizontal section of the spinal cord."[122] In this phenomenon of triple retraction (or triple flexion), Babinski insisted on the importance of foot flexion: "Foot flexion obtained by the stimulation of an area other than the plantar foot led us to recognize a pathological condition.... I propose a new expression, 'sign of the foot reflex flexion,' to indicate the pathological reflexes with which we are dealing."[123] Contrary to some authors, particularly Pierre Marie and Charles Foix, who considered the Babinski sign as part of the spinal automatism reflexes, Babinski defended the distinction between these two types of reflexes.[124] Several papers went in the same direction; however, future work proved that Marie and Foix were right.[125]

---

[121] J. Babinski, "De l'épilepsie spinale fruste" [On mild spinal epilepsy], *Rev Neurol (Paris)* 1906 (XIV): 287–289.

[122] On defense reflexes, see ibid.; Babinski, *Exposé des travaux scientifiques*, 56–58; J. Babinski, "Réflexes de défense. Étude clinique" [Defense reflexes. Clinical study], *Rev Neurol (Paris)* 1914–15 (15): 145–154; J. Babinski, "Réflexes de défense" [Defense reflexes], *Rev Neurol (Paris)* 1922 (38): 1049–1081. The quote is from J. Dejerine, A. Dejerine, and J. Mouzon, "Sur l'état des réflexes dans les sections complètes de la moelle épinière" [On the reflex status in complete section of the spinal cord], *Rev Neurol (Paris)* 1914 (II): 155–163.

[123] J. Babinski, "Réflexes de defense" [Defense reflexes], lecture delivered at the Royal Society of Medicine, London, with presentation of cases and cinematograph films, *Brain* 1922 (45): 149–184.

[124] P. Marie and C. Foix, "Sur le retrait réflexe du membre inférieur provoqué par la flexion forcée des orteils" [On the reflex withdrawal of the leg provoked by a toes forced flexion], *Rev Neurol (Paris)* 1910 (20): 121–123; P. Marie and C. Foix, "Les réflexes d'automatisme médullaire et le phénomène des raccourcisseurs. Leur valeur sémiologique, leur signification physiologique" [Defense flexor reflexes. Their semiological value and their physiological significance], *Rev Neurol (Paris)* 1912 (10): 656–676; R. Wartenberg, "Babinski reflex and Marie-Foix flexor withdrawal reflex. Historical note," *AMA Archives of Neurology and Psychiatry* 1951 (65): 713–716.

[125] Van Woerkom and Pastine both supported Babinski. W. Van Woerkom, "À propos des mouvements de retrait des membres inférieurs et du réflexe de Babinski" [On withdrawal movements of the inferior limbs and the Babinski reflex], *Rev Neurol (Paris)* 1913 (19): 407–408; C. Pastine, "Le signe de Babinski et les réflexes d'automatisme médullaire"

Babinski developed different techniques to demonstrate defense reflexes, particularly if they are doubtful; for example, one can stimulate "the thigh or leg integuments by faradization."[126] He showed that they may be provoked "not only by cutaneous stimulation but also by traction or pressure applied on the deeper parts." He made a detailed study of the defense reflexes in two patients presenting half a section of the spinal cord (Brown-Séquard syndrome), caused by stabbing with a knife.[127] He drew attention to the fact that "there may exist an increase in the defense reflexes, as in the toe phenomenon, in cases where the tendon reflexes are diminished or abolished; this exaggeration may be well pronounced."[128] Finally, he demonstrated the great value to neurosurgery of the study of the defense reflexes, adding to the information provided by his work on sensitivity. In fact, the limit of anesthesia gives only the superior limit of the compression, while the inferior limit is generally shown by the maximum of extension of the defense reflexes.[129]

[The Babinski sign and defense reflexes], *Rev Neurol (Paris)* 1913 (10): 403–406. Supporting Marie and Foix's idea, see Walshe, "The Babinski plantar response."

[126] J. Babinski, "Sur la transformation du régime des réflexes cutanés dans les affections du système pyramidal" [On the transformation of the status of cutaneous reflexes in pyramidal system diseases], *Rev Neurol (Paris)* 1904 (XII): 58–62.

[127] J. Babinski, J. Jarkowski, and J. Jumentié, "Syndrome de Brown-Séquard," *Rev Neurol (Paris)* 1911 (XXI): 649; J. Babinski, J. Jarkowski, and J. Jumentié, "Syndrome de Brown-Séquard par coup de couteau" [Brown-Séquard syndrome by knife stabbing], *Rev Neurol (Paris)* 1911 (XXII): 309–313; J. Babinski, S. Chauvet, and J. Jarkowski, "Sur un cas de syndrome de Brown-Séquard par coup de couteau" [On a case of Brown-Séquard syndrome by knife stabbing], *Rev Neurol (Paris)* 1913 (XXV): 857–861.

[128] J. Babinski, C. Vincent, and J. Jarkowski, "Des réflexes cutanés de défense dans la maladie de Friedreich" [On defense reflexes in Friedreich disease], *Rev Neurol (Paris)* 1912 (XXIII): 463–466.

[129] J. Babinski and J. Jarkowski, "Sur la possibilité de déterminer la hauteur de la lésion dans des paralysies d'origine spinale par certaines perturbations des réflexes" [On the possiblity of finding the level of a lesion in paraplegias of spinal origin by the modification of reflexes], *Rev Neurol (Paris)* 1910 (XIX): 666–668; J. Babinski and J. Jarkowski, "Sur la localisation des lésions comprimant la moelle. De la possibilité d'en préciser le siège et d'en déterminer la limite inférieure au moyen des réflexes de défense" [On the localization of compressing lesions of the spinal cord. On the possiblity of finding their level and their inferior limit with defense reflexes], oral presentation at the Académie de médecine, January 16, 1912; J. Babinski and A. Barré, "Compression de la moelle par tumeur extra-dure-mérienne. Valeur localisatrice des réflexes cutanés de défense" [Spinal cord compression by an extradural tumor. The value for localization of cutaneous defense reflexes], *Rev Neurol (Paris)* 1914 (XXVII): 268.

APPENDIX

On the different techniques used in searching for the Babinski sign

Sign of	Year	Techniques used to set off the big toe extension
Babinski Toe phenomenon	1896	Stimulation of the plantar foot
Strümpell	1899	Rubbing of the tibial crest
Schaefer	1899	Pinching of the Achilleus tendon
Oppenheim	1902	To press on the tibial crest
Babinski Toes abduction	1903	Stimulation of the plantar foot: "fan sign" of Dupré
Gordon	1904	Pressure on the calf muscles
Rossolimo	1908	Flick on the plantar face of the toes = toes flexion
Chaddock	1911	Skin stimulation below the external malleolar
Gordon	1911	Phenomenon of the fingers (equivalent at hand level of the Babinski sign) compression of the pisiforme bone = extension of the fingers
Trömner	1911	massage of the calf muscles
Austregesilo & Esposel	1912	stimulation of the thigh
Pierre Marie & Meige	1916	adduction reflex of the foot with a skin stimulation by a pin along the medial side of the foot, starting from the big toe to the heel
Egas Moniz	1916	Plantar flexion of the foot, with the leg flexed
Bing	1918	Pin pricking the dorsal face of the toe or foot
Gonda (-Allen)	1942	Plantar forced flexion of the distal phalanx of the fourth toe

(continued)

	Continued	
Sign of	*Year*	*Techniques used to set off the big toe extension*
Stransky	?	Strong adduction of the fifth toe followed by an abrupt slackening
Mendal Bechterew	?	percussion of the foot dorsal side in the area of the cuboïd bone = flexion of the four last toes
Hindfelt et al.	1976	"Crossed Upgoing Toe sign" = "CUT sign" forced flexion of the opposite hip
Throckmorton	?	Pressure on the dorsal face of the metatarsal-phalanx of the big toe
Cornell	?	"scratching the dorsum of the foot along the inner side of the extensor tendon of the great toe"
Hachinski	1992	"the upgoing thumb sign" equivalent of the Babinski sign in the hand
Szapiro	?	Put the four last toes in a plantar flexion, when the plantar foot is stimulated
Krawczyk	1996	Put the four last toes into dorsal extension during the stimulation of the plantar foot
Berger	2002	Lift up the bedsheet ("Babinski Bedsheet") or remove the sock

··· *twelve* ···

Cerebellar and Vestibular Symptomatology*

The description of cerebellar symptomatology was a major part of Babinski's work, and the neologisms he created (with one exception, *cerebellar catalepsy*) are even today commonly used in daily medical language, including terms such as *hypermetry, diadochokinesia,* and *asynergy*. Vestibular symptomatology, especially voltaic vertigo, also attracted his attention.

On the other hand, Babinski, not being involved in anatomoclinical studies, was completely uninvolved in the definition of some new syndromes that contemporary neurologists identified.[1] The most notable include Marie cerebellar hereditary ataxia (1893), Dejerine-Thomas olivopontocerebellar atrophy (1900), Holmes familial olivocerebellar atrophy (1907), Lejonne and Lhermitte olivorubrocerebellar atrophy (1909), and, later, Ramsay-Hunt dentorubro atrophy (1921), as well as Marie-Foix-Alajouanine syndrome (ataxia of the cerebellum in the elderly) (1922).[2]

---

* This chapter was written with the collaboration of Philippe Ricou, MD.
[1] R. Escourolle, F. Gray, and J. J. Hauw, "Les atrophies cérébelleuses" [Cerebellar atrophies], *Rev Neurol (Paris)* 1982 (138): 953–955.
[2] P. Marie, "Sur l'hérédo-ataxie cérébelleuse" [On hereditary cerebellar ataxia], *Semaine Médicale* 1893 (13): 444–447; J. Dejerine and A. Thomas, "L'atrophie-olivo-ponto-cérébelleuse" [Olivoponto cerebellar atrophy], *Nouvelle Iconographie de la Salpêtrière* 1900 (13): 330–370; G. M. Holmes, "A form of familial degeneration of the cerebellum," *Brain* 1907 (30): 466–489 (for a biography of Sir Gordon Holmes [1876–1965], see C. S. Breatnach, "Sir Gordon Holmes," *Medical History* 1975 [18]: 194–200, and J. M. S. Pearce, "Sir Gordon Holmes [1876–1965]," *Journal of Neurology, Neurosurgery and Psychiatry* 2004 [75]: 1502–1503); P. Lejonne and J. Lhermitte, "Atrophie

Cerebellar Symptomatology Before Babinski

Before Babinski, the cerebellum had largely been the subject of experimental work in animals. Marie-Jean-Pierre Flourens (1794–1867) demonstrated in the pigeon that cerebellar function controlled the coordination of movements. Many others, particularly Luigi Luciana (1840–1919), Sir David Ferrier (1843–1928), William Aldren Turner (1864–1945), J. S. R. Russell (1863–1939), François-Achille Longet (1811–1871), and Alfred Vulpian (1826–1887), demonstrated motor ataxia in the monkey and the dog following a cerebellar lesion.[3]

Guillaume Duchenne (1806–1875) talked to his patients or watched them silently for hours with scrupulous attention.[4] This technique of examination, sometimes called the "contemplative method," would be the one used later by Charcot, Dejerine, and Grasset. It was passed down afterward by Babinski and Foix. Duchenne gave a complete description of locomotor ataxia in a long report, published in 1858 and 1859 as abstracts in the *Archives de Médecine*, one year after a short paper at the Société de médecine de Paris. In 1864, he made the essential distinction between locomotor and cerebellar ataxias. He then drafted the cerebellar symptomatology: oscillations in all directions in the standing position and staggering similar to the one observed in drunkenness. He insisted on the absence of anxiety in the cerebellar patient, as opposed to the panic of the ataxic, "who is afraid of losing his equilibrium and whose glance, turned down or toward his legs, dares not to turn away because of the fear of falling." It was in regard to this distinction that Duchenne employed the famous aphorism "Clinical observation is much more preferable to vivisections, because with animals it is impossible to distinguish between the cerebellar staggering and lack of motor coordination."

Between Duchenne and Babinski, cerebellar symptomatology did not move forward very much. In Grasset's 1881 neurological textbook, there

---

olivo-rubro-cérébelleuse" [Olivorubrocerebellar atrophy], *Nouvelle Iconographie de la Salpêtrière* 1909 (22): 605–619; J. Ramsay-Hunt, "Dyssynergia cerebellaris myoclonica primary atrophy of the dentate system. A contribution to the pathology and symptomatology of the cerebellum," *Brain* 1921 (44): 490–538; P. Marie, C. Foix, and T. Alajouanine, "De l'atrophie cérébelleuse tardive à prédominance corticale" [Ataxia of the cerebellum in the elderly], *Rev Neurol (Paris)* 1922 (38): 849–885 and 1082–1111.

[3] This experimental work is set forth and analyzed in detail in L.-A. Tollemer, "Maladies du cervelet" [Cerebellar diseases], in J M. Charcot, Ch. Bouchard, and Ed. Brissaud, *Traité de médecine* (Paris: Masson, 1894), VI: 245–272; A. Thomas, *Le cervelet, étude anatomique, clinique et physiologique* [The cerebellum: an anatomical, clinical and physiological study] (Paris: G. Steinheil, 1897); J. D. Schmahmann, "Disorders of the cerebellum: ataxia, dysmetria of thought, and the cerebellar cognitive affective syndrome," *Journal of Neuropsychiatry and Clinical Neurosciences* 2004 (16): 367–378.

[4] P. Guilly, *Duchenne de Boulogne* (Paris: J. B. Baillière, 1936), 95, 145, 148.

was no reference to the cerebellum.[5] Hermann Nothnagel, professor at Iena University, in his 1885 book expressed the lack of consensus on cerebellar function and the symptomatology of cerebellar lesions. He considered disorders in movement coordination, especially the "staggering and unsteady walking" and "the violent vertigos[,] only as characteristic—but not pathognomonic—of the cerebellar lesions."[6]

Many authors, however, disputed for a long time the exact role of the cerebellum, or of the labyrinth, in the pathogenesis of vertigo. In the 1895 edition of his internal pathology textbook, Georges Dieulafoy (1839–1911) reduced cerebellar symptomatology to the staggering walk, considered at the same level as some nonspecific symptoms such as occipital headache, vertigo, vomiting, and eye troubles.[7] In his thesis, defended in 1897, two years before Babinski's first paper on the subject, André Thomas (1867–1963) made a detailed historical review of the question and concluded from his research that the cerebellum "is devoted to the maintenance of equilibrium in the different attitudes, movements, reflexes, automatic or voluntary: it is a reflex center of equilibration."[8]

Babinski's Contribution to Cerebellar Symptomatology

Even if other neurologists were involved in similar investigations, the importance of Babinski's contribution to the discovery of cerebellar symptomatology is beyond doubt.[9] "The clinical features of the now well-established cerebellar motor syndrome were defined by clinicians including Sanger Brown, Pierre Marie, Joseph François Babinski, and Gordon Holmes."[10]

The basis of Babinski's contribution in this field was the repeated examination of only one patient, Henri Mouninou, whom Babinski took care of

[5] J. Grasset, *Traité pratique des maladies du système nerveux* [A practical treatise on diseases of the nervous system] (Montpellier: Coulet, Delahaye & Lecrosnier, 1881).
[6] H. Nothnagel, *Traité clinique du diagnostic des maladies de l'encéphale basé sur l'étude des localisations* [Clinical treatise on the diagnosis of brain diseases based upon the study of localizations], trans. P. Kéraval (Paris: Delahaye et Lecrosnier, 1885). See also Grasset, *Traité pratique des maladies du système nerveux*.
[7] G. Dieulafoy, *Manuel de pathologie interne* [Manual on Internal pathology] (Paris: Masson, 1895), II:100–101.
[8] A. Thomas, *Le cervelet*; J. de Ajuriaguerra, "L'œuvre scientifique du Dr André-Thomas" [The scientific work of Dr. André Thomas], in *Jubilé du Dr André Thomas* [Paris: Masson et Cie, 1955), from *Rev Neurol (Paris)* 1955 (931): 1–28.
[9] E. J. Fine, C. C. Ionita, and L. Lohr, "The history of the development of the cerebellar examination," *Seminars in Neurology*, 2002 (22): 375–384.
[10] Schmahmann, "Disorders of the cerebellum."

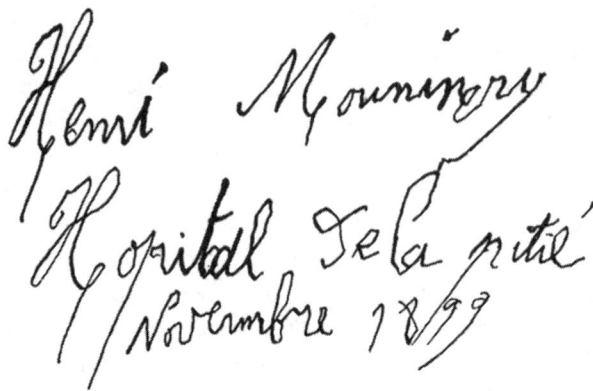

Figure 12-1 Example of handwriting by Mouninou, Babinski's cerebellar patient. (*Source:* From J. Babinski, *Oeuvre scientifique: recueil des principaux travaux* [Paris: Masson et Cie, 1934].)

in his department for more than twenty years (1899–1923).[11] Mouninou's postmortem examination was done by Jumentié, following the patient's expressed wish that this be done "so that Dr. Babinski can verify the exactness of the diagnosis he made during my life."[12] The diagnosis was in fact totally confirmed by the discovery of cerebellar necrotic lesions of vascular origin (Fig. 12-1).[13]

Cerebellar symptomatology did not appear in Babinksi's 1892 summary of his work to date.[14] In fact, his first paper on the subject was published in 1899; it concerned the description of cerebellar asynergy (reiterated in

---

[11] L. Rivet, "Joseph Babinski (1857–1932)," *Bull Mém Soc Méd Hôp Paris* 1932 (34): 1722–1733. In her thesis, Evelyne Fauconnet reported the following anecdote concerning Mouninou: "Concerned about the sexual desire of his patient, Babinski made arrangements with nurses in charge to take him once a week to a brothel, boulevard Blanqui, at the Doctor's expense. In return, he indirectly asked 'the ladies' what happened to the cerebellar syndrome in such circumstances!" E. Fauconnet, "Joseph Babinski, et la naissance de la neurochirurgie française" [Joseph Babinski and the birth of French neurosurgery], thesis for medical degree, School of Medicine, Rennes, 1985.

[12] Rivet, "Joseph Babinski."

[13] J. Babinski, "Syndrome cérébelleux" [Cerebellar syndrome], *Bulletin de l'Académie de Médecine*, April 23, 1925, No. 283 in J. Babinski, *Oeuvre scientifique: recueil des principaux travaux* [Scientific work: selection of main papers], ed. J. A. Barré, J. Chaillous, A. Charpentier, et al. (Paris: Masson et Cie, 1934), 293–294.

[14] J. Babinski, *Notice sur les travaux scientifiques du Dr. J. Babinski* [Note on scientific papers] (Paris: Masson, 1892).

1903).[15] Then came the description of adiadochokinesia in 1902.[16] The 1913 synthesis of his work to that date on the cerebellum successively analyzed asynergy (with the possibility of hemiasynergy and the description of Babinski-Nageotte syndrome), hypermetry (a term that he preferred to *dysmetry*), adiadochokinesia (a term proposed by Bruns, Babinski having suggested the word *diadochokinesia*), and cerebellar catalepsy.[17] The term *cerebellar ataxia* was proposed but not adopted. Hypotonia was not cited; it would be studied by Sir Gordon Holmes (1876–1965) with the Stewart-Holmes maneuver, first described in 1904.[18] At the London meeting in 1913,

[15] J. Babinski, "De l'asynergie cérébelleuse (présentations de malade et de photographies)" [On cerebellar asynergy (presentation of a patient and photographs)], *Rev Neurol (Paris)* 1899 (VII): 784–785 (abstract of the full paper "De l'asynergie cérébelleuse," *Rev Neurol [Paris]* 1899 [VII]: 806–816); J. Babinski, "Hémiasynergie," *Rev Neurol (Paris)* 1903 (XI): 557.

[16] J. Babinski, "Sur le rôle du cervelet dans les actes volitionnels nécessitant une succession rapide de mouvements (diadococinésie)" [On the role of cerebellum in voluntary movements necessitating a rapid succession of movements (diadokinesis)], *Rev Neurol (Paris)* 1902 (X): 1013–1015; J. Babinski, intervention of 2 lines (p. 1187) concerning the communication by C. M. Campbell and O. Crouzon, "Étude de la diadococinésie chez les cérébelleux" [Study on diadochokinesis in cerebellar patients], *Rev Neurol (Paris)* 1902 (X): 1186–1187.

[17] J. Babinski, *Exposé des travaux scientifiques* [Presentation of scientific papers] (Paris: Masson, 1913); J. Babinski and A. Tournay, "Symptômes des maladies du cervelet" [Symptoms of cerebellar diseases], *Rev Neurol (Paris)* 1913 (XXVI): 306; J. Babinski and A. Tournay, "Les symptômes des maladies du cervelet et leur signification" [Symptoms of cerebellar diseases and their significance], Congrès de Londres, August 1913. Reported by A. Barré in *Rev Neurol* (Paris), 1913, 26, 306–322; J. Babinski, "De l'équilibre volitionnel statique et de l'équilibre volitionnel cinétique (dissociation de ces deux modes de l'équilibre volitionnel, asynergie et catalepsie)" [On static and kinetic equilibrium (separation of these two voluntary equilibrium modes, asynergy and catalepsy)], *Rev Neurol (Paris)* 1902 (X): 470–474; J. Babinski and J. Jumentié, "Syndrome cérébelleux unilatéral" [Unilateral cerebellar syndrome], *Rev Neurol (Paris)* 1910 (XX): 604; J. Babinski and J. Jumentié, "Syndrome cérébelleux unilatéral" [Unilateral cerebellar syndrome], *Rev Neurol (Paris)* 1911 (XXI): 115–118; J. Babinski, "Quelques documents relatifs à l'histoire des fonctions de l'appareil cérébelleux et de leurs perturbations" [Some documents concerning the history of the functions of the cerebellum and of its disturbances], *Revue de Médecine Interne et de Thérapeutique* 1909 (1): 114–129; J. Babinski, "Asynergie et inertie cérébelleuses" [Asynergy and cerebellar inertia], *Rev Neurol (Paris)* 1906 (XIV): 685–686; J. Babinski, "Hémiasynergie et hémitremblement d'origine cérébello-protubérantielle" [Hemiasynergy and hemitremor of cerebello-pontine origin], *Rev Neurol (Paris)* 1901 (IX): 260–265, 422–424; J. Babinski and J. Nageotte, "Hémiasynergie, latéropulsion et myosis bulbaires avec hémianesthésie et hémiplégie croisées" [Hemiasynergy, lateropulsion and bulbar myosis with alternate hemiplegia and hemianesthesia], *Rev Neurol (Paris)* 1902 (X): 358–365.

[18] Thomas Grainger Stewart (1877–1957) was an English neurologist. T. G. Stewart and G. Holmes, "Symptomatology of cerebellar tumours; a study of forty cases," *Brain* 1904

a report by Babinski and Tournay and one by Rothmann gave detailed summaries of the contemporary knowledge of cerebellar symptomatology.[19]

Unrestrained Movements (Hypermetry)

Babinski described several techniques to show hypermetry during a neurological exam. These techniques, which are still part of a routine exam, are best described by using Babinski's exact words, which also demonstrate his clarity of expression.

> The patient, for instance, is asked to put his index finger (right or left) at the tip of his nose. Whereas a normal subject, whatever the speed of movement, is able to easily place without a shock the end of the finger exactly on the top of the nose and to keep it there, the patient with a cerebellar disorder cannot do so. His finger, after having followed in its trajectory the ordered direction and having touched the target, does not stop but goes beyond. The finger collides violently with the nose, slips or ricochets, and from there makes its way outside the target, toward the cheek and ear.
>
> The patient, being seated, is asked to place his hand in pronation, the palm placed on the knee of the same side. He is then asked to turn over his hand by a movement of supination, in such a way that its dorsal face comes to the same place over the knee. This movement, simple and easy for a normal subject, is not correctly carried out: the hand is pulled inside the thigh, and furthermore the supination movement is greater than necessary, the ulnar hand border reaching a higher level than the radial one.
>
> After having drawn a vertical line on the right side of a sheet of paper, the patient is asked to draw, from left to right, horizontal lines starting from any point but which should stop exactly at the vertical line; the hand crosses over the fixed limit. This exercise may be repeated from right to left, a less common movement.
>
> In the first step of walking, which generally cannot be executed without help, flexion of the thigh on the pelvis is more pronounced than normal, leading to an excessive raising of the foot; in the second step, the noise created by the plantar foot being applied violently on the ground shows the disproportionate extension of the thigh.
>
> The excessive flexion of the thigh on the pelvis may also be observed in another way: if the patient, lying on his back, tries to put the heel of one side on the knee of the other side, he places it beyond the target on the thigh; it is

---

(27): 522–549. The Holmes tremor, or rubro tremor, irregular and with a low frequency, is a combination of resting, postural, and active tremor, caused by lesions of the mesencephalon, near the red nucleus. M. Benedikt, "Tremblement avec paralysie croisée du moteur oculaire commun" [Tremor with an opposite paralysis of the third nerve], *Bull Méd (Paris)* 1889 (3): 547–548; G. Holmes, "On certain tremors in organic cerebral lesions," *Brain* 1904 (27): 325–337.

[19] Babinski and Tournay, "Symptômes des maladies du cervelet"; M. Rothmann, "Les symptômes des maladies du cervelet et leur signification" [Symptoms of cerebellar diseases and their significance], *Rev Neurol (Paris)* 1913 (XXVI): 322–331.

sometimes only after several attempts, with an excessive movement upward and downward, that the targeted point is reached.[20]

Babinski insisted on two essential points. One was that the patient must perform these movements rapidly. The other was that, contrary to what is observed in tabes, there is no aggravation of the disorder when the eyes are occluded. Babinski attributed the uncoordinated movements to some "excessive impulses, the effects of which cannot be corrected because of an insufficient action of braking." From this, he deduced that "the cerebellum is a regulator of movement, acting mainly as a brake."[21] He recalled that these disorders, named *dysmetry* by Luciani, had been observed in animals by physiologists and that the abrupt movements observed in some patients as reported by André Thomas in his thesis were not, strictly speaking, movements out of proportion.[22] Legitimately, Babinski concluded that "except for the isolated case of Huppert, the precise description and the full meaning of the uncoordinated movements or hypermetry—a term that I prefer to *dysmetry*—in the cerebellar disorders of man date from my work."[23]

Adiadochokinesia

The term *adiadochokinesia*, proposed by Bruns, was derived from the privative prefix *a-* and *diadochokinesia*, the latter a neologism (created by Babinski from two Greek words, the first meaning "successive" and the second "movement") that referred to the function of accomplishing successive movements. *Adiadochokinesia* therefore refers to the impossibility of executing a rapid succession of elementary movements, such as placing the hand alternately pronated or supinated (to use Babinski's words, "faire les marionettes" [make puppet-like movements]). As Babinski described it, "the cerebellar lesions are able in a way, without diminishing muscular strength, to create an inertia seen in the difficulty of starting the movement and stopping it in time."[24]

---

[20] J. Babinki, *Exposé des travaux scientifiques*, Paris, Masson et Cie, 1913, 136–137.
[21] Ibid., 139.
[22] Thomas, *Le cervelet*.
[23] Babinski indicated that it was only after his first report that he had been made aware that the existence of uncoordinated cerebellar movements had been already pointed out in 1878 by Karl-Hugo Huppert (1832–1904) in a paper that seems to have been unknown by the neurologists of that time. Babinski, *Exposé des travaux scientifiques*, 140.
[24] Babinski, "Sur le rôle du cervelet dans les actes volitionnels nécessitant une succession rapide de mouvements (diadococinésie)," 1013–1015.

Asynergy

Complex movements, such as standing up, walking, and carrying out on command various voluntary movements, necessitate good coordination between the different muscles involved, some tensing and others relaxing all in a controlled, synchronous, and harmonious way. This function is controlled by the cerebellum. Asynergy, as Babinski named it, is the disorder of this function.[25] He described several techniques that could serve to demonstrate it during a neurological exam.

When walking, "the patient is unable to associate the translatory motion of the trunk with the flexion of the thigh as is the case with a normal subject...: the trunk appears inert while the inferior limbs work." If the patient, when standing up, immobile and with no assistance, "tries to lean his head behind and to curve his trunk in the same direction like an arch, the inferior limbs stay quite immobile and do not carry out, or very partially the flexion movement of the leg on the foot and of the thigh on the leg, which a normal person does to maintain his equilibrium" (Fig. 12-2).

With the patient lying on his back, one may observe "a combined flexion of the thigh and trunk. If the patient, having lain down on his back and folded his arms on his chest, tries to sit up, he does not succeed. Furthermore, the thighs bend strongly toward the pelvis and the heels rise up noticeably above the floor, contrary to what is observed in a normal and vigorous patient."

The seated patient "is asked to place the tip of his toe toward a point located sixty centimeters above the floor. At first, the thigh remains flexed toward the pelvis, and the leg has only a slight extension on the thigh; then the leg's extension becomes more forceful and the toe reaches the target, but it is thrust with some abruptness. When the patient tries to resume his initial position, one first observes the leg becoming flexed on the thigh while the latter moves slightly. Then, when the leg becomes half flexed, there is a brutal extension of the thigh toward the pelvis and the foot lies flat on the floor."

Babinski pointed out that asynergy may be unilateral; in such cases, the asynergy occurs on the same side as the cerebellar lesion.[26]

---

[25] Babinski, "De l'asynergie cérébelleuse."
[26] Babinski, "Hémiasynergie et hémitremblement"; Babinski and Nageotte, "Hémiasynergie, latéropulsion et myosis bulbaires"; J. Babinski and J. Nageotte, "Lésions syphilitiques des centres nerveux. Foyers de ramollissement dans le bulbe. Hémiasynergie, latéropulsion et myosis bulbaires avec hémianesthésie et hémiplégie croisées" [Syphilitic lesions of the central nervous system. Softening areas in the medulla oblongata. Hemiasynergy,

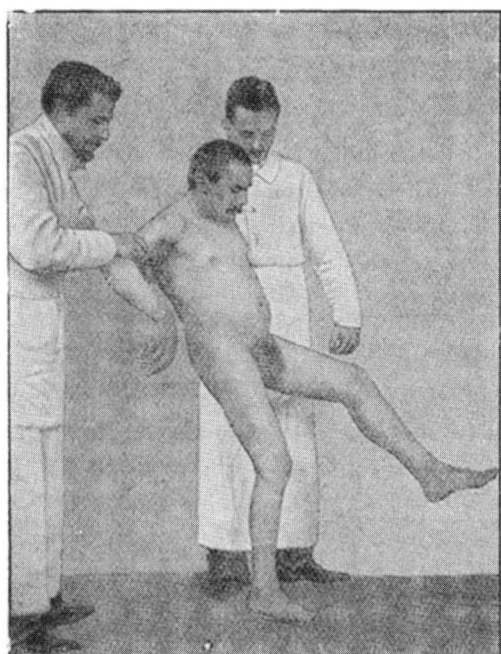

Figure 12-2 Attitude of patient with cerebellar syndrome while walking supported by two helpers. (*Source*: From J. Babinski, *Exposé des travaux scientifiques* [Paris: Masson et Cie, 1913].)

Cerebellar Catalepsy

Babinski gave the name of *cerebellar catalepsy* to the power of muscles, in the state of voluntary contraction, to stay still in certain positions for a long time "as if they were rigid, without, however, being in spasm."[27] The best way to reveal this phenomenon is to ask the patient to lie down on his back "with the thigh being flexed on the pelvis, the legs slightly flexed on the thighs, and the feet spread out one from the other." The position may be held for several minutes without the patient tiring: this remarkable fixity "is quite like a waxwork statue."

---

lateropulsion and bulbar myosis with alternate hemiplegia and hemianesthesia], *Nouvelle Iconographie de la Salpêtrière* 1902 (XV): 492–512.
[27] Babinski, "De l'équilibre volitionnel statique."

Babinski's Contribution to Vestibular Symptomatology

In the 1913 review of his work, Babinski paid particular attention to the distinction between cerebellar and vestibular symptomatologies. He attributed to vestibular lesions some disorders observed in cerebellar pathology, such as lateropulsion, spreading out of legs, drunken staggering, vertigo, or nystagmus, and he restricted as "proper to cerebellar disorders" only uncoordinated movements, asynergy, adiadochokinesia, and cerebellar catalepsy. He insisted that the location and importance of cerebellar lesions as well as the association with other lesions all have a direct influence on the presence or absence, intensity, and duration of these signs.

This having been said, Charbonnel underlined the fact that although Babinski was on target in posing the problem of the relationship between the cerebellar and vestibular symptomatologies, he had erroneously believed that cerebellar lesions were able to create "some signs that everyone looks at today as specifically vestibular," such as vertigo, nystagmus, index finger deviation, and equilibrium disorders.[28] Charbonnel explained Babinski's idea by the fact that "in 1913, the vestibular peripheral system was well known, which was not the case for the central one"; it was only later that neurophysiological research was able to clearly distinguish between cerebellar and vestibular symptoms.

Babinski's interest in voltaic vertigo was related to the same problem. From 1901 to 1913 he was completely involved with it; he published, alone or in collaboration with Vincent, Barré, and especially Weill, many reports and papers, some experimental (on pigeons and guinea pigs), others clinical.[29] Voltaic vertigo was created by the application of electrodes of a

---

[28] A. Charbonnel, "Liaisons et discrimination cérébello-vestibulaires" [Connections and discriminative functions in the cerebellovestibular system], in *Le cervelet* (Paris: Masson, 1958), 77–128.

[29] J. Babinski, C. Vincent, and A. Barré, "Vertige voltaïque. Nouvelles recherches expérimentales sur le labyrinthe du cobaye" [Voltaic vertigo. New experiments on the guinea pig labyrinth], *Rev Neurol (Paris)* 1913 (XXV): 410–413; J. Babinski, C. Vincent, and A. Barré, "Vertige voltaïque. Recherches sur le labyrinthe du cobaye" [Voltaic vertigo. Research on the guinea pig labyrinth], *Rev Neurol (Paris)* 1913 (XXVI): 351; J. Babinski, C. Vincent, and A. Barré, "Vertige voltaïque. Perturbation dans les mouvements des globes oculaires à la suite de lésions labyrinthiques expérimentales" [Voltaic vertigo. Pertubations in eyeball movements following experimental labyrinthic lesions], *Rev Neurol (Paris)* 1913 (XXV): 253–255; J. Babinski, "De l'influence des lésions de l'appareil auditif sur le vertige voltaïque" [On the influence of auditory system lesions on voltaic vertigo], *Comptes-rendus Hebdomadaires des Séances et Mémoires de la Société de Biologie* 1901 (52): 77–80, analyzed in *Rev Neurol (Paris)* 1901 (IX): 1170–1171 and in

voltaic apparatus on the temples or mastoid apophysis of a patient. It manifested itself by dizziness, nauseas, nystagmus, and head tilting (sometimes with head and even trunk rotation) on the side of the positive pole when the electrical current was interrupted. The question remained, however, whether the voltaic vertigo was provoked by electrical stimulation of the nervous system or of the labyrinth. Babinski demonstrated that the second hypothesis was the true one and that lesions in the auditory system significantly modify voltaic vertigo.[30] He concluded that this test was of interest in recognizing a vestibular disorder and could "eliminate the possibility of simulation (Fig. 12-3)."[31]

The Babinski-Weill test (blind walking or star walking) also aims at clinically showing a vestibular disorder. The patient, with his eyes closed, must take a step forward and backward in a straight line in the same direction several times; if there is a vestibular disorder, the direction of the movement deviates each time, in the form of a star.[32] In 1917 Henri Bourgeois gave a detailed description of this Babinski test, and in his report to the 8th International Neurological Meeting in 1927, Hautant recalled the important

---

Le Progrès Médical 1901 (XIII): 92; J. Babinski, "Sur la valeur sémiologique des perturbations dans le vertige voltaïque" [On the semiological value of disturbances in voltaic vertigo], *Rev Neurol (Paris)* 1902 (X): 474–475; J. Babinski, "Sur le mouvement d'inclination et de rotation de la tête dans le vertige voltaïque" [On the tilting and rotating of head movement in voltaic vertigo], *Comptes-rendus Hebdomadaires des Séances et Mémoires de la Société de Biologie* 1903 (LV): 513–515; J. Babinski, "Vertige voltaïque et lésions auriculaires" [Voltaic vertigo and auricular lesions], *Bulletins et Mémoires de la Société de Laryngologie, d'Otologie et de Rhinologie de Paris*, February 12, 1910; J. Babinski, "Du vertige voltaïque dans les affections du système vestibulaire" [On voltaic vertigo in vestibular system disturbances], *Rev Neurol (Paris)* 1911 (XXI): 780–783; J. Babinski, "Désorientation et déséquilibration provoquées par le courant voltaïque" [Disorientation and disequilibrium provoked by a voltaic current], *Bulletin Médical*, November 5, 1913; J. Babinski, "Désorientation et déséquilibration spontanées et provoquées par le courant voltaïque" [Disorientation and disequilibrium provoked by a voltaic current], *Archives d'Électricité Médicale*, December 10, 1913, 10–19. See also Babinski, *Exposé des travaux scientifiques*.

[30] J. Babinski, "Sur le mécanisme du vertige voltaïque" [On the mechanism of voltaic vertigo], *Comptes-rendus Hebdomadaires des Séances et Mémoires de la Société de Biologie* 1903 (LV): 350–353.

[31] Babinski, "Du vertige voltaïque dans les affections du système vestibulaire."

[32] J. Babinski and G. A. Weill, "Désorientation et déséquilibration spontanée et provoquée. La déviation angulaire" [Spontaneous and provoked disorientation and disequilibrium. Angular deviation], *Comptes-rendus Hebdomadaires des Séances et Mémoires de la Société de Biologie*, 1913 (I): 852–855; J. Babinski and G. A. Weill, "Mouvements réactionnels d'origine vestibulaire et mouvements contre réactionnels" [Reactive and counterreactive movements of vestibular origin], *Comptes-rendus Hebdomadaires des Séances et Mémoires de la Société de Biologie* 1913 (II): 98–100.

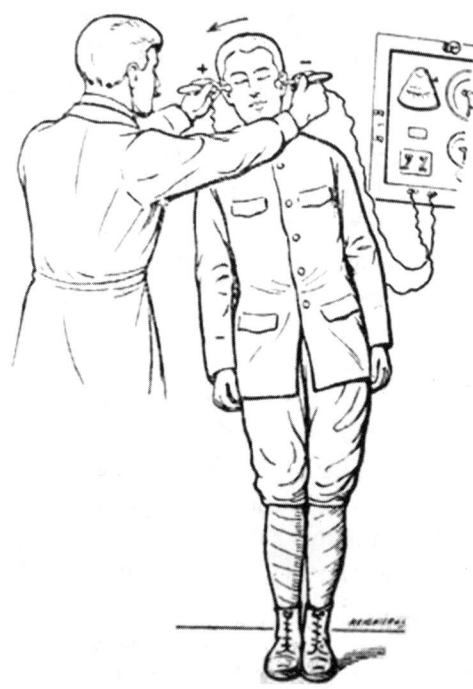

Figure 12-3 Electrodiagnostic according to Babinski. The patient normally tilts towards the positive pole. (*Source:* From H. Bourgeois, "Le vertige voltaïque dans les affections de l'oreille interne. Épreuve de Babinski," *Le Progrès Médical,* 1917 [34]: 279.)

contribution of Babinski to vestibular symptomatology, particularly the voltaic test, star walking, and the voltaic angular deviation.[33]

In his 1940 textbook, André Thomas expanded on Babinski's observations in his description of the respective place of the cerebellum and labyrinth in equilibrium:

> The labyrinthic system and the cerebellum control reactions, mainly activated by changing pose and movement, regarding which the body weight is a determining constant. The former governs reactions commanded by the head position while the latter controls partial reactions guided by segmental positions.

---

[33] H. Bourgeois, "Le vertige voltaïque dans les affections de l'oreille interne. Epreuve de Babinski" [Voltaic vertigo in inner ear diseases. The Babinski test], *Le Progrès Médical,* 1917 (34): 279; A. Hautant, "Rapport sur l'étude clinique de l'examen fonctionnel de l'appareil vestibulaire" [Report on the clinical study of the examination of functions of the vestibular apparatus], *Rev Neurol (Paris)* 1927 (I): 908–976.

However, the joint action of several segmental positions generates a global synergy in the body as a whole.³⁴

Cerebellar Symptomatology After Babinski

In the "Cerebellar Ataxia" chapter of the first edition of his textbook *Sémiologie* (1901), Dejerine did not quote any of Babinski's publications, although in the paragraph dedicated to what he named "galvanic vertigo," he briefly described the signs that Babinski would later call voltaic vertigo.³⁵ On the other hand, in the 1914 edition of *Sémiologie*,³⁶ Dejerine, even if significantly privileging references to Thomas, took into consideration Babinski's work, but without being truly enthusiastic. For example, in the section on dysmetry, he wrote:

> Babinski drew attention to the importance of uncoordinated movements with patients presenting a lesion of the cerebellar system, but none of his patients, the observations on which he published the case studies, presented a destructive lesion of the cerebellum: they corresponded to medullary or pontic lesions or to tumors compressing the cerebellar structures. Such observations are far from having the same physiological and clinical value for the lesions specific to the cerebellum, as observed in olivopontocerebellar atrophy.

The same reservation appeared later in the textbook when he criticized cerebellar catalepsy as described by Babinski: "Until now, these phenomena have not been studied in patients presenting exclusively cerebellar lesions, controlled by a detailed pathological examination."

In his 1911 textbook, Thomas dealt first with anatomical and physiological experimental data.³⁷ He then laid out very clearly the symptomatology of cerebellar disorders, including the most recent discoveries, particularly those coming from Babinski: hypermetry (the term Thomas preferred to *dysmetry*), adiadochokinesia, asynergy, and cerebellar catalepsy. In the last

---

³⁴ A. Thomas, *Équilibre et équilibration* [Equilibrium and equilibration] (Paris: Masson, 1940).

³⁵ J. Dejerine, "Sémiologie des affections du système nerveux" [Semiology of diseases of the nervous system], in C. Bouchard, *Traité de pathologie générale* (Paris: Masson, 1901, V :359–1168).

³⁶ J. Dejerine, *Sémiologie des affections du système nerveux* [Semiology of diseases of the nervous system] (Paris: Masson, 1914).

³⁷ A. Thomas, *La fonction cérébelleuse* [The cerebellar function], one volume in *L'encyclopédie scientifique* (Paris: Doin, 1911), analyzed in *Le Progrès Médical* 1911 (XXXI): 311.

part of the book, he considered the problems related to the interpretation of cerebellar functions in maintaining equilibration and regulating and coordinating voluntary movements. In 1914, Thomas published his animal experimental works on the cerebellum.[38]

Sir Gordon Holmes in 1917 carefully analyzed symptoms of the acute cerebellar lesions caused by bullet wounds, observed during World War I. Holmes recognized that

> it is impossible to deal with this subject without relying largely on Babinski's masterly analysis of the symptoms of cerebellar disease and on the careful descriptive work of other neurologists, especially André Thomas, who also attempted to establish a valuable correlation of these clinical symptoms with the disturbances that occur in animals after experimental injury.[39]

He insisted mainly on the hypotonia observed on the side of the cerebellar lesion and on the rebound phenomenon known as the Stewart-Holmes sign, but he also described cerebellar ataxia (underlining the fact that eye occlusion did not modify the symptoms), unsteady walking, decomposition of movement, asynergy, dysmetry, intentional tremor, and adiadochokinesia.

In 1922, in the section concerning the cerebellum in their *Nouveau traité de médecine* (A new treatise on medicine), Henri Claude and Joseph Lévy-Valensi reviewed all the known components of cerebellar symptomatology, clearly indicating the initial discoverers of the different signs, especially Babinski, Thomas, Jumentié, Holmes, and Stewart.[40]

The 185-page chapter written by André Thomas[41] in Roger, Widal, and Teissier's 1925 *Nouveau traité de médecine* (A new treatise on medicine; the title was the same as Claude and Lévy-Valensi's earlier work) was at the time and for many years afterward the most complete and well-documented text on the cerebellum. This exhaustive survey considered all aspects of the cerebellum, whether anatomical, physiological, clinical, or pathological. The author reviewed the signs of cerebellar pathology, giving in detail the techniques used to demonstrate them. He reserved a special place for hypotony, describing all the maneuvers capable of showing it, particularly

---

[38] A. Thomas and A. Durupt, *Localisations cérébelleuses* [Cerebellar localizations] (Paris: Vigot, 1914).

[39] G. Holmes, "The symptoms of acute cerebellar injuries due to gunshot injuries," *Brain* 1918 (40): 461–535.

[40] H. Claude and J. Lévy-Valensi, *Maladies du cervelet et de l'isthme de l'encéphale* [Cerebellar and brain stem diseases] (Paris: J. B. Baillière, 1922).

[41] A. Thomas, "Pathologie du cerveau et du cervelet" [Brain and cerebellar pathology], in G. H. Roger, F. Widal, and P. J. Teissier, *Nouveau traité de médecine* (Paris: Masson, 1925).

the Stewart-Holmes test. He described equilibrium disorders, hypermetry (which he preferred to continue to call dysmetry), intentional tremor, and cerebellar catalepsy. He noted that Babinski himself considered that "pure, perfect catalepsy is very rare; probably necessary for its development is the conjunction of particular conditions exceptionally combined." He also discussed adiadochokinesia, writing and speech disturbances (in relation to dysmetry, with the discontinuity of movement and adiadochokinesia), nystagmus (the presence of which is not always related to labyrinthic lesions), and asynergy (which he described in the conditional tense, as he was not fully convinced).[42]

The 22nd International Neurological Meeting, organized in June 1958 in Paris by the Société française de neurologie, had the cerebellum as its theme. In his general review of cerebellar symptomatology, François Lhermitte (1921–1998) noted the founding role of Babinski ("Joseph Babinski expanded a nascent symptomatology") but remarked that "the full bloom of cerebellar symptomatology was the work of two neurologists, André Thomas and Gordon Holmes, at the end of and after World War I." In fact, "muscular hypotony is the key symptom of cerebellar syndrome. Foreseen by Luciani in the animal, by Stewart and Homes in man, its discovery was by André Thomas and Gordon Holmes."[43]

Cerebellar syndrome, as it is taught today to medical students, is not very different from the one described so meticulously by André Thomas. It includes (1) hypotony (lumbar hyperlordosis, increase in limb dangling [flail sign of the hand, foot swinging sign], hyperlaxity, and pendular tendinous reflexes, with the Stewart-Holmes resistance test usually considered as "an essential element of the syndrome"), (2) cerebellar ataxia in the standing position and in walking, (3) pertubations in executing movements (dysmetry or hypermetry, asynergy, adiadochokinesia, writing disorders), (4) intentional cerebellar tremor, which is not really a true tremor but the consequence of asynergy, related to asynchronism of contraction of agonist and antagonist muscles, (5) cerebellar dysarthry (slow speech, scanned and plosive), due

---

[42] "According to Babinski, the cerebellum would play a fundamental role in the physiology of the kinetic associations; asynergy (absence or pertubation of synergy) would be a sign of cerebellar lesion. Here are some tests with which it would be easy to show asynergy with patients presenting a disorder of the cerebellar apparatus.... In summary, asynergy may be not be indicative of the disorder of a function that would consist in associating the different movements composing an act, but would be only the consequence of the other elementary perturbations of motility."

[43] F. Lhermitte, "Le syndrome cérébelleux. Etude anatomo-clinique chez l'adulte" [Cerebellar syndrome. An anatomical and clinical study in adults], in *Le cervelet* (Paris: Masson, 1958), 7–49.

to the noncoordination of the muscles responsible for phonation, and (6) potential oculomotor disturbances (ocular dysmetry, nystagmus).[44] Certain cognitivoaffective disorders are considered as possibly related to cerebellar lesions.[45]

Babinski's work on cerebellar symptomatology provided several diagnostic tests that are currently included in the basic neurological exam, all carrying the same names Babinski used: hypermetry (assessed with the technique of the finger on the nose and of the heel on the knee), adiadochokinesia (the "puppet" test), and asynergy (combined flexion of the thigh and trunk). Cerebellar catalepsy has disappeared. For unknown reasons, Babinski did not cite hypotony, although since Stewart and Holmes it has been considered of great importance in the diagnosis of cerebellar syndrome.

---

[44] J. de Recondo, *Sémiologie du système nerveux. Du symptôme au diagnostic* [Nervous system semeiology. From symptoms to diagnosis], 2nd ed. (Paris: Médecine-Sciences Flammarion, 2004); P. Trouillas, "Le syndrome cérébelleux" [Cerebellar syndrome], http://spiral.univ-lyon1.fr/polycops/NeuroInterFac/NeuroInterFac-3.5.html; "Syndrome cérébelleux," photocopied course document, Faculté Pitié-Salpêtrière, http://www.chups.jussieu.fr/polys/neuro/semioneuro/Poly.Chp.3.3.html.
[45] Schmahmann, "Disorders of the cerebellum."

··· *thirteen* ···

Babinski and the Birth of French Neurosurgery

A few days before Babinski's death in 1932, when his friend Jean Ferdinand Darier asked him what had been his greatest medical achievement, his answer was: "You may think it is the sign. I would rather say that the most important was showing the way to neurosurgery to de Martel and Vincent."[1]

Neurosurgery at the End of the Nineteenth Century

Sir William Macewen (1848–1924), from Glasgow, was probably the first to operate on a brain tumor when in 1879 he removed a frontal meningioma revealed by focal convulsions, a few months after having operated on a subdural hematoma.[2] Other attempts followed, but the choice of the site of trepanation remained a challenge, as it was based mainly on the observation of signs and symptoms. In 1884 Sir Rickman John Godlee (1849–1925), a nephew of Joseph Lister, operated on a lesion diagnosed by the neurologist Hughes Bennet (1848–1901), and in 1887 a tumor was recognized by Sir William Gowers and operated on by Victor Horsley, who at that time was at the National Hospital for the Paralyzed and the Epileptic in London

---

[1] C. Vincent, "J. Babinski (1857–1932)," *Rev Neurol (Paris)* 1932 (2): 441–446.
[2] W. Macewen, "Intracranial lesions: tumor of the dura mater," *Lancet* 1881 (2): 541–543.

and rapidly became one of the European pioneers of this new surgery.[3] In August 1890 he reported at the Tenth International Medical Congress in Berlin his operations on brain tumors, and in 1891 Sir Rupert Boyce, assistant to Horsley, gave a presentation at the French Congress of Surgery, held in Paris, on Horsley's trepanation technique.[4]

Such examples stimulated the interest of many specialists around the world, such as the neurologist Moses Allen Starr (1854–1932), the New York surgeon Charles McBurney (1845–1913), and William Williams Keen (1837–1932), who is credited with the first removal of a brain tumor in the United States, in Philadelphia in 1887.[5] In Germany, Ernst Von Bergman (1836–1907), a war surgeon, developed the technology of antisepsis after Lister. A generation later came Fedor Krause (1856–1937) and Hermann Oppenheim (1858–1919), who in 1899 demonstrated the value of X-rays, discovered a few years before by Wilhem Konrad Röntgen (1845–1922), in the diagnosis of a tumor of the hypophysis. In Italy, June 1, 1885 can be considered the birthdate of neurosurgery, as on that day in Rome, Francesco Durante (1844–1934), professor of surgery at the Royal University, successfully resected an olfactory groove meningioma, inspiring admiration worldwide.[6] Ludwig Martynovich Pussep (1875–1942) in Estonia was a pupil of the famous neurologist and psychiatrist Vladimir Bekhterev (1857–1927), who established the first operating room within the neurology department of the Russian Military Medical Academy in 1897.[7]

By the end of the century, about two hundred brain tumors had been operated on. However, the results were far from being satisfactory, as noted by David Ferrier (1843–1924) at the 1898 annual meeting of the British Medical Association; quoting the statistics collected by Allen Starr, he remarked that the recovery rate did not reach 40 percent, while mortality was close to

---

[3] R. C. Mulholland, "Historical perspective: Sir William Gowers, 1845–1915," *Spine* 1996, 721(9): 1106–1110; J. B. Lyons, "Sir Victor Horsley," *Medical History* 1967, 11(4): 361–373; V. Horsley, "Remarks on ten consecutive cases of operations upon the brain and cranial cavity to illustrate the details and safety of the method employed," *Br Med J* 1887 (1): 863–865.

[4] *Le Progrès Médical*, April 4, 1891, 278–282.

[5] M. A. Starr, *Brain Surgery* (New York: William Wood, 1893); W. W. Keen, "Three successful cases of cerebral surgery including the removal of a large intra cranial fibroma, resection of damaged brain tissue and resection of the cerebral cortex for the left hand. With remarks on the general technique for such operations," *Trans Am Surg Assoc* 1888 (6): 293–347, cited in *Le Progrès Médical*, April 5, 1890, 278.

[6] G. M. De Caro, A. Brunori, and R. Giuffre, "La neurochirurgia a Roma" [Neurosurgery in Rome, 1880–1970], *Ann Ital Chir* 1998 (69): 249–284.

[7] B. L. Lichterman, "Roots and routes of Russian neurosurgery (from surgical neurology towards neurological surgery)," *Journal of History of Neurosciences* 1998, 7(2): 125–135.

20 percent. His conclusions were rather pessimistic: "Treatment of intracranial tumors forms rather a melancholy chapter in therapeutics."[8]

News about neurosurgical developments made their way back to France, where *Le Progrès Médical* regularly referred to the operations performed by Victor Horsley; Charcot attended the 1881 International Medical Congress in London, where he discovered the physiological work of David Ferrier and was enthusiastic about Horsley's initial results. It is especially interesting to note that in 1887, in one of his weekly Tuesday lessons, Charcot spoke of the future of neurosurgery: "The operation is extremely simple; we should now follow the British surgeons, and when I see a case of motor partial seizure, I will refer it to one of my surgical colleagues; trepanation today does not carry a high risk and we have to think about it. You will see one day, everyone will be doing the same."[9]

Neurosurgery in France

Some French general surgeons, such as Paul Poirier (1857–1907), Félix Terrier (1837–1908), Paul Broca, Antony Chipault (1866–1920), Georges Marion (1869–1960), and Mathieu Jaboulay (1860–1913), began to be interested in cranial or spinal surgery around this time.

Paul Poirier, a professor of anatomy with whom Babinski had a cordial relationship, published in 1891 a book on cranioencephalic topography.[10] Félix Terrier reported at the Société de chirurgie in 1891 on craniotomy for Jacksonian convulsions, where the operation was followed by improvement in half of the cases.[11] Two years later, he published a book on trepanation.[12] But already some surgeons were complaining that they were consulted too late. As Paul Lucas-Championnière (1843–1913) noted: "If Horsley and Macewen and the American surgeons obtain more success, it is because the medical students have learned at the university to refer the patients earlier to surgery."[13]

---

[8] D. Ferrier, "Annual meeting: section of neurology," *Br Med J* 1898 (2): 964–970.

[9] J. M. Charcot, foreword in François François-Franck, *Leçons sur les fonctions motrices du cerveau* [Lessons on motor functions of the brain] (Paris: Doin, 1887).

[10] P. Poirier, *Topographie crânio-encéphalique. Trépanation* [Cranioencephalic topography. Trepanation] (Paris: Lecrosnier et Babe, 1891); review in *Le Progrès Médical* 1891 (XIII): 114–116. For more on Poirier's life, see his obituary in *Le Progrès Médical* 1907 (XXIII): 289–291.

[11] *Le Progrès Medical* 1891 (XIII): 471–472.

[12] F. Terrier and M. Peraire, *L'opération du trépan* [The trepaning operation] (Paris: Alcane, 1895).

[13] *Le Progrès Medical* 1891 (XIII): 487–488.

At the same time, Mathieu Jaboulay—an anatomist in Lyon, a brilliant general surgeon, and a pioneer in experimental kidney transplantation—had started to operate on brain tumors.[14] He took a broader approach to surgery of the nervous system, proposing operations for epilepsy or hydrocephalus and describing a technique of drainage of cerebral fluid into the temporal fossa muscle to treat subarachnoid space hypertension. His career was suddenly interrupted by his premature death in a railway accident.

In 1896, one year after Joseph Babinski took over the direction of a medical department at La Pitié, the first issue of the journal *Travaux de Neurologie Chirurgicale* appeared; this was the first journal devoted to surgery of the nervous system.[15] It was founded by Antony Chipault, who in 1894 had authored a monograph on surgery of the spinal cord and a year later had published an extensive book reviewing the state of neurosurgery at the time and describing the various approaches used for brain lesions.[16]

Also appearing in 1896 was Broca and Maubrac's book on cerebral surgery, in which the authors discussed head injuries, tumors, and brain abscesses; operative indications, trepanation technique, and cranial osteoplasty were also considered, as were the risks of cerebral surgery.[17] Maurice Auvray wrote his medical thesis in that same year, summarizing the first results of cranial surgery.[18]

Individual attempts at cranial surgery had been made before. Paul Broca, better known for his work on cerebral localization and speech mechanisms, was also interested, as a surgeon, in defining skull landmarks and underlying lesions. In a patient exhibiting a nonconfluent aphasia one month after injury, he determined by external measurements the projection of the speech area, permitting a trepanation over the region of the third frontal convolution in 1871. This case likely represents the first craniotomy based on cerebral localization; however, it remained little known, published in a nonmedical journal five years after the fact.[19]

[14] M. Jaboulay, "La trépanation décompressive (la mobilisation de la voûte du crâne)" [Decompressive craniotomy (movability of cranial vault)], *Lyon Medical* 1896, LXXXIII(38): 73–75.
[15] A. Chipault, *Travaux de neurologie chirurgicale* [Works in surgical neurology] (Paris: L. Bataille et Cie, 1896).
[16] A. Chipault, *Études de chirurgies médullaires, historique, chirurgie opératoire, traitement* [Studies on spinal cord surgery, history, operative techniques, treatment] (Paris: F. Alcan, 1894); A. Chipault, *Chirurgie opératoire du système nerveux* [Operative surgery of the nervous system], 2 vols. (Paris: Rueff et Cie, 1894–95).
[17] A. Broca and P. Maubrac, *Traité de chirurgie cérébrale* [Treatise on brain surgery] (Paris: Masson, 1896).
[18] M. Auvray, *Les tumeurs cérébrales* [Brain tumors] (Paris: Henri Jouve, 1896).
[19] P. Broca, "Diagnostic d'un abcès situe au niveau de la région du langage; trépanation de cet abcès" [Diagnosis of an abcess located in the speech area; trepanation of this abcess], *Rev Anthropol* 1876 (5): 244–248.

Despite these attempts, at the end of the nineteenth century neurologists were hesitant to refer their patients for surgery. As Antony Chipault describes it, "Neurologists, who have accepted with so much confidence operations that are rarely successful in brain abscesses because these kill rapidly, are reluctant to propose the same operations... in intracranial tumors because their evolution is slow and they do not want to cause a brutal end to a chronic affection." Forty years later, Clovis Vincent recalled this time in a speech marking the creation of the neurosurgical chair in Paris:

> The neurologist referred the patient to the surgeon with an incomplete or at times faulty diagnosis; on the other hand, the surgeon had not yet any knowledge of the brain's physiology or anatomical configuration on the living patient. Neither did he have the "soft touch" and cautionary approach so necessary; above all, the necessary technical facilities were not available to him.[20]

Chipault, however, was not completely discouraged, and he continued along his solitary path, helped by some well-known neurologists such as Pierre Marie. In 1894 Chipault described the anatomical relationship between spinal roots and spinal processes known as "Chipault laws."[21] In 1895, he advised physicians performing lumbar puncture to use the space between L5 and S1 rather than that between L4 and L5, as proposed by Heinrich Irenaeus Quincke (1842–1922).[22] In 1901, he showed that the epidural injection of cocaine offered an active anesthesia, allowing operations on rectum, perineum, and lower limbs without the inconvenience of the subarachnoid approach.[23] In 1903 he published in collaboration with several surgeons a new and important book on the state of surgery of the nervous system.[24] Unfortunately, Chipault suffered from a slowly progressive quadriplegia, forcing him to retire prematurely in 1905; he would die fifteen years later. His retirement can explain partially the delay in the development of neurosurgery in France.

---

[20] C. Vincent, "Leçon inaugurale pour la chaire de neurochirurgie" [Opening speech for the neurosurgical chair], *Presse Médicale* 1939 (1): 761–766.
[21] A. Chipault, "Rapport de l'origine des nerfs rachidiens avec les apophyses épineuses" [Relationships between spinal nerves and spinous processes], *Archives de Neurologie* 1895 (XXIX): 150–151.
[22] A. Chipault, "Manuel opératoire de la ponction vertébrale lombo-sacrée" [Operative technique manual for the sacro-lumbar puncture], *Archives de Neurologie* 1895 (XXIX): 472.
[23] A. Chipault, "Rachicocainisation" [Spinal injection of cocaine], *Le Progrès Médical* 1901 (XIII): 375–376.
[24] A. Chipault, *Etat actuel de la chirurgie nerveuse* [Present status of nervous system surgery], 3 vols. (Paris: J. Rueff, 1903).

However, despite many failures, a glimmer of hope appeared in some reports. Henri Duret (1849–1921), in an address to a surgical meeting in 1903, remarked: "Surgery for brain tumors is rare and difficult...patients die from the operation in 19 percent of the cases...but reviewing 344 cases operated, it appears that for more than half of them, there has been a clear improvement or even a complete cure."[25] Duret's report was considered a complete summary of existing knowledge at that time, and he was congratulated for it.[26] Dean of the Free Faculty of Medicine in Lille, he is especially known for his studies in Charcot's laboratory on cerebral vessels.[27] His name is attached to the brain stem hemorrhage in transtentorial herniation.[28]

Around the turn of the century, the pioneers of neurosurgery began to retire or turn their attention to other spheres of interest. Horsley became more interested in the social aspects of medicine than in neurosurgery; he died in 1916, during World War I, in a small hospital in Mesopotamia. Macewen retained a professorship of surgery at Glasgow University, but he worked alone as a general surgeon.

To develop and acquire new dimensions, surgery of the nervous system had to find new roads. The first to have understood that and realized it in practice was certainly Harvey Cushing (1869–1939).[29] He studied surgery under William Stewart Halsted (1852–1922), and he visited Emil Theodor Kocher (1841–1917) in Switzerland, Fedor Krause in Germany, and Victor Horsley in Great Britain, which gave him an interest in neurosurgery. He rapidly came to the conclusion that in order to be successful, he would have to devote all his time to this new field, from diagnosis to the operating theater and the postoperative period. While Cushing is considered the true founder of neurosurgery, two other names emerged in the United States at the beginning of the century: Charles Harrison Frazier (1870–1936), professor of clinical surgery at the University of Pennsylvania, described retrogasserian neurotomy and spinal cordotomy, and Charles Elsberg (1871–1948), the first chief of neurological surgery at the New York Neurological Institute, was

---

[25] H. Duret, *Tumeurs de l'encéphale: rapport au congrès de chirurgie* [Brain tumors: report to the congress on surgery] (Paris: F. Alcan, 1903), 393–407.

[26] *Le Progrès Médical* 1905 (XXI): 869.

[27] L. Tatu, T. Moulin, and G. Monnier, "The discovery of encephalic arteries. From Johann Jacob Wepfer to Charles Foix," *Cerebrovasc Dis* 2005 (20): 427–432.

[28] P. M. Parizel, S. Makkat, G. Jorens, et al., "Brain stem haemorrhage in descending transtentorial herniation (Duret hemorrhage)," *Intensive Care Medicine* 2002 (28): 85–88.

[29] E. Anderson and W. Haymaker, "Harvey Cushing (1869–1939)," in W. Haymaker and F. Schiller, eds., *The Founders of Neurology*, 2nd ed. (Springfield, Ill.: Charles C. Thomas, 1970), 543–549.

probably the surgeon who had the greatest experience in spinal cord tumors; Clovis Vincent considered Elsberg and Babinski the only men able to make a precise diagnosis of cord compression. Initially a disciple of Cushing before coming into conflict with him, Walter Dandy (1886–1946) was an exceptional surgeon, inventing in 1918 the technique of injecting air into the brain ventricles; his remarkable treatise on surgical technique remained in print for many years.[30]

Spinal Tumors

The fundamental problem with spinal tumors was how to obtain a precise and early diagnosis. Babinski, with his meticulous and almost obsessive method, tried to find objective signs that would allow recognition of brain and spinal tumors. But without a reasonable guarantee of success he would not accept the risks of surgery, and for almost ten years he did not refer any patient to a surgeon except for palliative operations.

It is not surprising that under these conditions, the neurological examination was first used to identify spinal lesions. Two successive papers insisted on the value of the neurological exam. The first was presented at the Academie de médecine.[31] The conclusions of the second one, presented at the Société de neurologie, are especially interesting, as they predicted localization and, eventually, etiology:

> While the topography of anesthesia generally permits the recognition of the superior limit of a spinal compression, the inferior one is generally determined by the level where the defense reflex is found. In a compression syndrome, if the distance between the anesthesia limit and defense reflex is important, the hypothesis of compression by an extradural tumor or by pachymeningitis is likely. On the other hand, if the two limits are identical or close, it is extremely probable that we are in the presence of an intradural tumor.[32]

An increasing number of spinal tumors were diagnosed at La Pitié; by this point Babinski was convinced of the value of surgery, and in 1911 he decided

---

[30] W. E. Dandy, *The Brain* (Hagerstown, Md.: W. F. Prior, 1966).

[31] J. Babinski, "Sur la localisation des lésions comprimant la moelle. De la possibilité d'en déterminer le siège au moyen des réflexes de défense" [On the localization of compressive lesions of the spinal cord. On the possibility of finding their level with defense reflexes], *Bull Acad Ntle Méd* 1910 (17): 371–374.

[32] J. Babinski and J. Jarkovski, "Sur la possibilité de déterminer la hauteur de la lésion dans les paraplégies d'origine spinale par certaines perturbations des réflexes" [On the possibility of finding the level of a lesion in paraplegias of spinal origin the modification of reflexes], *Rev Neurol (Paris)* 1910 (XIX): 666–668.

to refer his first patient to Horsley in London. In the same year, he referred another patient to a well-known French general surgeon, Paul Lecène (1878–1929); the operation, carried out on March 17, 1911, was for removal of a spinal meningioma. A year later, Thierry de Martel (1876–1940) operated on another tumor at the exact level predicted by the neurological exam.[33] In France it was the first such operation to be undertaken in a truly stepwise fashion, and the first results were reported in the medical thesis of André Gendron, a pupil of Babinski.[34] At an international meeting in Paris (June 8–9, 1923), where the topic was spinal cord compression, two reports were submitted: one on anatomy, etiology, and pathological anatomy, presented by Sir James Purves Stewart (1869–1949) and Georges Riddoch (1888–1947), the other on clinical pathology and treatment by Charles Foix (1882–1927). A few years later Babinski was able to report on thirteen cases (with five deaths, two stabilizations, and six showing marked improvement).[35]

At that time, the physician with the most extensive experience with spinal tumors was Charles Elsberg in the United States. As early as 1912, he reported on forty-three laminectomies. In 1916, he published his notable book on diagnosis and treatment of tumors of the spinal cord and its membranes, and in 1925 he brought out a textbook reporting on a hundred cases of confirmed tumors.[36]

The development of the contrast myelogram with lipiodol by Jean-Athanase Sicard (1872–1929) and Jacques Forestier (1890–1978) around the same time added an important diagnostic tool, even if some neurologists and neurosurgeons were initially skeptical about its usefulness.

Maurice Robineau (1870–1950), a general surgeon, *Chirurgien des Hôpitaux de Paris*, to whom Sicard referred his patients, rapidly obtained

---

[33] J. Babinski, T. de Martel, and J. Jumentié, "Tumeur méningée de la région dorsale supérieure; paraplégie par compression de la moelle. Extraction de la tumeur. Guérison" [Meningeal tumor of the superior thoracic region; paraplegia due to compression of the spinal cord. Removal of the tumor. Recovery], *Rev Neurol (Paris)* 1912 (23): 640–644; J. Babinski, P. Lecène, and F. Bourlot, "Tumeur méningée: paraplégie par compression de la moelle. Extraction de la tumeur, guérison" [Meningeal tumor: paraplegia due to the compression of the spinal cord. Removal of the tumor, recovery], *Rev Neurol (Paris)* 1912 (23): 1–4.

[34] A. Gendron, "Étude clinique des tumeurs de la moelle et des méninges spinales. Contribution à l'étude des localisations médullaires en hauteur" [A clinical study of spinal cord and meningeal tumors. A contribution to the study of level in spinal cord lesions], medical thesis, 1913, Paris.

[35] J. Babinski, "Sur le traitement des tumeurs juxta médullaires" [On the treatment of tumors close to the spinal cord], *Rev Neurol (Paris)* 1923 (39): 695–701.

[36] I. S. Weschler, "Charles Elsberg (1871–1948)," in W. Haymaker and F. Schiller, eds., *The Founders of Neurology*, 2nd ed. (Springfield, Ill.: Charles C. Thomas, 1970), 552–554.

excellent results in cerebral and spinal tumors. He was also a pioneer in France for trigeminal retrogasserian neurotomy. "For a long time, as did de Martel, he operated on brain and spinal cord tumors with means which today appear rudimentary. But his perfect anatomical knowledge of the nervous system, his skill, his caution, allowed him to obtain amazing results that converted neurologists who had not yet put their trust in this new field of surgery."[37]

Cerebral Tumors

The problem was much more complicated for brain tumors, as Joseph Babinski noted in 1910:

> It is known that in cases of brain tumor craniectomy is the only curative way...and it may show remarkable results. But it appears also from the cases already published that recoveries are rare if one considers all the conditions necessary for a direct operation to be successful: the existence of a neoplasm has to be proved and its location recognized; the tumor must be benign and not deeply situated, in order that its extirpation does not create too much brain damage.[38]

If we add to these rational limitations the fact that Babinski, always scrupulous and anxious, did not want to put a patient at risk for an uncertain result, it is possible to understand why for ten years cranial decompression was the only solution he proposed. If the limits of such a technique were clear, its action in controlling papilledema was nevertheless noteworthy. Babinski recognized, after Victor Horsley, the existence of a syndrome of pseudotumor, where cranial decompression was an extremely effective treatment. On the other hand, with inoperable tumors (which many tumors were considered to be at this time), craniectomy was able to stabilize intracranial hypertension for several weeks or months. Following Cushing's recommendations, Babinski advised performing it in the temporal region of the nondominant hemisphere. In the same article, he went back to the value of lumbar puncture in some cases of advanced papilledema, recognized too late for cranial decompression, a point that was already hardly disputed: however, Babinski tried to justify the usefulness of this technique: "The risks did not appear to

---

[37] A. Sicard, Leçon inaugurale [Opening lesson], Chair of Clinical Surgery of the Beaujon hospital, *La Presse Médicale*, January 2, 1957, 19–22.
[38] J. Babinski, "De la craniectomie décompressive" [On decompressive craniotomy], *Bull Médical*, April 20, 1910, 247–253.

be too great if some rules were followed: the patient should be placed in a horizontal position in order to subtract CSF very slowly, in a small amount, and to stop evacuation if the flow was too rapid."[39]

In 1910, the palliative method appeared to have limited indications, as emphasized by Horsley in an address to the German society of neurologists.[40] But brain surgery was beginning to take off in France. Just a year before, after a long period of hesitation, Babinski had proposed to a general surgeon, Antonin Gosset (1872–1944), in the case of a patient with severe papilledema and stupor, a direct approach on the frontal lobe based upon clinical signs; the side of approach was chosen according to the location of maximum papilledema and pain. No tumor was found. Two weeks later, after the patient's death, autopsy revealed a contralateral glioma. Babinski recognized very honestly his error, which was due to a false localization. At the same time, Jumentié and de Martel underlined the importance of clinical work for diagnosis.[41] Maurice Lannois (born in 1856), a neurologist from Lyon who worked with Jaboulay, reported two cases of direct approach to cerebellopontine angle tumors.[42]

During the March 29, 1911, session of the Société de chirurgie, several surgeons, including Lucas-Championnière, Delorme, Sieur, Walther, and Lejars (the last of whom had operated on a patient referred by Babinski), debated craniotomy.[43] The same year, the existence of an external cranial exostosis allowed Thierry de Martel to remove a frontal osteomeningioma.[44] This first success represented the beginning of a regular collaboration; in fact, for several years Babinski had been looking for a surgeon who would devote himself wholly to surgery of the nervous system. Clovis Vincent, at

---

[39] Résultats thérapeutiques de la ponction lombaire dans les névrites optiques d'origine intra-crânienne. [Therapeutic results of lumbar puncture in optic neuritis of intracranial origin]. *Bulletins et mémoires de la Société Française d'ophtalmologie*, May 1907, 590–597.

[40] V. Horsley, "Surgical versus the expectant treatment of intracranial tumor," *BMJ*, December 10, 1910, 1833–1835.

[41] J. Jumentié and T. de Martel, "Deux cas de tumeurs sous corticales diagnostiquées et localisées par la clinique" [Two cases of subcortical tumors clinically recognized and localized], *Rev Neurol (Paris)* 1910 (XIX): 529–532.

[42] M. Lannois and M. Durand "Deux cas de tumeurs de l'angle ponto-cérébelleux (tumeurs de l'acoustique opérées chirurgicalement)" [Two cases of cerebellopontine angle tumors (surgery on acoustic nerve tumors)], *Rev Neurol (Paris)* 1909 (XVII): 674.

[43] *Le Progrès Médical* 1911 (XXXI): 177.

[44] J. Babinski and T. de Martel, "Trépanation pour tumeur cérébrale. Ablation de la tumeur; grande amélioration" [Trepanation for brain tumor. Removal; marked improvement], *Rev Neurol (Paris)* 1909 (XVII): 665–667.

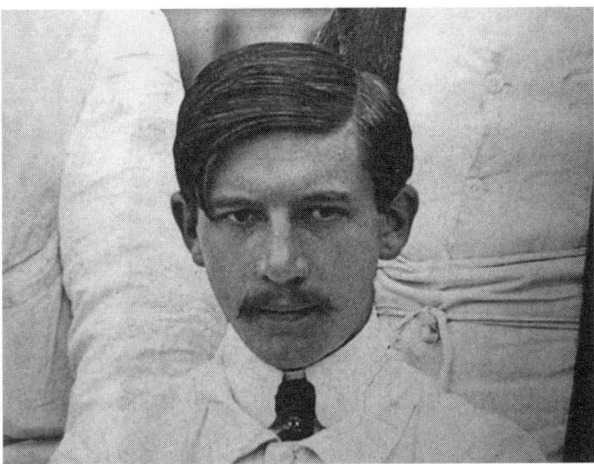

Figure 13-1 Clovis Vincent while a resident at the Salpêtrière Hospital in 1908–1909. (*Source*: Personal collection, J. Philippon.)

that time an assistant in neurology, suggested collaborating with de Martel, who had been his colleague during residency in 1904 (Figs. 13-1 and 13-2).

Vincent and de Martel made a curious duo inasmuch as they were opposite in so many ways. De Martel was the aristocratic son of the Comtesse de Martel de Janville (1850–1932), a woman of letters who was descended from the well-known revolutionary family of the Comte de Mirabeau (1749–1791). Clovis Vincent, the son of a general practitioner in rural France, was a hard worker with a very independent character. In 1910, the thirty-four-year-old de Martel, already a brilliant general surgeon with a strong competitive streak (he was an active sportsman, regularly practicing boxing), did not hesitate to enter the new field of neurosurgery, and he took his training very seriously. He wanted to improve his technique, so at Babinski's suggestion he went to London every week for a period of several months to attend Victor Horsley's Thursday-morning operative sessions, returning to Paris the next day to pursue his own work.

His deep gratitude to Babinski is clearly evident in an address to the Société de neurologie in 1928:

> Twenty years ago, among the French neurologists, J. Babinski understood all that surgery could offer to patients with brain and spinal cord tumors. He was the first supporter of neurosurgery in France and our leader.... Dr. Babinski chooses me as his surgeon; when he referred one of his patients to me and attended the operation from beginning to end, I sensed how much he regretted not being able to operate himself. Is this not normal? The neurologist dealt with and examined so many brains in every sense that he knew the

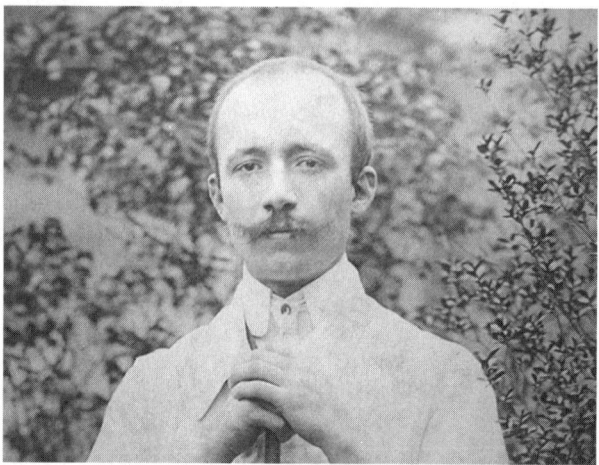

Figure 13-2 Thierry de Martel while a resident at the Salpêtrière Hospital in 1902–1903. (*Source*: Personal collection, J. Philippon.)

anatomy and physiology infinitely better than the general surgeon. Is he not more qualified to remove a tumor or to detect a lesion during an operation?

Convinced of this, for the last two years I have asked C. Vincent to assist in all my brain operations; I have taught him all that I know as a surgeon. He has done his best to return the favor in neurology. Together we are a team that works in perfect harmony, but sometimes the number of operations has obliged us to separate, with each working on his own; C. Vincent has already presented several patients whom he has operated upon and cured completely independently. I wanted particularly to say this in the presence of Dr. Babinski, who throughout so many years gave me much encouragement. It is without doubt a great satisfaction to him that I pass the scalpel to C. Vincent, his preferred pupil, and in doing so, I am serving French neurosurgery in the best way possible.

At the International Congress of Medicine in London in 1913, one of the topics was the treatment of cerebral tumors. After a general presentation by Bruns (from Hanover) and Tooth (from London),[45] Fedor Krause (from Berlin) reported on 154 cases of brain tumor, while de Martel was the only French surgeon to speak. In making a presentation on decompressive craniotomy, de Martel noted, "This technique has been established in collaboration with Joseph Babinski, who has been among the French neurologists the first ardent supporter of surgery of the nervous system." Some other great neurologists, such as Pierre Marie, began to refer neurological patients to de

---

[45] J. Bruns and M. H. Tooth, "Le traitement des tumeurs du cerveau" [Brain tumor treatment], *Rev Neurol (Paris)* 1913 (XXVI): 343–347.

Martel.⁴⁶ It is interesting to note that in the report presented at the Société de Neurologie, which included twenty five cases of cranial surgery, only three took a direct approach to the tumor, the others being palliative.⁴⁷

The War

On August 2, 1914, a general mobilization order was issued, and the team that had begun to be so productive was obliged to disband. Babinski maintained his activities at La Pitié, assuming at the same time the direction of a military neurological department at the Lycée Buffon. He quickly became involved in the challenge presented by the arrival of numerous wounded soldiers with affections or lesions of the nervous system, as can be seen by the fact that alone or in collaboration with Jules Froment, a neurologist from Lyon, he published in one year (1915) eighteen papers on nervous disorders related to traumatic nerve lesions.⁴⁸ He contrasted signs related to true nerve lesions with those caused by muscular or tendinous pathologies. He insisted on the distinction between hysterical or malingering manifestations and what he called those of "reflex origin," the organicity of which could be shown by the exaggeration of the reflexes under chloroform anesthesia and which were attributed to a sympathetic nervous system dysfunction (Fig. 13-3).

De Martel, remaining true to his ideals, managed to be assigned as a physician on the front line; for his courageous actions, he received the Legion of Honor and the War Cross. He was wounded, but as soon he recovered, he went to work on a hospital boat in the Dardanelles; a few months later, struck down by malaria, he was repatriated to Paris, but was far from being inactive, continuing to practice surgery and sharing his experience of war surgery.⁴⁹

---

⁴⁶ P. Marie, T. de Martel, and C. Chatelin, "Dix huit mois de chirurgie nerveuse dans le service du Professeur P. Marie à la Salpêtrière" [Eighteen months of surgery of the nervous system in the department of Professor P. Marie at the Salpêtrière Hospital], *Revue Neurol (Paris)* 1913 (XXVI): 132–134.

⁴⁷ T. de Martel and C. Chatelin, "Tumeur du lobe frontal droit. Opération en deux temps, ablation de la tumeur" [Right frontal lobe tumor. Operation in two phases, removal of the tumor], *Rev Neurol (Paris)* 1913 (XXV): 139–142.

⁴⁸ J. Babinski, "Sur les lésions des nerfs par blessure de guerre" [On nerve lesions by war wounds], *Rev Neurol (Paris)* 1915 (17–18): 273–279; J. Babinski and J. Froment, "Service de neurologie militarisé de l'hôpital de la Pitié" [Neurological military department at the Pitié Hospital], *Rev Neurol (Paris)* 1915 (23–24): 1151–1154.

⁴⁹ T. de Martel and C. Chatelin, *Les blessures du crâne et du cerveau* [Cranial and brain wounds] (Paris: Masson, 1917); S. Delaporte, "*Les médecins dans la Grande Guerre*

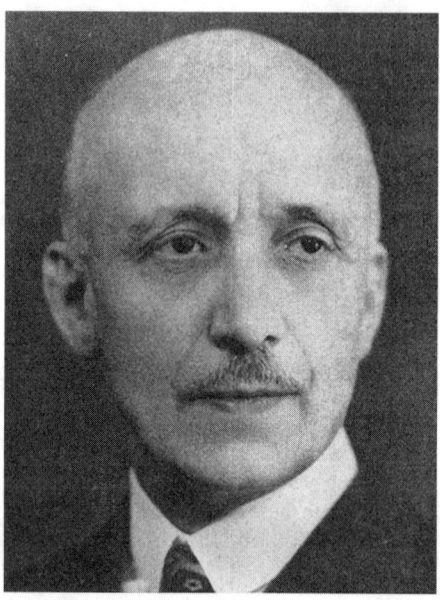

Figure 13-3   Thierry de Martel. (*Source*: Photographic collection, Assistance publique, Hôpitaux de Paris.)

Clovis Vincent also had an exemplary stint at the front; after being wounded and decorated, he was named chief of a neurological military center: trying to distinguish between the true patients and the hysterical or malingering, he sometimes used methods that have been criticized, including applying a light electric shock with a needle ("torpedoing," in military vocabulary). A soldier who had heard of the pain caused by this technique and was not willing to be treated this way struck Vincent in the face; the physician retaliated in a similar manner. The incident was widely reported in the press and raised the question of the right of patients to refuse to be treated. In the lawsuit that followed, Vincent was vindicated, as several medical authorities, including Babinski, testified on his behalf.

Toward the end of the war, Babinski went through periodic phases of discouragement, to the point where he considered leaving neurology altogether and working at the Pasteur Institute. Why did this happen? A letter to Babinski wrote to Moniz shows that he was deeply affected by what he

1914–1918 [Physicians during the First World War] (Paris: Bayard, 2003); H. Giroire, *Clovis Vincent 1879–1947, pionnier de la neurochirurgie française* [Clovis Vincent 1879–1947, a pioneer of French neurosurgery] (Paris: Olivier Perrin, 1972).

termed the folly of war. One should not forget that at the age of sixty, he was carrying a full patient load at the hospital, his private practice, and heavy responsibilities in directing the military neurological department at the Lycée Buffon. It is reasonable to think that he was, at least temporarily, attracted by the less stressful atmosphere at the Pasteur Institute. When the war ended and his assistants returned, he regained his enthusiasm for clinical work, and maintained it until his official retirement in 1923.

During this period of his life, he was primarily concerned with spinal cord compression, and he wrote four short papers on the topic between 1920 and 1926. The importance of a precise neurological examination was demonstrated by a case in which a small lesion (the size of a grape) was diagnosed at the level of the fifth and sixth cervical roots through the inversion of the radial reflex. Results presented in 1924 showed that only half of the patients who have been operated had clearly improved, but this was largely due to late diagnosis.[50]

Especially interesting was the attitude of Babinski the clinician toward opacification of the spinal space by lipiodol, the first radiological technique able to help the neurologist in determining the level of a compression.[51] While Clovis Vincent was hostile to the technique, at least at the beginning, Babinski displayed some interest.[52] Discussing a case with a negative result, however, Babinski noted that the technique was not able to rule out a compression. "If we do not take into account such a possibility, this interesting way of diagnosis would risk failing to recognize the existence of a lesion and delay the necessary operation."[53]

His enthusiasm grew when Egas Moniz presented the first results of cerebral angiography.[54] At a meeting of the Société de neurologie in 1927,

---

[50] J. Babinski and J. Jarkovski, "Quelques documents relatifs aux compressions de la moelle" [Some documents concerning spinal cord compressions], *Rev Neurol (Paris)* 1924 (6): 375–405.

[51] J. A. Sicard, J. Forestier, and L. Laplane, "Radiodiagnostic lipiodolé au cours des compressions rachidiennes" [Intraspinal injection of lipiodol for the diagnosis of spinal cord compressions], *Rev Neurol (Paris)* 1923 (6): 276.

[52] J. Babinski, "Sur l'épreuve du lipiodol comme moyen de diagnostic des compressions médullaires" [On the lipiodol technique for the diagnosis of spinal cord compressions], *Rev Neurol (Paris)* 1924 (1): 228–230.

[53] J. Babinski, "Paraplégie crurale par compression extradurale de la région dorsale. Opération, guérison (sur l'épreuve du lipiodol)" [Crural paraplegia caused by an extradural compression of the thoracic cord. Operation, cure (on the lipiodol technique)], *Rev Neurol (Paris)* 1926 (2): 587–595.

[54] E. Moniz, "L'encéphalographie artérielle, son importance dans la localisation des tumeurs cérébrales" [Arterial encephalography, its importance in the diagnosis of brain tumors], *Rev Neurol (Paris)* 1927 (1): 72–90.

Babinski said, "If future observations confirm definitively that the injections are harmless for the patients, all neurologists will be grateful to our distinguished colleague, due to his having provided a new method for the diagnosis of brain tumors, the localization of which is so difficult to determine."

Peripheral Nervous System

Babinski's studies of the peripheral nervous system were a perfect demonstration of his working method, in which clinical observation serves as the basis for a pathogenic hypothesis. In two cases of spasmodic torticollis (considered to be of psychological origin), he observed an extensive plantar response in one patient and the exaggeration of the tricipital reflex in another.[55] He concluded that "this affection is related, if not always at least sometimes, to an irritation of the pyramidal system, the nature of which I cannot pinpoint." He later went even further, suggesting that the variability of the spasm may correspond to a disturbance of the long tract in the vicinity of the striatum.[56]

He proposed as a treatment the surgical section of the peripheral spinal accessory nerve, recognizing at the same time that the results may be transient and surgery may be indicated only if medical treatment has been unsuccessful. He would return at the end of his hospital career to this technique, publishing a new article on it.[57]

Another question was raised by the transient effect of surgery due to the reinnervation of the muscles; he did not know the exact answer, but hypothesized the possibility of a double innervation, explaining the reappearance of the spasticity.

His last paper concerning neurosurgery was published in 1927, in collaboration with Thierry de Martel.[58] Even if he less regularly attended the monthly meetings of the neurological society after this time, he was still

---

[55] J. Babinski, "Sur un cas d'hémispasme (contribution à l'étude de la pathogénie) du torticolis spasmodique" [On a case of hemispasm (contribution to the pathogenesis of spasmodic torticollis)], *Rev Neurol (Paris)* 1900 (8): 142–147.

[56] J. Babinski, E. Krebs, and A. Plichet "Torticolis spasmodique avec lésion du système nerveux central" [Spasmodic torticollis with a central nervous system lesion], *Rev Neurol (Paris)* 1922 (38): 587–593.

[57] J. Babinski, "De la section du spinal externe dans le torticolis spasmodique" [On spinal accessory nerve section in spasmodic torticollis], *Rev Neurol (Paris)* 1924 (4): 453–455.

[58] J. Babinski and T. de Martel, "Tumeur de l'angle pontocérébelleux: amélioration rapide à la suite d'une extirpation intracapsulaire par morcellement" [Cerebellopontine

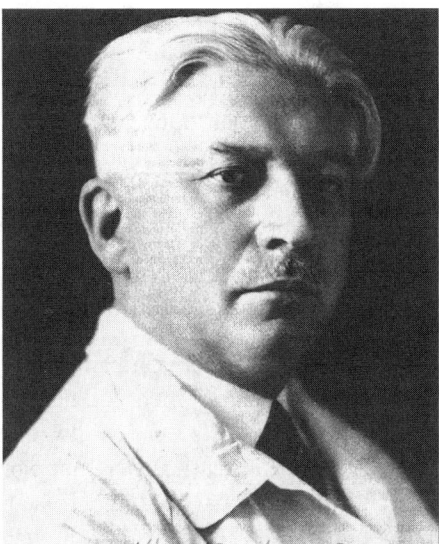

Figure 13-4 Clovis Vincent. (*Source*: Photographic collection, Assistance publique, Hôpitaux de Paris.)

interested in new techniques: for instance, he observed a transsphenoidal operation for pituitary tumor, which had been proposed by Cushing more than twenty years earlier but now had been made easier by the use of cranial X-rays, which allowed visualization of the bone modifications. In France, this technique became commonly used after World War I, and the advantages of different approaches were discussed at a meeting of the Société de biologie.

Before retiring completely from his professional life, Babinski had a last but important satisfaction: his pupil Clovis Vincent, having participated in de Martel's operations for several years, decided to specialize in neurosurgery, strongly encouraged by his old master. Vincent had been particularly impressed during a trip to the United States, where neurosurgery, as the field had been named by Cushing, had become a distinct field. Vincent wanted to make the same thing happen in France; a dispute with his old friend de Martel in 1929 did not prevent rapid progress toward this goal. Unfortunately, the creation of the first department of neurosurgery at La Pitié, under the direction of Vincent, took place in 1933, one year after Babinski's death; this department was given a chair in 1938 (Fig. 13-4).

angle tumor: rapid improvement following intracapsular removal by fragmentation], *Rev Neurol (Paris)* 1925: 371–374.

One may wonder about the exact place of Joseph Babinski in the birth of French neurosurgery. Undoubtedly, brain and spinal surgeries were performed years before he encouraged de Martel and Vincent. Chipault, who often goes unrecognized by French authors, unjustifiably so—for example, he was mentioned only briefly in Vincent's inaugural lesson—is considered as an important pioneer by American authors. Greenblatt, in his history of neurosurgery, remarks that "Chipault's two volumes, which contain more than 1,540 pages, are probably the most important compendium of operative neurosurgery as it was practiced in the two decades between 1875 and 1895."[59]

As mentioned earlier in this chapter, Chipault's early retirement only partially explains the delay in development of neurosurgery in France. Generally speaking, French neurologists were disillusioned by the high failure rate in brain surgery. Furthermore, they were not particularly interested in therapeutics, preferring the classical anatomoclinical method as taught by Laennec, Cruveilher, Charcot, and Vulpian, and were still passionately involved in the debate over hysteria.

Some neurologists did become interested in this new field. As noted above, Pierre Marie published in 1913 data on a series of nervous system operations on patients he had referred to de Martel. Babinski's particular merit was that he considered this type of surgery to be a separate field that required a surgical team exclusively devoted to its practice. De Martel was a brilliant general surgeon, but his hectic schedule and his other interests did not lend himself to such specialization. It was under the influence and encouragement of Babinski that Clovis Vincent shifted his professional orientation to neurosurgery, later becoming the first professor of neurosurgery in France. Relying on the rigor and precision in neurological diagnosis that he had learned from Babinski, Vincent was able to synthesize clinical neurology and surgical treatment. It is through Clovis Vincent that the first school of neurosurgery in France began, much as Babinski had envisaged and worked toward. If Vincent was the founder, Babinski was most certainly the pathfinder.

---

[59] S. Greenblatt, T. F. Dagi, and M. H. Epstein, *A history of neurosurgery in its scientific and professional contexts* (Park Ridge, Ill.: American Association of Neurological Surgeons, 1997).

··· *fourteen* ···

Babinski as Therapist

Babinski's interest in therapy was unusual at the beginning of the last century, a time when French medicine was more interested in clinical research than patient treatment. These evocative lines, taken from an article by Octave Mirbeau (1848–1917), appeared in the newspaper *Le Matin* on June 27, 1907:

> I timidly asked the professor after his lesson: "What about the treatment, sir?" "Well!... Yes, of course! Whatever you want... exactly what you want!" I wrote rapidly at random, a short prescription, and, showing to him: "Is it like that?" He did not even give a glance, and said to me, looking tired, irritated: "Naturally, of course!... It does not matter."[1]

Unlike the majority of his fellow neurologists, Babinski was deeply committed to therapeutics, as many of his biographers remark.[2] It was certainly not under the influence of Charcot that he acquired this interest: in fact, "Charcot did not care about cure or even treatment. Therapeutics was devoid of attraction; his prescriptions were generally limited to some hygienic precepts, associated with bromide or chloral and taking the waters in Lamalou."[3]

---

[1] Archives de la Préfecture de police de Paris, Box BA 1190.
[2] E. Krebs, "Nécrologie J. Babinski 1857–1932" [Obituary J. Babinski 1857–1932], *L'Encéphale* 1933 (1): 72–80; A. Charpentier, "Babinski (Joseph) (1857–1932)," in M. Genty, ed., *Les biographies médicales* [Medical biographies] (Paris: Librairie J. B. Baillière et fils, 1937–39), VI: 17–32; T. Ott in *Rev Neurol (Paris)* 1958 (98): 664.
[3] L. Daudet, *Les oeuvres dans les hommes* [Men as seen through their works] (Paris: Nouvelle Librairie Nationale, 1922), 197–243. Lamalou-les-Bains, located in the south of

By contrast, Babinski was anxious for his patients and upset by the absence of efficient treatment.[4] This marked interest is shown by the fact that almost all the forewords Babinski wrote concerned works with therapeutic consequences, such as the therapeutic use of lumbar puncture as a treatment for brain tumors, water cures, or prostheses and apparatuses.[5]

Sodium Salicylate, Morphine, Scopolamine

Babinski was one of the first to use sodium salicylate for the treatment of Basedow disease.[6] Observing the apparently positive effect of a high dose of morphine chlorhydrate in a patient addicted to morphine and presenting with tetanus, he tried to verify this fact by experiments on guinea pigs. These led him to the conclusion that "this drug may in some circumstances have

---

France, is a well-known spa, recommmended for rheumatic and neurological diseases; it was started by Charcot, to whom a street and a monument have been dedicated there.

[4] "With what a sad look, he dictated a prescription which he knew was only palliative, after having examined a child with a Heine-Medin myopathy. Returning home, he would talk of it again and call around to get additional information on the efficiency of new therapeutics such as electrical current or X-rays." A. Charpentier, *Un grand médecin, Joseph Babinski (1857–1932)* [A great physician, Joseph Babinski (1857–1932)] (Paris: Typographie François Bernouard, 1934).

[5] The exception is the foreword Babinski wrote for J.-M. Charcot, *Leçons du mardi à la Salpêtrière; notes de cours de MM. Blin, Charcot [Jean-Baptiste] et Colin* [Tuesday lessons at the Salpêtrière; course notes by MM. Blin, Charcot [Jean-Baptiste] and Colin] (Paris: C. Tchou pour la Bibliothèque des introuvables, 2002), 2 vols. For his other forewords, see O. Fontecilla and M. A. Sepulveda R., *Le liquide céphalo-rachidien. Études cliniques* [A clinical study of the cerebrospinal fluid] (Paris: Maloine, 1921) (Oscar Fontecilla was a former chief resident and substitute professor of neurology at the University of Chile and Marco A. Sepulveda R. was director of the laboratory of neurology and psychiatry at the University of Chile); E. Moniz, *Diagnostic des tumeurs cérébrales et épreuve de l'encéphalographie artérielle* [Diagnosis of brain tumors by the arterial encephalography method] (Paris: Masson et Cie, 1931); L. Lavielle and R. Lavielle, *Dax médical et thermal: études cliniques sur la station* [Clinical studies on the thermal waters of Dax] (Paris: Maloine, 1930); M. Chiray and J. Dagnan-Bouveret, *La prothèse fonctionnelle des paralysies et des contractures* [Functional prosthesis for paralysis and muscular spasm] (Paris: Maloine, 1919) (the foreword by Babinski is an appendix to this chapter); G. Bidou, *Nouvelle méthode d'appareillage des impotents* [A new method for fitting the disabled] (Paris: Presses Universitaires de France, 1923).

[6] J. Babinski, "Traitement de la maladie de Basedow par le salicylate de soude" [Treatment of Basedow's disease by sodium salicylate], *Rev Neurol (Paris)* 1901 (IX): 265.

a curative effect."[7] He recommended scopolamine for its beneficial effect, noted occasionally in Sydenham chorea and in Parkinson's syndromes.[8]

Mercury Treatment of Syphilis of the Nervous System

Despite the great uncertainties surrounding its efficacy and the seriousness of treatment complications, Babinski insisted on the value of the prolonged and intensive use of mercury in the treatment of syphilis.[9] He reported having performed thousand of injections of calomel (mercurous chloride) in patients with tabes and paralysis of the insane, without having noticed serious side effects.[10] "While some consider that the effects of this drug are useless and even harmful, others, and I am one of them, are convinced that mercury has beneficial effects, at least in some cases of tabes."[11]

He agreed with Alfred Fournier, first holder of the chair of cutaneous and syphilis diseases at the University of Paris, who wrote in 1893: "The cure of syphilis by mercury is a truth as dazzling as the light of day, which can only be ignored by the blind or by these, even worse, as in the sacred text, 'blind who have eyes but cannot see.'"[12] Vaquez too, in his *Précis de thérapeutique*, was still convinced of the value of mercury treatment.[13] Curiously, it does

---

[7] J. Babinski, "De l'action du chlorhydrate de morphine sur le tétanos" [On the effect of morphine chlorhydrale on tetanus], *Comptes-rendus Hebdomadaires des Séances et Mémoires de la Société de Biologie* 1897 (IV): 600–602.

[8] J. Babinski, "De l'action de la scopolamine sur la chorée de Sydenham" [On the effect of scopolamine on Sydenham chorea], *Rev Neurol (Paris)* 1907 (XV): 86; Krebs, "Nécrologie de J. Babinski 1857–1932."

[9] G. Tilles and D. Wallach, "Le traitement de la syphilis par le mercure. Une histoire thérapeutique exemplaire" [Syphilis treatment by mercury. A story of exemplary therapy], *Histoire des Sciences Médicales* 1996 (XXX): 501–510.

[10] J. Babinski, "À propos du procès-verbal. Sur les injections de sels mercuriels insolubles" [Concerning the minutes on injection of insoluble mercury salts], *Bulletins et Mémoires de la Société Médicale des Hôpitaux de Paris*, 1906 (XXIII): 1203–1204; J. Babinski, "Traitement hydrargyrique dans le tabès" [Mercurial treatment in tabes], *Rev Neurol (Paris)* 1920 (36): 695.

[11] J. Babinski, "Du traitement mercuriel dans la sclérose tabétique des nerfs optiques" [On mercurial treatment of optic nerve tabetic sclerosis], *Rev Neurol (Paris)* 1900 (VIII): 626–628.

[12] A. Fournier, *Traitement de la syphilis* [Treatment of syphilis] (Paris: Rueff, 1893), quoted in Tilles and Wallach, "Le traitement de la syphilis par le mercure."

[13] H. Vaquez, *Précis de thérapeutique* [A therapeutic handbook] (Paris: J.-B. Baillière, 1907).

not appear that Babinski accepted the revolution in the treatment of syphilis represented by the use of arsenic compounds, as proposed by Paul Ehrlich (1854–1915), such as 606 (salvarsan or Ehrlich salt) in 1909, then neosalvarsan in 1912.[14] These compounds were recommended by many neurologists in France and abroad, and their results were analyzed in the *Revue Neurologique*.[15] Although the use of these arsenic compounds was strongly opposed by Ernest Gaucher (1854–1919), holder after Alfred Fournier of the chair of cutaneous diseases and syphilis, Babinski denied any categorical opposition to these treatments: "If I defend the mercury treatment, I am not against the arsenic medication, far from it. These two types of treatment are by no means incompatible: the acquisition of a new weapon does not force us to leave an old one behind."[16] Others concurred; as Paul Ravaut (1872–1934) noted: "If mercury cyanate is excellent in the acute treatment, I prefer calomel by far for syphilis of the nervous system; I share completely the opinion of M. Babinski on this point and I understand why he defends with so much energy this old helpful technique."[17]

---

[14] Ehrlich was a famous German doctor and biologist, professor at the Berlin School of Medicine; his work on cell dyes led him to use them for destruction of microorganisms. He received the Nobel Prize in 1908 for his work on immunology.

[15] Many papers reporting the beneficial effect of arsenic in syphilis treatment were analyzed in different issues of the *Revue Neurologique*, especially between the years 1911 and 1914. For instance: G. Marinesco, "Sur quelques résultats obtenus avec le '606' dans le traitement des maladies nerveuses" [On some results obtained with salvarsan in the treatment of nervous diseases], *La Presse Médicale* 1911 (8); G. Marinesco and J. Minea, "L'emploi des injections de sérum salvarnisé 'in vitro' et 'in vivo' sous l'arachnoïde spinale et cérébrale dans le tabes et la paralysie générale" [Subarachnoid spinal and cerebral injection using salvarsan serum in tabes and paralysis of the insane], *Rev Neurol (Paris)* 1914 (XXVII): 336–347; M. P. Weil, "Sur un cas de méningite syphilitique incurable par le mercure et guérie par le dioxydiamidoarsenobenzol" [On a case of syphilitic meningitis resistant to mercury and cured by an arsenic compound], *Rev Neurol (Paris)* 1914 (XXVII): 762; J. Collins, "Syphilis and the nervous system," *Journal of the American Medical Association* 1913 (LXI): 860–866, analyzed in *Rev Neurol (Paris)* 1914 (XXVII): 33; H. Swift and A. Ellis, "Direct treatment of central nervous system syphilis," *Journal of Nervous and Mental Disease* 1913: 467–470, analyzed in *Rev Neurol (Paris)* 1914–1915 (XXVIII): 197–198.

[16] J. Babinski, intervention (pp. 695–697), "Du traitement hydrargyrique dans le tabes" [On mercurial treatment in tabes], concerning the report by J. A. Sicard (with discussions), "Syphilis nerveuse et son traitement" [Syphilis of the nervous system and its treatment], *Rev Neurol (Paris)* 1920 (XXXVI): 609–748.

[17] P. Ravaut, intervention (pp. 707–709), concerning the report by J. A. Sicard (with discussions), "Syphilis nerveuse et son traitement" [Syphilis of the nervous system and its treatment], *Rev Neurol (Paris)* 1920 (XXXVI): 609–748. Physician in chief at the Saint-Louis Hospital, member of the *Académie de médecine*, Ravaut wrote several books on syphilis.

Lumbar Puncture as a Treatment

Babinski recommended extractions of lumbar cerebrospinal fluid for incontinence, vertigo, and some auricular diseases, as well as for optic neuritis of intracranial origin.[18] With repeated lumbar punctures, he reported being able to cure a seven-year-old girl struck down by cerebrospinal meningitis.[19] He also reported a case of hemorrhagic meningitis with spasmodic paraplegia and an Argyll-Robertson sign that was cured by lumbar punctures and a mercury treatment.[20] In this case, Babinski noticed that the spinal fluid was greenish yellow and coagulated immediately, forming a clot containing lymphocytes. This syndrome of massive coagulation was described accurately for the first time in Froin's thesis in 1903 and was also the thesis subject in 1909 of Georges Aubry, who noted that the first documented case of this syndrome (later known as Froin syndrome) was the one discussed by Babinski.[21] Whatever the indications for lumbar puncture, Babinski insisted on the technical care required to avoid potential problems: patients should

---

[18] J. Babinski and J. Boisseau, "Traitement de l'incontinence d'urine par la ponction lombaire" [Treatment of urinary incontinence by lumbar puncture], *Bull. Mem. Soc. Méd. Hôp.Paris* 1904 (XXI): 413–417, and see also P. Gastinel, "La ponction lombaire thérapeutique" [Lumbar puncture as a treatment], *Le Progrès Médical* 1914 (2): 283; J. Babinski, "Traitement du vertige de Ménière par les ponctions lombaires" [Treatment of vertigo in Ménière's disease by lumbar puncture], *Rev Neurol (Paris)* 1908 (XVI): 1169; J. Babinski, "Ponction lombaire dans les névrites optiques d'origine intra-crânienne" [Lumbar puncture in optic neuritis of intracranial origin], *Rev Neurol (Paris)* 1907 (XV): 1281. "Lumbar puncture is effective on different ear diseases, either of labyrinthic origin with Ménière disease or associated middle ear and labyrinthic troubles, etc.... It may be ineffective if the labyrinthic lesions are too deeply situated. Until further notice, M. Babinski concluded that lumbar puncture remains indicated in these affections"; J. Babinski, "Traitement des affections auriculaires par la ponction lombaire" [Treatment of ear diseases by lumbar puncture], *Le Progrès Médical* 1903 (18): 328.

[19] J. Babinski, "Méningite cérébro-spinale subaigue, à polynucléaires. Ponctions lombaires. Guérison. (Présentation de malade)" [Subacute cerebrospinal meningitis. Cure by lumbar puncture. (Patient presentation)], *Bulletins et Mémoires de la Société Médicale des Hôpitaux de Paris* 1902 (XIX): 907–909.

[20] J. Babinski, "Méningite hémorragique fibrineuse; paraplégie spasmodique. Ponctions lombaires; traitement mercuriel—Guérison" [Hemorrhagic and fibrinous meningitis; spasmodic paraplegia. Lumbar punctures; mercurial treatment. Cure], *Bull. Mém. Soc. Méd. Hôp. Paris* 1903 (XX): 1083–1089.

[21] G. Froin, "Inflammations méningées avec réactions chromatique, fibrineuse et leucocytique du liquide céphalo-rachidien" [Meningeal inflammation with colored, fibrinous and leucocytic reactions of the cerebrospinal fluid], *Gazette des Hôpitaux*, September 3, 1903; G. Aubry, *Le syndrome de coagulation massive du liquide céphalorachidien* [Massive cerebrospinal fluid coagulation syndrome] (Paris: Steinheil, 1909).

be lying down, and extraction of cerebrospinal fluid has to be moderate (less than 8–10 cc) and done slowly (drop by drop), and bed rest is necessary for several days afterward.[22]

Electrotherapy

Babinski was interested in the use of electric treatment as a way of suppressing malingering and hysterical symptoms, but also as a treatment in other pathologies, particularly in trigeminal neuralgias.[23] "[Henri Babinski] studied with his brother, Dr. Babinski, the mechanical engineering of equipment for the treatment of specific diseases. His efforts were crowned with success, and the Legion of Honor rewarded [Henri's] works as an electrician as well as his long career as a prospector."[24]

The report of the cure of a melancholic patient by head faradization causing a voltaic vertigo led some authors to see Babinski as the precursor of electric shock treatment (sismotherapy).[25] Babinski was very cautious about the interpretation of the outcome of this case, admitting that the patient's recovery could be a pure coincidence; however, it seemed to him difficult

---

[22] J. Babinski and J. Chaillous, "Résultats thérapeutiques de la ponction lombaire dans les névrites optiques d'origine intra-crânienne" [Therapeutic results of lumbar puncture in optic neuritis of intracranial origin], *Société française d'ophtalmologie,* May 1907.

[23] J. Babinski, M. Delherm, and J. Jarkowski, "Sur l'association de deux courants en électro-diagnostic et en électrothérapie" [On the association of two types of current in electrodiagnosis and electrotherapy], *Rev Neurol (Paris)* 1913 (XXV): 462. Babinski reported the evolution of two facial palsies: "One, which was recent, has been cured by some sessions of faradic electrization; the other, which appeared earlier, necessitated the help of psychotherapy, as electrization did not seem to be efficient. For this reason, the patient has been hypnotized. By associating these two methods, the patient has been quite completely cured." J. Babinski, "Paralysie faciale hystérique" [Hysterical facial paralysis], *Bul. Mém. Soc. Méd. Hôp. Paris* 1892 (IX): 738. See also J. Babinski and M. Delherm, "Sur le traitement de la névralgie faciale par les courants voltaïques à intensité élevée" [On the treatment of facial neuralgia by high intensity voltaic currents], *Rev Neurol (Paris)* 1906 (XIV): 544–546.

[24] Alexis Rey, "Nécrologie de Henri Babinski" [Obituary of Henri Babinski], in *Bulletin de l'Association des anciens élèves de l'École des mines de Paris,* 1931, http://www.annales.org/archives/x/babinsky.html.

[25] J. Babinski, "Guérison d'un cas de mélancolie à la suite d'un accès provoqué de vertige voltaïque" [Cure of a melancholic patient following a provoked voltaic vertigo], *Rev Neurol (Paris)* 1903 (XI): 525–528; P. Cossa, "Babinski, précurseur des méthodes de choc électrique" [Babinski, a precursor in electric shock], *Annales Médico-Psychologiques* 1950 (I): 325–330.

"not to imagine a cause-and-effect relationship between electrization and patient cure.... I am not deceiving myself and I do not claim—far be it for me to pretend—that we have there an infallible way of curing melancholy; however, I would recommend, because of the absolute harmlessness of this technique, trying it routinely in similar cases and to use it several times on the same patient. The experiment should be tried even with the simple hope to speed up the cure, as it seems to have happened in our reported case."

Radiotherapy

In France, Babinski was the first to use radiotherapy, mainly for analgesic purposes, especially in the treatment of various spinal diseases.

In 1906, at a meeting of the Société médicale des hôpitaux de Paris, he presented the case of a fifteen-year-old child with a generalized contracture of the neck, trunk, and all four limbs in relation to a cervical cord compression caused by a hematoma or pachymeningitis, following a car accident.[26] After radiotherapy, the contracture rapidly disappeared, allowing the patient to walk again. The following year, he presented to the same society the case of a thirty-two-year-old woman with spastic paraplegia that had been markedly improved by radiotherapy on the thoracolumbar spine, whereas previous medical treatment had not shown results.[27] He also recalled that he had observed a case of Pott's disease where "radiotherapy seems to have had a positive influence." He concluded that "without being completely affirmative, I am inclined to believe that X-rays have a positive action."

In 1908, at a meeting of the Société de neurologie, he reported the case of a patient who had suffered for seven years from bilateral sciatica caused by vertebral spondylosis, making walking extremely difficult and painful.[28] Drug treatment, including salicylate of soda, was completely ineffective. The patient received twenty-two sessions of X-ray treatment on the lumbar spine.

---

[26] J. Babinski, "Contracture généralisée due à une compression de la moelle cervicale, très améliorée à la suite de l'usage de rayons X" [Generalized contracture related to a cervical spinal cord compression markedly improved by X-ray therapy], *Bulletins et Mémoires de la Société Médicale des Hôpitaux de Paris* 1906 (XXIII): 1205–1210.

[27] J. Babinski, "De la radiothérapie dans les paralysies spasmodiques spinales" [On the use of radiotherapy in spinal spastic paralysis], *Bulletins et Mémoires de la Société Médicale des Hôpitaux de Paris* 1907 (XXIV): 208–213.

[28] J. Babinski, "Spondylose et douleurs névralgiques très atténuées à la suite de pratiques radiothérapiques" [Spondylosis and neuralgic pain markedly relieved with radiotherapy], *Rev Neurol (Paris)* 1908 (XVI): 262–263.

Improvement was rapid, with a marked decrease in pain starting as early as the second session. By the end of the treatment, the patient was able to walk for one kilometer without pain, having left his walking stick behind. With his usual caution, Babinski concluded: "Is there any cause-and-effect relationship between the X-ray treatment, spondylosis, and neuralgia? I cannot say for certain, but tend to believe it."

In a paper written in 1911, he reported four cases of sciatica that had resisted all usual forms of treatment but had been cured completely following radiotherapy.[29] On this occasion, he was more positive than he had been previously and stated that "the disappearance of symptoms and the application of X-rays to the lumbosacral area is not a coincidence but a cause-and-effect relationship." The final paper by Babinski on the therapeutic effects of X-rays, in 1917, dealt with a case of crural neuralgia caused by a hydatid cyst.[30] However, later results did not confirm his optimism about the usefulness of radiotherapy in sciatica and other painful spinal diseases, with the exception of some instances of spinal tumor.

Neurosurgery

Babinski played a leading role in France in the development of neurosurgery. At the beginning, he advocated only decompressive techniques; later, however, he began to refer patients for ablative operations (see chapter 13). He was interested as well in surgical treatment of the peripheral nervous system, for instance recommending surgical section of the peripheral spinal accessory nerve in spasmodic torticollis.

Rehabilitation of the Handicapped

Babinski showed a continuing interest in the rehabilitation of handicapped patients. At a meeting of the heads of department at La Pitié in June 1907, he complained that patients in medical wards could not obtain

---

[29] J. Babinski, A. Charpentier, and J. Delherm, "Radiothérapie de la sciatique" [Radiotherapy in sciatica], *Rev Neurol (Paris)* 1911 (XXI): 525–528.
[30] J. Babinski and M.S. Grunspan, "Kyste hydatique. Névrite crurale. Disparition des douleurs à la suite de la radiothérapie" [Hydatid cyst. Crural neuralgia. Disappearance of pain following radiotherapy], *Bull. Mém. Soc. Méd. Hôp. Paris* 1917 (XLI): 105.

orthopedic apparatuses or prostheses.³¹ These were supplied only those surgical patients who had been operated on in the hospital. In 1919, he wrote the preface to a book by Maurice Chiray, chief of the neurological center of the Tenth Military Region, and his former student Jean Dagnan-Bouveret, on functional prostheses for paralysis and muscular contracture.³²

He also had a close professional relationship with Gabriel Bidou (1878–1959), "who for many years has agreed to make available to the patients of my department... his time, his knowledge, and his dedication."³³ The importance of Bidou, a pioneer in medical rehabilitation, should be emphasized.³⁴ After his medical studies in Lille, Bidou worked at the Orthopedic Institute in Berck as director of the mechanical therapy section, then from 1906 to 1920 at the Physical Therapy Institute in Grenoble. He then moved to Paris and became chief of the department of functional rehabilitation at the Salpêtrière (created in 1924 in Guillain's department) before leaving in 1929.³⁵ During this period, Bidou opened two private clinics devoted to functional recovery. Bidou proposed new concepts, perfected measurement tools, devised ingenious apparatuses, and incorporated into his daily practice both scientific and social considerations. He was a member of the Société des ingénieurs civils de France. Bidou wrote many books, the prefaces to which were contributed by well-known physicians: Henri Duret for his book on scoliosis, Georges Guillain for his work on the functional recovery of paralytics, Arsène d'Arsonval for his volume on mechanical therapy, and Joseph Babinski for his book on fitting the disabled with prostheses.³⁶

---

[31] Archives de l'Assistance Publique, Hôpitaux de Paris, Box 9L 128. In regard to that, it is interesting to note that Babinski, contrary to his colleagues Claisse and Walther, spoke very rarely at the meetings of the departments heads.

[32] Chiray and Dagnan-Bouveret, *La prothèse fonctionnelle des paralysies et des contractures*.

[33] In Babinski's foreword to Bidou, *Nouvelle méthode d'appareillage des impotents*.

[34] M. W. Thewlis, "1932—the death of Babinski," *Medical Times* 1972 (100): 40–44. See also this excellent monograph: J. M. Wirotius, *Histoire de la rééducation* [A history of rehabilitation], *Encycl Méd Chir* (Elsevier, Paris), "Kinésithérapie-Médecine physique-Réadaptation" [Physical therapy- rehabilitation], 26-005-1-A-10, 1999.

[35] G. Guillain and G. Bidou, "Sur la récupération fonctionnelle des grandes paralysies" [On functional recovery of severely paralyzed patients], *Académie de médecine*, May 4, 1926.

[36] G. Bidou, *La scoliose et son traitement* [Scoliosis and its treatment] (Paris: Maloine, 1913); G. Bidou, *Principes scientifiques de récupération fonctionnelle des paralytiques* [Scientific principles of functional recovery in paralytics] (Paris: Le Livre pour Tous, 1927); G. Bidou, *La thérapie mécanique* [Mechanical therapy] (Paris: Vuibert, 1929); Bidou, *Nouvelle méthode d'appareillage des impotents*.

In his foreword, Babinski was generous with his compliments:

> The book by Dr. Gabriel Bidou is not just a presentation of the different prosthetic means used today in orthopedics. As shown by his title, it is a study of new methods of equipment when motor disturbances responsible for disabilities are not manageable by other treatment. This volume, full of original ideas, represents twenty years of hard work. To bring to a successful conclusion such a task, one has to be at the same time physiologist, pathologist, and accomplished engineer, and show an ability to juggle different scientific concepts and eventually to modify one's orientation.
>
> This quality does not surprise me: it seems to be a family trait. For instance, a close relative of the author, an eminent man of letters, is, depending on the circumstances, a brilliant dramatic critic, a wise politician, and a clear-sighted military advisor. I do not think it necessary to analyze the work of M. Bidou and to show its great value. The reader will rapidly become aware of this, thanks to the clarity with which the ideas are laid out and to the beautiful illustrations. What I want to say is that I have been able to personally observe a number of positive results obtained through the techniques of M. Bidou, who for many years has agreed to make available to the patients of my department at La Pitié his time, his knowledge, and his dedication. While presenting M. Bidou to his readers, I take the opportunity offered to me to express my high regard for the conscientiousness and impartiality he has always shown and to congratulate him for the talent and cleverness with which he has increased the recovery of disabled patients by improving the existing techniques of equipment and by creating new ones.

Thermal Water Cures

Babinski provided a laudatory foreword to the book by Louis and René Lavielle that spoke highly of the therapeutic merits of the spa in Dax (Fig. 14-1). He wrote:

> The systematic use of the mud bath and of the hot springs in Dax constitutes, for many rheumatic patients, an effective treatment for pain and disabilities created by articular stiffness and deformation. This notion is based upon observations made for centuries, and which therefore has passed the proof of time.... To the stubborn skeptic who, despite the obvious, questions the beneficial effects of mud baths, the authors raise as an objection the good results obtained with this treatment in veterinary medicine... on the one hand they clarify the cases where the treatment, instead of being useful, is generally harmful and should be banned or postponed, and on the other hand, those in which, and the list is long, they offer good chances of improvement or cure.[37]

---

[37] Lavielle and Lavielle, *Dax médical et thermal.*

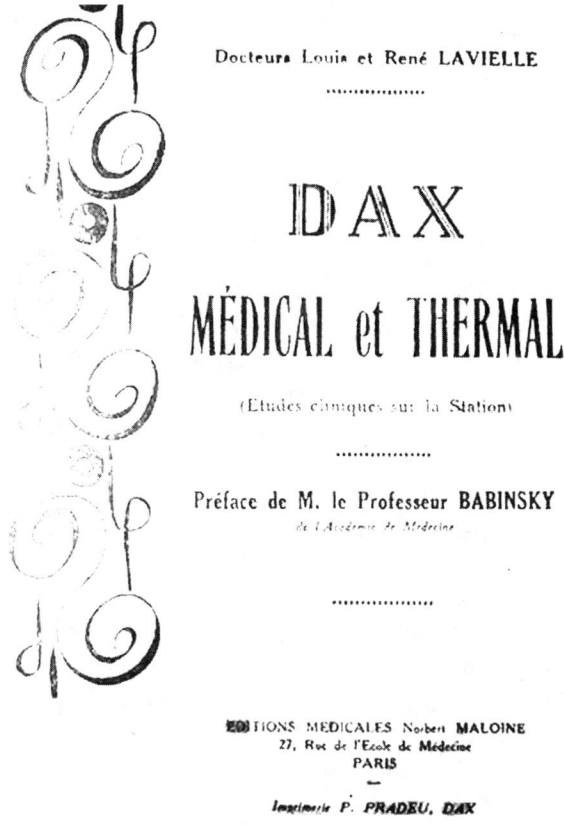

Figure 14-1 Cover of the book *Dax médical et thermal* (1930) by the Drs. Lavielle.

Project to Create Special Asylums for the "Partially Disabled"

Babinski's interest in treatment, especially for the underprivileged, is evident in his 1903 recommendation, at a meeting of the Société médicale des hôpitaux de Paris, for the creation of special asylums for chronic patients and the "partially disabled" (for example, those afflicted by heart disease, tabes, or epilepsy).[38] This might help solve the problem of hospital overloading, Babinski thought, and the "poor people deserving help because of their

---

[38] Charpentier, *Un grand médecin*; *Le Progrès Médical* 1903, 147.

weakness would find a place of refuge, while keeping their independence and not being exposed to dying of starvation."[39]

APPENDIXES

An Example of Babinski's Prescriptions (May 9, 1924)

1. In the morning, one hour before breakfast, and in the evening, before going to bed, take a pill of phenobarbital (five centigrams), dissolved in a small amount of water. This treatment may be followed for varying periods of time, according to results and tolerance.
2. For fifteen consecutive days each month, for a period of three months, take at mealtimes a pill of calcium glycerophosphate (0 gr. 50).
3. Avoid any cause of fatigue.
4. Avoid any fermented drink.[40]

Excerpt from Babinski's Foreword to La prothèse fonctionnelle des paralysies et des contractures by Maurice Chiray and Jean Dagnan-Bouveret

It is not necessary to introduce Dr. Chiray, one of the authors of the *Prothèse fonctionnelle*, to the medical audience. Resident in the Paris hospitals, then chief resident, and finally for several years head of a neurological center, he has been well known and appreciated for his interesting works.

His coworker, Jean Dagnan-Bouveret, died before the publication of this book. He died while serving his country, victim of an infectious disease that he contracted in an ambulance in the front of the battlefield. His demise has deeply saddened all who knew him. He had already accomplished important work, and he leaves the memory of a generous, fair personality.

The son of the famous painter, having in his heredity and increased by his education the love of beauty, early in his life he was captivated by literature, and after studies at the Sorbonne became a *professeur agrégé* in philosophy.

Having acquired great shrewdness and a precise and elegant style, he devoted himself to neurology and psychiatry, following the example of his mentor Professor Dumas. I had the privilege of having him as student; he became my friend, and I was able to appreciate his exceptional moral and intellectual qualities; he was a person of distinction, and a great future lay before him.

---

[39] A. Tournay, *La vie de Joseph Babinski* [The life of Joseph Babinski] (Amsterdam: Elsevier, 1967).

[40] C. Hamonet, "Note historique, la prescription médicale par Babinski" [Historical note, medical prescription by Babinski], *Journal de Réadaptation Médicale* 1999 (19): 29.

It may seem strange that this mind, passionately fond of difficult psychological problems, was so intrigued by a simple and practical problem, that of the functional prosthesis. This is but a new proof of his adaptability, and perhaps one can also detect the latent character trait that drove all of his investigations, as successful orthopedic research requires an inventive mind coupled with the capacity to get down to work at the practical level.

The team of Dagnan-Bouveret and Chiray, I must say, was a most fortunate alliance. They were both ingenious workaholics, though each made of a different metal, one having followed from the start of his studies the path of the medical competitions, the other becoming a physician after having first specialized in literature and philosophy. The finished product is a book full of facts, containing new ideas, a few of which need to be emphasized.

The authors clearly demonstrate the importance and the future of functional prostheses in dealing with paralysis due to peripheral nerve lesions or of the nervous centers, on the condition that they are adapted to each type of case. We have to get it through our heads that it is necessary to devise new prostheses of various types and specifications....

MM. Chiray and Dagnan-Bouveret have set forth in an extremely detailed manner the different types of apparatus required in the treatment of paralysis encountered during the world war. They have likewise brought to this study their extensive personal touch through reference to the numerous unique prostheses that they themselves devised and perfected at the Neurological Center of the Tenth Region.

This book is easy to read, thanks to the authors' clear and precise style and the illustrations that supplement the text. It is indeed very instructive and will become a valuable guide for orthopedists, surgeons, and neurologists: I cannot recommend it too strongly.

··· *fifteen* ···

Pithiatism Versus Hysteria*

When Jean-Martin Charcot selected Babinski as senior resident in 1885, Charcot's fame, international as well as national, was at its peak, especially in regard to hysteria. This became the main topic of his teaching, as shown by the large number of his lessons that are devoted to it.[1]

The importance of hysteria in the second half of the nineteenth century, particularly in France, is amazing. Since its description in Antiquity, hysteria had been considered a female illness associated with womb disorders and female sexuality. With a better knowledge of ovarian functions, the role of the womb in hysteria was challenged in the mid-1800s. Hysteria was no longer considered a sexual disorder, though it remained genital in nature and restricted to women. The notion that hysteria was a disorder of the nervous system and could occur in men, first suggested by figures such as Thomas Sydenham (1624–1669) and defended by Paul Briquet (1796–1881)[2] and then Charcot, would not be commonly accepted before the end of the century.

During this period growing attention was being given to the role of the cerebral cortex in brain function. Localization of brain functions, such as that of language by Paul Broca (1824–1880) and Karl Wernicke (1848–1905), placed the philosophical and religious debate on the relationship between mind and body within a scientific framework. Hysteria,

---

* This chapter was written by Christian Derouesné, MD.
[1] M. Gauchet and G. Swain, *Le vrai Charcot* [The real Charcot] (Paris: Calman-Levy, 1997), 72–73.
[2] P. Briquet, *Traité clinique et thérapeutique de l'hystérie* [Clinical and therapeutic treatise on hysteria] (Paris, Plon, 1859).

involving both mind and body, was obviously part of this debate. Charcot's studies on cerebral localization[3] and hysteria contributed to the emergence of neurology as a discipline but also were an essential part of this controversy, which was especially widespread in France on account of the ongoing and acute societal struggle between Monarchists and Catholics, on one hand, versus Republicans, Positivists, and Materialists, on the other. Hysteria was also closely linked to the conception of the role of women in society.[4]

Hysteria According to Charcot

Because Charcot's thoughts on hysteria were the starting point for Babinski, a brief overview of his ideas is essential if one wishes to understand the path that Babinski took (Fig. 15-1).

Charcot's ideas on the subject were developed in his lessons, which were actually clinical presentations of patients during which he included some general comments on recent developments in the field. The very popular lessons were attended by many French and foreign physicians, but also by nonprofessionals. During his residency (1885–1887) and thereafter until 1890, Babinski organized and attended the presentations, as shown in the 1887 painting by Pierre-André Brouillet (1857–1914). He collected the texts of the Tuesday lessons for publication and thus was very familiar with all aspects of them.

Despite the fact that a great deal of literature has been devoted to Charcot's work on hysteria, it must be said that he developed no general conception of the disorder that could be compared to Babinski's. In the lessons devoted to hysteria, many of Charcot's statements are repetitive or contradict each other. Moreover, the chronology of the lessons is not easy to establish, and Charcot's thought both is complicated and evolved over time. Therefore, different interpreters could emphasize different aspects of his work. In the twentieth century, when the interest in hysteria had decreased, many neurologists blamed Charcot for having gone off on the wrong track in his work on hysteria. On the other hand, many psychiatrists acknowledge Charcot

---

[3] J.-M. Charcot, *Leçons sur les localisations cérébrales* [Lessons on localizations in the brain] (Paris: Alcan, 1893).

[4] N. Edelman, *Les métamorphoses de l'hystérique. Du début du XIXe siècle à la Grande Guerre* [Metamorphosis of the hysteric. From the early 19th century to the First World War] (Paris: Éditions de la découverte, 2003).

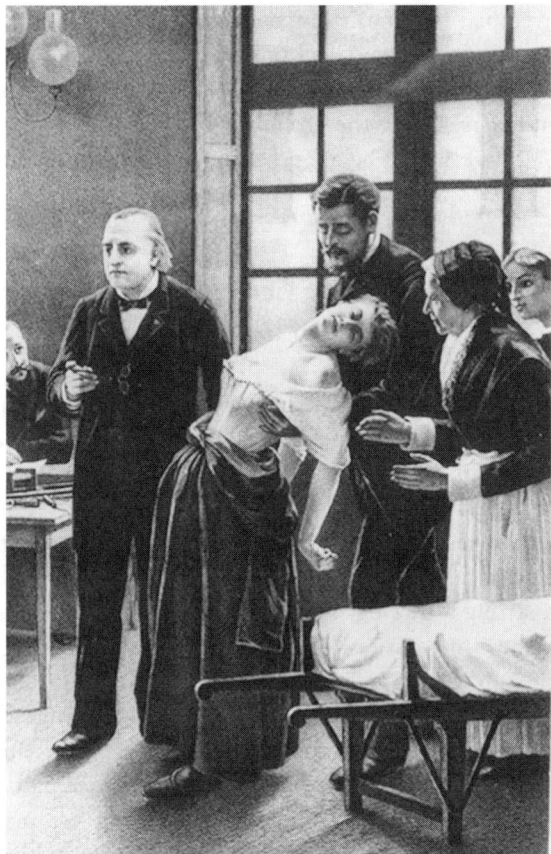

Figure 15-1 From left to right: Charcot, Blanche Wittman (hysterical patient), Babinski (chief resident), Ms. Bottard (head nurse), Ms. Ecary (nurse). (*Source*: From Une leçon du docteur Charcot à la Salpêtrière, engraving from the painting of André Brouillet, 1887.)

as the father of the psychological conception of hysteria, noting that both Sigmund Freud (1856–1939)[5] and Pierre Marie Félix Janet (1859–1947) recognized their debt to him.[6] More recently, Charcot's conception of hysteria has been considered a precursor to related cognitive theories.[7]

[5] S. Freud, "Charcot," *Wiener Medizine Wochenschrift 1893*, French translation in S. Freud, *Resultats, Idées et problèmes* (Paris: Presses Universitaires de France, 1984), 61–73
[6] P. Janet, "Quelques définitions de l'hystérie" [Some definitions of hysteria], *Archives de Neurologie* 1893 (25): 417–438, (26): 1–29.
[7] D. Widlöcher, "L'hystérie, cent ans après" [Hysteria, 100 years afterward], *Rev Neurol (Paris)* 1982(138): 1053–1060.

Charcot developed two main concepts on hysteria.[8] The first one is neurological. The second, psychological one, evolved later, but it never entirely replaced his initial premise. Shortly before his death, Charcot himself recognized this in his preface to the *Traité sur l'hystérie* by Georges Gilles de la Tourette (1857–1904), which he acknowledged as a faithful reflection of his thought.[9]

Hysteria as a Central Nervous System Disorder

As did Briquet, Charcot refuted the traditional concept of hysteria as being related to womb disorders, defending both its cerebral origin and the need for a clear description of the associated clinical phenomena. For Charcot, hysteria was an organic brain disorder, even if he very often pointed out the role of the ovaries and noted that ovary compression could either set off or stop a hysterical seizure. His insistence on the phenomenon of male hysteria was a strong argument for its cerebral origin, even if he proposed, paradoxically, the compression of the testicles as equivalent to that of the ovaries.

According to this concept, hysterical manifestations were due to a cerebral cortex lesion, which he called "dynamic" because, as in epilepsy, no brain changes could be shown by the currently available pathological techniques. Starting with this notion, Charcot insisted on two points: first, the modification of tendon jerk reflexes and its association with other neurological symptoms such as edema or visceral and circulatory disorders, and second, the similar or even identical aspects between some manifestations of hysteria and those of organic disorders. From 1878, Charcot used hypnosis and showed that hysterical symptoms could be both created and suppressed by hypnosis. He concluded that hysteria and hypnosis are of the same nature and are related to a special state of the central nervous system, resulting in specific clinical manifestations.[10] This idea was challenged by Hippolyte Bernheim (1840–1919), who claimed that hysteria and hypnosis were due to

---

[8] J.-M. Charcot, "De la contracture hystérique" [On hysterical contracture], *Leçons sur les maladies du système nerveux*, vol. 1 of *Oeuvres complètes* (Paris: Progrès médical, Bataille, 1892), 347–366.

[9] G. de la Tourette, *Traité clinique et thérapeutique de l'hystérie d'après l'enseignement de la Salpêtrière* [Clinical and therapeutic treatise on hysteria based on teaching at the Salpêtrière], vol. 1: *Hystérie normale ou interparoxystique* (Paris: Plon, 1891).

[10] S. Nicolas, *L'hypnose: Charcot face à Bernheim* [Hypnosis: Charcot Versus Bernheim] (Paris: L'Harmattan, 2004).

suggestion and consequently were not an organic disturbance of the cerebral cortex but a psychological disorder.[11]

Hysteria as a Psychological Disorder

In his preface to Pierre Janet's doctoral thesis, Charcot wrote: "Hysteria is, to a large extent, a mental disease."[12] This sentence and the role that Charcot assigned to psychological factors as a trigger of hysterical symptoms explains why Freud and Janet saw Charcot as the pioneer of the psychological nature of hysteria. The role of psychological factors was mainly developed in regard to the concept of traumatic hysteria.[13] Charcot pointed out the importance of emotion as the trigger mechanism for hysteria. But he noted that the clinical symptoms do not appear immediately after the trauma: there is a "phase of meditation," during which the subject is caught by a fixed idea and becomes paralyzed through autosuggestion. "The paralysis thus can be described as ideal, psychic, fueled by imagination (but not imaginary)."[14] Nevertheless, according to Charcot, psychology cannot be dissociated from the physiology of the central nervous system.[15]

The Etiology of Hysteria

Charcot associates hysteria and heredity in accordance with the major governing role attributed to heredity in the etiology of diseases at his time. Heredity may be direct (cases of hysteria in the same family) or indirect (any familial mental disorder). It results in a hysterical diathesis, expressed by hyperexcitability of the nervous system that leads to proneness to muscular cramps and adynamia. The symptoms occur following multiple predisposing conditions, whether physical or psychological. Charcot referred to two main precipitating factors, trauma and dreams. Finally, he pointed out the association of hysterical manifestations with organic disorders in some patients.

[11] H. Bernheim, *Hypnotisme, suggestion, psychothérapie* [Hypnotism, suggestion, psychotherapy], 3rd ed. (Paris: Doin, 1891).
[12] P. Janet, "Contribution à l'étude des accidents mentaux chez les hystériques" [A contribution to the study of mental accidents in hysterics], Thèse de médecine, Paris, 1893.
[13] J.-M. Charcot, "Leçon du mardi 17 janvier 1888" [Lesson of Tuesday, January 17, 1888], *Leçons du mardi 1887–1888* (Paris: Bureaux du Progrès médical, 1888).
[14] J.-M. Charcot, "Leçon du mardi 24 janvier 1888" [Lesson of Tuesday, January 24, 1888], *Leçons du mardi 1887–1888* (Paris: Bureaux du Progrès médical, 1888).
[15] J.-M. Charcot, "Leçon du mardi 17 janvier 1888" [Lesson of Tuesday, January 17, 1888], *Leçons du mardi 1887–1888* (Paris: Bureaux du Progrès médical, 1888); "what I call psychology is the rational functioning of the cerebral cortex." ["ce que j'appelle psychologie, c'est le fonctionnement rationnel de l'écorce cérébrale"]

Babinski as a Pupil of Charcot

Babinski's first papers on hysteria were directly inspired by Charcot's ideas and were devoted to some clinical manifestations that he would later exclude from hysteria, such as transfer of hemianesthesia through the action of a magnet, or muscular atrophy, or polyuria.[16]

Development of a Clinical Methodology

Unlike in Charcot's case, there are no extent manuscripts, notes, or letters that allow one to specifically follow Babinski's development of thought. His publications are the only source. In 1909, he wrote (Fig. 15-2):

> Beginning my neurological career at the Salpêtrière School where I had the honor to be the senior resident of Charcot from 1885 to 1887, I was at first imbued with the ideas on hysteria that were taught there at that time, and which were, until recently, almost unanimously accepted. I first accepted these ideas without reservation, but later, struck by some findings that I considered difficult to conciliate, gradually began to doubt their accuracy and decided that henceforth, I would monitor the exactitude of all facts with a rigorous analysis, without any preconceived opinion.[17]

Babinski's desire to clearly define the framework of hysteria appears as early as 1890.[18] When he distinguished between two types of hysterical manifestations, he asserted that some symptoms or syndromes may be directly attributed to hysteria because of their specific clinical characteristics (e.g., the major hysterical seizure or hysterical mutism), while others share clinical aspects with organic disorders.

---

[16] J. Babinski, "Recherches servant à établir que certaines manifestations de l'hystérie peuvent être transmises d'un sujet à l'autre sous l'influence de l'aimant" [Research to demonstrate that some nervous phenomenon may be transmitted from one patient to another one under the influence of a magnet], *Le Progrès Médical* 1886 (4): 1010–1011; "De l'atrophie musculaire dans les paralysies hystériques" [On muscular atrophy in hysterical paralysis], *Archives de neurologie* 1886 (12): 1–27; "Polyurie hystérique. Influence de la suggestion sur l'évolution du syndrome" [Hysterical polyuria. Influence of suggestion on the evolution of this syndrome], *Semaine médicale des Hôpitaux* 1891 (8): 568–574.
[17] J. Babinski, "Démembrement de l'hystérie traditionnelle" "Dismembering traditional hysteria," *La Semaine médicale* 1909 (29): 3–8.
[18] J. Babinski, "De la migraine ophtalmique hystérique" [On hysterical ophthalmic migraine], *Archives de neurologie* 1890 (20): 305–335.

> # SOCIÉTÉ DE NEUROLOGIE
> ## DE PARIS
>
> Séance du 7 Novembre 1901
>
> Présidence de M. le professeur Raymond, Président.
>
> SOMMAIRE
>
> Correspondance.
> Élections.
> Communications et présentations.
> I. MM. Feindel et Henry Meige. Torticolis mental surajouté à des mouvements hémichoréiformes. Guérison du torticolis. Amélioration générale. — II. M. Crestan. Une
>
> VII. — **Définition de l'Hystérie**, par M. J. Babinski.
>
> Malgré le grand nombre des travaux dont l'hystérie a été l'objet, les médecins ne semblent pas se faire tous une conception identique de cette névrose. Dans notre Société même, composée cependant de membres élevés pour la plupart à la même École, il y a eu plusieurs fois des discussions tendant à montrer qu'il y a de notables différences dans la manière dont, les uns et les autres, nous comprenons l'hystérie.
> Le désaccord tient sans doute à ce que les auteurs qui ont traité de l'hystérie n'en ont pas donné une définition suffisamment nette,

Figure 15-2 Definition of hysteria from Babinski's initial paper. (*Source*: From Revue Neurologique, 1901.)

While Charcot asserted that a diagnosis of hysteria could be made using indirect criteria such as the presence of permanent stigma (anesthesia, sensorial deficits such as concentric narrowing of the visual field, and so on), circumstances of occurrence, modality of onset, symptom progression, and the possibility of reproducing them under hypnosis, Babinski completely rejected this assumption and emphasized that diagnosis should be based only on specific clinical characteristics, whether for hysteria or organic diseases, because extrinsic characteristics are neither permanent nor reliable features. Babinski therefore directed his work toward identifying, on one hand, the specific clinical characteristics that allow one to distinguish hysteria from organic disorders and, on the other, the role of hypnosis and suggestion in the triggering of hysterical symptoms.

The Distinction Between Hysterical and Organic Symptoms

Charcot remained ambiguous regarding the distinction between symptoms of hysteria and those of organic disorders. For example, he clearly laid out the clinical characteristics of major hysterical seizures and those of epilepsy[19] and also described some specific features of hysterical anesthesia.[20] However, he could not distinguish hysterical paralysis, contracture, or hemianesthesia from organic manifestations on a purely clinical basis because, according to his neurological concept of hysteria, both were related to cerebral cortex disturbances.

Babinski tackled the question by trying to identify specific aspects of organic symptoms such as inversion of the plantar reflex, the toe phenomenon, and loss of the cremasteric and abdominal reflexes. At the same time, he searched for specificity in some hysterical manifestations and pointed to the absence of modification of deep tendon or cutaneous reflexes, lack of epileptoid jerk of the foot,[21] and circulatory disorders. He also described the specific topography of hysterical hemiplegia[22] or hemianesthesia.[23]

This clear distinction between the clinical symptoms of hysteria and those of organic disorders favored a purely psychological understanding of hysteria and in no way supported Charcot's idea of a dynamic lesion of the cerebral cortex. Babinski suggested two interpretations of the psychic causality: (1) the patient has lost the ability to evoke the "motor images", that is the image of movements, of the paralyzed limb segments, or (2) the patient's will is

---

[19] J.-M. Charcot, "De l'hystéro-épilepsie" [On hysterò-epilepsy], *Leçons sur les maladies du système nerveux,* vol. 1 of *Oeuvres complètes* (Paris: Progrès médical, Bataille, 1892), 367–385.

[20] J.-M. Charcot, "De l'hémianesthésie hystérique" "On hysteric hemianesthesia", *Leçons sur les maladies du système nerveux,* vol. 1 of *Oeuvres complètes* (Paris: Progrès médical, Bataille, 1892), 300–346.

[21] J. Babinski, "Contractures organiques et hystériques" [Hysterical and organic contractures], *Bulletins et Mémoires de la Société Médicale des Hôpitaux de Paris* 1893 (10): 327–343.

[22] J. Babinski, "Paralysie hystérique systématique (paralysie partielle ou systématique des fonctions motrices du membre inférieur gauche)" [Systematic hysterical paralysis (partial or systematic paralysis of the left inferior limb motor functions)], *Bulletins et Mémoires de la Société Médicale des Hôpitaux de Paris* 1892 (9): 533–538; J. Babinski, "Paralysie faciale hystérique" [Hysterical facial palsy], *Bulletins et Mémoires de la Société Médicale des Hôpitaux de Paris* 1892 (9): 867–870.

[23] Babinski and J. Jarkowski, "Étude comparative des limites de l'anesthésie organique et de l'anesthésie hystérique" [Comparative study on the edges in organic and hysteric anesthesia], *Rev Neurol (Paris)* 1912 (24): 144–145.

unable to execute certain movements. The reproduction of the paralysis by hypnosis shows that it is due to suggestion or autosuggestion. He wrote:

> Hysterical paralysis being a psychic disorder, the result of a disturbance of imagination or will, a product of the suggestion or autosuggestion can only give rise to phenomena that can be modified by imagination, will or suggestion. Therefore, hysterical paralysis does disturb neither muscular sensitivity nor reflexes. Autosuggestion has no influence on unconscious or subconscious movements.[24]

Hypnosis and Suggestion

The main difference between Babinski's thought and that of Charcot concerns the concept of hypnosis and suggestion. In his first publication on the transfer phenomenon, Babinski was completely in line with Charcot when he ruled out the role of suggestion. In 1891,[25] he still defended Charcot in the controversy between the Salpêtrière school and the Nancy school, led by Bernheim. Refuting Charcot's ideas, Bernheim asserted that hypnosis corresponds neither to a specific state of the nervous system nor to an artificial neurosis identical to hysteria. He stated that hypnosis is a physiological state, common to all people, and that suggestion is its one and only cause. As a consequence, hypnosis could be used for the treatment of many pathologies, including organic diseases, and should not be restricted to the treatment of hysteria, as claimed by Charcot.

Babinski moved progressively closer to Bernheim's ideas, though without acknowledging it. In 1892,[26] he made a distinction between "great hysteria" occurring in the "neuropathic aristocracy"—that is, subjects prone to the disease since birth—and "little hysteria," which can occur following minor trauma, simple emotion, or any ordinary circumstance. He wrote: "Hysteria is one of the most common disorders, and I think that there are few people who, under certain circumstances, cannot be subject to its consequences."

---

[24] J. Babinski, "Grand et petit hypnotisme" [Deep and light hypnosis], *Archives de neurologie* 1889 (19): 92–108, 253–269.

[25] J. Babinski, "Hypnotisme et hystérie. Du rôle de l'hypnotisme en thérapeutique" [Hypnosis and hysteria. On the therapeutic role of hypnosis], *Gazette Hebdomadaire de Médecine et de Chirurgie* 1891 (30): 350–360.

[26] J. Babinski, "Association de l'hystérie avec les maladies organiques du système nerveux, les névroses et diverses autres affections" [Association between hysteria and other organic diseases of the nervous system, neurosis and other disturbances], *Bulletins et Mémoires de la Société Médicales des Hôpitaux de Paris* 1892 (9): 777–795.

He only formally acknowledged his agreement with Bernheim in 1907[27] when he admitted having neglected the importance of suggestion in hypnotic and hysterical manifestations, and conceded that the "great hysteric crisis" and the permanent stigma were artifacts due to suggestion.

Parting with Charcot's School of Thought: Pithiatism

In 1901, Babinski presented the first clear definition of his concept of hysteria[28] which would be slightly modified in 1903:

Hysteria is a psychic state in which the subject is prone to autosuggestion. It results mainly in primary disorders and, incidentally, in secondary disorders. The specificity of the primary disorders is that they may be exactly reproduced by suggestion in some subjects and be made to disappear by the exclusive influence of persuasion. The characteristic of the secondary disorders is to be strongly dependant on primary disorders.[29]

He proposed, therefore, abandoning the term *hysteria*, ill-defined and etymologically unsuitable, and suggested as a substitute the term *pithiatism* (curable by persuasion). The pithiatic disorder is thus defined as a disorder created by suggestion and curable by persuasion. This definition gives operational criteria for the diagnosis of hysterical manifestations and disintegrates Charcot's concept of hysteria, which Babinski believed was far too extensive, by including three distinct conditions: organic disorders that could not be identified as such due to lack of sufficient knowledge about their clinical characteristics, undetected simulation, and real phenomena unmodified by suggestion or persuasion (such as vasomotor and trophic disorders). He considered it illogical to group different phenomena under the same label. Therefore, manifestations that cannot be modified by suggestion and persuasion should not be included under the term *pithiatism*, because

---

[27] J. Babinski, "Suggestion et hystérie. À propos de l'article de M Bernheim intitulé: 'Comment je comprends le mot hystérie,'" [Suggestion and hysteria. Concerning the paper by M Bernheim entitled: "How I understand the word hysteria"] *Bulletin médical* 1907(21): 272–276.

[28] J. Babinski, "La définition de l'hystérie" [Definition of hysteria], *Rev Neurol (Paris)* 1901 (9): 1074–1080.

[29] J. Babinski, "À propos de l'albuminurie prétendue hystérique" [On the so-called hysterical albuminuria], *Bulletin et Mémoires de la Société Médicale des Hôpitaux de Paris* 1903 (20): 1405–1409.

they are related either to unknown organic disorders or to simulation generated by the willful use of toxic or foreign substances.

The Physiopathic Disorders

This clear distinction between hysteria and vasomotor and reflex disorders was challenged by the pathology observed among soldiers during World War I. In 1915[30] Babinski published with Jules Froment the case of a soldier with a minor injury of the thigh who showed a marked limp that suggested a hysterical manifestation, but which was associated with a notable muscular atrophy of the thigh and important vasomotor disorders (Fig. 15-3). The persistence of hyperreactive tendon jerk reflexes and contracture under general anesthesia ruled out the diagnosis of hysteria. Numerous similar cases were thereafter observed in war pathology. These disorders, resulting from wounds or various limb trauma, can be characterized by contracture, paralysis, muscular atrophy, hypotonia, enhanced tendon reflexes, abolition of cutaneous reflexes, muscular and nervous hyperexcitability, various sensory disorders, cutaneous hypothermia, vasomotor disorders, trophic changes of skin, ligaments, or bone, and frequent tendinous, fibrotendinous, or muscular retraction.

Babinski suggested a link between these disorders and those previously described by Charcot and Vulpian following articular pathology, which were related to a reflex disorder implicating the sympathetic autonomous system. "These phenomena can be termed physiopathic to express, on the one hand, that no hysteria or other psychopathic disorder can create them and, on the other hand, although they are related to a physical, material change of the nervous system, they appear to result from a lesion that cannot be shown by the available investigative means."[31] These disorders are very resistant to the best therapeutic means, all the more so since they are frequently associated with organic and/or pithiatic disorders.

Babinksi's separation of physiopathic disorders from hysteria and simulation had strong implications in war psychiatry, because treatment, not to speak of disciplinary consequences, is very distinct in cases of hysteria, simulation, organic, or physiopathic disorders (Fig. 15-4).

---

[30] 30 J. Babinski and J. Froment, "Contribution à l'étude des troubles nerveux d'origine réflexe" [Contribution to the study of nervous disorders of reflex origin], *Rev Neurol (Paris)* 1915 (29): 925–933.

[31] J. Babinski and J. Froment, *Hystérie-pithiatisme et troubles nerveux d'origine réflexe en neurologie de guerre* [Hysteria or pithiatism and reflex nervous disorders in the neurology of war] (Paris: Masson, 1918).

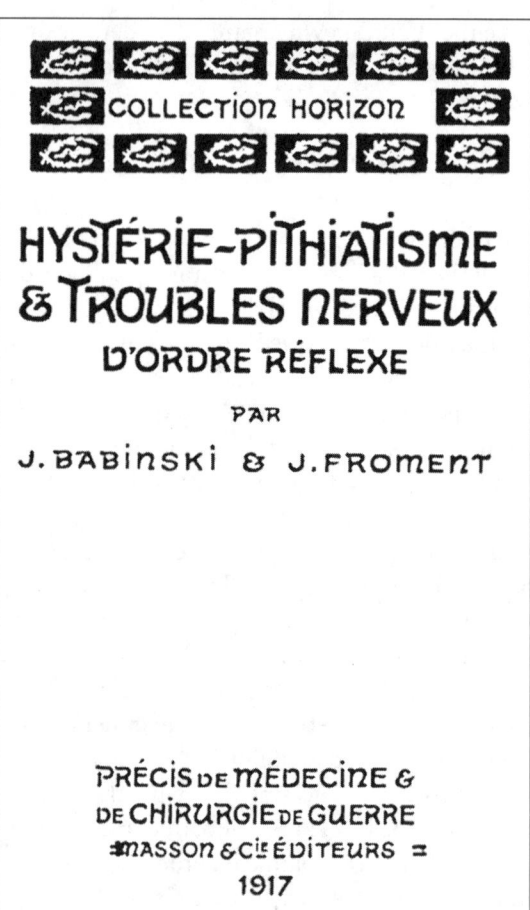

Figure 15-3 Cover of the first edition of Babinski and Froment's book. (*Source*: From J. Babinski and J. Froment, Hystérie-pithiatisme et troubles nerveux d'ordre réflexe en neurologie de guerre [Hysteria or pithiatism and reflex nervous disorders in the neurology of war]. [Paris: Masson et Cie, 1917].)

Pithiatism and Simulation

The relationship between hysteria and simulation is not clear in Babinski's thought. In several papers, he wrote that the clinical manifestations of hysteria and simulation cannot be distinguished. Moreover, "in many circumstances, hysterics behave as if they are partly in control of the disorder and as if their sincerity could be questioned.... Therefore, hysteria and simulation are very close, and I usually say that a hysteric is, in a way, a semi-simulator." This statement has been the source of a fundamental

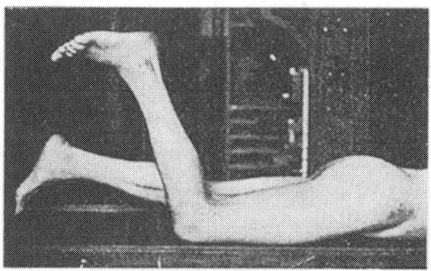
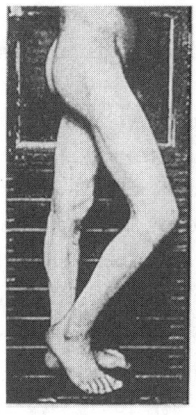
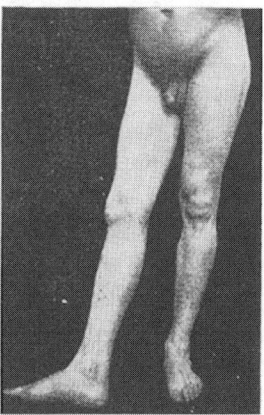

Figure 15-4 Nervous troubles of reflex origin. On the left: Contracture of the flexor muscles of the leg toward the thigh. At bottom right: contracture of the pelvic trochantric muscles with a paresis of the foot and toes. (*Source:* From J. Babinski and J. Froment, Hystérie-pithiatisme et troubles nerveux d'ordre réflexe en neurologie de guerre [Paris: Masson et Cie, 1917].)

ambiguity with regard to pithiatism, many authors making no distinction between pithiatism and simulation. This ambiguity had a particular impact on military psychiatry during World War I. The combat conditions and social attitudes of the time resulted in a considerable number of mental disorders during the war. The distinction between emotional stress and psychic trauma related to fighting, on one hand, and simulation, on the other, was a major concern for army physicians. The Société de neurologie de Paris and representatives of neurological military centers held a joint meeting on the topic in 1916.[32]

---

[32] "Réunion de la Société de neurologie de Paris avec les représentants des centres neurologiques militaires de France et des pays alliés" [Meeting of the Paris Neurological Society with representatives from the French and Allied military centers], *Rev Neurol (Paris)* 1916 (24): 449–563.

Babinski's theory of pithiatism was later criticized for resulting in excessive use of both chloroform anesthesia to distinguish pithiatism from simulation and methods that could be described as torture, such as extremely hot paraffin baths or faradization (electric therapy, termed "torpedoing" by Clovis Vincent, a pupil of Babinski's).[33] Some physicians chose to use them on the assumption that many soldiers would rather go back to the front rather than endure them again. Babinski's responsibility for these methods cannot be ruled out, although he pointed out many times that the main component of treatment should involve persuasion. According to Charpentier,[34] Babinski himself used electric stimulation at low intensity or even simulated. It is worth noting, however, that these methods were used in the German army as well as in the Allied armies.

The survey of the archives of the French Army Health Service during World War I shows considerable diversity among different army centers in the nosology and frequency of disorders classified as psychic. In the two centers for wounded soldiers directed by Babinski (his department at La Pitié and a center at the Lycée Buffon), the frequency of these disorders was low: at the Lycée Buffon it was 6 percent in 1915, 1.4 percent in 1916, and 3 percent in 1917. At La Pitié, the records show a frequency of 7.1 percent from August 1917 to February 1918.[35] In the same hospital, in the center directed by Achille Souques, psychic disorders were reported in 20 percent of the patients in 1915 and in between 5 and 15 percent from April 1917 to January 1919. In several provincial centers, the frequency of disorders classified as reflex or physiopathic was much higher than those labeled hysteria, which itself was no more frequent than the cases classified as depression or neurasthenia. The diagnosis of simulation was extremely rare. However, the uncertainty of the classifications and the fuzziness of the concepts can be seen in comments by Dr. Heitz, an army physician assistant of Babinski's at the Lycée Buffon center, who wrote that "physiopathic disorders are nearly always associated with psychiatric disorders, or pithiatism."

Pithiatism and the Controversy on Hysteria

In the early twentieth century, both the definition and nature of hysteria were subject to animated debates among neurologists and psychiatrists, as reflected

---

[33] P. Darmon, "Des suppliciés de la Grande Guerre: les pithiatiques" [The pithiatics, tortured in the First World War], *Histoire, économie et société* 2001 (20): 49–64.

[34] A. Charpentier, *Un grand médecin. J. Babinski (1857–1932)* [A great physician. J. Babinski (1857–1932)] (Paris: Typographie François Bernouard, 1934).

[35] Archives du Service de Santé des Armées, C 61.

in congresses and meetings held in Lausanne,[36] Amsterdam,[37] and Paris. The definition of hysteria given by Babinski in 1901 was used as the basis for discussion at the meeting of the Société de neurologie de Paris in 1908.[38] The consensus was that a number of clinical manifestations might be created and cured by suggestion; however, disagreements persisted among the participants. Some were reluctant to admit that hysterical stigmas were the result of medical suggestion or autosuggestion. Others faithful to the ideas of Charcot, such as Jules Dejerine, maintained that hysteria could be associated with reflex, trophic, or vasomotor disorders. Babinski repeatedly replied by demonstrating that such cases were due to diagnostic errors or simulation.[39]

A controversy also emerged over the significance of the term *suggestion*. According to Dejerine, suggestion involved the acceptance of any idea, true or false, and thus he argued that Babinski's stress on the role of suggestion made the notion of hysteria too broad. Babinski replied that according to the Littré dictionary, the term *suggestion* should only be applied to the acceptance of a false idea, and that *persuasion* more accurately described the therapeutic effect. He pointed out that while persuasion can be of some benefit in certain physical or psychological disorders, it results in the complete disappearance of symptoms only in hysteria. However, he recognized that in some cases, resistance to persuasion can be observed as a consequence of familial influence or search for material advantages.[40]

The main disagreement between Babinski and other participants concerned the role of emotion in the occurrence of hysterical symptoms and the question of mental change in hysterics. Some participants pointed out that even if the definition of pithiatism provided operational criteria for the diagnosis of hysterical disorders, it did not directly address the basic question of the nature of hysteria. Babinski replied that hysteria was defined only by natural ability to present hysterical symptoms. Albert Pitres (1848–1928) and Fulgence Raymond (1844–1910), Charcot's successor, considered

---

[36] "XVIIè Congrès des médecins aliénistes et neurologistes de France et des pays de langue française. Définition et nature de l'hystérie" [17th meeting of French and French-speaking alienists and neurologists. Definition and nature of hysteria], *Presse médicale* 1907 (15): 532–534.

[37] P. Hartenberg, "Les nouvelles idées sur l'hystérie" [New ideas on hysteria], *Presse médicale* 1907 (15): 469.

[38] "Discussion sur l'hystérie" [Discussion on hysteria], *Rev Neurol (Paris)* 1908 (16): 375–404, 494–519.

[39] J. Babinski, "Sur la fièvre et les troubles trophiques attribués à l'hystérie" [On fever and trophic disorders attributed to hysteria], *Rev Neurol (Paris)* 1909 (17): 207–209.

[40] J. Babinski, "Hystérie et pithiatisme" [Hysteria and pithiatism], *Exposé des travaux scientifiques* [Presentation of scientific papers] (Paris: Masson, 1913), 193–218.

pithiatism as a syndrome that could be observed not only in hysteria but also in other disorders, and thus it could not replace hysteria as a basic diagnostic definition.

Charcot often stressed the role of emotion as a precipitating factor for hysterical symptoms, and this idea was commonly accepted by participants at the 1909 joint meeting of the French societies of neurology and psychiatry that was devoted to the role of emotion in neurological diseases.[41] Babinski, in contrast to Dejerine, was strongly opposed to the role of emotion in the occurrence of hysterical symptoms[42]: "When a sincere, deep emotion shakes the human soul, there's no place left for hysteria." He proposed distinguishing acute emotions (*émotions-chocs*), associated with objective physiological changes, from the slow emotions that follow them. To demonstrate the absence of relationship between acute emotion and hysterical manifestations, he investigated individuals who had lived through various circumstances associated with severe stress (for example, unexpected bereavement, natural disaster, or combat stress). For Babinski, acute emotions resulted in psychic disorders that were very different from hysteria. His opinion was strengthened by the fact that during the war hysteria had not been observed at the front but only at the rear. Hysterical disorders are thus due to autosuggestion. They are linked to "a pathological need to exaggerate the manifestations of emotion and to make them more obvious for the spectators. For these manifestations to appear, the hysteric needs a public just as the actor must have an audience to play, and the effect on the people around him is certainly a contributing factor, if not to their first appearance, at least to partly determine their clinical aspects and duration."[43]

The most debatable point remained the patient's mental state. Most of the participants at the 1909 meeting believed that the main characteristic of hysteria was a specific mental state, a way of being (in Janet's words), or a trait of suggestibility. This particular mental state was considered to be the result of a specific hereditary predisposition. When accused by Oskar Vogt (1870–1959) of discarding the psychological theory of hysteria, Babinski replied: "If the subjects who present pithiatic disorders had a

---

[41] "Du rôle de l'émotion dans la genèse des accidents névropathiques et psychopathiques. L'émotion et l'hystérie" [On the role of emotion as the origin of neuropathological and psychopathological incidents. Emotion and hysteria], *Rev Neurol (Paris)* 1909 (18): 1591–1601.

[42] J. Babinski, "Émotion, suggestion et hystérie" [Emotion, suggestion and hysteria], *Rev Neurol (Paris)* 1907 (15): 752–754.

[43] J. Babinski and J. Dagnan-Bouveret, "Emotion et hystérie" [Emotion and hysteria], *Journal de Psychologie Normale et Pathologique* 1912: 92–146.

specific mental disorder, we would have a feature distinct from pithiatism that should be included in the definition. However, can you tell me what this characteristic is?"[44]

Babinski and Pierre Janet

Janet joined Charcot's department in 1889, after the end of Babinski's residency. In 1893, he published his own conception of hysteria. Closely following Charcot, he emphasized the importance of ideas in the development of hysterical paralysis, and he summarized the concept of paralysis by representation as described by Moebius. He demonstrated the similarity between hysteria and somnambulism in split personality disorder. Finally, he introduced the notion of "shrinkage of consciousness" to explain hysterical stigmas. Stigmas, in fact, differ from other hysterical symptoms because they have a negative character, suggesting a weakening of nervous functions. Hysteria, therefore, is "a kind of mental breaking up, characterized by a tendency toward a split personality." For Janet, hysteria was defined by a particular mental state: "Hysteria is first dependant on a specific mental state, an emotional state that localized phenomena according to the laws of emotion and suggestion. With this state, there is a tendency toward a dulling of the association centers, a tendency toward independent functioning."[45] Heredity is responsible for a background of a weak constitution and physical and psychological degeneration. Janet did not attend the debate on the definition of hysteria at the Société de neurologie de Paris in 1908, but a year later, at the debate on the role of emotion in neurological diseases, he contested Babinski's opinion on the absence of hysterical phenomena during acute emotions, arguing that they can occur secondarily (which, by the way, actually supports Babinski's theory). He criticized the importance of suggestion, maintaining that ideas alone were not sufficient to provoke hysterical symptoms. Babinski replied in 1912, along the lines of Theodule Ribot (1839–1916), that all ideas, even the most abstract, have some affective elements:

> Suggestion is only effective to an hysteric if she experiences it as immediately linked to her personality, interesting for her, and in a way imposing on her.... Similarly, the hysteric catches onto an idea and carries it out when this idea is especially relevant for her; it focuses her attention and, by its affective elements, is imperative, arousing an abnormal desire to surprise and attract

---

[44] Janet, "Quelques définitions de l'hystérie." [Some definitions of hysteria]
[45] Babinski and Dagnan-Bouveret, "Emotion et hystérie." [Emotion and hysteria]

attention, at least the infinite variety of motives which may arouse the easily influenced will of these patients.[46]

Babinski, Charcot, and Freud

During the period of Babinski's residency, Freud spent four months in Charcot's department at the Salpêtrière (from October 1885 to the end of February 1886). Relations between Freud and Babinski were not particularly warm. In a letter to his fiancée, Martha Bernays, dated January 27, 1886, Freud related that Charcot had asked him if he would agree to examine a patient with Babinski, and added, "Of course I did not have any objection." On this occasion, Babinski (apparently for the first time) invited Freud to lunch together in the residents' dining room. That afternoon, "from 16:00 to 19:00," they examined the patient together. "I wrote the anamnesis.... Next, the assistant (Babinski), who probably had no desire to confront me in this investigation, left and, in a quarter hour, not being a novice like him, I had found all and already given it to him. Other than that, he has always been polite with me. Tomorrow, we will present the case to Charcot."[47] Babinski never wrote about his relationship (or absence of relationship) with Freud; "I searched for the name of Freud in Babinksi's publications without any success," noted Schaltenbrand.[48]

The relations between Charcot and Freud, by contrast, were most cordial. Charcot did not meet Freud again after 1886, missing him at the Congress in Vienna in 1891, but they kept up a correspondence from 1888 to 1893.[49] Freud admired Charcot and translated into German the *Leçons du mardi*, published in June 1892. Charcot wrote on June 30: "Dear Dr. Freud, you've given me great pleasure these days. I read from beginning to end the first fascicle of the Tuesday lessons... it was like a dream: a pleasant dream. I deeply thank you, believe me, for the trouble you have taken." In the preface to the German edition, Freud devoted a paragraph to Babinski's preface, which itself, however, was not included:

> The French edition was prefaced by Dr. Babinski, in which this favorite pupil of Charcot points out, with legitimate pride, the nearly inexhaustible content

[46] Freud S. *Correspondance 1873–1939*, traduction A. Berman, Paris, Gallimard, 1966.
[47] Addresses from various Neurological Societies, Société Française de Neurologie, meeting of June 2, 1958 (Centennial of J. Babinski's birth), *Rev Neurol (Paris)*, 1958 (98): 640–668: Germany (G. Schaltenbrand).
[48] Mijolla A de. Letters from J.M. Charcot to Sigmund Freud (1886–1893). The sun-down of a God [Les lettres de Jean-Martin Charcot à Sigmund Freud (1886–1893). Le crépuscule d'un Dieu], *Revue Française de Psychanalyse* 1988: 702–725.
[49] From the French translation made by Véronique Leroux-Hugon and Pr Jean-Paul Poirier.

of investigations and lessons from the "Master" over several years, and how the study of his publications is a poor substitute for his oral teaching. It is thus justified to bring these improvised lessons to the public knowledge, and, in that way, to widen the circle of his pupils and listeners. And I think that those who had the opportunity, even for a short moment, to see the great scientist at work and to communicate with him, will be happy to abide by the opinion of Dr. Babinski.[50]

Charpentier mentions that Babinski, speaking to foreign physicians who attended demonstrations at his outpatient clinic, "showed the absurdity of Freudianism, which required each day for months the recollection, not without moral danger, of supposed repressed erotic dreams." Babinski was thus more radical than his colleague Dr. Trepsat, who, after using the Freudian method to cure a patient with facial twitches, wrote in 1922 that

> with a patient (at least a French or a Latin) one should do psychoanalysis, but without proclaiming it from the rooftops, even without telling the patient himself; one should always take into consideration this therapeutic means, use it sometimes and never talk about it.[51]

As an example of Babinski's attitude toward Freud, Babinski never referred to Freud's study on the clinical distinctions between hysterical and organic paralyses, made at Charcot's request and published in French in the *Archives de neurologie* in 1893.[52] In this study, Freud categorizes two types of paralysis according to the anatomic structures involved: the peripheral type, or paralysis by projection, which is partial, and paralysis by representation, which involves a complex motor apparatus and includes the cortical paralyses. Freud showed that hysterical paralyses differ from those of organic origin. The latter are more severe in the distal part of the limb than in the proximal part. They can be dissociated, but hysterical paralysis can be even more dissociated, involving only one function or one part of the limb; and, contrary to organic paralysis, limited hysterical paralyses may be complete. Freud concludes that these characteristics do not support the hypothesis of a dynamic lesion of the cerebral cortex. Hysterical paralyses belong to the paralysis-by-representation type but involve a particular type

---

[50] Trepsat Ch. "Traitement d'un tiqueur par la psychanalyse" [Treatment of a patient with tics through psychoanalysis], *Le Progrès Médical* 1922 (16): 182–184.
[51] S. Freud, "Quelques considérations pour une étude comparative des paralysies motrices organiques et hystériques" [Some considerations on a comparative study of organic and hysterical motor paralysis], *Archives de Neurologie* 1893 (26): 29–43.
[52] J. Breuer and S. Freud, "Le mécanisme psychique des phénomènes hystériques. Communication préliminaire" [The psychic mechanism of hysterical phenomena. Preliminary report], in *Études sur l'hystérie* (Paris: Presses Universitaires de France, 1956), 1–13.

of representation. "The hysteric behaves in her paralysis and other symptoms as if the anatomy does not exist, or that she has no knowledge of it." "I agree with Mr. Janet that it is the popular representation of the organs or the body that is involved in hysteric paralysis or anesthesia, etc." He added: "The paralyzed organ or the abolished function is associated in the subconscious with a strong affect, and the limb becomes free when this affect is subdued." Although the subject of this study was of major interest for him, Babinski never referred to this particular paper.

In contrast to Babinski and his colleagues from the Salpêtrière, Freud persisted in his convictions regarding the causality of hysteric symptoms. In a book he published with Breuer in 1892, he generalized Charcot's concept of traumatic hysteria by attributing all hysteric manifestations to psychic trauma.[53] However, according to Freud, the trauma is not a triggering factor; it is an external entity that, long after its occurrence, keeps playing an active role. The hysterical symptom is related either to the content of the memory or to the psychic state associated with the trauma.

Breuer further suggested that hysteria is due to a dissociation of the consciousness, a hypnoid state. This work is mentioned only in passing in Janet's 1893 paper on the definition of hysteria (where he misspells Breuer as "Brener") and in the thesis of Henri Cesbron, a pupil of Babinski's who mixes up the dissociation of consciousness and split personality.[54] The term *autosuggestion* is never analyzed by Babinski, Janet, or any of Charcot's other followers and is considered an explanation by itself.[55]

Freud, on the other hand, made a deep psychic analysis of hysterics the basis upon which he founded psychoanalysis. As of 1896, he rejected the official tenet that neuroses have a hereditary basis.[56] He maintained that trauma, to be a trigger of hysterical symptoms, should fulfill two conditions: it should be the determining link between the trauma and the symptom (e.g., a feeling of disgust associated with the trauma and vomiting as a symptom), and it should be of sufficient strength. Within this context, the trauma itself is only a reminiscence of an older sexual trauma: "Hysterical

---

[53] H. Cesbron, *Histoire critique de l'hystérie* [Hysteria: a critical history] (Paris: Asselin et Houzeau, 1909).
[54] D. Laplane and M. Bonduelle, "Le débat sur l'hystérie" [The debate on hysteria], *Rev Neurol (Paris)* 199 (155): 815–821.
[55] Freud S. "L'hérédité et l'étiologie des névroses" [Heredity and etiology of neurosis] (1896) In *Névroses, psychoses et perversions,* Paris, PUF, 1978, pp. 47–59.
[56] Freud S. "L'étiologie de l'hystérie" [The etiology of hysteria]. In *Névroses, psychoses et perversions,* Paris, PUF, 1978, pp. 83–112.

symptoms can only appear with the aid of memories. They are the offspring of active memories in the unconscious."[57]

Freud's work was ignored not just by Babinski but by most of his colleagues of the Salpêtrière school. In his report on psychoanalysis presented at the XVIIth International Congress of Medicine in London in 1913, Pierre Janet noted:

In opposition to [Freud's] excessive theses, ordinary psychic analysis, as carried out by old-school French psychiatrists, restricts the role of sexual traumatic memories, acknowledges the importance of other emotions and disorders, and mainly considers sexual disorders as the consequence of mental disorder rather than their cause. The big difference between psychoanalysis and psychological analysis is that the former is mainly a philosophy and a metaphysical approach, whereas neurology and psychiatry require at present further studies. Psychology can be accepted in medicine only if those who practice it give up immoderate ambitions and restrict themselves to summarizing the behavior and attitudes of patients using exact and well-defined terms, and connecting facts by a determinism that is as accurate as possible.[58]

Because of his notion of pithiatism, Babinski is often blamed for the negation of the concept of hysteria or its restriction to conversion disorders, and for betraying Charcot's ideas. Actually, in contrast to Bernheim, Babinski never denied the existence of hysteria, and he remained a follower of Charcot on two points: the need to distinguish hysterical manifestations from organic disorders, and the psychological nature of hysteria. However, if he developed the role of suggestion in the occurrence of symptoms, the mechanisms of autosuggestion remained unspecified. This is probably due to Babinski's basic distrust of psychology, as attested by his opposition to Janet's and Freud's work, and no doubt also is linked to his personality and his strong need for objective control.

According to Babinski, the diagnosis of hysteria must be based on a negative approach: the absence of signs or characteristics specific to organic diseases. Babinski brought to the medical world essential clarification in the definition of the conversion disorder, and was the first to provide accurate criteria to distinguish between hysterical symptoms and organic disorders. Moreover, Babinski can be credited with demonstrating that conversion

---

[57] Janet P. "La psycho-analyse" [Psychoanalysis]. Rapport au XVIIe Congrès international de médecine de Londres (6–13 August 1913), *Rev Neurol (Paris)*, 1913 (26): 371–372.
[58] Veith I. *Four thousand years of hysteria*. In Horowitz MJ. "Hysterical personality", New York, Aronson, 1977, pp. 7–94; Crimslik HL, Ron M. Conversion hysteria: history, diagnostic issues and clinical practice, *Cognitive Neuropsychiatry* 1999 (4):165–180.

disorders can be observed in various types of subjects, and also with establishing the therapeutic importance of suggestion (persuasion), whether only verbal or with the addition of various tools such as faradization or placebo administration. Modern psychiatry has likewise adopted his distinction between the psychic consequences of acute emotions and hysteria, as well as the diagnostic importance of the absence of reflex, trophic, or vasomotor disorders in hysteria.

Pithiatism After Babinski

Babinski's work on hysteria deeply influenced neurologists: the diagnosis of hysteria still depends on first eliminating the possibility of an organic disorder. Babinski's ideas are reflected in many studies on hysteria, particularly in reference to pithiatism, the role of suggestion, and the deleterious impact of medical intervention, but often with a lack of specific reference to Babinski's work.

> It has also been suggested that the development of conversion symptoms requires a powerful ally (the doctor in some cases) who helps to promote the sick role. The process of conveying information during consultation, investigation and treatment may be relevant in shaping and maintaining the symptoms in suggestible individuals.[59]

Contemporary manuals or textbooks of neurology differ in the importance they attribute to hysteria or hysterical symptoms. Some include a special chapter devoted to hysteria (though without any reference to Babinski).[60] In many neurological textbooks, however, no reference is made either to hysteria or to conversion disorders.

Pithiatism and Present Theories of Hysteria

Apart from the psychoanalytic theories, still very much alive, contemporary theories on hysteria point to its cognitive or social aspects. An important obstacle overcome by the concept of pithiatism comes from the relationship

---

[59] R. D. Adams and M. Victor, *Principles of Neurology* (New York: McGraw-Hill, 1977), 995–1001.
[60] E. R. Hilgard, "Neodissociation theory," in S. J. Lynn and J. W. Rhue, eds., *Dissociation: Clinical and Theoretical Perspectives* (New York: Guilford Press, 1994), 32–51, 312–329.

between hysteria, hypnosis, and simulation, as expressed by Babinski's term *semi-simulator*. Simulation, as opposed to hysteria, is conscious and intentional. The development of the cognitive neurosciences allows a better understanding of these phenomena. Consciousness is no longer considered a single entity. Some cognitive theories of consciousness and regulation of action propose explanations for hypnotic and hysterical phenomena based on Janet's concept of dissociation of psychic processes[61] or on Babinski's concept of autosuggestion.[62] The distinction between intentional simulation and hypnotic or hysterical manifestations remains difficult, but some data from neuropsychology or functional brain imagery favor the involvement of different brain mechanisms.[63]

Even if these data allow a better understanding of hysterical symptoms, they shed no light on the causal mechanisms. It is now well demonstrated that conversion disorders can be associated with different mental or personality disorders, as suggested by Babinski. While recognizing the particular psychic fragility of some subjects prone to pithiatism, he rejected the concept of hereditary degeneration sustained by Charcot and Janet. On the other hand, with its notions of suggestion and autosuggestion, the concept of pithiatism stresses the importance of social factors, which also play a major role in the modern conceptions of hypnosis and hysteria.[64]

In conclusion, it can be said that the work of Babinski, both in the ways it continued Charcot's work and in the ways it diverged from it, played a major role in the description and understanding of the neurological manifestations of hysteria. Although Babinski's comprehension of its psychological mechanisms was much more limited than today's understanding, one should not forget that hysteria, even today, remains a mysterious disorder.

---

[61] D. A. Oakley, "Hypnosis and suggestion in the treatment of hysteria," in P. W. Halligan, C. Bass, and J. C. Marshall, eds., *Contemporary Approaches to the Study of Hysteria: Clinical and Theoretical Perspectives* (Oxford: Oxford University Press, 2001), 312–329.

[62] P. Vuillemier, C. Chichero, F. Assal, et al., "Functional neuroanatomical correlates of hysterical sensorimotor loss," *Brain* 2001 (124): 1077–1090.

[63] D. A. Oakley, N. S. Ward, P. W. Halligan, et al., "Differential brain activations for malingered and subjectively 'real' paralysis," in P. W. Halligan, C. Bass, and D. A. Oakley, eds., *Malingering and Illness Deception* (Oxford: Oxford University Press, 2003), 267–284; P. Vuilleumier, "Hysterical conversion and brain function," *Progress in Brain Research* 2005 (150): 309–329.

[64] B. F. Malle, "The social cognition of intentional action," in in P. W. Halligan, C. Bass, and D. A. Oakley, eds., *Malingering and Illness Deception* (Oxford: Oxford University Press, 2003), 83–92.

··· *sixteen* ···

Neurology in the Time of Babinski

During Babinski's lifetime, neurology was progressively recognized in France as a distinct discipline with its own institutional framework. The starting point had been the creation in 1882 for Jean-Martin Charcot of the chair for the study of diseases of the nervous system at the Salpêtrière. However, the neurological scene was complex and widespread. Aside from Charcot's at the Salpêtrière, there were other neurological centers of equal importance, such as those at Bicêtre, Ivry, elsewhere at the Salpêtrière itself, in Villejuif, and naturally at La Pitié with Babinski. Leadership of these departments was often a stepping-stone to the Salpêtrière and possibly to the chair (Table 16-1).

From the beginning of his residency in 1880 until his retirement in 1922, Babinski was in continual contact with all the famous names in medicine throughout the Paris hospital system and especially in neurology. In 1896, when he took over as head of department at La Pitié, Victor Cornil, professor of pathological anatomy, was working at the Hôtel-Dieu, Gilles de la Tourette had a post at Hérold, Pierre Marie and alienist Désiré Bourneville were at Bicêtre (note that the *médecins alienists des Hôpitaux de Paris*, found only at the Bicêtre and Salpêtrière hospitals, were different from the *aliénists des asiles* assigned to psychiatric hospitals such as Ste. Anne and were recruited through a different competition system), Fulgence Raymond held the chair at the Salpêtrière, Jules Dejerine was working in another department (Jacquart) at the Salpêtrière, and Albert Gombault was in Ivry.[1]

---

[1] *Almanach national* (National almanac), 1896.

Table 16-1: Heads of neurological departments in Paris at the time of Babinski

Pitié	Bicêtre	Salpet (Jacquart)	Salpet (Cazalis)		Ivry	Paul-Brousse	Aliénist Salpet	Aliénist Bicêtre
		Vulpian then Luys	Charcot	1862 to 1882				
		Luys		1882			Legrand du Saulle	
				1883				
				1884				
				1885				
		Alix Joffroy	The Chair Charcot	1886				
				1887				
				1888				
	Dejerine			1889				
				1890				
				1891			Voisin J.	
				1892				
		Raymond	Brissaud	1893	Gombault			
				1894				Bourneville
				1895				
				1896				

	1897	1898	1899	1900	1901	1902	1903	1904	1905	1906	1907	1908	1909	1910	1911	1912	1913	1914	1915	1916	1917	1918
B																						
A	Pierre Marie							Dejerine							Raymond							
B																						
I																						
N																						
S																						
K																						
I																						
									Souques						Nageotte							
B																						
A	Souques							Pierre Marie							Dejerine				Sicard			
B																						
I																						
N																						
S																						
K																						
I																						

(continued)

Table 16-1: Continued

Pitié	Bicêtre	Salpet (Jacquart)	Salpet (Cazalis)		Ivry	Paul-Brousse	Aliénist Salpet	Aliénist Bicêtre
				1919				
			Pierre Marie	1920		Gustave Roussy		
		Souques		1921				
				1922	Clovis Vincent			
				1923				
			Guillain	1924		then	Nageotte	
				1925	Charles Foix			
		Crouzon		1926				
				1927		Jean Lhermitte		
				1928				
				1929				
				1930				
				1931				
	Alajouanine			1932				
				1933				
				1934	Haguenau			
				1935				

Thirteen years later, in 1909, Babinski was still at La Pitié; Pierre Marie, who had become professor of pathological anatomy, was at Bicêtre; Raymond and Dejerine were at the Salpêtrière; Gilles de la Tourette and Bourneville had passed away; Nageotte was at Bicêtre; Achille Souques was at Ivry; Edouard Brissaud was at the Hôtel-Dieu; and Gustave Roussy was head instructor in pathological anatomy at the medical school.[2]

The Chair for the Study of Diseases of the Nervous System

Jean-Martin Charcot had the responsibility of a department at the Salpêtrière from 1862 to his death in 1893; in 1882 he became the first holder of the chair for the study of diseases of the nervous system.[3]

After having graduated as a veterinarian from the Alfort school, Fulgence Raymond afterward started his medical studies.[4] A resident in 1871, Raymond was nominated *médecin des hôpitaux* in 1878 and successively occupied a position at the Hospice des Incurables, the St. Antoine Hospital, and Lariboisière, finally coming to the Salpêtrière in 1884; he succeeded Charcot in the chair in 1894, after Edouard Brissaud's interim period.[5] His inaugural lesson was a long and rousing eulogy of Charcot.[6]

Jules Dejerine was an associate professor and head of department at Bicêtre in 1887 before moving to the Salpêtrière in 1895, where he ran the second neurological unit (in Jacquart).[7] Professor of medical history and of internal medicine, he succeeded Raymond in the chair for nervous diseases on March 1, 1911. In 1888, he had married Augusta Klumpke, an American medical student and the first woman to pass the competitive examination to be a resident in the Paris hospitals (1887); Mrs. Dejerine would be an efficient teammate for her husband.[8] Dejerine's scientific papers are numerous.

---

[2] Ibid., 1909.
[3] M. Bonduelle, T. Gelfand, and C. G. Goetz, *Charcot: un grand médecin dans son siècle* [A great physician in his century] (Paris: Éditions Michalon, 1996). See also chapter 6.
[4] http://www.whonamedit.com/doctor.cfm/671.html.
[5] On Raymond's residency, see Table 16–1.
[6] *Le Progrès Médical* 1894 (XX): 399–407, 410.
[7] E. Gauckler, *Le professeur J. Dejerine (1849–1917)* (Paris: Masson et Cie, 1922); J. Hallion, "Allocution de M. Hallion, président à l'occasion du décès du Pr. Dejerine" [Obituary by M. Hallion, président, for Professor Dejerine], *Rev Neurol (Paris)* 1917 (I): 216–218 ; http://www.whonamedit.com/doctor.cfm/337.html.
[8] G. Roussy, "Eloge de Mme Dejerine-Klumpke" [Eulogy of Mrs. Dejerine-Klumpke (1859–1927)], *Rev Neurol (Paris)* 1927 (II): 635–642.

The most important deal with the description of Dejerine-Roussy disease, caused by a lesion in the posterior thalamus; Landouzy-Dejerine syndrome, or facio-scapulo-humeral muscular dystrophy (1885); and Dejerine-Sottas neuropathy (1893). Three of his books are especially important: his treatise on spinal cord diseases, written with André Thomas, and the two masterpieces of his anatomy of the central nervous system (where the participation of Mrs. Dejerine was of capital importance) and his book on the semiology of diseases of the nervous system.[9] Although the major part of his work deals with organic neurology, Dejerine late in his life turned to a new field. Like many other eminent neurologists of this time, and encouraged by his friendship with Paul-Charles Dubois (1848–1918) from Bern, Switzerland, he became interested in psychology, functional disorders, and hysteria. He published "Les manifestations fonctionnelles des psychonévroses" (The Psychoneuroses and their treatment by psychotherapy) with E. Gauckler in the *Nouveau Traité de Médecine* (1911). He was convinced that the personality of the psychotherapist is crucial in the relationship with the patient (Figs. 16-1 and 16-2).

At the end of his residency, Pierre Marie defended a thesis on Basedow disease and became chief resident under Charcot, with whom he described progressive muscular atrophy, named later Charcot-Marie-Tooth disease.[10] He was associate professor and head of a department at Bicêtre in 1895 and at the Salpêtrière in 1911, becoming a professor of pathological anatomy in 1907; he was also a member of the Académie nationale de médecine. At the age of sixty-four, he took over from Dejerine—whom he hated most implacably—in the chair of the Clinic of Nervous Diseases, which he held for six years, from 1917 to his retirement in 1923. He described acromegaly (Pierre Marie disease), hypertrophic pulmonary osteoarthropathy, hereditary cerebellar ataxy, hereditary cleidocranial dysostosis, and rhizomelic spondylosis. He worked on aphasia, though his ideas were opposed to those of Paul Broca and Karl Wernicke. With Edouard Brissaud, he started the *Revue de Neurologie*, in 1893, and the Société de neurologie de Paris, of which he was

---

[9] J. Dejerine and A. Thomas, *Traité des maladies de la moelle épinière* [Treatise on spinal cord diseases] (Paris: J. B. Baillière, 1902); J. Dejerine with the collaboration of Mme Dejerine-Klumpke, *Anatomie des centres nerveux* [Anatomy of the central nervous system], 2 vols. (Paris: Rueff, 1890–1901); J. Dejerine, *Sémiologie des affections du système nerveux* [Semiology of diseases of the nervous system] (Paris: Masson, 1914). The last of these was praised highly in *Le Progrès Médical* 1913 (supplement, 444): "Finally, this book represents, with its complete documentation, a perfect overview of the present neurological science."
[10] A. Tournay, "Nécrologie de M. Pierre Marie" [Obituary of M. Pierre Marie], *Rev Neurol (Paris)* 1941 (73): 618–621; J. Poirier and F. Chrétien, "Pierre Marie (1853–1940)," *J Neurol* 2000, 247(12): 983–984; G. Milian, *Le Progrès Médical* 1907 (XXIII): 884.

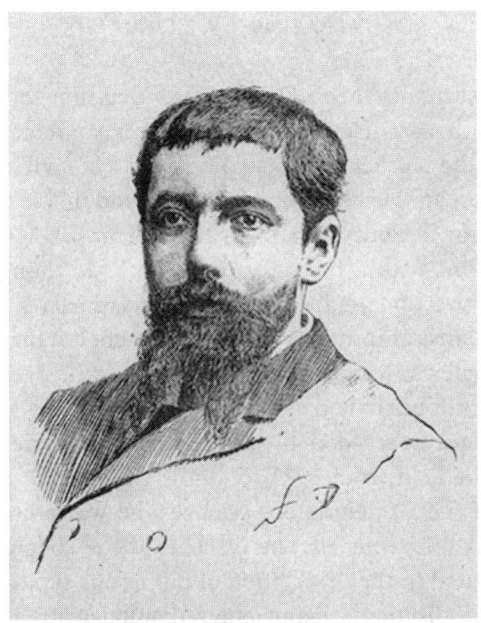

Figure 16-1 Jules Dejerine. (*Source*: From Horace Bianchon, Nos grands médecins d'aujourd'hui [Paris: Société d'éditions scientifiques, 1891].)

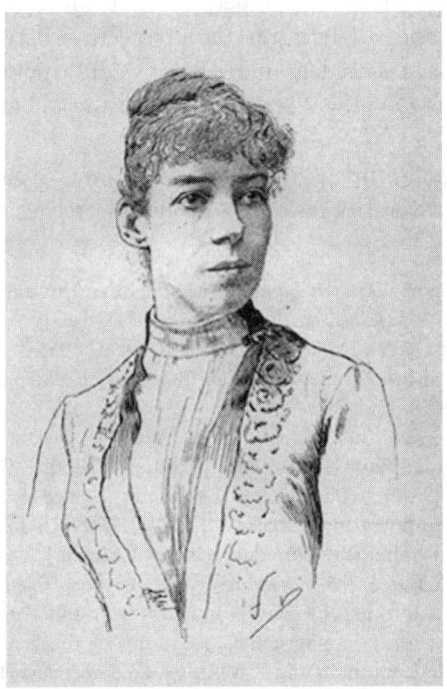

Figure 16-2 Augusta Dejerine-Klumpke. (*Source*: From Horace Bianchon, Nos grands médecins d'aujourd'hui [Paris: Société d'éditions scientifiques, 1891].)

the first general secretary. Léon Daudet described him thus: "Pierre Marie, kind, studious with a satisfactory scientific career, would, as Brissaud, swear on the words of the teacher. He looks like a perfect civil servant, punctual and meticulous, an affable librarian who could find in five minutes the book you are looking for."[11] Four years older than Babinski, Marie was in fact a contemporary of his within the hospital system, and though they were not really close, the two apparently had a good relationship. Marie once was invited by the Babinski brothers to a Sunday lunch, but made a serious mistake by adding water to his glass of great vintage wine; Henri murmured to Jo seph, "He will not be invited again" (Figs. 16-3 and 16-4)[12]

Georges Guillain succeeded his teacher Pierre Marie in the chair of Charcot, which he held from 1923 to 1947.[13] Member of the Académie de médecine and of the Académie des sciences, he was a commander in the Legion of Honor. With Léchelle, he discovered the colloidal benzoic reaction and participated in the description of numerous syndromes bearing his name, the most well-known being polyradiculoneuritis or Guillain-Barré syndrome (or Guillain- Barré-Strohl syndrome). He also published several books, including a work on neurology under conditions of war with Alexandre Barré, an anatomy of the central nervous system with Ivan Bertrand, a monograph on the Salpêtrière with Mathieu, and a biography of Charcot.[14] Alexandre Barré was the connection between Guillain and Babinski; he had been a resident under Babinski, to whom he remained very attached, and during World War I he had also worked for and got on very well with Guillain.

Théophile Alajouanine (1890–1980), while not a pupil of Babinski's, had met him on several occasions. Alajouanine relates that Babinski was

---

[11] L. Daudet, *Les oeuvres dans les hommes* [Men as seen through their works] (Paris: Nouvelle Librairie Nationale, 1922), 197–243.

[12] L. Rivet, "Joseph Babinski (1857–1932)," *Bull. Mém. Soc. Méd. Hôp. Paris* 1932 (34): 1722–1733; T. Alajouanine, "Le centenaire de Babinski" [Centenary of Babinski], *Sem Hôp Paris*, May 12, 1958, 1355–1364.

[13] Dossier Georges Guillain, Archives de l'Académie des sciences; P. Mollaret, "Nécrologie. Georges Guillain (1876–1961)" [Obituary. Georges Guillain (1876–1961)], *La Presse Médicale* 1961 (69): 1696–1706 ; M. Bonduelle, "Notice biographique de Georges Guillain" [Biographical notes on Georges Guillain (1876–1961)], *Rev Neurol (Paris)* 1977 (133): 661–666; www.whonamedit.com.doctor.cfm/1318.html.

[14] G. Guillain and J. A. Barré, *Travaux neurologiques de guerre* [Neurological work in war conditions] (Paris: Masson, 1920); G. Guillain and I. Bertrand, *Anatomie topographique du système nerveux central* [Topographical anatomy of the central nervous system] (Paris: Masson, 1926); G. Guillain and P. Mathieu, *La Salpêtrière* (Paris: Masson, 1925); G. Guillain, *Charcot, sa vie, son oeuvre* [J.-M. Charcot, his life and work] (Paris: Masson et Cie, 1955).

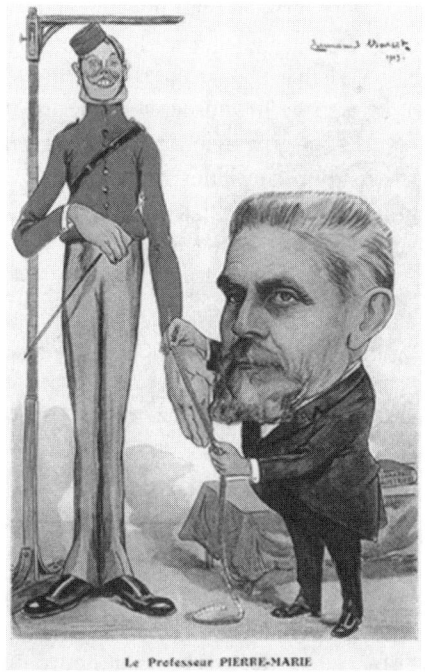

Figure 16-3 Pierre Marie. (*Source*: From Chanteclair, January 1910; personal collection, J. Poirier.)

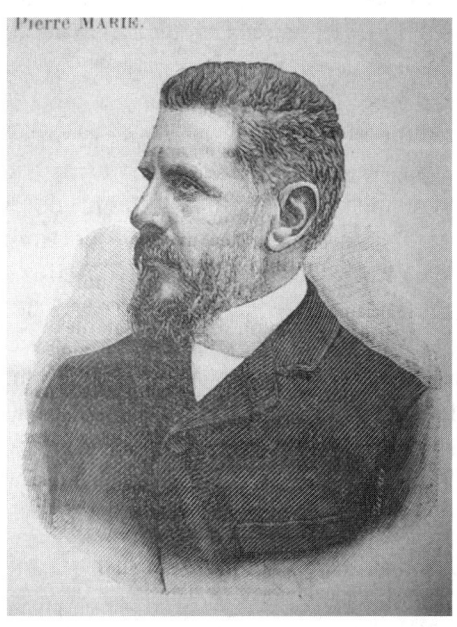

Figure 16-4 Pierre Marie. (*Source*: From Le Progrès Médical 1907 [XXIII]: 884.)

the president of the jury at his first competition for *médecin des hôpitaux*: "I always remember him, his chronometer in hand, measuring the time for the clinical test."[15] Alajouanine also deeply appreciated Babinski's great courtesy when he called upon the older man for a consultation on one of his patients.[16] A pupil of Guillain, Alajouanine held the chair from 1947 until 1959, when his own pupil Paul Castaigne, the last holder of the chair, succeeded him.[17]

Other Neurological Departments

A second neurological department, located in the Jacquart building at the Salpêtrière, was successively led by Alix Joffroy, Jules Bernard Luys (1828–1897), and Vulpian (before he moved to the Charité), then by Dejerine from 1895 to 1910; the last two holders were Pierre Marie and Achille Souques (1860–1944).

In the Bicêtre hospice, the department of neurology was successively run by Dejerine (with Sottas as resident from 1887 to 1895), then by Pierre Marie, and finally by Achille Souques, who left for the Salpêtrière in 1919. It was only in 1932 that neurology returned to Bicêtre with Alajouanine.

Babinski's department at La Pitié (first in the old Pitié, then in the new) was devoted to general medicine (see chapter 8). No neurologist preceded or succeeded him as head of department (see Table 16–1). Two of his very close pupils, Albert Charpentier and Auguste Tournay, practiced mainly neurology but had no official positions in the hospital system (see chapter 9).

In the Ivry hospice, the head of the department was Albert Gombault (1844–1904), who remained in that position until his death in 1904; he wrote his thesis on amyotrophic lateral sclerosis (1877), was a founding member of the Société de neurologie de Paris in 1899, and also was curator of the medical history museum (Musée Dupuytren). His neurological, neuropathological, and neurohistological works remain quite important. With authorization from the university he established an open course on histology in 1888.[18] He wrote, in collaboration with Claude Philippe, the fifth part of the *Traité d'histologie pathologique*, edited by Cornil and Ranvier.

---

[15] Alajouanine, "Le centenaire de Babinski."
[16] Ibid.
[17] T. Alajouanine, "Leçon inaugurale de la chaire de Clinique des maladies du système nerveux" [Opening speech for the chair of the Clinic for Nervous Diseases], Société de neurologie, November 21, 1947.
[18] *Le Progrès Médical* 1904 (XX): 222.

He published several papers, but his name is particularly linked to the neuritis of Gombault and Philippe.

Claude Philippe (1865–1903), resident first in Lyon and then in Paris, was Gombault's favorite pupil.[19] For six years he was head of the laboratory in Raymond's clinic, where Raymond showed him special attention: "Pupil of my colleague and friend Gombault, whom I consider as one of the best pathological anatomists of our time, he rapidly stood out from the others. A remarkable histologist, he was at the same time a great clinician, never separating one from the other."[20]

Achille Souques, a resident (receiving a gold medal) under Charcot the year the latter died, became chief resident with Brissaud, temporary head of the chair, then with Raymond who was named to the chair in 1894.[21] Nominated *médecin des hôpitaux* in 1898, he took over from Gombault as head of the department in Ivry in 1905, then succeeded Pierre Marie in 1911 at Bicêtre, and then in 1919 went to Jacquart at the Salpêtrière. He was a founding member of the *Revue Neurologigue* and a member of the Académie nationale de médecine. His scientific work is substantial, covering the main fields of neurology and especially semiology, Parkinson's disease, palilaly, and aphasia. His history of neurology in ancient Greece is a masterpiece of erudition.[22]

Jean-Athanase Sicard (1872–1929), pupil of Brissaud and Raymond, was a preferred disciple of Fernand Widal.[23] His thesis dealt with subarachnoid injections and the cerebrospinal fluid.[24] Professor of internal pathology, he succeeded Achille Souques at Ivry in 1911 and then went to Necker in 1919. His works in neurology are numerous and concern neurosyphilis, lethargic encephalitis, migraine, therapy of malaria, and neurology in war conditions. He perfected the use of alcohol injections in the treatment of facial neuralgia and sclerosing solutions in the varicose veins. Above all, with his pupil Jacques Forestier (1890–1978), physician in a hydrotherapic establishment and rheumatologist, he recommended in 1921 the use of an iodized oil (lipiodol

---

[19] R. Cestan, J. Oberthur, and C. Philippe, *Le Progrès Médical* 1903 (XVIII): 470–471.
[20] F. Raymond, quoted in ibid.
[21] "Achille Souques (1860–1944)," *Rev Neurol (Paris)* 1945 (77): 37.
[22] A. Souques, *Étapes de la neurologie dans l'Antiquité grecque (d'Homère à Galien)* [Neurological steps in the ancient Greek civilization (from Homer to Galen)] (Paris: Masson et Cie, 1936).
[23] http://www.whonamedit.com/doctor.cfm/920.html; L. Babonneix, "J.-A. Sicard (1872–1929)," *Rev Neurol (Paris)* 1929 (I): 161–164; E. Rist, *25 portraits de médecins français, 1900–1950* [25 portraits of French physicians, 1900–1950] (Paris: Masson, 1955), 97–104.
[24] J. A. Sicard, *Les injections sous-arachnoïdiennes et le liquide céphalo-rachidien. Recherches expérimentales et cliniques* [Subarachnoid injections and cerebrospinal fluid. Experimental and clinical research] (Paris: Georges Carré et C. Naud, 1900).

or pantopaque) impervious to X-rays.[25] Injected into the subarachnoid space, it allowed precise localization of an intraspinal tumor. He recommended its use for opacification of the bronchi and the urinary tract as well.

Clovis Vincent became head of the department in Ivry in 1921, leaving for Tenon in 1924 before returning to La Pitié (see chapter 13).

Charles Foix, a resident (receiving a gold medal) under Pierre Marie in Bicêtre, became head of the laboratory of Pierre Marie in the Salpêtrière (1912) and then served in World War I in the neurological center at Salonika, Greece.[26] As an associate professor, he succeeded Clovis Vincent at the Ivry hospice (1924), where his reputation attracted many foreign visitors.[27] Foix's scientific contribution is considerable, in terms of both quantity and quality. One may especially cite his precise description of the brain arteries, their territories, and the vascular syndromes related to their pathology; he also published a fine anatomy of the mesencephalon suboptic area (with Nicolesco), a craniocerebral topography (with Marie and Ivan Bertrand), and studies on cerebellar syndromes (with Marie and Thiers), cerebellar atrophy with cortical predominance (with Marie and Alajouanine), aphasias (with Marie), and centrolobar and symmetrical intracerebral sclerosis (with Pierre Marie and Julien Marie).[28] Charles Foix was also an author of prose and poetry. Babinski was deeply affected by the death of this young and brilliant neurologist, twenty-five years younger than himself.

The regional hospital Paul-Brousse was not in the strict sense a Paris hospital, as it was located in the southern Paris suburb of Villejuif; it was at first designated to take care of the elderly, disabled, and those with incurable diseases.[29] Dedicated in December 1913 by the president of the Republic, Raymond Poincaré, its first director was Professor Gustave Roussy. A resident under Dejerine and Pierre Marie, he was never a pupil of Babinski's.[30] In

---

[25] J. A. Sicard and J. Forestier, "Méthode radiographique d'exploration de la cavité epidurale par le lipiodol" [Radiological exploratory method of the epidural cavity using lipiodol], *Rev Neurol (Paris)* 1921 (28): 1264–1266. See the historical accounts in S.M. Wolpert, G. Di Chiro, and D. Schellinger, "CT of spinal cord after lumbar intrathecal introduction of Metrizamide (Computer assisted myelography)," *Am. J. of Neuroradiol* 2001(22): 219–221.

[26] C. Foix and G. Roussy, *Rev Neurol (Paris)* 1927 (I): 441–446; Rist, *25 portraits*, 49–56.

[27] http://cfx-jrs.aphp.fr/histoire/1900.html.

[28] P. Marie, C. Foix, and T. Alajouanine, "De l'atrophie cérébelleuse tardive à prédominance corticale" [On late predominantly cortical cerebellar atrophy], *Rev Neurol (Paris)* 1922, 38(7): 849–885, 38(8): 1082–1111.

[29] "Guérir du cancer et mourir de vieillesse: histoire de l'hospice Paul-Brousse de 1905 à 1975" [To be cured of cancer and die of old age: a history of the Paul Brousse hospice], *Asclepio* 1983 (XXXV): 317–326.

[30] Dossier Gustave Roussy, Archives de l'Académie des sciences; J. Poirier and F. Chrétien, "Gustave Roussy (1874–1948)," *J Neurol* 2000 (247): 888–889.

1907, he had defended his thesis (the board of examiners was chaired by Dejerine) on the thalamus and thalamic syndrome; this would later be named Dejerine-Roussy syndrome.[31] Named an associate professor of pathological anatomy in 1910, he then became professor of pathological anatomy after Letulle in 1925. Leaving neurology, he devoted himself to cancer, from both clinical and pathological points of view, and was a pioneer in the crusade against this disease. In 1919 he created at Paul-Brousse an outpatient clinic that rapidly became a reference center for cancer patients. The Institut du cancer was built in 1934–35 as the west wing of the hospital. Roussy became dean of the Faculty of Medicine in 1933 and then rector of the University of Paris in 1937. Like many others physicians of this time, Roussy was an "untiring worker who, every day for long hours, devoted himself to multiple and difficult tasks."[32] The victim of a smear campaign based upon a supposedly financial scandal, he was driven to suicide in 1948. The Institut du cancer was named after him in 1949.

At the beginning of the twentieth century, a neurological outpatient department was opened at the St. Joseph Hospital by Paul Berbez.[33] A resident in 1882, he was very much appreciated by Charcot, under whom he became chief resident after Pierre Marie; he wrote his thesis in 1887 on hysteria and trauma. Berbez appears in Brouillet's painting "A Lesson at the Salpêtrière," as does his younger brother Henry, at that time still a student under Charcot. He was a regular dinner guest at Charcot's home. In 1887, he played in *Macbeth* with Henri Meige, Babinski, and Jeanne and Jean Charcot. Despite being favored by Charcot, he had a modest career, writing very few papers.[34] He resigned from St. Joseph in 1911; André Thomas, with his two assistants Hecaen and Ajuriaguerra, succeeded him. Henri Schaeffer would arrive there in 1929.

The Clinical Chair for the Mind and Brain Diseases at the Ste. Anne Hospital

This chair was over a long period held in succession by three of Charcot's pupils: Benjamin Ball (1834–1893), first holder from 1877 to his death in 1893;

---

[31] G. Roussy, *La couche optique (étude anatomique, physiologique & clinique). Le syndrome thalamique* [The thalamus and thalamic syndrome (anatomical, physiological, and clinical study)] (Paris: G. Steinheil, 1907).

[32] Speech of Professor Cornil (Marseille) at the funeral of Gustave Roussy, Dossier Gustave Roussy, Archives de l'Académie des sciences.

[33] M. Bonduelle, personal communication.

[34] Bonduelle, Gelfand, and Goetz, *Charcot: un grand médecin dans son siècle*.

Alix Joffroy (1844–1908), from 1894 to 1908; and Gilbert Ballet (1853–1916), from 1909 to 1916.[35] Ballet's thesis was dedicated to anatomoclinical research.[36] Charcot's first chief resident when the chair for the study of diseases of the nervous system was created in 1882, Ballet was later professor of the history of medicine and a member of the Académie nationale de médecine. His extensive neurological and psychiatric work can be seen in his noteworthy volume on psychiatric disorders *Traité de pathologie mentale*, published in 1903.[37]

Next in the chair was Ernest Dupré (1862–1921), from 1916 to 1921.[38] From 1922 to 1939, Henri Claude (1872–1945) had the chair; he is known both as a psychiatrist and a neurologist, as seen in his description of certain brain stem syndromes and his perfection of an apparatus to measure cerebrospinal fluid and venous pressure.[39]

A student under Babinski in 1897–1898, Maxime Laignel-Lavastine (1875–1953) succeeded Henri Claude from 1939 to 1942. Joseph Lévy-Valensi (1879–1943) was nominated to the chair in 1942; prevented from practicing medicine because of the anti-Semitic decrees, he was arrested on September 5, 1943, during a mass roundup, taken to the camp of Drancy, and interned in Auschwitz on November 20 of that year. He was murdered five days later.[40]

Pupils of Charcot with an Academic Career Outside Neurology

Professor of internal medicine and member of the Académie nationale de médecine, Charles Bouchard (1837–1915) was also a member and president

---

[35] Joffroy was the first president of the Société de neurologie de Paris. A. Joffroy, "Discours donné par le Pr Joffroy" [Speech given by Professor Joffroy, Société de neurologie de Paris, meeting of July 6, 1899], *Rev Neurol (Paris)* 1899 (VII): 506–509; M. Klippel, "Hommage à Professeur Joffroy" [Homage to Professor Joffroy], *Rev Neurol (Paris)* 1908 (XVI): 1326–1327; M. Huet, "Discours donné par M. Huet, président à l'occasion de la mort du Professeur Gilbert Ballet" [Speech by M. Huet, president, on the occasion of the death of Professor Gilbert Ballet], *Rev Neurol (Paris)* 1916 (6): 896–898; J. Postel and D. F. Allen, "L'oeuvre historique de Gilbert Ballet (1853–1916)" [Historical works of Gilbert Ballet], http://www.bium.univ-paris5.fr/sfhm/histoire3.htm.
[36] G. Ballet, *Recherches anatomiques et cliniques sur le faisceau sensitif et les troubles de la sensibilité dans les lésions du cerveau* [Anatomical and clinical research on the sensory tract and sensory disturbances in brain lesions] (Paris: Delahaye et Lecrosnier, 1881).
[37] G. Ballet, *Traité de pathologie mentale* [Treatise on mental pathology] (Paris: Dom, 1903).
[38] André Breton did not like him very much, describing him without any affection as having a "naive face and stubborn expression." A. Breton, *Nadja* (Paris: Gallimard, 1928).
[39] H. Claude, "L'hypertension intracrânienne" [Intracranial hypertension], *Le Journal Médical Français*, May 1915; http://www.uic.edu/depts/mcne/founders/page0019.html.
[40] http://psychiatrie.histoire.free.fr/pers/bio/levy-valensi.htm.

of the Académie des sciences.⁴¹ On July 2, 1887, in honor of his election, his friends and pupils (Babinski was not present) offered a banquet at the Hôtel Continental. Joseph Landouzy (1845–1917) proposed the toast. In his response, Bouchard paid overly enthusiastic homage to Charcot as his "intellectual father."⁴² Quite aside from his conflictive and competitive relationship with Charcot and the ousting of Babinski at the *agrégation* in 1892, Bouchard was not unanimously admired. Léon Daudet painted a verbal portrait of the man:

> Bouchard, metaphysicist and fanciful clinician, ignorant creator of diseases caused by "slowdown" or "acceleration" of nutrition, originator of lethal and colorless diets that rival in fantasy the emptiness of those of Albert Robin. Sad, full of bitterness, with gold-colored glasses, a dull voice, and a suspicious look, Professor Bouchard gives to an observer the impression of unbelievable stupidity coupled with tremendous self-satisfaction.⁴³

Maurice Loeper (1875–1961), in the obituary he wrote of Bouchard, spoke doubtfully of the importance of his works: "Only the future will tell us what real merit shall be attached to it and what portion of truth it contains. It is possible that hypothesis occupies a too predominant place and is not always supported by undisputable facts; maybe we are more often surprised than convinced by the abundance of scientific arguments?"⁴⁴ But the strongest blow came in *Le Journal des Praticiens*, a real posthumous hatchet job that may have delighted Babinski and quenched his desire for revenge:

> Today when silence has over shadowed the memory of Professor Bouchard, his example should be recalled for a moment in order to remind to the medical world the errors in methodology that, followed stubbornly until the end, drove this intelligent man to the worst mistakes in the clinical and therapeutic fields.... He was arrogant and formal. The confidence he had in his own merit prevented him from using the classical methods of observation. He was not interested in clinical studies, or only if they confirmed his own interpretation. Another man might have corrected himself; becoming aware of the faulty starting point, he would have gone back to the beginning. Bouchard wandered even more astray. The atmosphere of flattery in which he was wallowing prevented him from even getting to the healthy climate that reflects the undisguised truth. Accepting compliments at face value, he persisted in his mistaken methodology.⁴⁵

---

[41] Dossier Charles Bouchard, Archives de l'Académie des sciences; P. Le Gendre, *Charles Bouchard, son œuvre et son temps (1837–1915)* [Charles Bouchard, his work and times (1837–1915)] (Paris: Masson et Cie, 1924).
[42] *Le Progrès Médical* 1887 (VI): 29–30.
[43] Daudet, *Les oeuvres dans les hommes*, 197, 243.
[44] *Le Progrès Médical* 1914 (suppléments): 623.
[45] *Journal des Praticiens* 1917, MLV.

Perhaps the supreme insult came in 1917:

> The work of Professor Bouchard is full of recurrent Krautism, cherishing himself and looking voluptuously to the German traits guiding his effort. Nothing except a memory remains of the poor devils who paid with their lives for their confidence in the naphtols.

If the name of Bouchard is still familiar to neurologists today, he owes this to his work on miliary aneurysms, described as Charcot-Bouchard aneurysms, although it remained a controversial topic for quite some time.[46]

Pupil, associate, and friend of Charcot, Georges-Maurice Debove (1845–1920) was present when his mentor died in the Morvan countryside.[47] Professor of medical pathology and of a medical clinic at la Charité, then in Beaujon, he became dean of the medical faculty from 1901 to 1907. After his thesis on lingual psoriasis, his work for the most part concerned nervous diseases and hysteria; he then shifted from neurology to the study of tuberculosis. An enthusiastic follower of bacteriological research, he discovered tuberculin in exudate and was in favor of overfeeding for tubercular patients. He was also interested in nutrition, obesity, gout, the fight against alcoholism, and many other topics, notably digestive tract pathology.

A pupil of Charcot and of Lasègue (1816–1883), Edouard Brissaud (1852–1909) temporarily (1893–1894) held the chair for the study of diseases of the nervous system after Charcot's death; he then became professor of the history of medicine (1899) and finally professor of medical pathology (1900).[48] A man of lively nature and a passionate defender of justice, motivated by generous ideas, Brissaud was a freethinker and fervent supporter of Dreyfus. He published an atlas of the brain drawn completely by hand—a monumental achievement that necessitated an incredible amount of work.[49] He was associate editor of six volumes of the *Traité de Médecine*.[50] In 1899,

---

[46] J.-M. Charcot and C. Bouchard, "Nouvelles recherches sur la pathogénie de l'hémorragie cérébrale" [New research on brain hemorrhage pathogenesis], *Arch Physiol Norm Pathol*. 1868 (1): 110–127, 643–665, 725–734; F. Dubas, "Bibliothèque idéale. Histoire de la controverse sur les anévrysmes miliaires de Charcot et Bouchard" [An ideal library. A history on the controversy about the miliary aneurysms of Charcot and Bouchard], *Rev Neurol (Paris)* 2006 (162): 400–405.

[47] M. Loeper, "Nécrologie de G.-M. Debove" [Obituary of G.-M. Debove], *Le Progrès Médical* 1920 (48): 517.

[48] www.whonamedit.com/doctor.cfm/1272 "Edouard Brissaud (1852–1909)," *Rev Neurol (Paris)* 1910 (1): 1–4.

[49] E. Brissaud, *Anatomie du cerveau de l'homme; morphologie des hémisphères cérébraux, ou cerveau proprement dit* [Human brain anatomy; brain hemisphere morphology] (Paris: Masson, 1893).

[50] J.-M. Charcot, C. Bouchard, and E. Brissaud, *Traité de médecine* [Treatise on medicine] (Paris: G. Masson, 1891–93).

he published his *Leçons sur les maladies nerveuses*.[51] With Pierre Marie, he founded the *Revue Neurologique*. Struck down by a brain tumor, despite an operation by the well-known British neurosurgeon Victor Horsley, he died in 1909, surrounded by the affection of his nearest and dearest.

Neurology in the Provinces

In 1899, the Société de neurologie de Paris was founded essentially, as its name implies, for neurologists of the capital; it is significant that half a century went by before it finally became the Société française de neurologie, in 1949.[52] In Babinski's time and for several decades afterward, the great names in French neurology were all based in Paris; some provincial physicians more or less specialized in neurological diseases, but their names and works remain generally unknown.

During its first meeting in 1899, the Société de neurologie de Paris designated nineteen provincial neurologists as corresponding members, and five others were named at the next meeting; however, for the most part these individuals did not contribute in any notable way to progress in neurology. Among the exceptions were Albert Pitres (1848–1928), pupil of Charcot, professor in Bordeaux; Hippolyte Bernheim (1837–1919), professor in Nancy famous for his work on hysteria; Joseph Grasset (1849–1918), professor in Montpellier; and Henri Duret (1849–1921), dean at the Free Faculty of Lille (See chapter 15 on Bernheim and chapter 13 on Duret).

Later, other provincial physicians trained in Paris became more well known. These include Cestan, pupil of Babinski and of Raymond, holder of the chair of psychiatry in Toulouse in 1913; and Barré, a pupil of Babinski's and associate of Guillain's who became professor of neurology in Strasbourg in 1919.

A Glance at World Neurology

Paris was not the center of the neurological and psychiatric world at the end of the nineteenth century and the beginning of the twentieth. While great neurologists and psychiatrists were found in many different countries, three

---

[51] E. Brissaud, *Leçons sur les maladies nerveuses* [Lessons on nervous sytem diseases] (Paris, 1899).

[52] M. Bonduelle, "Histoire de la Société française de neurologie: 1899–1974" [A history of the French Neurological Society: 1899–1974], *Rev Neurol (Paris)* 1999 (155): 785–801.

main schools outside of France led the field: those of England, Germany, and the United States (Table 16-2).

In Great Britain, the National Hospital (Queen's Square) was founded in 1860. As in Paris, neurology in England was concentrated in a single site, but in contrast to France and other countries, the hospital had no links with the university system.

Table 16-2: Some great names of the world neurology at the time of Babinski

Germany	Moritz Heinrich Romberg (1795–1873)	Romberg Sign
	Karl Westphal (1833–1890)	Bone and tendon reflexes Westphal's pseudosclerosis Edinger-Westphal nucleus
	Theodor Hermann Meynert (1833–1892)	
	Wilhelm Heinrich Erb (1840–1921)	Bone and tendon reflexes Erb-Goldflam syndrome Erb's myelitis
	Carl Wernicke (1848–1905)	Wernicke's aphasia Wernicke's encephalopathy
	Arnold Pick (1851–1924)	Pick's dementia
	Otto Ludwig Binswanger (1852–1929)	Binswanger's leucoencephalopathy
	Ludwig Edinger (1855–1918)	Edinger-Westphal nucleus
	Hermann Oppenheim (1858–1919)	
	Adolf Wallenberg (1862–1949)	Wallenberg's syndrome
	Alois Alzheimer (1864–1915)	Alzheimer's disease
	Korbinian Brodmann (1868–1918)	Localization in the cerebral cortex

(continued)

Table 16-2: Continued

	Oskar Vogt (1870–1959)	
	Otfrid Foerster (1873–1941)	
	Alfons Maria Jakob (1884–1931)	Creutzfeldt-Jakob disease
	Hans Gerhard Creutzfeldt (1885–1964)	Creutzfeldt-Jakob disease
Austria	Sigmund Freud (1856–1939)	Psychoanalysis
	Constantin von Economo (1876–1931)	Von Economo's encephalitis lethargica
Belgium	Arthur van Gehuchten (1861–1914) Ludo van Bogaert (1897–1988)	Van Bogart's disease
United Kingdom	Hughlings Jackson (1835–1911)	"The father of British neurology" Jacksonian epilepsy Jackson's laws
	Douglas Argyll Robertson (1837–1908)	Argyll-Robertson's sign
	Sir Byron Bramwell (1847–1931)	
	David Ferrier (1843–1924)	Brain localizations
	Sir William Richard Gowers (1845–1915)	Gowers haemoglobinometer Gowers bundle *A Manual of the Diseases of the Nervous System* (1886–1888) First removal of a spinal tumor with Horsley (1888)
	Sir Victor Horsley (1857–1916)	First removal of a spinal tumor with Gowers (1888)
	Henry Head (1861–1940)	Head-Holmes syndrome

(continued)

Table 16-2: Continued

	Samuel Kinnier-Wilson (1878–1937)	Wilson's disease
Ireland	Gordon Morgan Holmes (1876–1965)	
Italy	Giovanni Mingazzini (1859–1919)	Mingazzini's sign
Poland[1]	Samuel Goldflam (1852–1932)	Erb-Goldflam ssyndrome
	Edward Flatau (1869–1932)	
Portugal	Egas Moniz (1874–1955)	Lobotomy Angiography
Roumania	Gheorge Marinescu (1863–1938)	
Russia	Alexis Jakovlevich Kojevnikoff (1836–1902)	Partial constant epilepsy
	Ivan Petrovitch Pavlov (1849–1936)	Conditionned reflexes
	Sergei Korsakoff (1856–1900)	Korsakoff syndrome
	Wladimir Bechterew (1857–1927)	Rheumatoid spondylitis (Bechterew's disease)
	Grigorii Ivanovich Rossolimo (1860–1928)	Rossolimo's sign Child psychology
Switzerland	Constantin von Monakow (1853–1930)	Neuroanatomy
United States	Silas Weir Mitchell (1829–1914)	"One of the fathers of American neurology"
	William Alexander Hammond (1828–1900)	"One of the fathers of American neurology"
	George Huntington (1850–1916)	Huntington's chorea
	Harvey Cushing (1869–1939)	Founder of neurosurgery
	James Ramsay Hunt (1872–1937)	

John Hughlings Jackson (1835–1911) may be considered as the father of English neurology, but by the end of the century other famous names belonged to the staff of Queen's Square: Sir William Richard Gowers (1848–1915), neurosurgical pioneer Sir Victor Alexander Horsley, Charles E. Beavor (1854–1908), and Sir David Ferrier (1843–1928), who undertook exceptional studies on brain cortical function. The best-known is probably Gowers, whose book *Clinical Lectures on Diseases of the Nervous System* is a fundamental neurological textbook. Later on, other figures maintained the reputation of Queen's Square, including Samuel A. Kinnier-Wilson (1858–1937), who made his name in neurology with the publication of his doctoral thesis in 1912 on "progressive lenticular degeneration; a familial neurological disease associated with cirrhosis of the liver," later to be known as Wilson's disease. Sir Henry Head conducted pioneering work on the somatosensory system and sensory nerves.

Although English neurology was focused at the National Hospital, other centers were active: in Edinburgh, Byron Bramwell (1847–1931) did important work on diseases of the spinal cord (1882) and later on intracranial tumors (1888). Born in Dublin, Sir Gordon Morgan Holmes (1876–1965) published on the cerebellum at the same time as Babinski (1904); his contributions to the physiological approach to clinical disorders of the nervous system were extensive, focusing on somatosensory function and vision.

In Germany, the situation was somewhat different. There was little distinction between psychiatry and neurology (psychosis was considered a brain disease), and this overlap was illustrated by the fact that such great figures as Carl Wernicke in Breslau and Karl Westphal (1833–1890) in Berlin were both neuropsychiatrists. The first example of a true neurologist was probably Hermann Oppenheim, a direct contemporary of Babinski's. Having begun his career in psychiatry, he later made important contributions to neurology, and his textbook *Lehrbuch der Nervenkrankheiten*, translated into several languages, was an important reference. He ended his career as professor of neurology at the University of Berlin.

William H. Erb, the holder of a chair in internal medicine in Leipzig, favored the separation of neurology from psychiatry. He described the knee-jerk reflex and a special form of myelitis. His successor was given the first official chair of neurology in Heidelberg in 1911.

Additional departments of neurology were also created in large municipal hospitals, so several German experts obtained prominence simultaneously. Ludwig Edinger (1855–1918), professor of neurology at Frankfurt, may be considered the founder of modern comparative anatomy of the nervous system.

Due to political tensions between the two countries, exchanges between German and French neurology remained rare except for Otfrid Foerster, who attended Babinski's lessons but was essentially a disciple of Dejerine, with whom he worked from 1897 to 1899.

Mention should be made of the importance of basic neurosciences in Germany and especially that of neuropathology: after Aloïs Alzheimer (1864–1915), professor of psychiatry and founder of the Munich school of neuropathology, of importance were Franz Nissl (1860–1919) and Arnold Pick (1851–1924), who described lobar cortical atrophy.

In the United States, neurology developed separately in different universities on the East Coast (Philadelphia, New York, Boston). A special military hospital for nervous diseases was established in Philadelphia in 1862 by Silas Weir Mitchell (1829–1934); having served in the Civil War, he published in 1864 a landmark book on gunshot wounds affecting the nerves. His friend William A. Hammond (1828–1900), surgeon general of the army in 1862, used his experiences during the war to improve field hospitals; appointed professor of psychiatry and nervous diseases at the College of Physicians and Surgeons of New York in 1874, he published several books on neurology between 1871 and 1876. The same year a chair of neurology was established at the University of Pennsylvania for Horatio C. Wood (1841–1920). His successor, Charles K. Mills (1845–1931), devoted himself entirely to neurology, and his work on cerebral localization was only part of his numerous contributions to neurology. William J. Spiller (1863–1940) spent four years in Europe after graduation, studying internal medicine and neurology in Germany and in France under Dejerine, before returning to the University of Pennsylvania. He worked there with Charles Harrison Frazier, one of the pioneers in neurosurgery

In New York the Neurological Institute was founded in 1909 and linked to Columbia University. Following Edward C. Seguin (1843–1898), the professor of nervous diseases was Moses S. Starr (1854–1932) who also studied in Europe, particularly in German laboratories. Charles A. Elsberg became the first chief of neurological surgery. James Ramsay Hunt (1872–1937), after having studied in Paris, Vienna, and Berlin, returned to New York in 1900 to work at Cornell Medical School; he was appointed professor of neurology at Columbia University in 1924.

In Boston the neurological tradition was established by James G. Putman (1846–1918). In 1870, he went to Europe to learn about electrotherapeutics and neurology. Upon his return to the United States, he experimented with hypnosis and psychotherapy and was aware of Freud's work. Harvey Cushing, the father of neurosurgery, was appointed professor at Harvard in 1912 and became the director of Peter Bent Brigham Hospital.[53] The creation

---

[53] On Cushing, see chapter 13.

of the American Neurological Society in 1875, three years after the New York Neurological Society, represented probably the first national association of neurologists in the world.

Aside from these three major poles, neurology benefited from important contributions from scientists in other countries, such Arthur van Gehuchten and Ludo van Bogaert (1897–1988) in Belgium, Giovanni Mingazzini (1859–1919) in Italy, and Alexis J. Kojevnikoff (1836–1902), Ivan P. Pavlov (1849–1936), Sergei Korsakoff (1856–1900), and Vladimir Bekhterev in Russia.[54]

---

[54] Fulgence Raymond made a professional trip to Russia in 1889 (F. Raymond, "[L'étude des maladies du système nerveux en Russie. Rapport adressé à M. le ministre de l'Instruction publique" [A study of the diseases of the nervous system in Russia. Report to the Secretary of State for Education] (Paris: G. Doin, 1889).

··· seventeen ···

Babinski's Public Image

Joseph Babinski's public image, already positive during his career, retains an international impact 150 years after his death. Although this recognition concerns mainly the Babinski sign, which accounts for more than half of the bibliographical references, the fraternal dedication and culinary talents of his brother, which form an integral part of his life story, are reflected as well. There is still some mystery concerning his private life, his father's revolutionary activities, the exotic countries where his father and brother spent several years, and even the exceptional gourmet qualities of Ali-Bab. Too, the authenticity of many anecdotes involving Babinski is sometimes difficult to confirm. To try to develop a more complete picture of how he is remembered, we can look at the contents of official speeches, the hagiographic writings of his pupils, commemorative celebrations, the mention he receives in encyclopedias and history books, and sites named after him.

Well Recognized and Admired During His Life

Twenty years after his failure in the *agrégation* competition, he was greeted with a standing ovation from a worldwide assembly of neurologists at the London meeting in 1913. The same year, the professors of the University of

Lvov in Poland proposed his candidacy for the Nobel Prize, but his scientific contribution was considered too dated by the committee.[1]

In 1925, at the twenty-fifth anniversary of the founding of the Société de neurologie de Paris, Guillain expressed the society's gratitude for Babinski's significant scientific contributions and for the glory he had brought to his country.[2] Louis Dartigues relates that in 1931, during the inaugural lesson of the chair of the history of medicine, Laignel-Lavastine paid rousing tribute to J. Babinski, present in the audience.[3] The thunderous applause was even greater when he added, referring to the unsuccessful *agrégation* in 1892, "Let us give him a special welcome in this place where he should have taught."[4] Few of his contemporaries had as many adulators among Paris hospital and university circles: in that respect, as probably in others, he was Charcot's foremost rival.

Administrative authorities are less dithyrambic. When Babinski became a *médecin honoraire des hôpitaux de Paris* in 1922, Henri Roger briefly recounted the highlights of Babinski's professional life to members of the Conseil de surveillance de l'Assistance publique (its advisory board).[5] Roger spoke of him as being "well known as a master in the field of neurological diseases" and someone who "has always helped the administration and contributed his enlightened dedication." These words appear particularly banal since two other physicians (whose names have been altogether forgotten by posterity) retiring at the same time were described with quite similar words. The advisory board expressed its appreciation in standard terms for all that these eminent teachers had done during their careers and regretted that they had reached the time for retirement.

While we would not assert that Babinski was strongly affected by the "name syndrome," he was probably not completely immune to it.[6] In this condition, as described by Blanchard in 1898, the patient—usually a physician—has an irresistible impulse to describe a disease, or a part of it, and rushes to give it his own name. In fact, Babinski quite rapidly referred to the toe phenomenon as the Babinski sign.[7] His name is attached not only

---

[1] A. Gasecki and V. Hachinski, "On the names of Babinski," *Canadian Journal of Neurological Sciences* 1996 (23): 76–79.

[2] G. Guillain, "Discours du professeur G. Guillain, président de la Société" [Speech of Professor G. Guillain, president of the society], *Revue Neurol (Paris)* 1925 (1): 1155–1158.

[3] L. Dartigues, *Faisceau scriptural* [Scriptural Light], vol. 3 (Paris: G. Doin, 1932).

[4] A. Segal and A. Lellouch, "Maxime Laignel-Lavastine (1875–1953)," http://www.bium.univ-paris5.fr/sfhm/histoire5.htm.

[5] Conseil de surveillance de l'Assistance publique [Advisory board of the Assistance publique], meeting of October 26, 1922, 143–144.

[6] Blanchard, "Le syndrome du baptême" [The name syndrome], *Le Progrès Médical* 1898 (VIII): 504–505.

[7] J. Babinski, *Exposé des travaux scientifiques* [Presentation of scientific papers] (Paris: Masson, 1913).

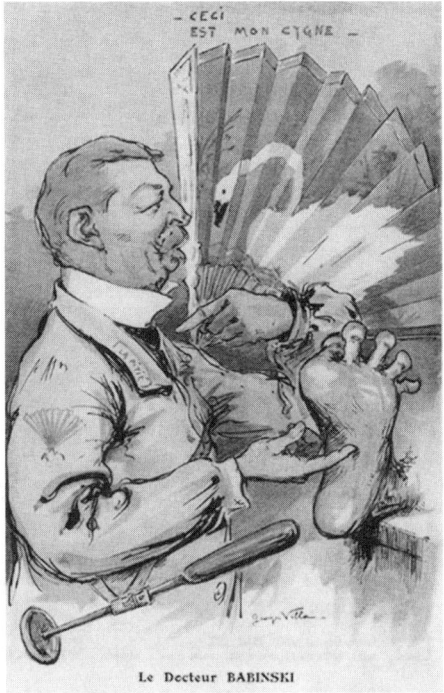

Figure 17-1 Caricature of Joseph Babinski in 1911. (*Source*: From *Chanteclair*, October 1911; personal collection, J. Poirier.)

to the sign but also to a number of different syndromes: Babinski, Babinski-Frolich, Babinski-Nageotte, Babinski-Froment, Babinski-Vaquez, and Anton-Babinski, as well as a variant of the hammer reflex (see chapters 10 and 15) (Figs. 17-1 and 17-2).

His reputation went well beyond the medical frontier, as reflected in two cartoons published in the satirical review *Chanteclair*, the first in 1911 making a play on his "swan sign" (*cygne* and *signe* being homophones in French) and the second in 1933, a few weeks after his death.[8] Babinski's name surfaces from time to time in the general press, especially in conjunction with the infamous episode of the *agrégation* and with the dramatic suicide at his private office of one of his patients.[9] Journalists also announced his conferences and followed the evolution of his work, especially in *Le Figaro*, where the Académie de médecine's weekly sessions were regularly reported on. In 1903 his paper on the treatment of some ear diseases and vertigo was

---

[8] *Chanteclair*, October 1911 and January–February 1933.
[9] *Le Temps*, Sunday, June 28, 1903, cited in *Annales médico-psychologiques* 1903: 346–347.

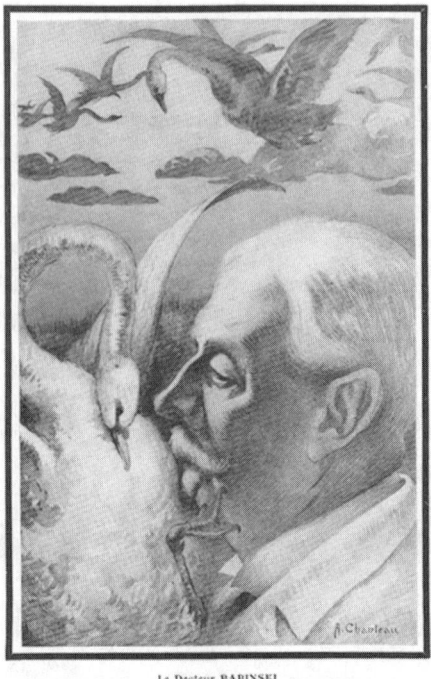

Le Docteur BABINSKI
(1857-1932)

Figure 17-2 Caricature of Joseph Babinski in 1933. (*Source:* From Chanteclair, January–February 1933; personal collection, J. Poirier.)

reported in *Le Petit Parisien*, a daily with quite high circulation, resulting in a considerable increase in his private outpatient practice (Fig. 17-3).[10]

His Posthumous Reputation

After Babinski's death, which occurred in the same year as that of Emile Chauffard (1855–1932), professor of internal medicine, Mr. Bompard, vice president of the Conseil de Surveillance de l'Assistance publique, offered a short review of their hospital careers, following which the director general concluded: "Medical science as a whole and the Assistance Publique in

[10] J. Babinski, "Sur le traitement des affections de l'oreille et en particulier du vertige auriculaire par la rachicentèse" [On the treatment of auricular diseases, especially auricular vertigo, by lumbar puncture], *Annales des maladies de l'oreille et du larynx* 1904 (XXX): 849.

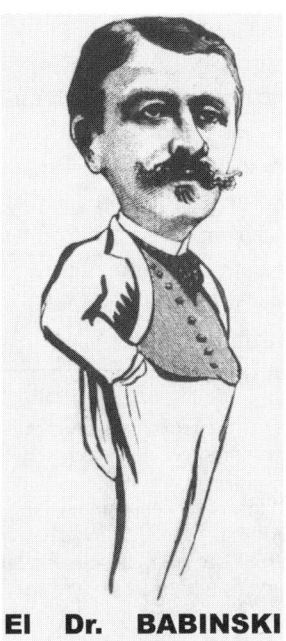

El Dr. BABINSKI

Figure 17-3 Caricature of Joseph Babinski, (*Source*: From Tribuna Medica, 19, courtesy of National Library of Medicine, Bethesda, Maryland.)

particular have just experienced a substantial loss with the passing of Dr. Babinski and Professor Chauffard, two scientists of great merit."[11]

A notice of Babinski's funeral appeared in *Le Figaro*, and obituary articles—all much more laudatory than the administration's comments—were numerous in France, Poland, Great Britain, and the United States (though coverage in the *New England Journal of Medicine* was rather measured: "as a clinical neurologist and teacher Babinski held a high place in Paris for many years, although somewhat overshadowed by Pierre Marie and Jules Dejerine").[12]

---

[11] M. Loeper, "Nécrologie. A. Chauffard" [Obituary: A. Chauffard], *Le Progrès Médical* 1932 (46): 1947; Conseil de surveillance de l'assistance publique [Advisory board of the Assistance publique], meeting of November 29, 1932, 206–207.

[12] A. Charpentier, "Babinski," *Le Figaro*, October 30, 1932, 2; G. Guillain, "Babinski (1857–1932)," *La Presse Médicale* 1932 (9): 1705–1707; E. Krebs, "Nécrologie J. Babinski," *L'Encéphale* 1933 (XXV): 72–80; L. Le Sourd, "Le docteur Joseph François Félix Babinski (1857–1932)," *Gazette des Hôpitaux* 1932 (92): 1681; M. Loeper, "Babinski," *Le Progrès Médical* 1932 (45): 1885; L. Rivet, "Joseph Babinski (1857–1932)," *Bull. Mém. Soc. Méd. Hôp. Paris* 1932 (34): 1722–1733; H. Vaquez, "Joseph Babinski (1857–1932)," *Bulletin de l'Académie de Médecine* 1932 (3): 1265–1273; C. Vincent, "J. Babinski" (1857–1932), *Rev Neurol (Paris)* 1932 (2): 441–446; *Paris Médical* 1932 (86): 449; A. Baudoin, *Semaine des Hôpitaux de Paris* 1932: 557–561; *Revue Médicale française* 1932: 839; A. Gasecki,

Several foreign neurologists, representing noted scientific societies, sent messages of condolences to the Société de neurologie de Paris: Egas Moniz (Lisbon), Södebergh (Goteborg), Medea (Milan), Izzedin (Istanbul), the president and the secretary of the Société de neurologie de Buenos-Aires, Professor G. Marinesco, neurologists from Brazil, the general secretary of the Royal Society of Medicine in London (of which Babinski was an honorary member), Jean Saucier in the name of the Montreal Neurological Society, Professor Minkovski in the name of the Zurich Society of Psychiatry and Neurology, and Professor Russetzki in the name of the Clinique des Maladies Nerveuses in Kazan.[13]

The press was no less enthusiastic:

[An] internationally famous neurologist...A great scientist, with a sharp mind and a welcoming personality, Babinski will leave behind him unanimous regrets.[14]

This great clinician will take a place, beside his master Charcot, as a founder of modern neurology....A great figure of French medicine disappears.[15]

One of the greatest among the French neurologists.[16]

Specialized in neurology, to which he contributed so well.[17]

All weep on the grave of this thaumaturgist who, with a punch or a stick, restored their ruined brains.[18]

With Babinski has disappeared one of the greatest and most noble figures of French contemporary medicine....It can be said without any undue emphasis that the name of Babinski is written in the golden book of science....A passionate research scientist, with an exceptional talent for observation and an acute critical mind, he was only interested in the pursuit of truth, affirming nothing before being absolutely certain that he was right....All the sharpness of his genius for observation was revealed in his steel-blue look, as penetrating as a blade, the apparent coldness of which from time to time would lighten

---

"Jozeph Babinski wspoltworca wspolcaesnej neurologii i neurochirurgii" [Jozef Babinski co-founder of contemporary neurology and neurosurgery], *Neurologia i Neurochirurgia Polska* 1997 (31): 641–656 (obituaries in Polish journals were written by Artwinski, Orsechoski, Krzeminski, Bychoski and Pienkowski); "Death of Dr. Babinski," *British Medical Journal*, 1932: 892; A. F. Hurst, "Dr. Babinski," *British Medical Journal* 1932: 988; "Babinski," *Lancet* 1932 (2): 1122; J. Fulton, "Joseph François Babinski 1857–1932," *Archives of Neurology and Psychiatry* 1933 (29): 168–174; J. Fulton, "Science in the clinic as exemplified by the life and work of Joseph Babinski," *Journal of Nervous and Mental Diseases* 1933 (77): 121–133; "Deaths," *Journal of the American Medical Association* 1932 (99): 2045–2046; quote from "Joseph F. Babinski, 1857–1932," *New England Journal of Medicine* 1932 (27): 898–899.

[13] Société de neurologie de Paris, meeting of December 1, 1932, in *Rev Neurol (Paris)* 1932 (II): 661–662; meeting of January 5, 1933, in *Rev Neurol (Paris)* 1933 (I): 60–61.

[14] *Siècle Médical*, November 1, 1932.

[15] *Le Temps*, October 30, 1932.

[16] *Le Temps*, October 31, 1932.

[17] *Débats*, October 29, 1932.

[18] *Aux Ecoutes*, November 5, 1932.

with a spark of irony. But behind this impassive screen, due in great part to excessive shyness, what generosity and true kindness did abide!...They will be missed for a long time. Their memory will remain forever.[19]

The word *genius* is a highly significant term, often incorrectly used, which should only describe an exceptional skill, and more especially the innate gifts of the great creative minds. It is judiciously that we use this word for J. Babinski....All those who have worked with him remember his extreme meticulousness, his constant hesitations and objections, continuously looking back on results that were seemingly well established; in short, the ferment of doubt and anxiety, observed in so many creative minds, that represents the most reliable token of perfection....No physician since the great Laennec, at least in the clinical field, has brought such a decisive and complete contribution to his specialty....In the different and successive steps of a neurological investigation, the clinician starts with Babinski, keeps on with Babinski, and finishes with Babinski....It is to Babinski that French neurology owes the position it had in the world, which means the first.[20]

Among his pupils the two wordiest hagiographers, functioning almost as official biographers, are Auguste Tournay and especially Albert Charpentier. The latter wrote, as the introduction to his book dedicated to the life of Babinski, a poetic tribute.[21]

Other pupils were more discreet but nevertheless devoted to the memory of their master. For Clovis Vincent, Babinski was "one of the greatest physicians of the century and probably of all times; the sign is unforgettable."[22] Monier-Vinard emphasized "the talent of a rigorous and patient observation" and concluded that "we are indebted to him to have given the unshakeable foundations of the contemporary structure of neurology."[23] Krebs, on the occasion of the acceptance of an award from the Babinski fund, addressed the Société de neurologie with these words: "For those who had the privilege to have been students of a venerable master who has passed away, it is not difficult to recall his memory because he remains so present in their heart, their minds, and even their efforts to always try to be motivated by his own sense of perfection."[24] In his inaugural lesson in 1947, Alajouanine—who was not one

---

[19] L. Daudet, "Babinsky" [sic], *Action française,* October 30, 1932.

[20] "Psychologie et thérapeutique. Un neurologue de génie: Babinski" [Psychology and therapeutics. Babinski, a neurologist of genius] *Le Temps,* November 18, 1932.

[21] A. Tournay, "Allocution du président sortant" [Speech of the past president, Société de neurologie de Paris, meeting of January 9, 1941], *Rev Neurol (Paris)* 1941 (73): 24–26; A. Charpentier, *Un grand médecin. J. Babinski (1857-1932)* [A great physician. J. Babinski] (Paris: Typographie Francois Bernouard, 1934].

[22] Vincent, "J. Babinski (1857-1932)."

[23] M. Monier-Vinard, "Discours de M. Monier-Vinard, président" [Speech of M. Monier-Vinard, president], *Rev Neurol (Paris)* 1939 (71): 54–56.

[24] E. Krebs, "Du diagnostic et des indications opératoires dans les complications récentes et tardives des traumatismes cérébraux fermés" [On diagnosis and operative indications

of his pupils—gave him the same place as Pierre Marie, Souques, and Dupré, and on the occasion of his centenary evoked "the brilliant observer, the semiologist beyond comparison,...a kind of divinity in neurology (this word does not appear too strong)."[25] Baruk, who likewise did not figure among his students, is full of admiration, speaking of him as "one of the greatest geniuses in modern psychiatry."[26] In a compendium published in 1947, Babinski was included among a group of "famous physicians."[27] Humorists in their own way joined in this flattery: for instance, Georges Pérec wrote of an imaginary patient in 1966: "They would take his pulse, pull his tongue, measure his intellect and look at his toes to see how is his Babinski (oh! I get my revenge, because I am quite sure that you don't know what a Babinski sign is! Don't hold out any hope that I will tell you)."[28]

The Subject of Repeated Commemorations

> Some malcontents will probably think that we have too many commemorations, mainly for the pleasure of talking. But is it not the duty of every country to honor their scientific celebrities? Let us not be ungrateful sons! We shall not and cannot in any way break the chain which links the past to the present and the present to the future.[29]

The centenary of Babinski's birthday was the occasion for numerous speeches and papers in France and other countries, delivered during the 22nd International Neurological Congress, organized by the Société française de neurologie in Paris, June 2–4, 1958. Raymond Garcin analyzed Babinski's work in detail.[30] Sir Francis Walshe was full of praise for him, describing him as "an unsurpassable artist in the use of the semiological method" and emphasizing "his acute sense of observation as a rare talent for detecting

in early and late complications of closed head injuries], *Rev Neurol (Paris)* 1939 (71): 369–388.

[25] T. Alajouanine, "Le centenaire de Babinski" [The Babinski centenary], *Semaine des Hôpitaux de Paris* 1958 (22): 1355–1364.
[26] H. Baruk *Des hommes comme nous* [Men like us] (Paris: Robert Laffont, 1976).
[27] A. Plichet, "Babinski (1857–1932)" in R. Dumesnil and F. Bonnet-Roy, eds., *Les médecins célèbres* [Famous physicians] (Genève: Éditions d'Art Lucien Mazenod, 1947), 250–251.
[28] G. Pérec, *Quel petit vélo chromé au fond de la cour?* [And the little chrome bike at the back of the yard?] (Paris: Denoel, 1966).
[29] G. Roussy, "Centenaire de Vulpian" [Centenary of Vulpian], *Rev Neurol (Paris)* 1927 (II): 1159–1160.
[30] R. Garcin, "L'œuvre de Babinski" [Babinski's work], *Rev Neurol (Paris)* 1958 (98): 619–631.

new or unusual things as the most common. As a clinical observer, he has always seemed to me unmatched among the neurologists of his time."[31] The Polish tribute was given by Jerzy Chorobski (Warsaw). Representatives of the neurological societies of many countries—Belgium (Van Gehuchten), Chile, Denmark, Germany (G. Schaltenbrand), Hungary, Italy (V. Néri), the Netherlands, Norway, Portugal, Romania, Spain, Switzerland, Turkey, United States (Sir Percival Bailey), and Uruguay—expressed their admiration, with the speakers competing in their laudatory remarks: Babinski was hailed as the "father of neurological semiology," "the brilliant clinician," "this scientist of genius" "whose name will always be written in golden letters in the history of medicine," "the immortal merits of Joseph Babinski… the magnificent work of this great scientist."[32]

> He has been the creator of modern neurological semiology as it is performed at the patient's bedside.… If Babinski seems sometimes forgotten, this is only an illusion; his work is not a museum piece in the history of medicine, but reborn every day during a neurological exam performed somewhere in the world.[33]

On this same occasion of his birthday centennial, Jean Lhermitte spoke in praise of him at the Académie de medicine, finding just the right words for his qualities: his scientific work is "a jewel in neurology," and "if one were to imagine that one day the name of Babinski as well as his writings were to disappear from history, those consulting his clinical observations would easily see that they were not like those of Charcot and would search in the sky of neurology the path of a great lost star."[34]

The 1st International Congress of the Neurological Sciences, held in Brussels July 21–28, 1957, was dedicated to the memory of the well-known Belgian neurologist Arthur Van Gehuchten (1861–1914), from Louvain, but the organizers emphasized that 1957 was also the centennial of the birth of three men who had made significant contributions to the neurological sciences: Sir Charles Sherrington (1857–1952), Joseph Babinski, and Sir Victor Horsley. In honor of these three distinguished scientists, a medal was created by the artist A. Crommelynck, with Van Gehuchten on one side and the names of the other three on the reverse.

---

[31] F. Walshe, "Où situer Babinski dans la neurologie moderne" [What is the place of Babinski in modern neurology], *Rev Neurol (Paris)* 1958 (98): 632–636.
[32] *Rev Neurol (Paris)* 1958 (98): 640–668.
[33] *Rev Neurol (Paris)* 1958 (98): 664.
[34] J. Lhermitte, "J. Babinski (1857–1932)," *Bulletin de l'Académie nationale de médecine* 1957: 727–740.

In 1996, the centenary of the Babinski sign was celebrated with dignity in the neuroscience world, and the present volume was conceived to mark the 150th anniversary of his birth in 2007.[35]

A Limited Place in the Books of History, Neurology, and Medicine

Babinski's devotion to medicine, to the exclusion of any involvement in political or local affairs, does not naturally lead to inclusion of his name in books of general history. In fact, as was the case for Charcot, Dejerine and Marie, he does not appear in the *Dictionnaire des intellectuels français,* although Émile Duclaux, Bourneville and Brouardel were cited[36] Maurice Agulhon fails to include him, along with Claude Bernard, Charcot, and Pasteur, in *La République*.[37]

The same can be said for books on the general history of medicine, perhaps because Babinski's work was completely devoted to neurological semiology and has not radically changed the course of medical science. Unlike the great Parisian neurologists Charcot, Dejerine, and Marie, Babinski gave his name not to a disease but only to a sign and—in association with others—to some rare syndromes. For example, in the three thick volumes of the monumental *Histoire de la médecine* by Laignel-Lavastine, Babinski is briefly cited half a dozen times, and his work is summarized in five lines (quite relevant, however).[38] In *L'histoire de la médecine*, Bariéty and Coury consider him "as probably the greatest of all the semiologists in neurology," but only twenty lines (in a book of 1,217 pages) are allotted to him.[39] *L'histoire de la médecine et des médecins* by Jean-Charles Sournia only mentions Babinski's name as a pupil of Charcot, along with Marie and—curiously, given the hostility

---

[35] M. G. Sahadevan, "A hundred years of the Babinski reflex," *Journal of the Royal College of Physicians of London* 1996 (30): 83.

[36] J. Julliard and M. Winock, eds., *Dictionnaire des intellectuels français* [Dictionary of French intellectuals], new ed. (Paris: Seuil, 2002).

[37] M. Agulhon, *La République* (Paris: Hachette, 1990).

[38] M. Laignel-Lavastine, ed., *Histoire générale de la médecine, de la pharmacie, de l'art dentaire et de l'art vétérinaire* [A general history of medicine, pharmacy, dentistry and veterinary science] (Paris: A. Michel, 1936/1949). "Babinski's neurology, as described by Guillain, deeply differs from that of Charcot. It is completely oriented toward an early diagnosis by means of the search for objective signs, the cutaneous plantar response being the type universally acknowledged. Babinski has described the cerebellar syndrome, specified the exact localization of spinal compressions, and opened the way to modern neurosurgery." (T. III, p. 340–341)

[39] M. Bariety and C. Coury, *Histoire de la médecine* [A history of medicine] (Paris: Fayard, 1963).

between the two men—Dejerine and his wife.[40] The index of Jacques Léonard's *La médecine entre les pouvoirs et les savoirs* (Medicine between power and knowledge), rich in physicians' names, has only one citation for Babinski; it refers to a simple note about hypnotism, where Babinski has the same place as Gilles de la Tourette, lost among numerous others.[41] Babinski was probably not far enough along in his career and not yet well enough known to figure in *Nos grands médecins d'aujourd'hui* (Our great physicians of today), appearing in 1891. In fact, the great majority of the selected personalities in this volume were born between 1830 and 1840, belonging to the generation preceding that of Babinski.[42] On the other hand, in 1979, Birch wrote fifty-six biographical notes of physicians "whose names are often on the tip of our tongue every day and used in current medical practice," and Babinski appeared with eight other French physicians: Broca, Calmette, Charcot, Dupuytren, Fallot, Guérin, Ménière, and Raynaud.[43] Babinski's name does not appear in the index of *The Cambridge World History of Human Disease*, with its 1,176 pages, although Charcot and Dejerine are cited.[44]

More recently, with François Dagognet, who praises "his clinical subtlety," epistemology has taken an interest in Babinski.[45] However, in the final analysis Babinski is most often quoted in the history of neurology and neurological journals published in French, Polish, and English. In the neurological section of the chapter on the great clinicians of the nineteenth century in *Histoire du diagnostic médical* (History of medical diagnosis) by R. Villey, Babinski, with three pages, is given more attention than Charcot and Jackson (two and a half pages each), Duchenne (two pages), and Dejerine (a page and a half).[46] In the 467 pages of *The Doctrine of the Nerves: Chapters in the History of Neurology*, the place devoted to Babinski is limited to two

---

[40] J. C. Sournia, *Histoire de la médecine et des médecins* [A history of medicine and of physicians] (Paris: Larousse, 1991).

[41] J. Léonard, *La médecine entre les pouvoirs et les savoirs* [Medicine between power and science] (Paris: Aubier Montaigne, 1981), 336.

[42] H. Bianchon (pseudonym of Maurice de Fleury), *Nos grands médecins d'aujourd'hui* [Great physicials of today] (Paris: Société d'éditions scientifiques, 1891).

[43] C. A. Birch, *Names We Remember. 56 Eponymous Medical Biographies* (Beckenham: Ravenswood, 1979), 9–10.

[44] K. F. Kiple, ed., *The Cambridge World History of Human Disease* (Cambridge: Cambridge University Press, 1993).

[45] "Joseph Babinski has transformed our body into a signal station, discovering in it a multitude of information of which he had favored the emergence." F. Dagognet, "Le grand déchiffreur: J. Babinski" [The great decipherer: J. Babinski], in *Savoir et pouvoir en médecine* [Knowledge and power in medicine] (Le Plessis Robinson: Synthélabo, 1998), 99–103.

[46] R. Villey, *Histoire du diagnostic médical* [A history of medical diagnosis] (Paris: Masson, 1976), 166–168.

citations and only one phrase concerning the Babinski sign.[47] Dejerine is not better considered: only the thalamic syndrome of Dejerine-Roussy is mentioned. Pierre Marie is not even cited, nor is Nageotte, and Ranvier is limited to three lines and Charcot but a few; on the other hand, Duchenne's contribution is described in ten pages.

Baruk was upset by the fact that Babinski's work is not well enough known and that his place among the founders of neurology is often shadowy.[48] More recently, Professor Trelles, trained in the French school after Babinski (he was a student of Lhermitte), published a paper on the main stages of neurological thought in the *Revista de neuropsiquiatria* and quotes only Charcot, Jackson, von Monakow, and Goldstein, leaving out Babinski.[49]

In American journals, some articles are more enthusiastic about the importance of Babinski:

> He is certainly one of the most original, astute and forceful of living neurology. He seems to combine Gallic brilliance with the methodological thoroughness of the German and by some is considered the greatest French neurologist. Having true scientific insight, the fruit of his labor was rarely without value. Deprived of his contributions on the reflexes on spinal and brain stem localization, on cerebellar disorders, hysteria, and many other things, modern neurology would be far from being what it is.[50]

Georges Guillain relates that shortly before his death, Babinski showed him an article in a foreign journal where the portraits of Westphal, Argyll Robertson, and Babinski had been placed together to illustrate the three essential signs of neurological semiology.[51] What remains today of these three signs?

His Place in Encyclopedias

In encyclopedia, notices concerning Joseph Babinski are generally descriptive and sober, though at times there is some excess. As one might anticipate, he

---

[47] J. D. Spillane, *The Doctrine of the Nerves: Chapters in the History of Neurology* (Oxford: Oxford University Press, 1981).
[48] H. Baruk, "Babinski (1857–1932)," *Revue philosophique de la France et de l'étranger* (Paris: Presses Universitaires de France, 1959), 459–465.
[49] Oscar Trelles (1904–1990), Peruvian neurologist and politician, was the founder of the *Revista de neuro-psiquiatria*. He described Lhermitte–Trelles syndrome (lymphoblastic infiltration of the peripheral nervous system). He was prime minister of Peru from July 28 to December 31, 1963 (http://www.whonamedit.com/doctor.cfm/2166.html).
[50] *Science and Learning in France: The Society for American Fellowships in French Universities*, vol. 1, Chicago, 1917.
[51] Guillain, "J. Babinski (1857–1932)."

is particularly well treated in books with a Polish connection: in the *Grande Encyclopedie de Pologne* (2004) he receives thirty-one lines, while neither Charcot, Dejerine, or Pierre Marie is cited; moreover, it is indicated that he had a close link with Poland, that some of his works were published in Polish, and that he was the "co-creator of world neurology."[52] The Babinski sign is especially emphasized, with a paragraph of its own. Babinski is generally considered a "French neurologist, clinician and teacher; son of a Polish immigrant" or a "French neurologist of Polish origin," and occasionally as a "Polish neurologist who has practiced in France."[53] It is noted that he was a member of the Académie nationale de médecine and that he had been nominated professor *honoris causa* at Vilnius University in 1925. Two Polish encyclopedias have notices on four French neurologists: with nineteen and thirteen lines, respectively, Babinski is more privileged than Charcot (seventeen and six lines), Dejerine (eight and four lines), or Pierre Marie (seven and five lines).[54] Two others have only notices on Charcot (six and four lines) and Babinski (a little better treated, with twelve and six lines).[55] Five others write about Babinski (from six to thirty-one lines), but Charcot, Dejerine, or Pierre Marie are not cited.[56] Some other Polish encyclopedia have no comments on Babinski.[57] The preeminent French biographical dictionary gives

---

[52] Jaroslaw Marek Rymkiewicz, ed., *Wielka Encyklopedia Polski* [*The Grand Polish Encyclopedia*], 2 vols. (Krakow: Wydawnictwo Tyszard Kluszczynski, 2004).

[53] *Wielka Encyklopedia Powszechna Pwn* [*The Grand Universal Encyclopedia*] (Warsaw: Panstwowe Wydawnictwo Naukowe Pwn, 1978–1993); *Mala Encyklopedia Powszechna Pwn* [*The Condensed Universal Encyclopedia*] (Warsaw: Wydawnictwo Naukowe Pwn, 1997); Stanislawa Lama, ed., *Ilustrowana Encyklopedja Trzaski, Everta i Michalskiego* (Warsaw: Nakladem Ksiegarni Trzaski, Everta i Michalskiego) [*Traska, Evert and Michalski Illustrated Encyclopaedia*, directed by Stanislaw Lam, 5 volumes, Warsaw, Evert and Michalski], 1927.

[54] Wydanie Drugie, ed., *Encyklopedia Powszechna Pwn*, 4 vols., (Warsaw: Pwn [*Universal Encyclopaedia PWN*, by Wydanie Drugie, Warsaw, 4 vol., PWN] 1983; *Nowy Leksykon* [*New Lexicon*] Pwn (Warsaw: Wydawnictwo Naukowe Pwn, 1998).

[55] Lama, ed., *Ilustrowana Encyklopedja Trzaski*; *Mala Encyklopedia Powszechna*. It is interesting to note that in this last encyclopedia, Joseph Babinski was given six lines, Charcot four, while there was none for Dejerine or Pierre Marie. Josef Brudzinski (1874–1917), the Polish neurologist who discoverd the eponymic sign in meningitis, received fifteen lines.

[56] Mieczyslaw Szymczak, ed., *Slownik Jezyka Polskiego*, 3 vols. (Warsaw: Wydawnictwo Naukowe Pwn, 1993) [*Polish Language Dictionary*, Pr Dr Mieczyslaw Szymczak (ed. by), 3 vol., Warsaw, National Scientific Editions, 1993]; *Encylopedia Polski* (Krakow, 1996); Rymkiewicz, ed., *Wielka Encyklopedia Polski*; *Wielka Ilustrowana Encyklopedja Powszechna* (Krakow: Wydawnictwo Gotenberga); *Wielka Encyklopedia Powszechna Pwn* (Warsaw: Panstwowe Wydawnictwo Naukowe Pwn, 1978–1993).

[57] Stanislas Lam, ed., *Nowa Ksiazka* [TK] (Warsaw: Nakladem Ksiegarni Trzaski, Everta i Michalskiego, 1935); Stanislas Lam, ed., *Podreczna Encyclopedia Powszechna* (Paryzu: Ksiegarnia Polska W.), 1954; Witold Doroszewski, ed., *Slownik Jezyka Polskiego* (Warsaw: Panstwowe Wydawnictwo Wiedza Powszechna, 1958); *Encyklopedia Wiedsy*

about the same treatment to Dejerine (five lines), Pierre Marie (six lines), and Babinski (six lines, without taking into consideration his brother); there is no entry for Gilles de la Tourette, Vaquez, or Darier.[58]

If we look comparatively at the places given to Jean-Martin Charcot, Jules Dejerine, Pierre Marie, and Joseph Babinski in five international encyclopedias (excluding the French and Polish ones, discussed above), one may note that Charcot, with one exception, is always noted (receiving from eight lines to one and a half columns), Dejerine never, Marie only once (but with a column and a half), and Babinski twice.[59]

His Name on Street Signs in Paris and Poland

Rue du Docteur Babinski, opened by the city of Paris in 1946, 352 meters long and 12 meters in width, was restructured in 1966 when the circular highway was completed. It starts at avenue de la Porte Montmartre and ends at avenue de la Porte de Saint-Ouen; its naming dates from a decree on April 25, 1965.[60] No particular recognition of Babinski's merits is to be found there. As pointed out by Fierro, between 1965 and 1970 Paris named streets "honoring members of the resistance movement,... battles or fighters of Free France,... we add to the mania of dates,... we honor the Allied forces.... The remaining depend on a cultural sprinkling within which are mixed writers, painters, engineers, some politicians, and a handful of physicians," including André Lemierre, Antonin Gosset, Henri Mondor, Antoine Béclère, and Babinski. In all, about a hundred doctors of the nineteenth and twentieth centuries have a street in Paris named after them, such as Charcot, Chantemesse, Bourneville, Charles Robin, Dejerine, Pinel, Fernand Widal, Vulpian, and so on (Fig. 17-4).[61]

---

o Ksiazce (Wroclaw: 1971); *Encyklopedia Katolicka* [Catholic Encyclopaedia], (Lublin: 1973); *Encyklopedia Staropolska*, 2 vols. (Warsaw: Panstwowe Wydawnictwo Naukowe, 1990) [Cultured Encyclopaedia, 2 vol., Warsaw, National Scientific Editions]; *Maly ilustrowany Leksykon, Pwn*, Warszawa, Wydawnictwo Naukowe Pwn, 1997 [*Brief Illustrated Lexicon*, PWN, Warsaw, National Scientific Editions PWN, 1997].

[58] P. Robert, ed., *Le grand Robert des noms propres* [The great Robert dictionary of proper nouns] (Paris: Le Robert, 1989).

[59] *Lietuviskoji Tarybine Enciklopedija*, 9 vols. (Vilnius: Leidykla Mosklas, 1976); *Chambers' Encyclopaedia. A dictionary of universal knowledge*, 10 vols. (London: William and Robert Chambers Ltd., 1901); C. C. Gillispie, ed., *Dictionary of scientific biography*, 8 vols. with supp. (New York: Charles Scribner's Sons, 1981).

[60] "Nomenclature officielle des voies de Paris" [Official nomenclature of Paris streets], http://www.v1.paris.fr/Carto/Nomenclature/2819.nom.html.

[61] A. Fierro, *Histoire et mémoire du nom des rues de Paris* [History and memory of Paris street names] (Paris: Parigramme, 1999).

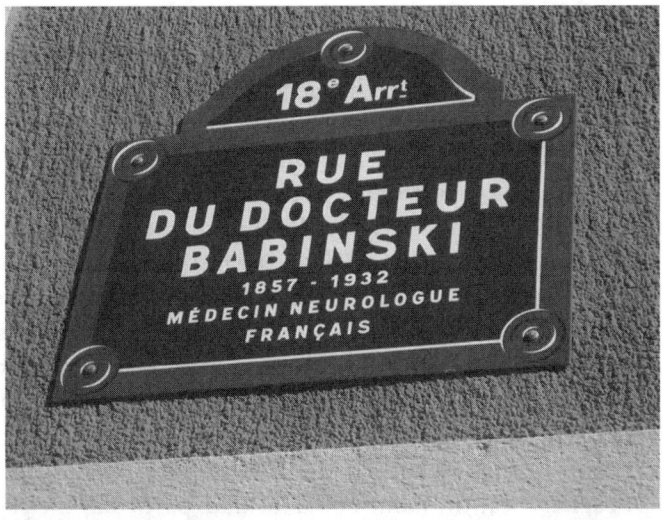

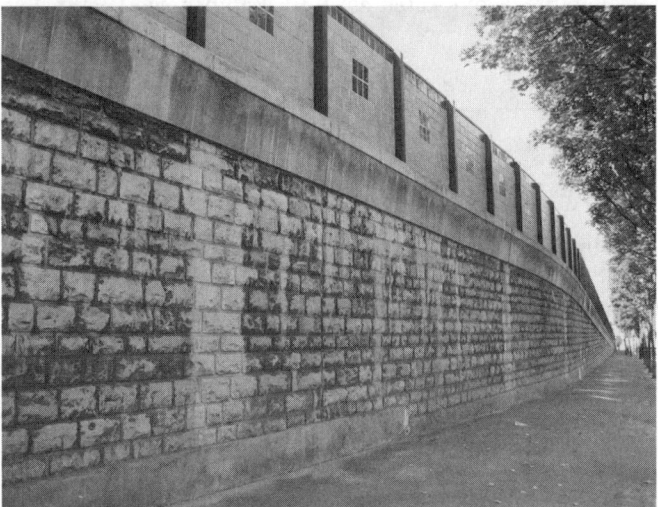

Figure 17-4 Rue du docteur Babinski, [Doctor Babinski street] Eighteenth Arrondissement, Paris. (*Source*: Personal collection, J. Poirier.)

Perhaps reasonably well known by tourists due to the presence of a modest hotel and of a fast-food restaurant, rue du Docteur Babinski is without character; its importance does not correspond to that of the man it is supposed to honor. In France there are numerous examples of streets dedicated to a pair, either married (rue des Docteurs Dejerine, in Paris) or fraternal (streets named after the brothers Périer and Flaviens in Paris, Chappes in Lyon, Lumières in Mulhouse, and Montgolfiers in Belfort), and one may regret—considering the close relationship between Henri and Joseph Babinski and of the fame in different fields of the two brothers—that the street was not named after both Babinski brothers.

At the Salpêtrière Hospital, in the Jacquart Division, the Rochefoucauld ward took the name of Babinski in 1934, as was also the case in 1949 for the lecture room in the department of Dr. Moreau at the Bicêtre hospital.[62] The Babinski Building, constructed between 1993 and 1996 in the new part of the Salpêtrière by the architect Pierre Riboulet (1928– 2003), comprises several clinical and technical departments: the Institut de Myologie (jointly administered by the Association française contre les myopathies and the Assistance publique Hôpitaux de Paris), a lecture hall named after Babinski, and specialized units for neurosurgery, neuroradiology, ophthalmology, and ENT. In Paris, the Tenon hospital has a ward named after Babinski (modernized in 1998–2000), as does the department of gerontology in the Charles Foix hospital in Ivry, in the suburbs of Paris. In Poland, numerous hospitals bear the name of Babinski, in particular the psychiatric ward Josefa Babinskiego, located at 29 ul. Babinskiego (Babinski Street) in Krakow (Fig. 17-5).[63]

Epilogue

For Alajouanine, Babinski will leave

> the memory of an important body of work, a great figure, a great name. A great work which brought a deep and durable change to neurological semiology. A great figure as the example of a constant and persevering search, for more efficiency in the diagnosis and treatment of the nervous diseases. A great name who is a celebrity in French neurology, certain of lasting as long as neurological science, of which he has been one of the leaders.[64]

How does Babinski differ from his contemporaries? Why is he better known than Georges Gilles de la Tourette, Pierre Marie, Achille Souques, or Jules Dejerine? Babinski's myth, quite well implanted in France and

---

[62] Conseil de surveillance de l'Assistance publique, meeting of November 8, 1934, 207–208; Ward denominations in different hospitals, reported by M. Ravina, at the Conseil de surveillance, meeting of March 31, 1949, 214–217.

[63] L. Babinski, "Sylwetka Jozefa Babinskiego na tle jego zycia codziennego" [Joseph Babinsky, day by day], *Neurol Neurochir Pol* 1969 (XIX): 543–546. In Polish, *Babinskiego* is the genitive of *Babinski*.

[64] T. Alajouanine, "Le centenaire de Babinski" [The Babinski centenary], *Semaine des Hôpitaux de Paris* 1958 (22): 1355–1364.

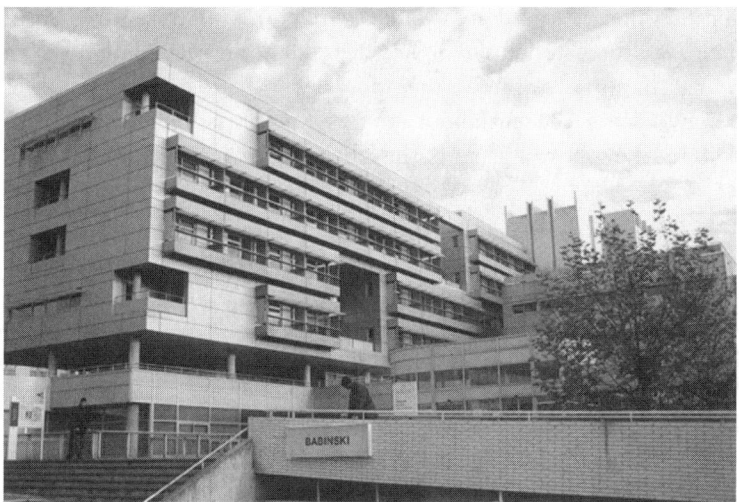

Figure 17-5 Babinski Building at the Salpêtrière Hospital in Paris. (*Source*: Personal collection, J. Poirier.)

Poland, seems related to several factors, which can be summarized as follows.

1. From the start of the nineteenth century, French physicians became almost exclusively interested in clinical studies, "the good milk of the French clinic," and in semiology, while having deep reservations about laboratory investigations. Babinski was first and foremost a clinician in the French style, as shrewdly observed by the daily *Le Temps*:

Babinski appears above all as a clinician: it is a French predilection. Physicians from other countries are able, as much and even more than we do, to distinguish themselves in physical, chemical, histological research, in the laboratory or in pathological anatomy. The French doctor is excellent in the clinic, which is the examination of the living man in his bed; he makes the best possible use of this direct observation, without the help of any apparatus, depending only upon his senses limited to themselves; Babinski was a born clinician, gifted with this apparently simple and ordinary quality, which is in fact so rare. He knew how to observe; he displayed perceptiveness, attention, ingenious shrewdness, and, even more, implacable rigor and a never-tiring perseverance. His genius was built upon infinite patience. But what he described was perfectly observed: it was "acquired forever.[65]

[65] "Psychologie et thérapeutique. Un neurologue de génie: Babinski" [Psychology and therapeutics. A neurologist of genius], *Le Temps*, November 18, 1932.

The obituary that appeared in the *Lancet* also points out this fact: "Throughout his life he was a master clinician, less dependant on neuropathology and the laboratory than many of his contemporaries."[66] In 1927, in connection with a paper by Clovis Vincent about surgery for intraspinal tumors, Babinski spoke about the subordination of the laboratory investigations to the clinical exam:

> It never occurred to me to question the interest of the Sicard-Forestier technique concerning the diagnosis and localization of the spinal cord compressions: I use it in the cases where surgery is indicated. It is for me a way to control the results of the clinical examination. But I want to recall that this clinical exam has always led me until now, as much yesterday as today, to a localization sufficiently precise from a surgical point of view, and the number of my patients is quite considerable.[67]

This attitude should be qualified by the fact that at the end of his career Babinski showed great enthusiasm for the technique of cerebral angiography, invented by his pupil Egas Moniz (see chapter 13). One should remember nevertheless that Babinski never tried to develop for the brain functions, as he did for the spinal cord, a semiology that would have helped in the localization of brain tumors.

2. The bedside examination of the patient, born at the same time as the medical school of Paris at the beginning of the nineteenth century, was highly praised, contrary to the theoretical and verbose speeches of the university professors. In Babinski's time this clinical examination was still important. Through his work, his discoveries, and his charisma, Joseph Babinski, merely a hospital practitioner who had failed the *agrégation* and so was without the prestigious title of professor, illustrates perfectly the revenge of the hospital on the university.

Other factors to be borne in mind include:

1. The media impact of *La gastronomie pratique* and the devotion of Ali-Bab to his brother certainly played a role in building the reputation of Joseph Babinski.

[66] "Babinski," *The Lancet* 1932 (2): 1122.
[67] J. Babinski, intervention of 13 lines (p. 498) concerning a paper by Clovis Vincent, "La chirurgie des tumeurs intramédullaires en France en 1913. Sur un cas rapporté par Gendron, opéré avec succès par Th. De Martel" [Surgery on spinal cord tumors in France in 1913: on a case reported by Gendron, successfully operated on by T. De Martel], *Rev Neurol (Paris)* 1927 (I): 491–498.

2. Binational patriotism, especially noticeable in the Babinski family, was viewed with favor in France and Poland, where the sentiments of national pride have been particularly accentuated by the historical circumstances both populations have endured. It may be that the very positive image of Babinski is fundamentally a French-Polish construction and is not yet fully reflected at the international level.
3. The passionate activism of Babinski's hagiographers has certainly had a far from negligible impact. Very few of his colleagues have had as many verbose and efficient supporters as Tournay, Charpentier, Plichet, Vaquez, and others.

When celebrating in 1951 the 150th anniversary of the founding of the medical residency program within the Paris hospital system, Henri Mondor included Babinski in the honor list among the great names in French medicine:

> by selecting some of the best, how am I to judge in the name of all the former residents for whom I am speaking today?...; let us recall for a moment Pierre Marie, Babinski, Widal, Chauffard, Gilbert, Achard, Ch. Richet, Darier, Marfan, Ch. Foix, Cl. Vincent who have joined their great masters Jaccoud, Charcot, Dieulafoy, Cruveilhier, Hayem.[68]

Joseph Babinski, this blue-eyed, good-looking giant, was not a genius nor a god, but a man, a great man—at the same time a great clinician and a great consultant, a great Frenchman and a great Pole. Why should he not be recognized for eternity as "just a man, as every man, equal to all and better than none"?[69]

---

[68] H. Mondor, "Discours prononcé à la Sorbonne en 1951 à l'occasion du Cent-Cinquantenaire de l'Internat des Hôpitaux de Paris" [150 years of the residency program. Speech delivered at the Sorbonne at the commemoration festivities], *La Presse Médicale,* 1952 (60), fasc. 62: 1305–1308.

[69] J.-P. Sartre, *Les mots* [Words] (Paris: Gallimard, Collection Folio, 1964), 214.

Bibliography[1]

Archival Sources

Archives nationales, Paris

Brunel G. Les sources de l'histoire de la Pologne et des Polonais dans les Archives françaises. Paris, Direction des Archives de France, 2003.
Favier J. (ed. by) Etat général des fonds, T. IV, Paris, Archives Nationales, 1980.
Laszuk A. (ed. by) Miedzy Sekwana a Wisla. Zroda do dziejow Francji I stosunkow polsko-francuskich w archiwach polskich, Warszawa, 2002.
Walichnowski T. (ed. by) Balcanica, Guide to the Polish archives relative to the history of the Balkan Countries, Warsaw, Polish Scientific Publishers, 1979.

Dossiers de Légion d'honneur:

Joseph Babinski (L0085063), Jules Bucquoy (L0388034), Victor Cornil (L0592034), Jean-Ferdinand Darier (L0661042), Louis Delherm (L0712076), Georges Gilles de la Tourette (L1134076), Jean Jarkowscki (*sic*) (L1355013), Louis-Charles Malassez (L1702053), Pierre Marie (L1741017), Pierre Marquès (L1749049), Charles-Emile Picard (L2144015), Louis Ranvier (L2266021), Fulgence Raymond (L2273064), Clovis Vincent (L2710023), Alfred Vulpian (L2742047).

Dossiers de naturalisation:

microfilm 595; microfilm 605.

Cartons:

AB/XlV, Thèses et mémoires universitaires, Inventaire par Pascal R. David.

---

[1] Bibliographical references are given here in a complete formulation (precise date, volumes, and issue numbers when possible).

AB/XIX/3779, dossier 4 : Dictionnaire des polonais ayant participé à la Commune de Paris, par Julien Grossbart, dactylographié.
AJ/A6/303-1: Faculté de médecine 1876.
AJ/16/451, 453, 454: Lycée Louis-le-Grand (1862–1863, 1868–1873, 1874–1880).
AJ/16/4699: Registre de déclarations d'ouverture d'écoles secondaires libres 1850–1924.
AJ/16/4733: Enseignement secondaire libre. Notices annuelles d'inspection. Ecole polonaise (17è arrondissement), directeur, 1874–1875 à 1882–1883.
AJ/16/6350: Concours du clinicat 1874–1908.
AJ/16/6498: Etudiants étrangers 1860–1933. Etudiants polonais. Listes des étudiants bénéficiant de la gratuité des droits d'inscription et d'examens (1864–1874).
AJ/16/6550: Service militaire 1872–1914. Situation des étudiants en médecine vis à vis du service militaire.
AJ/16/6686: Assistance publique 1841–1881. Stages hospitaliers des étudiants 1841–1885.
AJ/16/6864: Dossiers des étudiants de la Faculté de médecine, classés par année d'obtention de la Thèse, et dans chaque année, par ordre alphabétique, année 1885.
AJ/16/6717: Registre de délivrances des diplômes 1881–1885.
AJ/16/6718: Registre de délivrances des diplômes 1885–1890.
AJ/16/6864: Dossiers des étudiants de la faculté de médecine, classés par année d'obtention de la Thèse, et dans chaque année, par ordre alphabétique, 1885.
F/14/11409 à 11425: Dossiers d'ingénieurs, de sous-ingénieurs, de contrôleurs des mines, en fonction de 1842 à 1919. Répertoire nominatif inclus dans l'inventaire dactylographié de F/14/11400 à F/14/12855

Archives of the Assistance publique-Hôpitaux de Paris

Cartons:

672 Foss 2: Etats du personnel médical des établissements hospitaliers 1897–1924.
751 Foss: collection de photos.
761 Foss 1–72: Personnel médical : concours et prix (1861, 1863, 1872, 1873–1914), 1932.
774 Foss 1–37: Externes et internes en médecine dans les hôpitaux de l'Assistance publique : fiches nominatives de suivi et d'évaluation pédagogique 1880–1920.
791 Foss 38-3 Archives de l'AP, Nominations de médecins; avis de nomination. Correspondances 1890–1895.
Fonds Fosseyeux, Liasse 680: Concours pour la nomination des élèves en médecine et en chirurgie.
D 617: Etat du personnel médical 1898–1936.
9 L 1: Généralités. Activité et fonctionnement.
9 L 128: La Pitié. Activité et fonctionnement de l'établissement.
9 L 129: La Pitié. Services hospitaliers.
9 L 145: La Pitié. Personnel médical.
449 W 1–24: Etats nominatifs du personnel médical des hôpitaux et hospices (médecins, pharmaciens, internes, externes), 1874–1910.

Registers:

La Pitié. Registres d'inscription des employés et gens de service: 1 K 14 (1901–1902), 1 K 16 (1905–1906), 1 K 18 (1908–1910), 1 K 19 (1910–1911), 1 K 20 (1911–1912), 1 K 22 (1914–1916), 1 K 24 (1918–1919), 1 K 25 (1919–1920), 1 K 26 (1921–1923).
2 K 15 à 2K 19: La Pitié. Registres des appointements (1892–1895) à (1904–1907).
2 K 20: Hôpital de la Pitié. Registres des appointements.
Hôpital de la Pitié. Registre des entrées: 1 Q 2/28 (1890), 1 Q 2/164 (1895), 1 Q 2/169 (1900), 1 Q 2/174 (1905), 1 Q 2/179 (1910), 1 Q 2/188 (1915), 1 Q 2/189 (1915), 1 Q 2/195 (1920), 1 Q 2/196 (1920).
3 Q 2/79: Hôpital de la Pitié. Registre des décès 1897–1899.

538 W/297: Hôpital de la Pitié. Registre des décès 1905–1907.
538 W/308: Hôpital de la Pitié. Registre des décès 1921–1922.
449W1-24 (24 registres) Etats nominatifs du personnel médical des hôpitaux et hospices (médecins, pharmaciens, internes, externes), 1874–1910.

Minutes of the Conseil de surveillance de l'Assistance publique:

Conseil de surveillance de l'Assistance publique, meeting of March 7, 1895, 1L30, pp. 481–482.
Dr Babinski: demande de consultation spéciale, meeting of October 31, 1895, pp. 30–32.
Honorariat de M. le docteur Bucquoy, meeting of January 31, 1895, pp. 393–394.
Obituary of Doctor Guibout, former *Médecin des Hôpitaux, Procès-Verbaux,* meeting of January 10, 1895, p. 246.
Conseil de surveillance de l'Assistance publique, meeting of November 14, 1895.
Décès de M. le docteur Constantin Paul, médecin de l'hôpital de la Charité, meeting of April 16, 1896, pp. 495–496.
Au sujet de la mort de M. le Professeur Cornil, médecin honoraire des hôpitaux, meeting of May 14, 1908, p. 531.
Ouverture de l'hôpital de la Nouvelle Pitié, meeting of June 29, 1911, p. 717.
Démolition des bâtiments de l'ancienne Pitié, meeting of November 30, 1911, p. 240.
Mort de M. le Dr. Bucquoy, meeting of July 1, 1920, pp. 669–670.
Admission à l'honorariat de MM. Les docteurs Babinski, Richardière et Florant, médecins des hôpitaux; Bar et Potocki, accoucheurs des hôpitaux; Chaslin, médecin du service des aliénés, meeting of October 26, 1922, pp. 143–144.
Création d'un service de neuro-chirurgie à la Pitié, meeting of November 12, 1931, p. 240.
Au sujet du décès de M. le docteur Babinski et de M. le professeur Chauffard, meeting of November 10, 1932, pp. 206–207.
Dénomination d'un pavillon à l'hôpital de la Pitié, meeting of May 18, 1933, p. 584.
M. Crouzon, sur la nécessité de créer un service de neuro-chirurgie à la Salpêtrière, meeting of October 19, 1933, pp. 7–12.
Au sujet du décès de M. le docteur Pierre Bazy, chirurgien honoraire des hôpitaux, meeting of January 11, 1934, p. 342.
Attribution du nom de Dejerine à la salle d'opérés du service de neurochirurgie de la Pitié, meeting of January 25, 1934, p. 364.
Babinski, dénomination des salles à la Salpêtrière, meeting of November 8, 1934, pp. 207–208.
Situation des neurochirurgiens des hôpitaux et du Professeur de la Clinique de neuro-chirurgie en ce qui concerne leur participation aux jurys du concours, meeting of November 15, 1948, pp. 13–16.
Dénomination de salles dans différents hôpitaux, meeting of March 31, 1949, pp. 214–217.
Dénomination de deux salles à l'hospice de Bicêtre, meeting of October 10, 1957, p. 165.

Commission du Vieux-Paris:

Visite de la Pitié, Rapport de M. Tesson, 1903, pp. 118–126.
Conservation de l'ancienne chapelle de la Pitié, 1911, pp. 108–111.
Conservation de l'ancienne chapelle de la Pitié, 1912, p. 27 et 61–63.
Les boiseries de la Pitié transférées au musée Carnavalet, 1914–1915, p. 48.
Fouilles rue de Lacépède, sur une partie des terrains occupés par l'ancienne Pitié, 1914–1915, pp. 40–41.

Archives of the Ministère des Affaires étrangères, Paris

Série Mémoires et Documents:
Pologne 36–37. Réfugiés polonais: dossiers communs à plusieurs individus 1831–1852.
Pologne 38–45. Réfugiés polonais: dossiers individuels 1824–1852.
Pologne 46. Réfugiés polonais: dossiers individuels 1852–1857.

Archives of the Préfecture de Police de Paris

"Docteurs 1843–1895": Listes des docteurs de Paris.
EB/58 et EB/96: Théâtre de l'Opéra.
DA 309–310: choléra de 1884.
DA 312–313: choléra de 1892.

Archives de Paris

Annuaire statistique de la ville de Paris, Vè année, 1884. Paris, Imprimerie municipale, 1886.
Annuaire statistique de la ville de Paris, XXIè année, 1900. Paris, Masson et Cie, 1902.

Archives and library of the Ecole des Mines de Paris

Comptes-rendus de voyage de MM. Les élèves 1876 (1), N° 169 Babinski (CR 1876/169).
Journaux de voyage de MM. Les élèves 1877, N° 579 Babinski (J 1877/579).
Compte-rendus des séances du Conseil de l'Ecole.

Archives of the Evêché de Pontoise, France

Carton "Paroisse de Montmorency".
Registres des actes de sépulture, Paroisse de Montmorency, annnées 1897, 1899, 1931, 1932.

Musée de l'Assistance publique-Hôpitaux de Paris

Dossier "microtome de Babinski".
Dossier Clovis Vincent.

Archives de l'Académie des Sciences, Paris

Dossiers Pierre Bazy, Charles Bouchard, Jean-Martin Charcot, Victor Cornil, Antonin Gosset, Léon Guignard, Georges Guillain, Paul Janet, Charles Laubry, Jean Nageotte, Emile Picard, Charles Potain, Louis Ranvier, Gustave Roussy, Alfred Vulpian, Fernand Widal.

Archives—Bibliothèque—Musée Paris Opera

Opera.Arch.19,336: Service médical. Arrêtés de nomination des médecins de l'Opéra, 1880–1900.
Opera.Arch.20/381: Service médical, 1912.

Archives of the Pasteur Institute, *Paris*

Dossiers biographiques: Henri Baruk, Jean Charcot, Albert Charrin, Jean Clunet, Georges Guillain, Maurice Letulle, Ignace Meyerson, Joseph Pilinski, Edouard Pozerski, Edouard Rist.
Cartons: André Chantemesse, Edouard Pozerski.

Museum of the Pasteur Institute, *Paris*

Registre d'inscriptions au "Cours de Monsieur Roux" de 1898.
Photographie de groupe du "Cours de Monsieur Roux" de February–March 1898.

Archives of the Collège de France, *Paris*

Dossiers Albert Charrin, Charles Malassez, Jean Nageotte, Eugène Suchard.
Cdf 22 Enseignement et recherche, art 13, liasse 39; art 14, liasses 40 et 41 (Ranvier).

Archives of the Mairies de Paris

Mairie du 8è arrondissement: Actes de décès de Joseph et d'Henri Babinski.

Archives of the Ministère de la Défense, *Paris*

Direction de la mémoire, du patrimoine et des archives, Service historique de la Défense: recherches concernant Aleksander Babinski.

Archives of the Service de Santé des armées (Val-de-Grâce, Paris)

Cartons C 61.

Libraries

Bibliothèque des Neurosciences Jean-Martin Charcot, Université Paris-6
Bibliothèque Nationale de France, Paris
Bibliothèque Inter-Universitaire de Médecine, Université Paris–5

Bibliothèque Historique de la Ville de Paris
Bibliothèque Sainte-Geneviève, Paris
Bibliothèque Polonaise de Paris
Bibliothèque de l'Académie nationale de médecine, Paris

Joseph Babinski Papers [2]

Société anatomique (from 1882 to 1889)

Babinski J. Pièces d'un malade qui, durant la vie, avait présenté les symptômes de cirrhose du foie, *Société Anatomique de Paris* meeting of January 13, 1882, *Bulletins de la Société Anatomique de Paris*, 1882, LVIIè année, 4è série, T. VII, p. 28.

Babinski J. Cancer du rein développé chez une femme opérée d'une squirrhe du sein, *Société Anatomique de Paris* meeting of February 10, 1882, *Bulletins de la Société Anatomique de Paris*, 1882, LVIIè année, 4è série, T. VII, p. 113.

Babinski J. Tuberculose pulmonaire – Angine et laryngite tuberculeuses – Ulcération tuberculeuse de la lèvre, *Société Anatomique de Paris* meeting of April 10, 1882, *Bulletins de la Société Anatomique de Paris*, 1882, LVIIè année, 4è série, T. VII, pp. 236–238.

Babinski J. Kystes multiples du foie et des reins – Urémie, *Société Anatomique de Paris* meeting of June 9, 1882, *Bulletins de la Société Anatomique de Paris*, 1882, LVIIè année, 4è série, T. VII, pp. 341–344.

Babinski J. Occlusion intestinale due à un calcul biliaire enclavé dans le rectum, *Société Anatomique de Paris* meeting of February 16, 1883, *Bulletins de la Société Anatomique de Paris*, 1883, LVIIIè année, 4è série, T. VIII, pp. 117–118 (Analysis *in Le Progrès Médical*, 1883, T.XI, n° 37 (15 September), pp. 736–737).

2. Babinski J. Ramollissement cérébral, *Société Anatomique de Paris* meeting of March 2, 1883, *Bulletins de la Société Anatomique de Paris*, 1883, LVIIIè année, 4è série, T. VIII, pp. 140–143 (Analysis *in Le Progrès Médical*, 1883, T.XI, n° 39 (29 September), pp. 770–771).

3. Babinski J. Kyste hydatique du cerveau, *Société Anatomique de Paris* meeting of March 2, 1883, *Bulletins de la Société Anatomique de Paris*, 1883, LVIIIè année, 4è série, T. VIII, 1883, pp. 143–146 (Analysis *in Le Progrès Médical*, 1883, T.XI, n° 41 (October 13), p. 808).

4. Babinski J. Epithélioma tubulé de la peau de la région fessière développé au dépens du corps muqueux de Malpighi, *Société Anatomique de Paris* meeting of May 4, 1883, *Bulletins de la Société Anatomique de Paris*, 1883, LVIIIè année, 4è série, T. VIII, pp. 232–233.

5. Babinski J. Deux cas d'épithélioma pavimenteux ayant vraisemblablement pour point de départ un kyste dermoïde de l'ovaire, *Société Anatomique de Paris* meeting of May 4, 1883, *Bulletins de la Société Anatomique de Paris*, 1883, LVIIIè année, 4è série, T. VIII, pp. 234–236, (Analysis *in Le Progrès Médical*, 1884, T.XII, n° 2 (January 12), p. 29).

Babinski J. Rapport sur la candidature de M. Charrin à la place de membre-adjoint, *Société Anatomique de Paris* meeting of November 30, 1883, *Bulletins de la Société Anatomique de Paris*, 1883, LVIIIè année, 4è série, T. VIII, 1883, pp. 482–484 (Analysis *in Le Progrès Médical*, 1884, T.XII, n° 24 (June 14), p. 480).

Babinski J. A propos d'une tumeur présentée par M. Ballue comme un épithéliome corné du maxillaire inférieur, M. Babinski dit "qu'il s'agit plutôt d'un épithéliome lobulé, muqueux: il existe fort peu d'éléïdine." *Société Anatomique de Paris* meeting of January 23, 1885, *Bulletins de la Société Anatomique de Paris*, 1885, LVè année, 4è série, T. X, 1885, p. 52, (Analysis *in Le Progrès Médical*, 1885, T.II, 2è série, n° 39 (September 26), p. 235).

[2] The references with bold numbers correspond to the numbers used in L'*Oeuvre scientifique* published in 1934. The references with a grey frame correspond to Babinski's interventions during discussion and not to a full paper. The references surrounded by a frame are analyses of Babinski papers written by several contributors.

Babinski J. Examen histologique de la tumeur présentée dans la dernière séance par M. Mérigot. *Société Anatomique de Paris* meeting of November 6, 1885, *Bulletins de la Société Anatomique de Paris*, 1885, LVè année, 4è série, T. X, 1885, p. 464.

Babinski J. Coupes de moelle offrant un type de *sclérose combinée*. *Société Anatomique de Paris* meeting of January 8, 1886, *Bulletins de la Société Anatomique de Paris*, 1886, LXIè année, 4è série, T. XI, p. 17.

Babinski J. Rapport sur la candidature de M. Hallé, *Société Anatomique de Paris* meeting of November 5, 1886, *Bulletins de la Société Anatomique de Paris*, 1886, LVIè année, 4è série, T. XI, pp. 648–649.

Babinski J. M. Babinski montre des préparations de figures nouvelles trouvées par lui dans les muscles striés de l'homme à l'état normal. Ces pièces ont déjà fait l'objet d'une communication à la Société de Biologie, *Société Anatomique de Paris* meeting of November 5, 1886, *Bulletins de la Société Anatomique de Paris*, 1886, LXIè année, 4è série, T. XI, p. 753.

Babinski J. Rapport sur la candidature de M. Guillet au titre de membre adjoint de la Société anatomique *Société Anatomique de Paris* meeting of July 1887, *Bulletins de la Société Anatomique de Paris*, 1887, LXIIè année, 5è série, T. I, pp. 496–497.

Babinski J. Arthropathies des ataxiques, *Société Anatomique de Paris* meeting of October 1887, *Bulletins de la Société Anatomique de Paris*, 1887, LXIIè année, 5è série, T. I, pp. 624–626.

19. Babinski J. Ataxie locomotrice – Arthropathie tabétique – Rhumatisme chronique, *Société Anatomique de Paris* meeting of November 11, 1887, *Bulletins de la Société Anatomique de Paris*, 1887, LXIIè année, 5è série, T. I, pp. 669–672.

Babinski J. Maladie pyocyanique – Arthropathies expérimentales, *Société Anatomique de Paris* meeting of July 12, 1889, *Bulletins de la Société Anatomique de Paris*, 1889, LXIVè année, 5è série, T. Iii, p. 468.

Société de Biologie *(from 1886 to 1905, with three papers in 1913)*

14. Babinski J. Atrophie musculaire d'origine cérébrale, avec intégrité des cornes antérieures de la moelle et des nerfs moteurs, *Société de Biologie*, meeting of February 20, 1886, *Comptes-rendus hebdomadaires des Séances et Mémoires de la Société de Biologie*, 1886, T. III, 8è série, pp. 76–78.

Babinski J. Recherches servant à établir que certains phénomènes nerveux peuvent être transmis d'un sujet à un autre sous l'influence de l'aimant, *Société de Biologie*, meeting of November 6, 1886, *Comptes-rendus hebdomadaires des Séances et Mémoires de la Société de Biologie*, 1886, T. III, 8è série, pp. 475–477, resumé in *Le Progrès Médical*, 1886, T.IV, 2è série, n° 46 (November 13, 1886), p. 996.

17. Babinski J. Sur la présence dans les muscles striés de l'homme d'un système spécial constitué par des groupes de petites fibres musculaires entourées d'une gaine lamelleuse, *Société de Biologie*, meeting of December 18, 1886, *Comptes-rendus hebdomadaires des Séances et Mémoires de la Société de Biologie*, 1886, T. III, 8è série, pp. 629–631.

18. Babinski J. Tabès bénins, *Société de Biologie*, meeting of May 28, 1887, *Comptes-rendus hebdomadaires des Séances et Mémoires de la Société de Biologie*, 1887, T. IV, 8è série, pp. 336–340.

21. Babinski J, Onanoff. Myopathie progressive primitive. Sur la corrélation qui existe entre la prédisposition de certains muscles à la myopathie et la rapidité de leur développement (Travail du laboratoire de M. le Prof. Charcot à la Salpêtrière). *Société de Biologie*, meeting of February 11, 1888, *Comptes-rendus hebdomadaires des Séances et Mémoires de la Société de Biologie*, 1888, T. V, 8è série, pp. 145–151.

22. Babinski J, Charrin. De la paralysie pyocyanique. Etude clinique et anatomique, *Société de Biologie*, meeting of March 10, 1888, *Comptes-rendus hebdomadaires des Séances et Mémoires de la Société de Biologie*, 1888, T. V, 8è série, pp. 257–259.

25. Babinski J, Charrin. Arthropathies expérimentales. Paralysie pyocyanique, meeting of July 27, 1889, *Comptes-rendus hebdomadaires des Séances et Mémoires de la Société de Biologie*,

1889, T. I, 9è série, pp. 545–547, résumé in *Le Progrès Médical*, 1889, T.X, 2è série, n° 35 (August 31, 1889), pp. 223–224).

Babinski J. Migraine ophtalmique hystérique, *Société de Biologie*, meeting of July 27, 1889, *Comptes-rendus hebdomadaires des Séances et Mémoires de la Société de Biologie*, 1889, T. I, 9è série, pp. 547–549, résumé in *Le Progrès Médical*, 1889, T.X, 2è série, n° 35 (August 31, 1889), pp. 223–224).

42. Babinski J, Zachariades. Paraplégie crurale par mal de Pott dorsal. Névrites périphériques des membres inférieurs, *Société de Biologie*, meeting of November 9, 1895, *Comptes-rendus hebdomadaires des Séances et Mémoires de la Société de Biologie*, 1895, T. II, 10è série, pp. 722–725, résumé in *Le Progrès Médical*, 1895, T.II, 3è série, n° 47 (November 23, 1895), p. 378 and in *Rev Neurol Paris)*, 1896, T. IV, n° 3 (February 15), pp. 87–88.

43. Babinski J. Sur le réflexe cutané plantaire dans certains affections organiques du système nerveux central, *Société de Biologie*, meeting of February 22, 1896, *Comptes-rendus hebdomadaires des Séances et Mémoires de la Société de Biologie*, 1896, T. III, 10è série, n° 48, pp. 207–208, résumé in *Le Progrès Médical*, 1896, T.III, 3è série, n° 9 (February 29, 1896), p. 137 and in *Rev Neurol (Paris)*, 1896, T. IV, n° 13 (July 15), p. 415.

44. Babinski J. Relâchement des muscles dans l'hémiplégie organique, *Société de Biologie*, meeting of May 9, 6, *Comptes-rendus hebdomadaires des Séances et Mémoires de la Société de Biologie*, 1896, T. III, 10è série, pp. 471–472. Résumé in *Rev Neurol (Paris)*, 1896, T.IV, n° 15 (August 15), p. 467 and in *Le Progrès Médical*, 1896, T.III, 3è série, n° 20 (May 16, 1896), pp. 310–311.

47. Babinski J. De l'action du chlorhydrate de morphine sur le tétanos, *Société de Biologie*, meeting of June 19, 1897, *Comptes-rendus hebdomadaires des Séances et Mémoires de la Société de Biologie*, 1897, T. IV, 10è série, pp. 600–602, résumé in *Le Progrès Médical*, 1897, T.V, 3è série, n° 26 (June 26, 1897), pp. 407–408 and in *Rev Neurol (Paris)*, 1897, T. V, n° 22 (November 30), p. 656.

Babinski J. Des phénomènes des orteils, *Société de Biologie*, meeting of June 25, 1898, *Comptes-rendus hebdomadaires des Séances et Mémoires de la Société de Biologie*, 1898, 10è série, T. V, pp. 669–700, résumé in *Rev Neurol (Paris)*, 1898, T. VI, n° 21 (November 15), pp. 781–782.

52. Babinski J. De la contractilité électrique des muscles striés après la mort, *Société de Biologie*, meeting of May 6, 1899, *Comptes-rendus hebdomadaires des Séances et Mémoires de la Société de Biologie*, 1899, T. I, 11è série, pp. 343–346, résumé in *Le Progrès Médical*, 1899, T.IX, 3è série, n° 20 (May 20, 1899), p. 319 and in *Rev Neurol (Paris)*, 1899, T.VII, n° 22 (30 November), p. 827.

67. Babinski J. De l'influence des lésions de l'appareil auditif sur le vertige voltaïque, *Société de Biologie*, meeting of January 26, 1901, *Comptes-rendus hebdomadaires des Séances et Mémoires de la Société de Biologie*, 1901, T. 52, pp. 77–80. Analysis in *Rev Neurol (Paris)*, 1901, T. IX, n° 23 (December 15), pp. 1170–1171 et in *Le Progrès Médical*, 1901, T. XIII, n° 6 (February 9), p. 92.

92. Babinski J. Sur le mécanisme du vertige voltaïque, *Société de Biologie*, meeting of March 14, 1903, *Comptes-rendus hebdomadaires des Séances et Mémoires de la Société de Biologie*, 1903, T. LV, pp. 350–353, résumé in *Le Progrès Médical*, 1903, T. XVII, n° 13 (March 28, 1903), p. 225.

94. Babinski J. Sur le mouvement d'inclination et de rotation de la tête dans le vertige voltaïque, *Société de Biologie*, meeting of April 25, 1903, *Comptes-rendus hebdomadaires des Séances et Mémoires de la Société de Biologie*, 1903, T. LV, pp. 513–515. Résumé in *Le Progrès Médical*, 1903, T. XVII, n° 18 (May 2, 1903), p. 327.

120. Babinski J, Nageotte J. Note sur un cas de tabes à systématisation exceptionnelle, Société de Biologie, meeting of October 14, *Comptes-rendus hebdomadaires des Séances et Mémoires de la Société de Biologie*, 1905, T. 57, pp. 280–283, résumé in *Le Progrès Médical*, 1905, T. XXI, n° 43 (October 28), p. 704.

203. Babinski J, Weill GA. Désorientation et déséquilibration spontanée et provoquée. La déviation angulaire, *Société de Biologie*, April 26, 1913, *Comptes-rendus hebdomadaires des Séances et Mémoires de la Société de Biologie*, 1913, (65è année), T. I, pp. 852–855.

206. Babinski J, Weill GA. Mouvements réactionnels d'origine vestibulaire et mouvements contre-réactionnels, *Société de Biologie*, July 19, 1913, *Comptes-rendus hebdomadaires des Séances et Mémoires de la Société de Biologie*, 1913, (65è année), T. II, pp. 98–100.

Archives de Neurologie
(from 1886 to 1895)

15. Babinski J. De l'atrophie musculaire dans les paralysies hystériques, *Archives de Neurologie (Paris)*, 1886, n° 34 et 35: 1–27. Résumé in *Annales Médico-Psychologiques*, 1891, T. I, p. 133.
20. Babinski J. Sur une déformation particulière du tronc causée par la sciatique, *Archives de Neurologie (Paris)*, 1888, n° 43. Résumé in *Annales Médico-Psychologiques*, 1891, T. II, p. 463.
23. Babinski J. Grand et petit hypnotisme, *Archives de Neurologie (Paris)*, 1889, n° 49 et 50, 17, 92–108; 253–269. Résumé in *Annales Médico-Psychologiques*, 1892, T. II, pp. 302–303.
27. Babinski J. De la migraine ophtalmique hystérique. *Archives de Neurologie (Paris)*, 1890; 20: 305–335. Résumé in *Annales Médico-Psychologiques*, 1893, T. I, p. 294.

Société Médicale des Hôpitaux de Paris (from 1890 to 1928)

Babinski J. Intervention of 5 lines (p. 949) on the paper by M. Debove "Paralysie des deux nerfs moteurs oculaires communs d'origine hystéro-traumatique", *Société Médicale des Hôpitaux de Paris*, meeting of December 12, 1890, *Bulletins et Mémoires de la Société Médicale des Hôpitaux de Paris*, 1890, T. VII, 3è série, pp. 948–949.

28. Babinski J. Intervention of 41 lines (pp. 95–96) on the paper by M. A. Joffroy "Nouvelle autopsie de maladie de Morvan. Syringomyélie", *Société Médicale des Hôpitaux de Paris*, meeting of February 27, 1891, *Bulletins et Mémoires de la Société Médicale des Hôpitaux de Paris*, 1891, T. VIII, 3è série, pp. 92–97.

Babinski J. Intervention of 19 lines (p. 198) on the paper by M. A. Laveran "D'une forme atténuée de la rage observée pendant le cours du traitement par les inoculations préventives", *Société Médicale des Hôpitaux de Paris*, meeting of April 25, 1891, *Bulletins et Mémoires de la Société Médicale des Hôpitaux de Paris*, 1891, T. VIII, 3è série, pp. 191–200.

31. Babinski J. Polyurie hystérique. Influence de la suggestion sur l'évolution de ce syndrome, *Société Médicale des Hôpitaux de Paris*, meeting of November 13, 1891, *Bulletins et Mémoires de la Société Médicale des Hôpitaux de Paris*, 1891, T. VIII, 3è série, pp. 568–574.
33. Desnos[3], Babinski J. Sur un fait de syringomyélie (présentation de malade), *Société Médicale des Hôpitaux de Paris*, meeting of December 11, 1891, *Bulletins et Mémoires de la Société Médicale des Hôpitaux de Paris*, 1891, T. VIII, 3è série, pp. 652–656.
34. Babinski J. Paralysie hystérique systématique (paralysie partielle ou systématique des fonctions motrices du membre inférieur gauche), *Société Médicale des Hôpitaux de Paris*, meeting of July 8, 1892, *Bulletins et Mémoires de la Société Médicale des Hôpitaux de Paris*, 1892, T. IX, 3è série, pp. 533–538.
35. Babinski J. Paralysies hystériques systématiques; Paralysie faciale hystérique, *Société Médicale des Hôpitaux de Paris*, meeting of October 28, 1892, *Bulletins et Mémoires de la Société Médicale des Hôpitaux de Paris*, 1892, T. IX, 3è série, pp. 706–716, résumé in *Le Progrès Médical*, 1892, T.XVI, 2è série, n° 46 (November 12, 1892), p. 409.
35. Babinski J. A l'occasion du Procès-Verbal, Paralysie faciale hystérique, *Société Médicale des Hôpitaux de Paris*, meeting of November 4, 1892, *Bulletins et Mémoires de la Société Médicale des Hôpitaux de Paris*, 1892, T. IX, 3è série, p. 738, résumé in *Le Progrès Médical*, 1892, T.XVI, 2è série, n° 46 (November 12, 1892), pp. 414–415.

---

[3] The only Babinski's paper where he does not appear as the first author! Desnos was then chief-physician at La Charité Hospital and Vice-President of the *Société Médicale des Hôpitaux de Paris*.

Babinski J. Intervention de 92 lines (pp. 745-748) M. A. Chauffard "Lèpre systématisée nerveuse, simulant la syringomyélie", *Société Médicale des Hôpitaux de Paris*, meeting of November 4, 1892, *Bulletins et Mémoires de la Société Médicale des Hôpitaux de Paris*, 1892, T. IX, 3è série, pp. 738-749, résumé in *Le Progrès Médical*, 1892, T.XVI, 2è série, n° 46 (November 12, 1892), pp. 414-415.

36. Babinski J. Association de l'hystérie avec les maladies organiques du système nerveux, les névroses et diverses autres affections, *Société Médicale des Hôpitaux de Paris*, meeting of November 11, 1892, *Bulletins et Mémoires de la Société Médicale des Hôpitaux de Paris*, 1892, T. IX, 3è série, pp. 775-795.

37. Babinski J. Des crampes musculaires dans le choléra et dans d'autres états pathologiques, *Société Médicale des Hôpitaux de Paris*, meeting of December 2, 1892, *Bulletins et Mémoires de la Société Médicale des Hôpitaux de Paris*, 1892, T. IX, 3è série, pp. 845-848, résumé in *Le Progrès Médical*, 1892, T.XVI, 2è série, n° 50 (December 10, 1892), p. 488.

38. Babinski J. Paralysie faciale hystérique, *Société Médicale des Hôpitaux de Paris*, meeting of December 16, 1892, *Bulletins et Mémoires de la Société Médicale des Hôpitaux de Paris*, 1892, T. IX, 3è série, pp. 867-870, résumé in *Le Progrès Médical*, 1892, T.XVI, 2è série, n° 52 (December 24, 1892), p. 519.

40. Babinski J. Contractures organique et hystérique, *Société Médicale des Hôpitaux de Paris*, meeting of May 5, 1893, *Bulletins et Mémoires de la Société Médicale des Hôpitaux de Paris*, 1893, T. X, 3è série, pp. 327-343, résumé in *Le Progrès Médical*, 1893, T.XVIII, 2è série, n° 19 (May 13, 1893), p. 368 and in *Rev Neurol (Paris)*, 1893, T. I, n° 11 (June 15), p. 307.

41. Babinski J. Sur les scléroses systématiques, dites primitives, de la moelle, *Société Médicale des Hôpitaux de Paris*, meeting of January 19, 1894, *Bulletins et Mémoires de la Société Médicale des Hôpitaux de Paris*, 1894, T. XIX, 3è série, pp. 21-30, résumé in *Le Progrès Médical*, 1894, T.XIX, 2è série, n° 4 (January 27, 1894), p. 66.

45. Babinski J. Hémiatrophie de la langue (présentation de malade), *Société Médicale des Hôpitaux de Paris*, meeting of July 31, 1896, *Bulletins et Mémoires de la Société Médicale des Hôpitaux de Paris*, 1896, T. XIII, 3è série, pp. 671-675, résumé in *Le Progrès Médical*, 1896, T.IV, 3è série, n° 34 (August 22, 1896), p. 133.

Babinski J. Intervention of 25 lines (p. 794) on the paper by M. Ricochon "Paralysie de l'hypoglosse", *Société Médicale des Hôpitaux de Paris*, meeting of November 20, 1896, *Bulletins et Mémoires de la Société Médicale des Hôpitaux de Paris*, 1896, T. XIII, 3è série, pp. 791-794.

46. Babinski J. Abolition due réflexe de tendon d'Achille dans la sciatique, *Société Médicale des Hôpitaux de Paris*, meeting of December 18, 1896, *Bulletins et Mémoires de la Société Médicale des Hôpitaux de Paris*, 1896, T. XIII, 3è série, pp. 887-889.

49. Babinski J. De quelques mouvements associés du membre inférieur paralysé dans l'hémiplégie organique, *Société Médicale des Hôpitaux de Paris*, meeting of July 30, 1897, *Bulletins et Mémoires de la Société Médicale des Hôpitaux de Paris*, 1897, T. XIV (3è série), pp. 1098-1103, Analysis in *Rev Neurol (Paris)*, 1898, T. VI, n° 5 (March 15), p. 151.

Babinski J. Spasme associé du peaucier du cou du côté sain dans l'hémiplégie organique, *Société Médicale des Hôpitaux de Paris*, meeting of July 30, 1897, *Bulletins et Mémoires de la Société Médicale des Hôpitaux de Paris*, 1897, T. XIV, 3è série, pp. 1103-1104, Analysis in *Rev Neurol (Paris)*, 1898, T. VI, n° 5 (March 15), p. 151.

50. Babinski J. Sur le réflexe du tendon d'Achille dans le tabès, *Société Médicale des Hôpitaux de Paris*, meeting of October 21, 1898, *Bulletins et Mémoires de la Société Médicale des Hôpitaux de Paris*, 1898, T. XV, 3è série, pp. 679-684, résumé in *Le Progrès Médical*, 1898, T. VIII, 3è série, n° 44 (October 29, 1898), p. 301.

51. Babinski J. Sur une forme de paraplégie spasmodique consécutive à une lésion organique et sans dégénération du système pyramidal, *Société Médicale des Hôpitaux de Paris*, meeting of March 24, 1899, *Bulletins et Mémoires de la Société Médicale des Hôpitaux de Paris*, 1899, T. XVI, 3è série, pp. 342-354.

Babinski J. Sur la ponction lombaire contre la céphalée des brightiques (concerning the minutes), *Société Médicale des Hôpitaux de Paris*, meeting of May 10, 1901, *Bulletins et Mémoires de la Société Médicale des Hôpitaux de Paris*, 1901, T. XVIII, 3è série, pp. 443-444. Analysis in *Rev Neurol (Paris)*, 1901, T. IX, n° 19 (October 15), p. 963.

Babinski J. Intervention of 17 lines (p. 474) on the paper by M. Pierre Marie "Sur la ponction lombaire contre la céphalée des brightiques", *Société Médicale des Hôpitaux de Paris*, meeting of May 17, 1901, *Bulletins et Mémoires de la Société Médicale des Hôpitaux de Paris*, 1901, T. XVIII, 3è série, p. 474.

74. Babinski J, Charpentier. De l'abolition des réflexes pupillaires dans ses relations avec la syphilis, *Société Médicale des Hôpitaux de Paris,* meeting of May 17, 1901, *Bulletins et Mémoires de la Société Médicale des Hôpitaux de Paris,* 1901, T. XVIII, 3è série, pp. 502-506, résumé in *Le Progrès Médical,* 1901, T. XIII, 3è série, n° 21 (May 25, 1901), p. 345.
75. Babinski J, Nageotte. Contribution à l'étude du cytodiagnostic du liquide céphalo-rachidien dans les affections nerveuses, *Société Médicale des Hôpitaux de Paris,* meeting of May 24, 1901, *Bulletins et Mémoires de la Société Médicale des Hôpitaux de Paris,* 1901, T. XVIII, 3è série, pp. 537-548, résumé in *Le Progrès Médical,* 1901, T. XIII, 3è série, n° 22 (June 1, 1901), p. 358, and *Contribution à l'étude du cytodiagnostic du liquide céphalo-rachidien dans les affections nerveuses,* Tours, Maretheux, 1901.
78. Babinski J. Des troubles pupillaires dans les anévrismes de l'aorte, *Société Médicale des Hôpitaux de Paris,* meeting of November 8, 1901, *Bulletins et Mémoires de la Société Médicale des Hôpitaux de Paris,* 1901, T. XVIII, 3è série, pp. 1121-1124, résumé in *Le Progrès Médical,* 1901, T. XIV, 3è série, n° 46 (November 16, 1901), p. 391 and in *Rev Neurol (Paris),* 1902, T. X, n° 10 (May 30, 1902), p. 459.

Babinski J. A propos du Procès-Verbal : De l'inégalité pupillaire dans les anévrismes, *Société Médicale des Hôpitaux de Paris,* meeting of November 15, 1901, *Bulletins et Mémoires de la Société Médicale des Hôpitaux de Paris,* 1901, T. XVIII, 3è série, pp. 1155-1156 and résumé in *Rev Neurol (Paris),* 1902, T. X, n° 10 (May 30, 1902), pp. 459-460.

Babinski J. Discussion sur la communication de M. Huchard et M. Bergouignan "Anévrisme latent de la crosse de l'aorte avec pneumonie massive et nécrosante gauche par compression du nerf pneumogastrique gauche", *Société Médicale des Hôpitaux de Paris,* meeting of November 15, 1901, *Bulletins et Mémoires de la Société Médicale des Hôpitaux de Paris,* 1901, T. XVIII, 3è série, p. 1183, résumé in *Le Progrès Médical,* 1901, T. XIV, 3è série, n° 47 (November 23, 1901), p. 410.

Babinski J. Signe d'Argyll-Robertson et syphilis (à propos du procès-verbal), *Société Médicale des Hôpitaux de Paris,* meeting of February 28, 1902, *Bulletins et Mémoires de la Société Médicale des Hôpitaux de Paris,* 1902, T. XIX, 3è série, pp. 149-150.
83. Babinski J. Tabès hérédo-syphilitique (tabès héréditaire) (présentation de malades). *Société Médicale des Hôpitaux de Paris,* meeting of October 24, 1902, *Bulletins et Mémoires de la Société Médicale des Hôpitaux de Paris,* 1902, T. XIX, 3è série, pp. 884-889, résumé in *Le Progrès Médical,* 1902, T. XVI, 3è série, n° 44 (1 November 1902), p. 284.
84. Babinski J. Méningite cérébro-spinale subaigue, à polynucléaires. Ponctions lombaires. Guérison (présentation de malade), *Société Médicale des Hôpitaux de Paris,* meeting of October 31, 1902, *Bulletins et Mémoires de la Société Médicale des Hôpitaux de Paris,* 1902, T. XIX, 3è série, pp. 907-909, résumé in *Le Progrès Médical,* 1902, T. XVI, 3è série, n° 46 (November 15, 1902), p. 395.

Babinski J. Discussion sur la communication de M. Triboulet "Réflexes tendineux dans les méningites cérébro-spinales", *Société Médicale des Hôpitaux de Paris,* meeting of November 7, 1902, *Bulletins et Mémoires de la Société Médicale des Hôpitaux de Paris,* 1902, T. XVIII, 3è série, p. 912.
86. Babinski J. De l'influence de la ponction lombaire sur le vertige voltaïque et sur certains troubles auriculaires (présentation de malade). *Société Médicale des Hôpitaux de Paris,* meeting of November 7, 1902, *Bulletins et Mémoires de la Société Médicale des Hôpitaux de Paris,* 1902, T. XIX, 3è série, pp. 918-921.
90. Babinski J. Projet de création d'asiles spéciaux pour les demi-infirmes, *Société Médicale des Hôpitaux de Paris,* meeting of February 20, 1903, *Bulletins et Mémoires de la Société Médicale des Hôpitaux de Paris,* 1903, T. XX, 3è série, pp. 208-211.

Babinski J. A propos du Procès-Verbal, *Société Médicale des Hôpitaux de Paris,* meeting of February 27, 1903, *Bulletins et Mémoires de la Société Médicale des Hôpitaux de Paris,* 1903, T. XX, 3è série, p. 234.
93. Babinski J. Du traitement des affections auriculaires par la ponction lombaire, *Société Médicale des Hôpitaux de Paris,* meeting of April 24, 1903, *Bulletins et Mémoires de la Société Médicale des Hôpitaux de Paris,* 1903, T. XX, 3è série, pp. 450-458, résumé in *Le Progrès Médical,* 1903, T. XVII, 3è série, n° 18 (May 2, 1903), p. 328.
99. Babinski J. Méningite hémorragique fibrineuse; paraplégie spasmodique. Ponctions lombaires; traitement mercuriel - Guérison, *Société Médicale des Hôpitaux de Paris,* meeting of October 23, 1903, *Bulletins et Mémoires de la Société Médicale des Hôpitaux de Paris,* 1903, T. XX, 3è série, pp. 1083-1089, résumé in *Le Progrès Médical,* 1903, T. XVIII, 3è série, n° 44 (October 31, 1903), pp. 291-292.

100. Babinski J. Sur l'albuminurie prétendue hystérique, *Société Médicale des Hôpitaux de Paris*, meeting of November 27, 1903, *Bulletins et Mémoires de la Société Médicale des Hôpitaux de Paris*, 1903, T. XX, 3è série, p. 1334.

101. Babinski J. Intervention of 35 lines (pp. 1344–1345) on the paper by Balzer et Fouquet à propos d'une observation de "pemphigus hystérique", *Société Médicale des Hôpitaux de Paris*, meeting of November 27, 1903, *Bulletins et Mémoires de la Société Médicale des Hôpitaux de Paris*, 1903, T. XX, 3è série, pp. 1339–1345.

104. Babinski J. A propos du procès-verbal. A propos de l'albuminurie prétendue hystérique (deuxième communication), *Société Médicale des Hôpitaux de Paris*, meeting of December 11, 1903, *Bulletins et Mémoires de la Société Médicale des Hôpitaux de Paris*, 1903, T. XX, 3è série, p. 1405, résumé in *Le Progrès Médical*, 1904, T. XIX, 3è série, n° 1 (January 2, 1904), p. 7.

107. Babinski J, Boisseau. Traitement de l'incontinence d'urine par la ponction lombaire, *Société Médicale des Hôpitaux de Paris*, meeting of April 29, 1904, *Bulletins et Mémoires de la Société Médicale des Hôpitaux de Paris*, 1904, T. XXI, 3è série, pp. 413–417, résumé in *Le Progrès Médical*, 1904, T. XIX, 3è série, n° 19 (May 7, 1904), p. 311.

129. Babinski J. A propos du procès-verbal. Sur les injections de sels mercuriels insolubles, *Société Médicale des Hôpitaux de Paris*, meeting of November 30, 1906, *Bulletins et Mémoires de la Société Médicale des Hôpitaux de Paris*, 1906, T. XXIII, 3è série, pp. 1203–1204.

128. Babinski J. Contracture généralisée due à une compression de la moelle cervicale, très améliorée à la suite de l'usage des rayons X, *Société Médicale des Hôpitaux de Paris*, meeting of November 30, 1906, *Bulletins et Mémoires de la Société Médicale des Hôpitaux de Paris*, 1906, T. XXIII, 3è série, pp. 1205–1210, résumé in *Le Progrès Médical*, 1906, T. XXII, 3è série, n° 49 (December 8, 1906), pp. 889–890.

133. Babinski J. De la radiothérapie dans les paralysies spasmodiques spinales, *Société Médicale des Hôpitaux de Paris*, meeting of March 1, 1907, *Bulletins et Mémoires de la Société Médicale des Hôpitaux de Paris*, 1907, T. XXIV, 3è série, pp. 208–213, résumé in *Le Progrès Médical*, 1907, T. XXIII, 3è série, n° 11 (March 16, 1907), p. 169.

145. Babinski J. A propos du procès-verbal. Sur les prétendus troubles trophiques de la peau dans l'hystérie, *Société Médicale des Hôpitaux de Paris*, meeting of December 6, 1907, *Bulletins et Mémoires de la Société Médicale des Hôpitaux de Paris*, 1907, T. XXIV, 3è série, pp. 1379–1383.

163. Babinski J. Quelques remarques sur la ponction rachidienne et la ponction céphalique comparées entre elles, *Société Médicale des Hôpitaux de Paris*, meeting of July 30, 1909, *Bulletins et Mémoires de la Société Médicale des Hôpitaux de Paris*, 1909, T. XXVII, 3è série, pp. 338–340.

172. Babinski J, Barré. Contribution à l'étude de la syphilis familale (recherches à l'aide de la méthode de Wassermann), *Société Médicale des Hôpitaux de Paris*, meeting of May 20, 1910, *Bulletins et Mémoires de la Société Médicale des Hôpitaux de Paris*, 1906, T. XXIX, 3è série, pp. 595–598, résumé in *Le Progrès Médical*, 1910, n° 23 (4 June 1910), p. 328.

176. Babinski J. Inversion du réflexe du radius, *Société Médicale des Hôpitaux de Paris*, meeting of October 14, 1910, *Bulletins et Mémoires de la Société Médicale des Hôpitaux de Paris*, 1910, T. XXX, 3è série, pp. 185–186, résumé in *Le Progrès Médical*, 1910, n° 43 (October 22, 1910), p. 579.

189. Babinski J, Gendron A. Leucocytose du liquide céphalo-rachidien au cours du ramollissement de l'écorce cérébrale, *Société Médicale des Hôpitaux de Paris*, meeting of March 22, 1912, *Bulletins et Mémoires de la Société Médicale des Hôpitaux de Paris*, 1912, T. XXXIII, 3è série, pp. 370–374.

195. Babinski J, Jumentié J. Contribution à l'étude de l'hémorragie méningée, *Société Médicale des Hôpitaux de Paris*, meeting of May 31, 1912, *Bulletins et Mémoires de la Société Médicale des Hôpitaux de Paris*, 1912, T. XXXIII, 3è série, pp. 744–749, résumé in *Le Progrès Médical*, 1912, n° 23 (June 8, 1912), p. 290.

205. Babinski J, Enriquez E, Durand G. Pseudo-coxalgie et appendicite, *Société Médicale des Hôpitaux de Paris*, meeting of July 18, 1913, *Bulletins et Mémoires de la Société Médicale des Hôpitaux de Paris*, 1913, T. XXXV, 3è série, pp. 191–199, résumé in *Le Progrès Médical*, 1913, n° 30 (July 26, 1913), p. 401.

232. Babinski J, Heitz J. Oblitérations artérielles et troubles vaso-moteurs d'origine réflexe ou centrale. Leur diagnostic différentiel par l'oscillométrie et l'épreuve du bain chaud, *Société Médicale des Hôpitaux de Paris*, meeting of April 14, 1916, *Bulletins et Mémoires de la Société Médicale des Hôpitaux de Paris*, 1916, T. XL, 3è série, pp. 570–575. Analysis in

Journal des Praticiens, 30è année, April 22, 1916, n° 17, p. 270 and in *Rev Neurol (Paris)*, 1916, T. XXIX, n° 11-12 (November-December 1916), p. 429.

235. Babinski J, Froment J. Névrite irradiante ou contracture d'ordre réflexe, *Société Médicale des Hôpitaux de Paris*, meeting of May 12, 1916, *Bulletins et Mémoires de la Société Médicale des Hôpitaux de Paris*, 1916, T. XL, 3è série, pp. 677-680.

243. Babinski J, Heitz J. Hyperthermie locale du membre supérieur après résection d'un anévrysme axillaire, chez un blessé présentant une paralysie complète du plexus brachial du même côté, *Société Médicale des Hôpitaux de Paris*, meeting of December 22, 1916, *Bulletins et Mémoires de la Société Médicale des Hôpitaux de Paris*, 1916, T. XL, 3è série, p. 2324.

Babinski J, Melle Grunspan, Kyste hydatique. Névrite crurale. Disparition des douleurs à la suite de la radiothérapie, *Société Médicale des Hôpitaux de Paris*, meeting of January 19, 1917, *Bulletins et Mémoires de la Société Médicale des Hôpitaux de Paris*, 1917, T. XLI, 3è série, p. 105. [Cette note annoncée pour paraître dans le prochain Bulletin n'a pas été retrouvée]. Résumé in *Journal des Praticiens*, 1917, p. 62.

286. Babinski J. Hystérie-Pithiatisme, A propos du procès-verbal (à propos de la communication de MM. Tinel, Baruk et Lamache intitulée : Crise de catalepsie hystérique et rigidité décérébrée), *Société Médicale des Hôpitaux de Paris*, meeting of November 16, 1928, *Bulletins et Mémoires de la Société Médicale des Hôpitaux de Paris*, 1928, T. LII, 3è série, pp. 1507-1521.

La RevueNeurologique
(from 1895 to 1928)

Babinski J. Cited in the paper by A. Mathieu "La polyurie hystérique", *Rev Neurol (Paris)*, 1893, T. I, n° 11, p. 307, communication à la *Société Médicale des Hôpitaux de Paris*, Résumé in *Archives de Neurologie*, 1895, T.XXIX, n° 96 (February), p. 130.

Babinski J. [...] coïncider le syndrome de Basedow et certains symptômes du myxoedème, *Congrès des aliénistes et Neurologistes de France et des pays de langue française*, meeting of 2 August, *Rev Neurol (Paris)*, 1895, T. III, n° 16 (August 30), p. 484. Résumé in *Archives deNeurologie*, 1895, T.XXX, n° 103 (September), p. 242. Résumé in *Le Progrès Médical*, 1895, T.II, n° 32 (August 10), p. 88.

Babinski J. Intervention of several lines p. 787, on the paper by Dejerine et Bernheim "Sur un cas de paralysie radiale par compression, suivi d'autopsie", *Société de Neurologie de Paris*, meeting of November 9, *Rev Neurol (Paris)*, 1899, T. VII, n° 21 (November 15), pp. 785-788.

53. Babinski J. Du "phénomène des orteils" dans l'épilepsie, *Société de Neurologie de Paris*, meeting of July 6, 1899, *Rev Neurol (Paris)*, 1899, T. VII, n° 13 (July 15, 1899), pp. 512-513.

55. Babinski J. De l'asynergie cérébelleuse (Présentations de malade et de photographies), *Société de Neurologie de Paris*, meeting of 9 November, *Rev Neurol (Paris)*, 1899, T. VII, n° 21 (November 15), pp. 784-785. [Il s'agit du résumé de l'article publié in extenso dans le n° 22, référence suivante].

Babinski J. De l'asynergie cérébelleuse, *Rev Neurol (Paris)*, 1899, T. VII, n° 22 (November 30), pp. 806-816.

56. Babinski J. Sur le prétendu réflexe antagoniste de Schaefer, *Société de Neurologie de Paris*, meeting of January 11, 1900, *Rev Neurol (Paris)*, 1900, T. VIII, n° 1 (January 15, 1900), pp. 52-53.

Babinski J. Intervention of a line ("le réflexe du tendon d'Achille était-il également aboli ?") p. 59, on the paper by Klippel "Tabes de la région dorsale, avec lésions ascendantes et descendantes. Anatomie pathologique et symptômes", *Société de Neurologie de Paris*, meeting of 11 January, *Rev Neurol (Paris)*, 1900, T. VIII, n° 1 (15 January), pp. 57-60.

57. Babinski J. Sur un cas d'hémispasme (contribution à l'étude de la pathogénie du torticolis spasmodique), *Société de Neurologie de Paris*, meeting of 1 February, *Rev Neurol (Paris)*, 1900, T. VIII, n° 3 (February 15, 1900), pp. 142-147.

Babinski J. Intervention of 9 lines p. 152, on the paper by R. Touche (Brévannes) "Deux cas de ramollissement du cervelet (pseudo-sclérose en plaques cérébelleuses. Chorée cérébelleuse", *Société de Neurologie de Paris*, meeting of 1 February, *Rev Neurol (Paris)*, 1900, T. VIII, n° 3 (February 15, 1900), pp. 149-152.

58. Babinski J. Intervention of 33 lines pp. 340-341, on the paper by Souques "Tabes conjugal", *Société de Neurologie de Paris*, meeting of April 5, *Rev Neurol (Paris)*, 1900, T. VIII, n° 7 (April 15, 1900), pp. 338-341.

Babinski J. Intervention of 6 lines p. 345, on the paper by Melle Pesker "Affection spasmodique congénitale et familiale", *Société de Neurologie de Paris*, meeting of April 5, *Rev Neurol (Paris)*, 1900, T. VIII, n° 7 (April 15, 1900), pp. 343-345.

60. Babinski J. Sur la paralysie du mouvement associé de l'abaissement des yeux, *Société de Neurologie de Paris*, meeting of June 7, 1900, *Rev Neurol (Paris)*, 1900, T. VIII, n° 11 (June15), pp. 525-531.

61. Babinski J. Tumeur du corps pituitaire sans acromégalie et avec arrêt de développement des organes génitaux, *Société de Neurologie de Paris*, meeting of 7, 1900, *Rev Neurol (Paris)*, 1900, T. VIII, n° 11 (June 15), pp. 531-533.

Babinski J. Intervention of 6 lines p. 536, on the paper by Vires et Calmette (communiqué par M. Souques) "Recherches sur le phénomène des orteils (signe de Babinski)", *Société de Neurologie de Paris*, meeting of June 7, *Rev Neurol (Paris)*, 1900, T. VIII, n° 11 (June 15, 1900), pp. 535-536. ["...ces Messieurs déclarent que ce signe n'a qu'une valeur bien minime..."]

62. Babinski J. Sur une forme de pseudo-tabes (névrite rétrobulbaire infectieuse et troubles dans les réflexes tendineux), *Société de Neurologie de Paris*, meeting of July 5, 1900, *Rev Neurol (Paris)*, 1900, T. VIII, n° 13 (July 15, 1900), pp. 622-625.

Babinski J. Intervention of 4 lines p. 622, on the paper by J. Piltz (de Varsovie) "Sur quelques nouveaux symptômes pupillaires dans le tabes dorsal", *Société de Neurologie de Paris*, meeting of 5 July, *Rev Neurol (Paris)*, 1900, T. VIII, n° 13 (July 15, 1900), p. 622 and in extenso pp. 593-597.

63. Babinski J. Association de tabes et de lésions syphilitiques, *Société de Neurologie de Paris*, meeting of July 5, 1900, *Rev Neurol (Paris)*, 1900, T. VIII, n° 13 (July 15, 1900), pp. 625-626.

64. Babinski J. Du traitement mercuriel dans la sclérose tabétique des nerfs optiques, *Société de Neurologie de Paris*, meeting of July 5, 1900, *Rev Neurol (Paris)*, 1900, T. VIII, n° 13 (July 15, 1900), pp. 626-628.

Babinski J. Intervention of 25 lines pp. 630-631, on the paper by Léopold Lévi "Trépidation épileptoïde hystérique ou hémiplégie organique avec trépidation épileptoïde sans contractures", *Société de Neurologie de Paris*, meeting of July 5, 1900, *Rev Neurol (Paris)*, 1900, T. VIII, n° 13 (July 15, 1900), pp. 628-631.

65. Babinski J. Intervention pp. 746-747, on the paper by Pierre Marie et Switalski (Lemberg) "Du tabes avec cécité", Section de Neurologie du XIIIè Congrès International de Médecine (2è Congrès International de Neurologie), Paris, 2-9 August 1900, meeting of August 4, *Rev Neurol (Paris)*, 1900, T. VIII, pp. 745-747.

66. Babinski J. Sur les scléroses combinées, Section de Neurologie du XIIIè Congrès International de Médecine (2è Congrès International de Neurologie), Paris, 2-9 August 1900, meeting of August 6, *Rev Neurol (Paris)*, 1900, T. VIII, pp. 758-759.

Babinski J. Intervention of 2 pages pp. 771-772, on the paper by MM. Ferrier (de Londres) et Roth (de Moscou) "Le diagnostic de l'hémiplégie organique et de l'hémiplégie hystérique", Section de Neurologie du XIIIè Congrès International de Médecine (2è Congrès International de Neurologie), Paris, 2-9 August 1900, meeting of August 8, *Rev Neurol (Paris)*, 1900, T. VIII, pp. 769-772.

Babinski J. Intervention of 5 lines p. 1006, on the paper by Léopold Lévi "Signe de Babinski dans la fièvre typhoïde", *Société de Neurologie de Paris*, meeting of November 8, 1900, *Rev Neurol (Paris)*, 1900, T. VIII, n° 21 (November 15, 1900).

Babinski J. Intervention of 2 lines p. 1115, on the paper by Léopold Lévi et Follet "Myoclonie et spondylose rhizomélique", *Société de Neurologie de Paris*, meeting of December 6, 1900, *Rev Neurol (Paris)*, 1900, T. VIII, n° 23 (December 15, 1900), pp. 1111-1115.

Babinski J. Intervention of 5 lines p. 57, on the paper by Léopold Lévi et Follet "Trépidation épileptoïde dans la tuberculose pulmonaire", *Société de Neurologie de Paris*, meeting of January 10, 1901, *Rev Neurol (Paris)*, 1901, T. IX, n° 1 (January 15, 1901), pp. 54-57.

Babinski J. Intervention of 4 lines p. 62, on the paper by Touche "Syringomyélie à forme sensitive. Douleurs spontanées. Coexistence de pachyméningite cervicale", *Société de Neurologie de Paris*, meeting of January 10, 1901, *Rev Neurol (Paris)*, 1901, T. IX, n° 1 (January 15, 1901), pp. 59-62.

69. Babinski J. Intervention of 13 lines p. 155, on the paper by Gilbert Ballet "Trois cas de gliomatose cérébrale", Société de Neurologie de Paris, meeting of February 7, 1901, Rev Neurol (Paris), 1901, T. IX, n° (February 15,1901), pp. 154–155.
70. Babinski J. Hémiasynergie et hémitremblement d'origine cérébello-protubérantielle, Société de Neurologie de Paris, meeting of February 7, Rev Neurol (Paris), 1901, T. IX, n° 5 (March 15), pp. 260–265.
71. Babinski J. Traitement de la maladie de Basedow par le salicylate de soude, Société de Neurologie de Paris, meeting of February 7, Rev Neurol (Paris), 1901, T. IX, n° 5 (March 15), p. 265.
68. Babinski J. Stase papillaire guérie par la trépanation, Société de Neurologie de Paris, meeting of 7 February, Rev Neurol (Paris), 1901, T. IX, n° 5 (March 15), pp. 266–267.
Babinski J. Intervention of 4 lines p. 282, on the paper by Félix Allard et René Monod "Pied bot paralytique simulant le pied de Friedreich", Société de Neurologie de Paris, meeting of March 7, Rev Neurol (Paris), 1901, T. IX, 5 (March 15), pp. 280–282.
Babinski J. Intervention of 14 lines p. 285, on the paper by E. Brissaud et F. Monod "Paralysie générale à évolution anormale", Société de Neurologie de Paris, meeting of March 7, Rev Neurol (Paris), 1901, T. IX, n° 5 (March 15), pp. 282–285.
72. Babinski J. Hémiasynergie et hémitremblement d'origine cérébello-protubérantielle, meeting of April 18, Rev Neurol (Paris), 1901, T. IX, n° 8 (April 30), pp. 422–424.
Babinski J. Intervention d'une page et demie pp. 433–434, on the paper by Pierre Marie "Spasme névropathique d'élévation des yeux", Société de Neurologie de Paris, meeting of April 18, 1901, Rev Neurol (Paris), 1901, T. IX, n° 8 (April 30, 1901), pp. 428–434.
Babinski J. Intervention of 20 lines p. 436, on the paper by G. Guillain "Aphasie hystérique", Société de Neurologie de Paris, meeting of April 18, 1901, Rev Neurol (Paris), 1901, T. IX, n° 8 (April 30, 1901), p. 436.
73. Babinski J. Sur le réflexe du tendon d'Achille, Société de Neurologie de Paris, meeting of May 2, Rev Neurol (Paris), 1901, T. IX, n° 9 (May 15, 1901), pp. 482–484.
Babinski J. Intervention of 4 lines p. 562, on the paper by M. Sherb (d'Alger) "De la rareté des accidents nerveux chez les arabes syphilitiques", Société de Neurologie de Paris, meeting of June 6, 1901, Rev Neurol (Paris), 1901, T. IX, n° 11 (June 15, 1901), pp. 560–562.
76. Babinski J. Sur le spasme du peaucier du cou, Société de Neurologie de Paris, meeting of July 4, Rev Neurol (Paris), 1901, T. IX, n° 14 (July 30), pp. 693–696.
Babinski J. Intervention d'une line p. 953, on the paper by Faisans et Audistère, "Pseudomyxoedème syphilitique précoce", Société Médicale des Hôpitaux de Paris, meeting of May 16, 1901, pp. 449–458, Rev Neurol (Paris), 1901, T. IX, n° 19 (October 15), pp. 952–953.
77. Babinski J. Définition de l'hystérie, Société de Neurologie de Paris, meeting of November 7, Rev Neurol (Paris), 1901, T. IX, n° 21 (November 15), pp. 1074–1080.
Babinski J. Intervention of 9 lines p. 1194–1195, on the paper by E. Brissaud et Félix Allard, "Un cas de myopathie avec récations électriques normales", Société de Neurologie de Paris, meeting of December 5, 1901, Rev Neurol (Paris), 1901, T. IX, n° 23 (December 15), pp. 1192–1195.
Babinski J. Intervention d'une page et demie p. 1211–1212, on the paper by Grasset et Calmette (de Montpellier), communiqué par Pierre Marie, "De la flexion du tronc dans le décubitus dorsal (acte de se mettre sur son séant)", Société de Neurologie de Paris, meeting of December 5, 1901, Rev Neurol (Paris), 1901, T. IX, n° 23 (December 15), pp. 1207–1212.
Babinski J. Intervention of 5 lines p. 56, on the paper by Raymond et Cestan, "Examen histologique d'une sclérose en plaques ayant déterminé une paralysie des mouvements associés des globes oculaires", Société de Neurologie de Paris, meeting of January 9, 1902, Rev Neurol (Paris), 1902, T. X, n° 1 (January 1902), pp. 52–56.
79. Babinski J. Intervention de une page et demie pp. 58–60, on the paper by E. Brissaud, "Variations de la gravité du tabes", Société de Neurologie de Paris, meeting of January 9, 1902, Rev Neurol (Paris), 1902, T. X, n° 1 (January 1902), pp. 56–62.
Babinski J. Intervention of 2 lines p. 164, on the paper by Lortat-Jacob, "Polynévrite avec phénomène des orteils", Société de Neurologie de Paris, meeting of February 6, 1902, Rev Neurol (Paris), 1902, T. X, n° 3 (February 15, 1902), pp. 162–164.
Babinski J. Intervention of 12 lines p. 272, on the paper by Pierrre Marie, "Un cas de ramollissement ancien énorme dans le doMaine de la sylvienne. Absence d'hémianesthésie. Réflexe plantaire en flexion", Société de Neurologie de Paris, meeting of March 13, 1902, Rev Neurol (Paris), 1902, T. X, n° 6 (March 31, 1902), pp. 271–272.

Babinski J. Intervention of 13 lines p. 272, on the paper by Pierrre Marie et G. Guillain, "Vitiligo et symptômes tabétiformes", *Société de Neurologie de Paris*, meeting of March 13, 1902, *Rev Neurol (Paris)*, 1902, T. X, n° 6 (March 31, 1902), pp. 273-274.

Babinski J. Intervention of 30 lines pp. 277-278, on the paper by Joffroy et Schrameck, "Des rapports de l'irrégularité pupillaire et du signe d'Argyll-Robertson", *Société de Neurologie de Paris*, meeting of March 13, 1902, *Rev Neurol (Paris)*, 1902, T. X, n° 6 (March 31, 1902), pp. 275-279.

Babinski J. Intervention of 4 lines p. 285, on the paper by Marato et A. Charpentier, "Choix d'une région analgésique pour les injections de calomel", *Société de Neurologie de Paris*, meeting of March 13, 1902, *Rev Neurol (Paris)*, 1902, T. X, n° 6 (March 31, 1902), p. 285.

Babinski J. Intervention of 3 lines p. 354, on the paper by P. Marie et G. Guillain, "Mouvements athétoïdes de nature indéterminée", *Société de Neurologie de Paris*, meeting of April 17, 1902, *Rev Neurol (Paris)*, 1902, T. X, n° 8 (April 30, 1902), pp. 352-355.

Babinski J. Intervention of 5 lines p. 357, on the paper by Brissaud, "Diagnostic différentiel entre la polynévrite et la poliomyélite", *Société de Neurologie de Paris*, meeting of April 17, 1902, *Rev Neurol (Paris)*, 1902, T. X, n° 8 (April 30, 1902), pp. 355-358.

80. Babinski J. et Nageotte J. Hémiasynergie, latéropulsion et myosis bulbaires avec hémianesthésie et hémiplégie croisées, *Société de Neurologie de Paris*, meeting April 17, 1902, *Rev Neurol (Paris)*, 1902, T. X, n° 8 (April 30), pp. 358-365.

Babinski J. Intervention of 13 lines pp. 466-467, on the paper by M. Leredde, "Sur les affections parasyphilitiques et leur traitement", *Société de Neurologie de Paris*, meeting of May 15, 1902, *Rev Neurol (Paris)*, 1902, T. X, n° 10 (May 30, 1902), pp. 466-467.

81. Babinski J. De l'équilibre volitionnel statique et de l'équilibre volitionnel cinétique (dissociation de ces deux modes de l'équilibre volitionnel, asynergie et catalepsie), *Société de Neurologie de Paris*, meeting of May 15, 1902, *Rev Neurol (Paris)*, 1902, T. X, n° 10 (May 30), pp. 470-474.

82. Babinski J. Sur la valeur sémiologique des perturbations dans le vertige voltaïque, *Société de Neurologie de Paris*, meeting of May 15, 1902, *Rev Neurol (Paris)*, 1902, T. X, n° 10 (May 30), pp. 474-475.

Babinski J. Intervention of 19 lines p. 478, on the paper by O. Crouzon et A. Dobrovici, "Un cas d'association hystéro-organique : hémispasme glosso-labié et hémiplégie hystérique chez un tabétique", *Société de Neurologie de Paris*, meeting of May 15, 1902, *Rev Neurol (Paris)*, 1902, T. X, n° 10 (May 30, 1902), pp. 477-478.

Babinski J. Intervention of 2 lines p. 479, on the paper by H. Lamy, "Paralysie amyotrophique du membre supérieur droit", *Société de Neurologie de Paris*, meeting of May 15, 1902, *Rev Neurol (Paris)*, 1902, T. X, n° 10 (May 30, 1902), pp. 478-479.

Babinski J. Intervention of 3 lines pp. 536-537, on the paper by Dejerine et André Thomas, "Examen histolologique d'un cas de névrite interstitielle hypertrophique et progressive de l'enfance, suivi d'autopsie", *Société de Neurologie de Paris*, meeting of June 5, 1902, *Rev Neurol (Paris)*, 1902, T. X, n° 11 (June 15, 1902), pp. 534-537.

Babinski J. Intervention of 5 lines p. 540, on the paper by Max Egger, "De la sensibilité du squelette", *Société de Neurologie de Paris*, meeting of June 5, 1902, *Rev Neurol (Paris)*, 1902, T. X, n° 11 (June 15, 1902), p. 540 [publié in extenso in n° 12 (June 30, 1902), pp. 549-554].

Babinski J. Intervention of 13 lines (p. 532), on the paper by M. Dejerine et André Thomas, *Société de Neurologie de Paris*, meeting of June 5, 1902, "Présentation d'un malade atteint de surdité verbale pure, de toubles de l'équilibre et de la vue", *Rev Neurol (Paris)*, 1902, T. X, n° 11 (15 June), pp. 527-532.

Babinski J. Intervention of 14 lines (p. 628) on the paper by M. Dejerine, "Présentation d'un malade atteint de surdité verbale pure, de toubles de l'équilibre et de la vue", *Société de Neurologie de Paris*, meeting of July 3, 1902, *Rev Neurol (Paris)*, 1902, n° 13 (July 15), à propos du procès-verbal, pp. 627-629.

Babinski J. Intervention of 8 lines (pp. 638-639) and of 2 lines (p. 639) on the paper by Vaquez, Laubry. "Tachycardie d'origine indéterminée", *Société de Neurologie de Paris*, meeting of 3 July, *Rev Neurol (Paris)*, 1902, T. X, n° 13 (15 July), pp. 635-639.

Babinski J. Intervention of 6 lines (p. 642) on the paper by Allard F. "Présentation d'un malade atteint de myopathie amélioré par le traitement électrique", *Société de Neurologie de Paris*, meeting of 3 July, *Rev Neurol (Paris)*, 1902, T. X, n° 13 (July 15), pp. 641-642.

Babinski J. Intervention of 2 lines (p. 1187), on the paper by Campbell CM, Crouzon O. "Etude de la diadococinésie chez les cérébelleux", *Société de Neurologie de Paris*, meeting of 4 December, *Rev Neurol (Paris)*, 1902, T. X, n° 23 (December 15), pp. 1186-1187.

85. Babinski J. Sur le rôle du cervelet dans les actes volitionnels nécessitant une succession rapide de mouvements (diadococinésie), *Société de Neurologie de Paris* meeting of 6 November (indiqué p. 1059), *Rev Neurol (Paris)*, 1902, T. X, n° 21 (November 15), pp. 1013–1015.

Babinski J. Intervention of 12 lines p. 1056, on the paper by Launois PE, Roy P. "Gigantisme et infantilisme", *Société de Neurologie de Paris*, meeting of November 6, *Rev Neurol (Paris)*, 1902, T. X, n° 21 (15 November), pp. 1054–1058.

Babinski J. Intervention of 7 lines (pp. 1064–1065), on the paper by Brissaud. "Syndrome de la sclérose en plaques chez deux frères", *Société de Neurologie de Paris*, meeting of 6 November, *Rev Neurol (Paris)*, 1902, T. X, n° 21 (November 15), pp. 1063–1065.

Babinski J. Intervention of 9 lines (p. 1071), on the paper by Dufour H. "Paralysie pseudo-bulaire constituée en l'espace de huit heures par deux ictus chez un jeune homme de 28 ans. HypoThesis sur le signe des orteils de Babinski", *Société de Neurologie de Paris*, meeting of 6 November, *Rev Neurol (Paris)*, 1902, T. X, n° 21 (November 15), pp. 1069–1072.

88. Babinski J. De l'épilepsie spinale, *Société de Neurologie de Paris*, meeting of 15 January, *Rev Neurol (Paris)*, 1903, T. XI, pp. 111–112.

89. Babinski J. Intervention de 2 pages (p. 235–237) à propos de la communication de Ballet G, Delherm L. "Clonus du pied chez un neurasthénique", *Société de Neurologie de Paris*, meeting of 5 February, *Rev Neurol (Paris)*, 1903, T. XI, pp. 234–238.

Babinski J. Intervention of 5 lines (p. 240), on the paper by Armand-Delille P, Camus J. "Examen du liquide céphalo-rachidien dans le tabès", *Rev Neurol (Paris)*, 1903, T. XI, p. 240.

Babinski J. Intervention de 6 + 7 lines (p. 325), à propos de la communication de Dejerine. "Un cas de paraplégie flasque d'origine syphilitique, avec abolition des réflexes tendineux, exagération du réflexe cutané plantaire, signe de Babinski et intégrité de la sensibilité", *Société de Neurologie*, meeting of 5 March, *Rev Neurol (Paris)*, 1903, T. XI, n° 6 (March 30), pp. 323–326.

91. Babinski J. Lymphocytose dans le tabès et la paralysie générale, *Société de Neurologie de Paris*, meeting of March 5, *Rev Neurol (Paris)*, 1903, T. XI, n° 6 (March 30), p. 341.

Babinski J. Intervention of 16 lignes (pp. 436–437), on the paper by Hauser G, Beauvy. "Paraplégie spasmodique avec trépidation spinale et signe de Babinski de nature vraisemblablement hystérique", *Société de Neurologie de Paris*, meeting of April 2, *Rev Neurol (Paris*, 1903, T. XI, n° 8 (April 30), pp. 435–437.

95. Babinski J. Guérison d'un cas de mélancolie à la suite d'un accès provoqué de vertige voltaïque. *Société de Neurologie de Paris*, meeting of May 7, *Rev Neurol (Paris)*, 1903, T. XI, n° 10 (May 30), pp. 525–528 [republié in Cossa P. Babinski, précurseur des méthodes de choc électrique, *Annales Médico-Psychologiques*, 108è année, T. I, March 1950, pp. 325–330].

Babinski J. Hémiasynergie, *Rev Neurol (Paris)*, 1903, T. XI, p. 557.

96. Babinski J. Pseudo-tabès spondylosique, *Rev Neurol (Paris)*, 1903, T. XI, p. 645.

97. Babinski J. De l'abduction des orteils (Présentation de malade, *Société de Neurologie de Paris*, meeting of July 2, 1903), *Rev Neurol (Paris)*, 1903, T. XI, pp. 728–729.

Babinski J. Trépidation épileptoïde et hémiparésie chez une hystérique, *Rev Neurol (Paris)*, 1903, T. XI, p. 733.

98. Babinski J. Névrite radiale, *Rev Neurol (Paris)*, 1903, T. XI, p. 734.

103. Babinski J. Intervention of 15 lines (p. 1197) on the paper by Camus et Chiray "Tabès juvénile hérédo-syphilitique et crises gastriques", *Rev Neurol (Paris)*. 1903, T. XI, pp. 1195–1198.

102. Babinski J. De l'abduction des orteils (signe de l'éventail) (Présentation de malade, Société de Neurologie de Paris, meeting of December 3, 1903), *Rev Neurol (Paris)*, 1903, T. XI, pp. 1205–1206.

106. Babinski J. Sur la transformation du régime des réflexes cutanés dans les affections du système pyramidal, *Société de Neurologie de Paris*, meeting of January 7, 1904, *Rev Neurol (Paris)*, 1904, T. Xii, n° 2 (January 30), pp. 58–62.

Babinski J. Intervention of 4 lines (p. 95) and of 20 lines (p. 96), à propos de la communication "Sur la transformation du régime des réflexes cutanés dans les affections du système pyramidal", *Rev Neurol (Paris)*, 1904, T. XII, pp. 94–96.

Babinski J. Intervention of 2 lines (p. 98), on the paper by Dejerine, Chiray. "Paraplégie spasmodique de l'enfance avec paralysie unilatérale de l'iris due probablement à l'hérédo-syphilis", *Rev Neurol (Paris)*, 1904, T. XII, n° 2 (January 30), pp. 96–98.

Babinski J. Intervention de 8 pages (échange de lettres avec Van Gehuchten), à propos du Procès-Verbal de la meeting of January 7, 1904, "Sur la transformation du régime des réflexes cutanés dans les affections du système pyramidal", *Rev Neurol (Paris)*, 1904, T. XII, n° 10, May 30, pp. 481–489.

Babinski J. Intervention of 35 lines (pp. 633–634), on the paper by Brissaud, Grenet H. "Tremblement cloniforme et clonus vrai", *Société de Neurologie de Paris*, meeting of June 2, 1904, *Rev Neurol (Paris)*, T. Xii, n° 13 (June 30), pp. 632–634.

Babinski J. Intervention of 4 lines (p. 776), on the paper by Souques. "Des troubles auditifs dans les tumeurs cérébrales", *Société de Neurologie de Paris*, meeting of July 9, 1904, *Rev Neurol (Paris)*, 1904, T. XII, n° 14 (July 30), p. 776.

109. Babinski J. Maladie bleue. Cyanose de la papille. Hémiplégie consécutive à la coqueluche, *Société de Neurologie de Paris*, meeting of November 3, 1904, *Rev Neurol (Paris)*, 1904, T. XII, n° 22 (November 30), pp. 1143–1146.

110. Babinski J. Myopathie hypertrophique consécutive de la fièvre typhoïde (dissociation de diverses propriétés des muscles), *Société de Neurologie de Paris*, meeting of 1 December 1904, *Rev Neurol (Paris)*, 1904, T. XII, n° 24 (December 30), pp. 1181–1186. Discussion pp. 1209–1211, avec intervention de Babinski de 2 pages (pp. 1210–1211).

Babinski J. Intervention de 1 page (pp. 1206–1207), on the paper by Massary E, Tessier JP. "Torticolis mental ou torticolis spasmodique (Torticolis-tic ou torticolis-spasme", *Société de Neurologie de Paris*, meeting of 1 December 1904, *Rev Neurol (Paris)*, 1904, T. XII, n° 24 (December 30), pp. 1204–1207.

111. Babinski J. Hémiplégie spasmodique infantile (paralysie post-spasmodique), *Société de Neurologie de Paris*, meeting of 1 December 1904, *Rev Neurol (Paris)*, 1904, T. XII, n° 24 (December 30), pp. 1212–1214.

Babinski J. Intervention of 8 lines (p. 114), on the paper by Léopold Lévi et Bonniot. "Un cas de syndrome de Benedikt. Pathogénie du tremblement", *Société de Neurologie de Paris*, meeting of January 12, 1905, *Rev Neurol (Paris)*, 1905, T. XIII, n° 2 (January 30), pp. 112–114.

113. Babinski J. Sur un cas de névrite dû peut-être à l'usage d'engrais artificiels (D'une particularité de la réaction de dégénérescence), *Société de Neurologie de Paris*, meeting of January 12, 1905, *Rev Neurol (Paris)*, 1905, T. XIII, n° 2 (January 30), pp. 116–118.

114. Babinski J. Formes latentes des affections du système pyramidal, *Société de Neurologie de Paris*, meeting of January 12, 1905, *Rev Neurol (Paris)*, 1905, T. XIII, n° 2 (January 30), pp. 118–120.

115. Babinski J. De la flexion combinée de la cuisse et du tronc dans la chorée de Sydenham, *Société de Neurologie de Paris*, meeting of January 12, 1905, *Rev Neurol (Paris)*, 1905, T. XIII, n° 2 (January 30), p. 120.

Babinski J. Intervention of 2 lines (p. 128), on the paper by Brissaud et Bauer. "Paralysie de l'hypoglosse, du spinal et de quelques ramifications du facial après ablation d'une adénite rétro-maxillaire", *Société de Neurologie de Paris*, meeting of January 12, 1905, *Rev Neurol (Paris)*, 1905, T. XIII, n° 2 (January 30), pp. 125–129.

Babinski J. Intervention of 5 lines (p. 133), on the paper by Gilbert Ballet. "Note sur le clonus du pied par irritation de voisinage du faisceau pyramidal, sans lésion de ce faisceau", *Société de Neurologie de Paris*, meeting of January 12, 1905, *Rev Neurol (Paris)*, 1905, T. XIII, n° 2 (January 30), pp. 132–133.

Babinski J. Intervention of 8 lines (p. 250), on the paper by Raymond et Guillain. "Névrite ascendante consécutive à une plaie de la paume de la main", *Société de Neurologie de Paris*, meeting of February 2, 1905, *Rev Neurol (Paris)*, 1905, T. XIII, n° 4 (February 28), pp. 248–251.

117. Babinski J. Hémispasme facial périphérique, *Société de Neurologie de Paris*, meeting of April 6, 1905, *Rev Neurol (Paris)*, 1905, T. XIII, n° 8 (April 30), pp. 443–450. Reproduit in *Nouvelle Iconographie de la Salpêtrière*, 1905, T. XVIII, n° 4 (July–August), pp. 419–423.

118. Babinski J. Thermo-asymétrie d'origine bulbaire, *Société de Neurologie de Paris*, meeting of April 6, 1905, *Rev Neurol (Paris)*, 1905, T. XIII, n° 8 (April 30), p. 452. *Société de Neurologie de Paris*, meeting of May 11, 1905, *Rev Neurol (Paris)*, 1905, T. XIII, n° 10 (May 30), pp. 568–572.

Babinski J. Intervention of lines (p. 550), on the paper by Pierre Marie. "Maux perforants buccaux chez deux tabétiques, dus au port d'un dentier", *Société de Neurologie de Paris*, meeting of May 11, 1905, *Rev Neurol (Paris)*, 1905, T. XIII, n° 10 (May 30), pp. 549–551.

119. Babinski J. Spasme du trapèze droit et tic de la face, *Société de Neurologie de Paris*, meeting of July 6, 1905, *Rev Neurol (Paris)*, 1905, T. XIII, n° 14 (July 30), pp. 752–754.

121. Babinski J. Hyperexcitabilité électrique du nerf facial dans la paralysie faciale, *Société de Neurologie de Paris*, meeting of November 9, 1905, *Rev Neurol (Paris)*, 1905, T. XIII, n° 22 (November 30), pp. 1098-1101.

Babinski J. (communiqué par), M. Acchioté (de Constantinople), Un cas de névrite du radial, probablement gonococcique, *Société de Neurologie de Paris*, meeting of November 9, 1905, *Rev Neurol (Paris)*, 1905, T. XIII, n° 22 (November 30), pp. 1123-1124.

Babinski J. Intervention of 12 lines (p. 1214), on the paper by A. Souques. "Intérêt clinique et médico-légal d'un cas d'hémiplégie traumatique tardive", *Société de Neurologie de Paris*, meeting of December 7, 1905, *Rev Neurol (Paris)*, 1905, T. Xiii, n° 24 (December 30), pp. 1212-1214.

122. Babinski J. De l'influence de l'obscuration sur le réflexe des pupilles à la lumière et de la pseudo-abolition de ce réflexe, *Société de Neurologie de Paris*, meeting of December 7, 1905, *Rev Neurol (Paris)*, 1905, T. XIII, n° 24 (30 December), pp. 1214-1218.

Babinski J. A propos du Procès-verbal du meeting of November 9, 1905 de la *Société de Neurologie de Paris*, au sujet de la communication de M. Babinski sur l'*Hyperexcitabilité électrique du nerf facial dans la paralysie faciale*, *Société de Neurologie de Paris*, meeting of 11 January 1906, *Rev Neurol (Paris)*, 1906, T. XIV, n° 2 (January 30), p. 79.

Babinski J. Intervention of 23 lines (pp. 185-186) on the paper by J. Dejerine et M. Norero, "Epilepsie spinale vraie et clonus de la rotule chez une hystérique anorexique ayant été atteinte d'une hémiplégie gauche actuellement guérie", *Société de Neurologie de Paris*, meeting of 1 February, *Rev Neurol (Paris)*, 1906, T. XIV, n° 4 (February 28), pp. 182-186.

Babinski J. Intervention of 23 lines (p. 283) on the paper by Henri Lamy, "Difficultés de diagnostic entre l'hémiplégie organique et l'hémiplégie hystérique à propos d'un cas", *Société de Neurologie de Paris*, meeting of 1 March 1906, *Rev Neurol (Paris)*, 1906, T. XIV, n° 6 (March 30), pp. 281-283.

123. Babinski J. De l'épilepsie spinale fruste, *Société de Neurologie de Paris*, meeting of 1 March 1906, *Rev Neurol (Paris)*, 1906, T. XIV, n° 6 (March 30), pp. 287-289.

124. Babinski J, Delherm. Sur le traitement de la névralgie faciale par les courants voltaïques à intensité élevée, *Société de Neurologie de Paris*, meeting of June 7, 1906, *Rev Neurol (Paris)*, 1906, T. XIV, n° 12 (June 30), pp. 544-546.

Babinski J. Intervention of 7 lines (p. 551) on the paper by M. Albert Charpentier, "Méningite chronique syphilitique conjugale", *Société de Neurologie de Paris*, meeting of June 7, 1906, *Rev Neurol (Paris)*, 1906, T. XIV, n° 12 (June 30), pp. 550-551.

Babinski J. Intervention of 4 lines (p. 553) on the paper by M. Henri Claude, "Troubles vasomoteurs de nature hystérique", *Société de Neurologie de Paris*, meeting of June 7, 1906, *Rev Neurol (Paris)*, 1906, T. XIV, n° 12 (June 30), p. 553.

Babinski J. Intervention of 6 lines (p. 559-560) on the paper by M. Pierre Marie, "Forme spéciale de névrite interstitielle hypertrophique progressive de l'enfance", *Société de Neurologie de Paris*, meeting of June 7, 1906, *Rev Neurol (Paris)*, 1906, T. XIV, n° 12 (June 30), pp. 557-560.

Babinski J. Intervention of 40 lines (pp. 676-677) on the paper by Brissaud, Sicard, Tanon, "Essais de traitement de certains cas de contractures, spasmes et tremblements des membres par l'alcoolisation locale des troncs nerveux", *Société de Neurologie de Paris*, meeting of July 5, 1906, *Rev Neurol (Paris)*, 1906, T. XIV, n° 14 (July 30), pp. 675-677. Mémoire in *Rev Neurol (Paris)*, 1906, T. XIV, n° 14 (July 30), pp. 633-640.

126. Babinski J. Asynergie et inertie cérébelleuses, *Société de Neurologie de Paris*, meeting of 5 July, *Rev Neurol (Paris)*, 1906, T. XIV, n° 14 (July 30), pp. 685-686.

127. Babinski J. De la paralysie par compression du faisceau pyramidal, sans dégénération secondaire (contribution au diagnostic précoce des néoplasmes intracraniens), *Société de Neurologie de Paris*, meeting of 5 July, *Rev Neurol (Paris)*, 1906, T. XIV, n° 14 (July 30), pp. 693-697.

Babinski J. Intervention of 31 lines (pp. 1086-1087) on the paper by A. Sauvineau, "La mydriase hystérique n'existe pas", *Société de Neurologie de Paris*, meeting of 8 November, *Rev Neurol (Paris)*, 1906, T. XIV, n° 22 (November 30), pp. 1086-1087. Mémoire in *Rev Neurol (Paris)*, 1906, T. XIV, n° 22 (November 30), pp. 1017-1022.

Babinski J. Intervention of 21 lines (pp. 1080-1081) on the paper by Henri Claude, "A propos d'un cas d'œdème de la Mayn supposé hystérique", *Société de Neurologie de Paris*, meeting of 8 November, *Rev Neurol (Paris)*, 1906, T. XIV, n° 22 (November 30), pp. 1080-1081.

130. Babinski J. Lésion bulbaire unilatérale : thermo-asymétrie et vaso-asymétrie; hémianesthésie alterne à forme syringomyélique, *Société de Neurologie de Paris*, meeting of 6 December, *Rev Neurol (Paris)*, 1906, T. XIV, n° 24 (December 30), pp. 1177-1182.

Babinski J. Intervention of 9 lines (p. 1187) on the paper by F. Raymond et E. Huet, "Tabès probable avec atrophie des muscles de la nuque, d'une partie des muscles de la ceinture scapulaire et des membres supérieurs. – Malformations familiales du squelette des avant-bras. – Appareil de contention pour remédier à l'insuffisance des muscles extenseurs de la tête sur le cou", *Société de Neurologie de Paris*, meeting of 6 December, *Rev Neurol (Paris)*, 1906, T. XIV, n° 24 (December 30), pp. 1182-1188.

Babinski J. Allocution de M. J. Babinski, Président, *Société de Neurologie de Paris*, meeting of January 10, 1907, *Rev Neurol (Paris)*, 1907, T. XV, n° 2 (January 30), p. 78.

131. Babinski J. De l'action de la scopolamine sur la chorée de Sydenham, *Société de Neurologie de Paris*, meeting of 10 January, *Rev Neurol (Paris)*, 1907, T. XV, n° 2 (January 30), p. 86.

Babinski J. Intervention of 7 lines (p. 195), on the paper by A. Souques "Sclérose combinée tabétique avec atrophie musculaire progressive du type Aran-Duchenne. (Sclérose combinée amyotrophique)", *Société de Neurologie de Paris*, meeting of 7 February, *Rev Neurol (Paris)*, 1907, T. XV, n° 4 (February 28), pp. 193-196.

Babinski J. Intervention of 7 lines (p. 312), on the paper by Gilbert Ballet "Sur un syndrome caractérisé par des troubles myotoniques de la musculature des yeux, de la langue et des membres supérieurs survenu accidentellement chez deux malades âgés l'un de 54 ans, l'autre de 40 ans", *Société de Neurologie de Paris*, meeting of March 7 (addendum at the meeting of January 7), *Rev Neurol (Paris)*, 1907, T. XV, n° 6 (March 31), pp. 308-312.

Babinski J. Intervention of 5 lines (p. 403), on the paper by Henri Lamy "Monoplégie du membre supérieur survenue subitement chez un vieillard artérioscléreux (distribution radiculaire supérieure de la paralysie)", *Société de Neurologie de Paris*, meeting of April 11, *Rev Neurol (Paris)*, 1907, T. XV, n° 8 (April 30), pp. 410-403.

Babinski J. Allocution de M. Babinski, président, à l'occasion du décès de M. Féré, membre titulaire, *Société de Neurologie de Paris*, meeting of May 2, *Rev Neurol (Paris)*, 1907, T. XV, n° 10 (May 10), pp. 510-511.

136. Babinski J. Intervention of 18 lines (p. 519), on the paper by F. de Lapersonne et Cerise "Tumeur cérébrale. Mort 60 heures aorès une ponction lombaire", *Société de Neurologie de Paris*, meeting of 2 May, *Rev Neurol (Paris)*, 1907, T. XV, n° 10 (May 30), pp. 517-519.

Babinski J. Intervention of 17 lines (p. 620), on the paper by Klippel et Monier-Vinard "Œdème chronique unilatéral", *Société de Neurologie de Paris*, meeting of June 6, *Rev Neurol (Paris)*, 1907, T. XV, n° 12 (June 30), pp. 618-622.

Babinski J. Intervention of 4 lines (p. 629), on the paper by Aynaud (Service du professeur Dejerine à la Salpêtrière) "Un cas de névrite ascendante", *Société de Neurologie de Paris*, meeting of June 6, *Rev Neurol (Paris)*, 1907, T. XV, n° 12 (June 30), pp. 628-629.

141. Babinski J. Emotion, suggestion et hystérie, *Société de Neurologie de Paris*, meeting of July 4, *Rev Neurol (Paris)*, 1907, T. XV, n° 14 (July 31), pp. 752-754.

138. Babinski J. De l'abduction des doigts dans l'hémiplégie organique, *Société de Neurologie de Paris*, meeting of July 4, *Rev Neurol (Paris)*, 1907, T. XV, n° 14 (July 31), p. 754.

139. Babinski J. De la pronation de la main dans l'hémiplégie organique, *Société de Neurologie de Paris*, meeting of July 4, *Rev Neurol (Paris)*, 1907, T. XV, n° 14 (31 July), p. 755.

140. Babinski J. Sur le réflexe cutané plantaire, *Société de Neurologie de Paris*, meeting of July 4, *Rev Neurol (Paris)*, 1907, T. XV, n° 14 (July 31), p. 755.

Babinski J. Intervention of 2 lines (p. 772), on the paper by Henri Claude "Examen des centres nerveux dans deux cas d'hystérie", *Société de Neurologie de Paris*, meeting of July 4, *Rev Neurol (Paris)*, 1907, T. XV, n° 14 (July 31), p. 769-772.

142. Babinski J. Intervention de 3 pages (p. 899-902), à propos de la communication de Henri Claude "Définition et nature de l'hystérie", XVIIè Congrès des médecins aliénistes et neurologistes de France et des pays de langue française, Genève-Lausanne, August 1-6 1907, *Rev Neurol (Paris)*, 1907, T. XV, n° 16 (August 30), pp. 882-902.

143. Babinski J. Section de la branche externe du spinal dans le toricolis dit mental, *Société de Neurologie de Paris*, meeting of November 7, *Rev Neurol (Paris)*, 1907, T. XV, n° 22 (November 30), pp. 1208-1213.

Babinski J. Intervention of 14 lines (p. 1304), on the paper by Félix Rose et F. Lemaître "Deux cas de syringomyélie avec signe d'Argyll Robertson", *Société de Neurologie de Paris*, meeting of December 5, *Rev Neurol (Paris)*, 1907, T. XV, n° 24 (December 30), pp. 1300-1304.

144. Babinski J. Intervention of 17 lines (p. 1322), on the paper by Raymond "A propos du pemphigus hystérique", *Société de Neurologie de Paris*, meeting of December 5, *Rev Neurol (Paris)*, 1907, T. XV, n° 24 (December 30), p. 1322.
147. Babinski J. Intervention of two pages (pp. 82–83) and of 30 lines (pp. 84–85), à propos du Procès-verbal de la dernière séance "Sur le prétendu pemphigus hystérique", *Société de Neurologie de Paris*, meeting of January 9, *Rev Neurol (Paris)*, 1908, T. XVI, n° 2 (January 30), pp. 82–86.
148. Babinski J. Instabilité hystérique (pithiatique) des membres et du tronc, *Société de Neurologie de Paris*, meeting of 5 March, *Rev Neurol (Paris)*, 1908, T. Xvi, n° 6 (March 30), pp. 259–262.
149. Babinski J. Spondylose et douleurs névralgiques très atténuées à la suite de pratiques radiothérapiques, *Société de Neurologie de Paris*, meeting of March 5, *Rev Neurol (Paris)*, 1908, T. XVI, n° 6 (March 30), pp. 262–263.
151. Babinski J, Clunet J. Tumeurs méningées unilatérales. Hémiplégie siégeant du même côté que les tumeurs, *Société de Neurologie de Paris*, meeting of July 2, *Rev Neurol (Paris)*, 1908, T. XVI, n° 13 (July 15), pp. 707–710.
153. Babinski J. Quelques remarques sur le mémoire de M. Alfred Gordon, intitulé : "Troubles vaso-moteurs et trophiques de l'hystérie", *Rev Neurol (Paris)*, 1908, T. XVI, n° 20 (October 30), pp. 1089–1090.

Babinski J. Traitement du vertige de Ménière par les ponctions lombaires, *Rev Neurol (Paris)*, 1908, T. XVI, n° 21 (November 15), p. 1169.

Babinski J. Intervention of 5 lines (p. 91), on the paper by Claude et Félix Rose "Syndrome de compression médullaire chez une grande hystérique (Association hystéro-organique ou manifestation purement hystérique ?", *Société de Neurologie de Paris*, meeting of January 9, *Rev Neurol (Paris)*, 1908, T. XVI, n° 2 (January 30), p. 91.

Babinski J. Intervention of 5 lines (p. 259), on the paper by Max Egger (travail du service du Pr Raymond) "Contribution à l'étude de l'ataxie. Ataxie périphérique et ataxie centrale sans anesthésie", *Société de Neurologie de Paris*, meeting of March 5, *Rev Neurol (Paris)*, 1908, T. XVI, n° 6 (March 30), pp. 257–259.

Babinski J. Intervention of 19 lines (p. 325–326), on the paper by Sicard et Descomps "Troubles consécutifs à la section de la branche externe du spinal", *Société de Neurologie de Paris*, meeting of April 2, *Rev Neurol (Paris)*, 1908, T. XVI, n° 7 (April 15), pp. 324–326.

Babinski J. Intervention of 3 lines (p. 331), on the paper by J. Dejerine et Melle Landry "Un cas de spasme glottique, avec râle trachéal, datant de 14 ans, chez une hystérique", *Société de Neurologie de Paris*, meeting of April 2, *Rev Neurol (Paris)*, 1908, T. XVI, n° 7 (April 15), pp. 328–332.

Babinski J. Intervention of 6 lines (p. 445), on the paper by Klippel et Pierre Weil "Aphasie ou démence", *Société de Neurologie de Paris*, meeting of May 7, *Rev Neurol (Paris)*, 1908, T. XVI, n° 9 (May 15), pp. 442–445.

Babinski J. Intervention of 9 lines (p. 556), on the paper by C. Vincent "Syndrome thalamique avec troubles cérébelleux et vaso-asymétrie", *Société de Neurologie de Paris*, meeting of June 4, *Rev Neurol (Paris)*, 1908, T. XVI, n° 11 (June 15), pp. 553–556.

Babinski J. Intervention of 5 lines (p. 680), on the paper by Sicard et Gy "Le creux sus-claviculaire dans la paralysie de la branche externe du spinal", *Société de Neurologie de Paris*, meeting of July 2, *Rev Neurol (Paris)*, 1908, T. XVI, n° 13 (July 15), pp. 679–680.

Babinski J. Intervention of 5 lines (p. 685), on the paper by Raymond et Sézary "Aphasie hystérique", *Société de Neurologie de Paris*, meeting of July 2, *Rev Neurol (Paris)*, 1908, T. XVI, n° 13 (July 15), pp. 683–685.

Babinski J. Intervention of 15 lines (p. 696–697), on the paper by Klippel, Serguéeff et Pierre Weil "Hémiplégie cérébrale avec troubles marquées de la sensibilité", *Société de Neurologie de Paris*, meeting of July 2, *Rev Neurol (Paris)*, 1908, T. XVI, n° 13 (July 15), pp. 694–697.

Babinski J. Intervention of 7 lines (p. 1231, numérotée à tort 2031), of 11 lines (p. 1233–1234, incorrectly numbered 2033–2034) and of 5 lines (p. 1237, wrongly numbered 2037), on the paper by Ch. Achard et Ch. Foix "Tabes fruste", *Société de Neurologie de Paris*, meeting of November 5, *Rev Neurol (Paris)*, 1908, T. XVI, n° 22 (November 30), pp. 1230–1238 (numérotées à tort 2030–2038).

Babinski J. Discussions sur l'hystérie, *Société de Neurologie de Paris*, meeting of April 9, 1908, *Rev Neurol (Paris)*, 1908, T. XVI, n° 8 (April 30), pp. 375–404. Interventions of Babinski: p. 383 (4 + 3 lignes), 384 (22 lignes), 385 (1 + 2 + 2 lignes), 386–387 (56 lignes), 389 (6 lines), 390 (3 + 8 + 2 lines), 391 (4 lines), 393 (1 + 27 lines), 394 (3 + 2 lines), 397 (9 +

2 lines), 398 (2 + 2 + 2 + 8 lines), 399 (23 lines), 400 (6 + 8 lines), 401 (2 + 2 lines), 402 (15 lines).

Babinski J. Communications concernant l'hystérie, *Société de Neurologie de Paris*, meeting of May 7, 1908, *Rev Neurol (Paris)*, 1908, T. XVI, n° 9 (May 15), pp. 453–464. Interventions de Babinski : p. 458 (20 lines), 462 (13 lines).

Babinski J. Deuxième discussion sur l'hystérie, *Société de Neurologie de Paris*, meeting of May 14, 1908, *Rev Neurol (Paris)*, 1908, T. XVI, n° 10 (May 30), pp. 494–519. Interventions de Babinski: p. 496 (10 + 3 + 2 lines), 497 (3 lines), 498 (14 lines), 500 (16 lines), 504 (13 lines), 505 (5 lines), 506 (7 + 19 lines), 507 (5 lines), 506 (7 + 19 lines), 507 (4 + 2 lines), 509 (15 lines), 510 (10 lines), 511 (4 + 9 lines), 514 (7 lines), 516 (4 lines), 517 (4 + 16 lines), 518 (16 lines), 519 (8 lines).

152. Babinski J, Tournay A. Section du cubital et du médian à la partie inférieure de l'avant-bras. Causes d'erreur dans l'exploration de la sensibilité, *Société de Neurologie de Paris*, meeting of July 2, *Rev Neurol (Paris)*, 1908, T. XVI, n° 13 (July 15), pp. 688–690.

154. Babinski J. Quelques remarques sur le mémoire de M. Valobra intitulé : "Contribution à l'étude des gangrènes cutanées spontanées chez les hystériques", *Rev Neurol (Paris)*, 1909, T. XVII/XVIII, n° 14 (July 30), p. 918 et *Nouvelle Iconogaphie de la Salpêtrière*, an XXI, n° 6, November-December 1908, pp. 506–509.

Babinski J. Intervention of 9 lines (p. 96) on the paper by Brissaud et Bauer "Méningo-myélite chronique syphilitique apparue 30 ans après le chancre infectant", *Société de Neurologie de Paris*, meeting of January 7, *Rev Neurol (Paris)*, 1909, T. XVII, n° 2 (January 30), pp. 94–96.

Babinski J. Intervention of 4 lines (p. 98) on the paper by Bauer et Gy "Maladie de Friedreich et hérédo-ataxie cérébelleuse dans une même famille. Maladie de Triedreich avec lymphocytose rachidienne", *Société de Neurologie de Paris*, meeting of January 7, *Rev Neurol (Paris)*, 1909, T. XVII, n° 2 (January 30), pp. 97–99.

Babinski J. Intervention of 16 lines (p. 107) on the paper by F. Soca (Montevideo) "Sur la fièvre hystérique", *Société de Neurologie de Paris*, meeting of January 7, *Rev Neurol (Paris)*, 1909, T. XVII, n° 2 (January 30), pp. 103–109.

158. Babinski J. A propos du Procès-verbal "Sur la fièvre et les troubles trophiques attribués à l'hystérie", *Société de Neurologie de Paris*, meeting of February 5, *Rev Neurol (Paris)*, 1909, T. XVII, n° 4 (February 28), pp. 207–209.

157. Babinski J. Monoplégie brachiale organique, mouvements actifs et mouvements passifs, *Société de Neurologie de Paris*, meeting of February 5, *Rev Neurol (Paris)*, 1909, T. XVII, N° 4 (February 28), pp. 218–220.

Babinski J. Intervention of 7 lines (p. 221) on the paper by M. Néri (Naples) (communiqué par M. Babinski) "Résumé d'observations faites sur des survivants de la catastrophe de Messine", *Société de Neurologie de Paris*, meeting of January 7, *Rev Neurol (Paris)*, 1909, T. XVII, n° 4 (February 28), p. 221.

159. Babinski J. Deux cas de tumeur cérébrale, *Société de Neurologie de Paris*, meeting of 4 March, *Rev Neurol (Paris)*, 1909, T. XVII, n° 6 (March 30), p. 383 [texte publié à la prochaine séance].

Babinski J. Intervention of 22 lines (p. 645–646) and of 9 lines (p. 647) on the paper by Ch. Achard et Ch. Foix "Tabes fruste avec arthropathie", *Société de Neurologie de Paris*, meeting of 6 May, *Rev Neurol (Paris)*, 1909, T. XVII, n° 10 (May 30), pp. 643–647.

160. Babinski J. Deux cas de tumeur cérébrale du lobe frontal, *Société de Neurologie de Paris*, meeting of May 6, *Rev Neurol (Paris)*, 1909, T. XVII, n° 10 (May 30), pp. 665–667.

Babinski J. Intervention of 23 lines (p. 939) on the paper by Sicard "Traitement du torticolis mental de Brissaud (lunettes hémianopsiantes)", *Société de Neurologie de Paris*, meeting of July 1, *Rev Neurol (Paris)*, 1909, T. XVII, n° 14 (July 30), pp. 938–940.

Babinski J. Intervention of 20 lines (p. 1420) on the paper by André-Thomas et Jumentié "Sur la nature des troubles de la motilité dans les affections du cervelet. Dysmétrie. Tremblement kinétique et statique. Mouvements cloniques. Perturbations des réactions d'équilibration. Asynergie", *Société de Neurologie de Paris*, meeting of November 4, *Rev Neurol (Paris)*, 1909, T. XVIII, n° 22 (November 30), p. 1420.

Babinski J. Intervention of 35 lines (p. 1422–1423) on the paper by A. Souques "Trépanation crânienne décompressive suivie d'aphasie transitoire et d'amélioration durable, dans un cas de tumeur cérébrale", *Société de Neurologie de Paris*, meeting of November 4, *Rev Neurol (Paris)*, 1909, T. XVIII, n° 22 (November 30), pp. 1422–1423.

Babinski J. Intervention de 2 lines (p. 1516) on the paper by F. de Lapersonne et A. Cantonnet "Signe d'Argyll Robertson unilatéral avec coexistence, du même côté, d'un syndrome oculo-sympathique incomplet", *Société de Neurologie de Paris*, meeting of December 2, *Rev Neurol (Paris)*, 1909, T. XVIII, n° 23 (December 15), pp. 1515-1517.

Babinski J. Intervention of 5 et 3 lines (p. 1575), of 14 lines (p. 1591), of 13 lines (p. 1591-1592), of 26 lines (p. 1594-1595), of 24 lines (p. 1599), of 3 lines (p. 1600), of 5 lines (p. 1601), of 5 lines (p. 1632), of 13 lines (p. 1633), of 20 lines (p. 1636) et de 5 lines (p. 1637) at the *Société de Neurologie de Paris* et *Société de Psychiatrie de Paris*, annual December 9-16, 1909 and January 13, 1910, "Du rôle de l'émotion dans la genèse des accidents névropathiques et psychopathiques", meeting of December 9, *Rev Neurol (Paris)*, 1909, T. XVIII, n° 23 (December 15), pp. 1549-1687.

Babinski J. Intervention of 8 lines (p. 236) on the paper by E. Long "Deux observations anatomocliniques de syndrome thalamique", *Société de Neurologie de Paris*, meeting of February 10, *Rev Neurol (Paris)*, 1910, T. XIX, n° 4 (February 28), pp. 236-239.

Babinski J. Intervention of 3 lines (p. 250) on the paper by A. Souques "Abolition de certains réflexes dans la sclérose en plaques", *Société de Neurologie de Paris*, meeting of February 10, *Rev Neurol (Paris)*, 1910, T. XIX, n° 4 (February 28), pp. 248-250.

Babinski J. Intervention of 8 lines (p. 388) on the paper by Scheffer et de Martel "Syndrome d'hypertension cérébrale très amélioré par la trépanation décompressive", *Société de Neurologie de Paris*, meeting of March 10, *Rev Neurol (Paris)*, 1910, T. XIX, n° 6 (March 30), pp. 388-389.

Babinski J. Intervention of 9 lines (p. 388) on the paper by André-Thomas "Chorée persistante peut-être congénitale. Signes de perturbation du faisceau pyramidal", *Société de Neurologie de Paris*, meeting of March 10, *Rev Neurol (Paris)*, 1910, T. XIX, n° 6 (March 30), pp. 384-388.

164. Babinski J, Martel (de) Th. Trépanation pour tumeur cérébrale. Ablation de la tumeur. Grande amélioration, *Société de Neurologie de Paris*, meeting of December 2, *Rev Neurol (Paris)*, 1909, T. XVIII, n° 23 (December 15), pp. 1521-1522.

166. Babinski J. Hypotonicité musculaire et réaction de dégénérescence, *Société de Neurologie de Paris*, meeting of February 10, *Rev Neurol (Paris)*, 1910, T. XIX, n° 4 (February 28), pp. 239-240.

169. Babinski J. Crâniectomie décompressive, *Société de Neurologie de Paris*, meeting of April 14, *Rev Neurol (Paris)*, 1910, T. XIX, n° 8 (April 30), p. 528.

171. Babinski J, Jarkowski J. Sur la possibilité de déterminer la hauteur de la lésion dans des paralysies d'origine spinale par certaines perturbations des réflexes, *Société de Neurologie de Paris*, meeting of May 12, *Rev Neurol (Paris)*, 1910, T. XIX, n° 10 (May 30), pp. 666-668.

168. Babinski J, Barré, Jarkowski J. Remarques sur la persistance de zones sensibles à topographie radiculaire dans des paraplégies médullaires avec anesthésie, *Société de Neurologie de Paris*, meeting of February 10, *Rev Neurol (Paris)*, 1910, T. XIX, n° 4 (February 28), pp. 241-247.

Babinski J, Barré, Jarkowski J. Sur la persistance de zones sensibles à topographie radiculaire dans des paraplégies médullaires avec anesthésie (deuxième note), *Société de Neurologie de Paris*, meeting of April 14, *Rev Neurol (Paris)*, 1910, T. XIX, n° 8 (April 30), pp. 532-537.

Babinski J. Intervention of 8 lines (p. 539-540) on the paper by Henri Claude et Pierre Merle "Un nouveau cas de sclérose en plaques avec agnosie tactile", *Société de Neurologie de Paris*, meeting of April 14, *Rev Neurol (Paris)*, 1910, T. XIX, n° 8 (April 30), pp. 538-541.

Babinski J. Intervention de 1 ligne (p. 756) in l'analyse par Zylberblast de la communication de Bychovski "Un cas de maladie des tics", *Société de Neurologie de Varsovie*, meeting of April 16, 1910, *Rev Neurol (Paris)*, 1910, T. XIX, n° 12 (June 30), p. 756.

Babinski J. Intervention of 7 lines (p. 119-120) on the paper by Sicard et Marcel Bloch : "Bi-spasme facial. Alcoolisation des branches de division du nerf facial", *Société de Neurologie de Paris*, meeting of July 7, *Rev Neurol (Paris)*, 1910, T. XX, n° 14 (July 10), pp. 119-121.

174. Babinski J. De la dégénération et de la régénération du sterno-mastoïdien et du trapèze à la suite de la section de la branche externe du spinal, *Société de Neurologie de Paris*, meeting of July 7, *Rev Neurol (Paris)*, 1910, T. XX, n° 14 (July 30), pp. 128-130.

Babinski J. Intervention of 16 lines (p. 533) and 10 lines (p. 534) à propos de la communication de A. Barré et Flandin : "Fracture spontanée de la tête humérale avec dislocation de l'épaule et arthropathie à type tabétique du poignet, sans tabes", *Société de Neurologie de Paris*, meeting of November 10, *Rev Neurol (Paris)*, 1910, T. XX, n° 22 (November 30), pp. 531-535.

Babinski J. Intervention of 7 lines (p. 602) on the paper by Henri Claude et E. Velter : "Syringomyélie cervicale. Inversion du réflexe du radius", *Société de Neurologie de Paris*, meeting of 1er December, *Rev Neurol (Paris)*, 1910, T. XX, n° 23 (December 15), pp. 601-602.

Babinski J. Intervention of 6 lines (p. 610) on the paper by A. Barré : "Maux perforants multiples et arthropathie tarsienne à type tabétique sans tabes", *Société de Neurologie de Paris*, meeting of December 1, *Rev Neurol (Paris)*, 1910, T. XX, n° 23 (December 15), pp. 608-610.

177. Babinski J. Paraplégie spasmodique organique avec contracture en flexion et contractions musculaires involontaires, *Société de Neurologie de Paris*, meeting of January 12, 1911, *Rev Neurol (Paris)*, 1911, T. XXI, n° 2 (January 30), pp. 132-136.

Babinski J, Jumentié J. Syndrome cérébelleux unilatéral, *Société de Neurologie de Paris*, meeting of January 12 (addendum to the meeting of December 1 1910), *Rev Neurol (Paris)*, 1911, T. XXI, n° 2 (January 30), pp. 115-118.

182. Babinski J. Du vertige voltaïque dans les affections du système vestibulaire, *Société de Neurologie de Paris*, meeting of June 1, *Rev Neurol (Paris)*, 1911, T. XXI, n° 12 (June 30), pp. 780-783.

Babinski J. Intervention of 5 lines (p. 124) on the paper by Henri Claude et A. Baudoin : "Un cas de pseudo-tumeur cérébrale. Valeur des signes dits "de localisation"", *Société de Neurologie de Paris*, meeting of January 12, 1911, *Rev Neurol (Paris)*, 1911, T. XXI, n° 2 (January 30), pp. 112-126.

Babinski J. Intervention of 4 lignes (p. 132) on the paper by R. Gauducheau et M. Ferry (travail du service du Pr Dejerine) : "Un cas de monoplégie crurale d'origine cérébrale avec accès d'épilepsie partielle débutant par le gros orteil", *Société de Neurologie de Paris*, meeting of January 12, 1911, *Rev Neurol (Paris)*, 1911, T. XXI, n° 2 (January 30), pp. 129-132.

Babinski J. Intervention of 14 lines (p. 250-251) on the paper by Henri Claude: "Sur la paraplégie avec contracture en flexion", *(à propos du Procès-verbal of the meeting of January 12)*, *Société de Neurologie de Paris*, meeting of February 2, 1911, *Rev Neurol (Paris)*, 1911, T. XXI, n° 4 (February 28), pp. 249-251.

Babinski J. Intervention of 18 lines (p. 377-378) on the paper by Souques et de Martel: "De la mort rapide à la suite des crâniectomies décompressives", *Société de Neurologie de Paris*, meeting of March 2, 1911, *Rev Neurol (Paris)*, 1911, T. XXI, n° 6 (March 30), pp. 377-378.

Babinski J. Intervention of 20 lines (p. 392) on the paper by L. Alquier et B. Klarfeld : "Huit cas de tumeurs juxta ou intraprotubérantielles avec autopsie. Etude des signes de localisation", *Société de Neurologie de Paris*, meeting of March 9, 1911, *Rev Neurol (Paris)*, 1911, T. XXI, n° 6 (March 30), pp. 391-392.

Babinski J. Intervention of 21 lines (p. 511-512) on the paper by A. Souques: "Inversion du réflexe tendineux du triceps brachial dans l'hémiplégie associée au tabes", *Société de Neurologie de Paris*, meeting of April 6, 1911, *Rev Neurol (Paris)*, 1911, T. XXI, n° 8 (April 30), pp. 510-512.

Babinski J. Intervention of 4 lines (p. 525) on the paper by Dr Thomas (du Raincy) et A. Barré: "Influence heureuse du traitement mercuriel sur l'arthropathie tabétique", *Société de Neurologie de Paris*, meeting of April 6, 1911, *Rev Neurol (Paris)*, 1911, T. XXI, n° 8 (April 30), pp. 522-525.

179. Babinski J, Charpentier, Delherm. Radiothérapie de la sciatique, *Société de Neurologie de Paris*, meeting of April 6, 1911, *Rev Neurol (Paris)*, 1911, T. XXI, n° 8 (April 30), pp. 525-528.

180. Babinski J, Jarkowski J, Jumentié J. Syndrome de Brown-Séquard, *Société de Neurologie de Paris*, meeting of May 4, *Rev Neurol (Paris)*, 1911, T. XXI, n° 10 (May30), p. 649 [sera publié ultérieurement comme mémoire original].

181. Babinski J, Jarkowski J. Sur l'excitabilité idio-musculaire et sur les réflexes tendineux dans la myopathie progressive primitive, *Société de Neurologie de Paris*, meeting of June 1, *Rev Neurol (Paris)*, 1911, T. XXI, n° 12 (June 30), pp. 778-780.

Babinski J. Du vertige voltaïque dans les affections de l'appareil vestibulaire, *Société de Neurologie de Paris*, meeting of June 1, *Rev Neurol (Paris)*, 1911, T. XXI, n° 12 (June 30), pp. 780-783.

Babinski J. Intervention of 41 lines (p. 177-178) on the paper by M. Noïca (de Bucarest): "A propos de l'article de M. Babinski "paralysie spasmodique organique avec contracture en flexion et contractions involontaires"", *Société de Neurologie de Paris*, meeting of July 6, 1911, *Rev Neurol (Paris)*, 1911, T. XII, n° 14 (July 30), pp. 173-178.

185. Babinski J. Modification des réflexes cutanés sous l'influence de la compression par la bande d'Esmarch, *Société de Neurologie de Paris*, meeting of November 9, 1911, *Rev Neurol (Paris)*, 1911, T. XXII, n° 22 (November 30), pp. 651-652.

Babinski J. 7 interventions of 10 lines (p. 762), 7 lines (p. 765), 15 lines (p. 766), 18 lines (p. 769-770), 26 lines (pp. 770-771), 6 lines (p. 776), 58 lines (pp. 778-779), dans la séance spéciale (December 14, 1911) de la *Société de Neurologie de Paris* "Sur la délimitation du tabes", *Rev Neurol (Paris)*, 1911, T. XXII, n° 24 (December 30), pp. 721-812.

184. Babinski J, Jarkowski J. Réapparition provoquée et transitoire de la motilité volitionnelle dans la paraplégie, *Société de Neurologie de Paris*, meeting of November 9, 1911, *Rev Neurol (Paris)*, 1911, T. XXII, n° 22 (November 30), pp. 652-653.

183. Babinski J, Jarkowski J, Jumentié J. Syndrome de Brown-Séquard par coup de couteau, *Rev Neurol (Paris)*, 1911, T. XXII, n° 17 (September 15), pp. 309-313.

186. Babinski J, Lecène P, Baclot[4]. Tumeur méningée; paraplégie crurale par compression de la moelle. Extraction de la tumeur. Guérison, *Société de Neurologie de Paris*, meeting of November 9, *Rev Neurol (Paris)*, 1911, T. XXII, n° 22 (November 30), p. 653 *[Cette communication sera publiée dans un prochain numéro]*.

Babinski J. Contractures tendino-réflexes et contractures cutanéo-réflexes, *Société de Neurologie de Paris*, meeting of May 9, 1912, *Rev Neurol (Paris)*, 1912, T. XXIII, n° 10 (May 30), p. 727. *[cette communication sera publiée dans les comptes-rendus de la prochaine séance]*.

193. Babinski J, Chaillous J, Martel (Th. de).Stase papillaire bilatérale; cécité presque complète; crâniectomie décompressive sans incision de la dure-mère: guérison, *Société de Neurologie de Paris*, meeting of April 25, *Rev Neurol (Paris)*, 1912, T. XXIII, n° 8 (April 30), pp. 638-640.

187. Babinski J, Jumentié J, Jarkowski J. Pachyméningite cervicale hypertrophique, *Société de Neurologie de Paris*, meeting of January 25, *Rev Neurol (Paris)*, 1912, T. XXIII, n° 3 (February 15), pp. 221-222. [in extenso in *Nouvelle Iconographie de la Salpêtrière*, n° **198**].

Babinski J, Lecène P, Bourlot. Tumeur méningée. Paraplégie crurale par compression de la moelle. Extraction de la tumeur : guérison, *Rev Neurol (Paris)*, 1912, T. XXIII, n° 1 (January 15), pp. 1-4. *[Presented at the Société de Neurologie de Paris, séance de November 1911]*

192. Babinski J, Martel (Th. de), Jumentié J. Tumeur méningée de la région dorsale supérieure; paraplégie crurale par compression de la moelle; extraction de la tumeur, guérison, *Société de Neurologie de Paris*, meeting of April 25, 1912, *Rev Neurol (Paris)*, 1912, T. XXIII, n° 8 (April 30), pp. 640-644.

188. Babinski J, Vincent, Jarkowski J. Des réflexes cutanés de défense dans la maladie de Friedreich, *Société de Neurologie de Paris*, meeting of March 7, *Rev Neurol (Paris)*, 1912, T. XXIII, n° 6 (March 31), pp. 463-466.

194. Babinski J. Contracture tendino-réflexe et contracture cutaneo-réflexe, *Société de Neurologie de Paris*, meeting of May 9, 1912, *Rev Neurol (Paris)*, 1912, T. XXIV, n° 14 (July 30), pp. 77-80,

Babinski J. Modification des réflexes cutanés sous l'influence de la compression par la bande d'Esmarch (à propos d'un travail du docteur Onorio de Almeida), *Société de Neurologie de Paris* meeting of July 11, 1912, *Revue Neurologique (Paris)*, 1912, T. XXIV, n° 14 (July 30), p. 147.

Babinski J. 7 intervention of 14 lines (p. 773) et 7 lines (p. 776), à propos de la communicatin de J. Dejerine et E. Long "Examen histologique d'un cas de section complète de la moelle cervicale inférieure, d'origine traumatique", *Société Neurologique de Paris*, meeting of December 12, 1912, *Rev Neurol (Paris)*, 1912, T. XXIV, n° 24 (December 30), pp. 769-776.

196. Babinski J, Jarkowski J. Etude comparative des limites de l'anesthésie organique et de l'anesthésie psychique, *Société de Neurologie de Paris*, meeting of 11 July, *Rev Neurol (Paris)*, 1912, T. XXIV, n° 14 (July 30), pp. 144-147.

199. Babinski J. Contracture liée à une irritation des cornes antérieures de la moelle dans un cas de syringomyélie, *Société de Neurologie de Paris*, meeting of January 9, *Rev Neurol (Paris)*, 1913, T. XXV, n° 1 (January 15), pp. 129-130. [Publié in extenso *Société de Neurologie de Paris*, meeting of 6 February, addendum to the meeting of January 9, *Rev Neurol (Paris)*, 1913, T. XXV, n° 4 (February 28), pp. 246-249].

Babinski J. Intervention of 10 lines (p. 134), on the paper by Pierre Marie et Ch. Foix "Le réflexe d' "allongement croisé" du membre inférieur et les réflexes d'automatisme médullaire", *Société de Neurologie de Paris*, meeting of January 9, *Rev Neurol (Paris)*, 1913, T. XXV, n° 2 (January 30), pp. 132-134.

---

[4] Baclot (sic), pour Bourlot.

200. Babinski J, Vincent Cl, Barré A. Vertige voltaïque. Perturbation dans les mouvements des globes oculaires à la suite de lésions labyrinthiques expérimentales, *Société de Neurologie de Paris,* meeting of February 6, *Rev Neurol (Paris),* 1913, T. XXV, n° 4 (February 28), pp. 253-255.
201. Babinski J, Vincent Cl, Barré A. Vertige voltaïque. Nouvelles recherches expérimentales sur le labyrinthe du cobaye, *Société de Neurologie de Paris,* meeting of March 6, *Rev Neurol (Paris),* 1913, T. XXV, n° 6 (March 30), pp. 410-413.
202. Babinski J, Chauvet (Stephen), Durand (Gaston). p. 436, Un cas de crises gastriques tabétiformes liées à l'existence d'un petit ulcus juxta-pylorique, *Société de Neurologie de Paris,* meeting of March 6, *Rev Neurol (Paris),* 1913, T. XXV, n° 6 (March 30), pp. 436-438.

Babinski J, Delherm, Jarkowski J. Sur l'association de deux courants en électro-diagnostic et en électrothérapie, Congrès pour l'avancement des sciences, section d'électricité médicale, Nîmes, August 1-6, 1912, *Rev Neurol (Paris),* 1913, T. XXV, n° 7 (April 15), p. 462.

Babinski J. Intervention of 10 lines (p. 845), on the paper by M.L. Alquier "Trente cas de Basedowisme fruste ou névrose vaso-motrice", *Société de Neurologie de Paris,* meeting of June 5, *Rev Neurol (Paris),* 1913, T. XV, n° 12 (June 30), pp. 132-134. In extenso *Rev Neurol (Paris),* 1913, T. XXV, n° 12 (June 30), pp. 795-804.

204. Babinski J, Chauvet (Stephen), Jarkowski J. Sur un cas de syndrome de Brown-Séquard par coup de couteau, *Société de Neurologie de Paris,* meeting of May 8, *Revue Neurologique. (Paris),* 1913, T. XXV, n° 10 (May 30), p. 702 et communication in extenso *Société de Neurologie de Paris,* meeting of June 5, addendum to the meeting of May 8, *Rev Neurol (Paris),* 1913, T. XXV, n° 12 (June 30), pp. 857-861.
212. Babinski J, Enriquez E, Jumentié J. Compression de la moelle par tumeur extra-dure-mérienne, paraplégie intermittente, *Société de Neurologie de Paris,* meeting of February 13, *Rev Neurol (Paris),* 1913, T. XXV, n° 5 (March 15), p. 356 et, in extenso, *Rev Neurol (Paris),* 1914, T. XXVII, n° 3 (February 15), pp. 169-172. *[malade opérée par Gosset]*

Babinski J. Intervention of 20 lines (pp. 114-115), on the paper by André Thomas et A. Durupt (travail du laboratoire du Pr. Dejerine, hospice de la Salpêtrière "Des troubles observés chez le chien et le singe à la suite de lésions limitées du cervelet. Contributions à l'étude des localisations cérébelleuses", *Société de Neurologie de Paris,* meeting of July 10, *Rev Neurol (Paris),* 1913, T. XXVI, n° 15 (July 30), pp. 111-115.

210. Babinski J, Jarkowski J. Sur les mouvements conjugués, *Société de Neurologie de Paris,* meeting of November 6, 1913, *Rev Neurol (Paris),* 1913, T. XXVI, n° 22 (November 30), p. 623; *Rev Neurol (Paris),* 1914, T. XXVII, n° 2 (January 30), pp. 73-76.

Babinski J, Tournay A. "Symptômes des maladies du cervelet", Premier rapport, XVIIè Congrès International de Médecine, Londres, August 6-12, 1913, Travaux de la sectionde Neuropathologie (section XI), Compte-rendu analytique par A. Barré, *Rev Neurol (Paris),* 1913, T. XXVI, n° 18 (September 30), pp. 306-322.

Babinski J, Vincent Cl, Barré A. "Vertige voltaïque. Recherches sur le labyrinthe du cobaye", XVIIè Congrès International de Médecine, Londres, August 6-12, 1913, Travaux de la sectionde Neuropathologie (section XI), *Rev Neurol (Paris),* 1913, T. XXVI, n° 18 (September 30), p. 351.

Babinski J. Intervention of 11 lines (p. 616), on the paper by Georges Guillain and Jean Dubois "Le signe de Babinski provoqué par l'excitation des téguments de tout le côté hémiplégié dans un cas d'hémiplégie infantile", *Société de Neurologie de Paris,* meeting of April 2, *Rev Neurol (Paris),* 1914, T. XXVII, n° 8 (April 30), pp. 614-616.

Babinski J. Intervention of 10 lines (p. 602), on the paper by Dupré et Heuyer "Chorée chronique intermittente à début infantile", *Société de Neurologie de Paris,* meeting of April 2, *Rev Neurol (Paris),* 1914, T. XXVII, n° 8 (April 30), pp. 595-604.

Babinski J. Intervention of 8 lines (p. 607), on the paper by O. Crouzon, C. Chatelin and Mme Athanassiu-Benisti "Sclérose en plaques ou pseudo-sclérose en plaques? affection organique ou affection psychonévropathique", *Société de Neurologie de Paris,* meeting of April 2, *Rev Neurol (Paris),* 1914, T. XXVII, n° 8 (April 30), pp. 604-607.

213. Babinski J. Contribution à l'étude des troubles mentaux dans l'hémiplégie organique cérébrale (anosognosie), *Société de Neurologie de Paris,* meeting of June 11, 1914, *Rev Neurol (Paris),* 1914, T. XXVII (1 semester), n° 12 (June 30), pp. 845-848.

Babinski J, Barré A. Compression de la moelle par tumeur extra-dure-mérienne. Valeur localisatrice des réflexes cutanés de défense, *Société de Neurologie de Paris,* meeting of January 29, *Rev Neurol (Paris),* 1914, T. XXVII, n° 4 (February 28), pp. 262-268.

Babinski J, Barré A. Hématomyélie après laminectomie simple, *Société de Neurologie de Paris*, meeting of May 28, *Rev Neurol (Paris)*, 1914, T. XXVII, n° 11 (June 15), pp. 784-785.

Babinski J, Barré A. Myasthénie. Altérations à type Paget des os du crâne. Lésions de certaines glandes à sécrétion interne, *Rev Neurol (Paris)*, 1914, T. XXVII, n° 11 (June 15), pp. 786-787.

Babinski J, Enriquez E, Jumentié J. Compression de la moelle par tumeur extra-dure-mérienne; paraplégie intermittente; opération extractive, *Rev Neurol (Paris)*, 1914, T. XXVII, n° 3 (February 15), pp. 169-172.

Babinski J, Gautier Cl. Pseudo-tabès et filariose sanguine, *Société de Neurologie de Paris*, meeting of June 11, *Rev Neurol (Paris)*, 1914, T. XXVII, n° 12 (June 30), pp. 856-857.

Babinski J, Lecéne P, Jarkowski J. Paraplégie crurale par néoplasme extra-dure-mérien. Opération. Guérison, *Rev Neurol (Paris)*, 1914, T. XXVII, n° 12 (June 30), pp. 801-805 (and Société Neurologique de Paris, meeting of June 11, p. 844 [intervention de De Martel]).

217. Babinski J. Réflexes de défense. Etude clinique, *Rev Neurol (Paris)*, 2è semestre 1914-1915, T. XXVIII, n° 15 (March 1915), pp. 145-154.

214. Babinski J. Sur les lésions des nerfs par blessures de guerre, *Rev Neurol (Paris)*, 2è semestre 1914-1915, n° 17-18 (May-June 1915), "Neurologie de guerre", pp. 274-279, (*Société de Neurologie de Paris*, meeting of January 7, 1915, p. 381).

215. Babinski J. De la paralysie radiale due à la compression du nerf par des béquilles (association organo-hystérique), *Société de Neurologie de Paris*, meeting of February 4, 1915, *Rev Neurol (Paris)*, 2è semestre 1914-1915, T. XXVIII, n° 17-18 (May-June 1915), "Neurologie de guerre", pp. 408-409.

216. Babinski J. Lenteur de la secousse faradique. Lenteur de la secousse tendino-réflexe. Fusion anticipée des secousses faradiques, *Société de Neurologie de Paris*, meeting of March 4, 1915, *Rev Neurol (Paris)*, 2è semestre 1914-1915, T. XXVIII, n° 17-18 (May-June 1915), pp. 444-445.

218. Babinski J. Névrite crurale paraissant due à une compression de nerf par bandage herniaire, *Société de Neurologie de Paris*, meeting of March 18, 1915, *Rev Neurol (Paris)*, 2è semestre 1914-1915, T. XXVIII, n° 17-18 (May-June 1915), p. 454.

219. Babinski J. Quelques observations sur les lésions des nerfs, *Société de Neurologie de Paris*, meeting of March 18, 1915, *Rev Neurol (Paris)*, 2è semestre 1914-1915, T. XXVIII, N° 17-18 (May-June 1915), pp. 455-456.

220. Babinski J. Lésion du nerf crural. Abolition de l'excitation faradique et voltaïque du quadriceps crural. Guérison rapide, *Société de Neurologie de Paris*, meeting of May 6, *Rev Neurol (Paris)*, 2è semestre 1914-1915, T. XXVIII, n° 19 (July), pp. 553-554. (p. 1012: simple renvoi).

221. Babinski J. Excitation faradique bilatérale de la plante du pied, *Société de Neurologie de Paris*, meeting of May 6, *Rev Neurol (Paris)*, 2è semestre 1914-1915, T. XXVIII, n° 19 (July), pp. 561-562, (p. 1030 : simple renvoi).

222. Babinski J. Lésion spinale par éclatement d'obus à proximité sans blessure ni contusion. Syndrome de Brown-Séquard, *Société de Neurologie de Paris*, meeting of June 3, 1915, *Rev Neurol (Paris)*, 2è semestre 1914-1915, T. XXVIII, n° 19 (July), pp. 581-583.

223. Babinski J. De l'extension paradoxale de la main provoquée par la faradisation unipolaire de la partie antéro-inférieure de l'avant-bras, *Société de Neurologie de Paris*, meeting of July 1, 1915, *Rev Neurol (Paris)*, 2è semestre 1914-1915, T. XXVIII, n° 20-21 (August-September 1915), p. 720, (p. 1030 : simple renvoi).

Babinski J. De la flexion paradoxale de la main provoquée par la faradisation unipolaire de la partie postéro-supérieure de l'avant-bras, *Société de Neurologie de Paris*, meeting of July 1, 1915, *Rev Neurol (Paris)*, 2è semestre 1914-1915, T. XXVIII, n° 20-21 (August-September 1915), pp. 722-723, (p. 1030 : simple renvoi).

225. Babinski J, Froment J. Service de neurologie militarisé de l'hôpital de la Pitié. Troubles consécutifs aux lésions des nerfs. Troubles nerveux consécutifs aux lésions des centres nerveux. Accidents hystériques. Troubles nerveux d'origine réflexe. *Rev Neurol (Paris)*, 2è semestre 1914-1915, T. XXVIII, n° 23-24 (November-December 1915) "Neurologie de guerre", pp. 1151-1154.

228. Babinski J, Froment J. Contribution à l'étude des troubles nerveux d'ordre réflexe. Examen pendant l'anesthésie chloroformique. *Société de Neurologie de Paris*, meeting of November 4, 1915, Paris*Rev Neurol (Paris)*, 2è semestre 1914-1915, T. XXVIII, n° 23-24 (November-December 1915) "Neurologie de guerre", pp. 925-933 (et p. 1276, annonce de la publication de cette communication dans le même numéro).

227. Babinski J, Froment. Sur une forme de contracture organique d'origine périphérique et sans exagération des réflexes, *Société de Neurologie de Paris*, meeting of November 4, 1915, *Rev Neurol (Paris)*, 2è semestre 1914-1915, T. XXVIII, n° 23-24 (November-December 1915) "Neurologie de guerre", p. 1276.

Babinski J. Intervention of 15 lines (p. 327), on the paper by M. Delorme, "Les Traumatismes des nerfs par les projectiles et les opérations qu'ils réclament" (*Bulletins et Mémoires de l'Académie de Médecine*, n° 3, 4, 5, p. 97, 132, 160, meetings of January 19 and 26, and February 2), *Société de Neurologie de Paris*, meeting of April 2, *Rev Neurol (Paris)*, 2è semestre 1914-1915, T. XXVIII, n° 17-18 (May-June 1915) "Neurologie de guerre", p. 327.

Babinski J. Annonce de l'intervention sur la communication de M. Dejerine, "sur l'abolition du réflexe cutané plantaire dans certains cas de paralysies fonctionnelles accompagnées d'anesthésie", *Société de Neurologie de Paris*, meeting of February 4, 1915, *Rev Neurol (Paris)*, 2è semestre 1914-1915, T. XXVIII, n° 17-18 (May-June 1915) "Neurologie de guerre", p. 405.

Babinski J. Intervention de 2 pages (pp. 450-452), *in* "Discussion sur les troubles nerveux dits fonctionnels observés pendant la guerre", *Société de Neurologie de Paris*, meetings of February 18 and March 4, 1915, *Rev Neurol (Paris)*, 2è semestre 1914-1915, T. XXVIII, n° 17-18 (May-June 1915) "Neurologie de guerre", pp. 447-453.

Babinski J. Intervention de 2 pages (pp. 527-529) on the paper by M. Dejerine, "sur l'abolition du réflexe cutané plantaire dans certains cas de paralysies fonctionnelles accompagnées d'anesthésie (hystéro-traumatisme)", *Rev Neurol (Paris)*, 2è semestre 1914-1915, T. XXVIII, n° 19 (July 1915), pp. 521-529.

Babinski J. Intervention of 21 lines (pp. 1225-1226) on the paper by Henry Meige, "De certaines boîteries observées chez les "blessés nerveux". Remarques morphologiques et physiologiques, *Société de Neurologie de Paris*, meeting of October 7 1915, *Rev Neurol (Paris)*, 2è semestre 1914-1915, T. XXVIII, n° 23-24 (November-December 1915) "Neurologie de guerre", pp. 939-947.

Babinski J. Lésion du nerf crural. Abolition de l'excitabilité faradique et voltaïque quadriceps crural. Guérison rapide, *Société de Neurologie de Paris*, meeting of May 6, 1915, *Rev Neurol (Paris)*, 2è semestre 1914-1915, T. XXVIII, n° 19 (July 1915), pp. 553-554.

Babinski J, rapporteur. Les caractères des troubles moteurs (paralysies, contractures, etc.) dits "fonctionnels" et la conduite à tenir à leur égard. Réunion de la *Société de Neurologie de Paris* avec les représentants des Centres neurologiques militaires de France et des pays alliés, (April 6 and 7, 1916), *Rev Neurol (Paris*, 1916, T. XXIX, N° 4-5 (April-May), pp. 450, 521-572.

Babinski J. Intervention of 14 lines (p. 404) on the paper by Laignel-Lavastine et Paul Courbon "Amaurose par éclatement d'obus avec méningite syphilitique", *Société de Neurologie de Paris*, meeting of March 2, 1916, *Rev Neurol (Paris)*, 1916, T. XXIX, n° 3 (March 1916), pp. 402-405.

231. Babinski J, Froment J. Des troubles vaso-moteurs et thermiques d'ordre réflexe, *Société de Neurologie de Paris*, meeting of March 2, *Rev Neurol (Paris)*, 1916, T. XXIX (1), n° 3 (March), pp. 410-414.

Babinski J. Intervention of 30 lines (p. 464) à propos du rapport de Pierre Marie "La conduite à tenir vis-à-vis des blessures du crâne", *Société de Neurologie de Paris*, meeting of April 6-7, 1916, *Rev Neurol (Paris)*, 1916, T. XXIX, n° 4-5 (April-May 1916), pp. 453-476.

Babinski J. Intervention of 10 lines (p. 507) à propos du rapport de M.A. Pitres (de Bordeaux) "La valeur des signes cliniques permettant de reconnaître dans les blessures des nerfs périphériques A. La section complète d'un nerf, B. Sa restauration fonctionnelle", *Société de Neurologie de Paris*, meeting of April 6-7, 1916, *Rev Neurol (Paris)*, 1916, T. XXIX, n° 4-5 (April-May 1916), pp. 476-520.

233. Babinski J, Froment J. Troubles nerveux d'ordre réflexe ou syndrome d'immobilisation. *Société de Neurologie de Paris*, meeting of May 4, 1916, *Rev Neurol (Paris)*, 1916, T. XXIX, n° 6 (June 1916), pp. 914-918.

234. Babinski J, Froment J. Abolition du réflexe cutané plantaire. Anesthésie associée à des troubles vaso-moteurs et à de l'hypothermie d'ordre réflexe, *Société de Neurologie de Paris*, meeting of May 4, 1916, *Rev Neurol (Paris)*, 1916, T. XXIX, n° 6 (June 1916), pp. 918-921.

Babinski J. Intervention of 18 lines (p. 105) on the paper by Clovis Vincent "Au sujet de l'hystérie et de la simulation", *Société de Neurologie de Paris*, meeting of June 29, 1916, *Rev Neurol (Paris)*, 1916, T. XXIX, n° 7 (July 1916), pp. 104-107.

240. Babinski J, Hallion, Froment J. La lenteur de la secousse musculaire obtenue par percussion et sa signification clinique. Etude par la méthode graphique, *Société de Neurologie de Paris*, meeting of June 29, 1916, *Rev Neurol (Paris)*, 1916, T. XXIX, n° 7 (July 1916), pp. 109-112.

Babinski J. Interventions of 26 lines (p. 508) and of 43 lines (pp. 509-510) à propos de la communication de A. Souques, J. Mégevand, Melles Naïditch et Rathaus, "Troubles de la température locale, à propos d'un cas de paralysie dite réflexe du membre inférieur", *Société de Neurologie de Paris*, meeting of October 12, 1916, *Rev Neurol (Paris)*, 1916, T. XXIX, n° 11-12 (November-December 1916), pp. 505-513.

Babinski J. Intervention of 36 lines (pp. 535-536) on the paper by Jean Courjon "A propos des paralysies dites réflexes", *Société de Neurologie de Paris*, meeting of November 9, 1916, *Rev Neurol (Paris)*, 1916, T. XXIX, n° 11-12 (November-December 1916), pp. 531-537.

Babinski J, Froment J (Service de neurologie militarisé de la Pitié). Contractures et paralysies d'ordre réflexe, *Rev Neurol (Paris)*, 1916, T. XXIX, n° 11-12 (November-December 1916), pp. 638-642.

237. Babinski J, Froment J (Service de neurologie militarisé de la Pitié). Hystérie-Pithiatisme, *Rev Neurol (Paris)*, 1916, T. XXIX, n° 11-12 (November-December 1916), pp. 642-643.

238. Babinski J, Froment J (Service de neurologie militarisé de la Pitié). Paralysies organiques, *Rev Neurol (Paris)*, 1916, T. XXIX, n° 11-12 (November-December 1916), pp. 643-645.

239. Babinski J. Réformes, incapacités, gratifications dans les névroses, *Rev Neurol (Paris)*, 1916, T. XXIX, n° 11-12 (November-December 1916), pp. 753-756.

Babinski J. Intervention of 7 lines (pp. 786-787) on the paper by Grasset "Les névroses et psychonévroses de guerre; conduite à tenir à leur égard", *Société de Neurologie de Paris*, meeting of December 15, 1916, *Rev Neurol (Paris)*, 1916, T. XXIX, n° 11-12 (November-December 1916), pp. 767-788.

242. Babinski J, Froment J. Parésie réflexe de la Main gauche, troubles vaso-moteurs et sudoraux bilatéraux, *Société de Neurologie de Paris*, meeting of November 9, 1916, *Rev Neurol (Paris)*, 1916, T. XXIX, n° 11-12 (November-December 1916), pp. 542-544.

244. Babinski J. Fusion anticipée des secousses faradiques dans les muscles de la plante du pied, *Société de Neurologie de Paris*, meeting of January 11, 1917, *Rev Neurol (Paris)*, 1917 (1er semestre), n° 1 (January), pp. 43-44.

Babinski J, Dubois. *Société de Neurologie de Paris*, April 5, 1917, *Rev Neurol (Paris)*, 1917 (1er semestre), n° 4-5 (April-May), p. 232 [no title].

246. Babinski J, Heitz J. A propos d'un cas de claudication intermittente par endartérite oblitérante, *Société de Neurologie de Paris*, meeting of May 3, 1917, *Rev Neurol (Paris)*, 1917, XXIVè année, n° 4-5 (April-May), pp. 257-258.

247. Babinski J, Heitz J. Paraplégie organique. Troubles vaso-moteurs au membre supérieur droit, avec méiopragie et sans modification locale des réflexes osso-tendineux, *Société de Neurologie de Paris*, meeting of May 3, 1917, *Rev Neurol (Paris)*, 1917, XXIVè année, 1er semestre, n° 4-5 (April-May), pp. 258-259.

Babinski J, Froment J. A propos de la communication de Roussy et Boisseau sur le pronostic et le traitement des troubles physiopathiques, *Société de Neurologie de Paris*, meeting of June 7, 1917, *Rev Neurol (Paris)*, 1917 (1er semestre), n° 6 (June), pp. 527-537.

249. Babinski J, Froment J. Hypotonie et laxité articulaire dans les affections organiques et physiopathiques du système nerveux, *Société de Neurologie de Paris*, meeting of November 8, 1917, *Rev Neurol (Paris)*, 1917, 24è année, 2ème semestre, n° 10-11-12 (October-November-December), pp. 257-258.

250. Babinski J. (Travaux en collaboration avec J. Froment et J. Heitz. Service de neurologie militarisé de la Pitié et de l'hôpital Buffon). Le syndrome physiopathique, *Rev Neurol (Paris)*, 1917, n° 10-11-12 (October-November-December), pp. 347-351.

253. Babinski J, Heitz J. De la claudication intermittente après ligature de l'artère principale du membre inférieur, *Société de Neurologie*, meeting of March 7, 1918, *Rev Neurol (Paris)*, 1918 (1er semestre), T. 34, n° 3-4 (March-April), pp. 175-178.

Babinski J. Intervention of 34 lines (pp. 205-206) on the paper by Clovis Vincent "Sur le pronostic des troubles réflexes", *Société de Neurologie de Paris*, meeting of April 11, 1918, *Rev Neurol (Paris)*, 1918, 1er semestre, T. 34, n° 3-4 (March-April), pp. 197-206.

254. Babinski J, Moricand I. Un cas de réflexe achilléen contralatéral homogène, *Société de Neurologie de Paris*, meeting of April 11, 1918, *Rev Neurol (Paris)*, 1918 (1er semestre), T. 34, n° 3-4 (March-April 1018), pp. 214-216.

Babinski J, Froment J. Les signes objectifs de la paralysie de l'adducteur du pouce, *Société de Neurologie de Paris*, meeting of June 6, 1918, *Rev Neurol (Paris)*, 1918 (1er semestre), T. 34, n° 5-6 (May-June), pp. 484-487.

255. Babinski J, Moricand I. Note sur un nouveau cas de réflexe achilléen contralatéral chez un homme porteur d'un spina bifida occulta, *Société de Neurologie de Paris*, meeting of July 11, 1918, *Rev Neurol (Paris)*, 1918 (1er semestre), T. 34, n° 5-6 (May-June), pp. 516-518.

Babinski J, Dubois. *Société de Neurologie de Paris*, meeting of January 10, 1918, *Rev Neurol (Paris)*, 1918 (1er semestre), T. 34, n° 1-2 (January-February), p. 58 [ni titre ni texte].

Babinski J. *Société de Neurologie de Paris*, meeting of July 11, 1918, *Rev Neurol (Paris)*, 1918 (1er semestre), T. 34, n° 5-6 (May-June), p. 526 [ni titre ni texte].

257. Babinski J. Anosognosie. *Société de Neurologie de Paris*, meeting of December 5, 1918, *Revue Neurologique (Paris)*, 1918, T. 34, n° 11-12 (November-December), pp. 365-367.

Babinski J. Intervention dans des "discussions" [pas de texte], *Société de Neurologie de Paris*, meeting of December 4, 1919, *Rev Neurol (Paris)*, 1919, T. 35, n° 12 (December), p. 948.

Babinski J. Intervention of 3 lines (p. 626) [sur l'influence des races dans le tabes] à propos du rapport de J.A. Sicard (avec les discussions) "Syphilis nerveuse et son traitement", *Réunion neurologique annuelle de la Société de Neurologie de Paris* consacrée à "Formes cliniques de la syphilis nerveuse et leur traitement" (July 9-10, 1920), *Rev Neurol (Paris)*, 1920, T. XXXVI, n° 7 (July 1920), pp. 609-748.

275. Babinski J. Intervention (pp. 695-697) "Du traitement hydrargyrique dans le tabes", à propos du rapport de J.A. Sicard (avec les discussions) "Syphilis nerveuse et son traitement", *Réunion neurologique annuelle de la Société de Neurologie de Paris* consacrée à "Formes cliniques de la syphilis nerveuse et leur traitement" (July 9-10, 1920), *Rev Neurol (Paris)*, 1920, T. XXXVI, n° 7 (July 1920), pp. 609-748.

260. Babinski J, Jarkowski J. Etude de la raideur musculaire dans un cas de syndrome parkinsonien consécutif à une encéphalite léthargique. Réaction des antagonistes, *Société de Neurologie de Paris*, meeting of June 3, 1920, *Rev Neurol (Paris)*, 1920, T. 36, n° 6 (June 1920), pp. 564-570.

261. Babinski J, Jarkowski J. Sur une forme de syncinésie dans l'hémiplégie organique, *Société de Neurologie de Paris*, meeting of July 1 1920, *Rev Neurol (Paris)*, 1920, T. 36, n° 7 (July 1920), pp. 760-761.

262. Babinski J, Jarkowski J. Etude des troubles moteurs dans un cas de choréo-athétose double, *Société de Neurologie de Paris*, meeting of July 1, 1920, *Rev Neurol (Paris)*, 1920, T. 36, n° 7 (July 1920), pp. 761-764.

259. Babinski J, Jarkowski J. Contribution à l'étude de l'anesthésie dans les compressions de la moelle dorsale, *Société de Neurologie de Paris*, meeting of April 15, 1920, *Rev Neurol (Paris)*, 1920, T. 36, n° 9 (September 1920), pp. 865-871.

265. Babinski J. Torticolis spasmodique, *Société de Neurologie de Paris*, meeting of April 7, 1921, *Rev Neurol (Paris)*, 1921, T. 37, n° 4 (April 1921), pp. 367-371.

263. Babinski J, Jarkowski J. De la surréflectivité hyperalgésique, *Société de Neurologie de Paris*, meeting of February 3, 1921 *(Rev Neurol (Paris))*, 1921, T. 37, n° 2, February 1921, pp. 194, 433-438), sera publié ultérieurement comme manuscrit original : *Rev Neurol (Paris)*, 1921, T. 37, n° 5 (May 1921), pp. 433-438.

266. Babinski J. Syndromes parkinsoniens. Traitement, *Société de Neurologie de Paris*, meeting of May 5, 1921, *Rev Neurol (Paris)*, 1921, T. 37, n° 5 (May 1921), p. 462.

Babinski J. Spasme facial post-encéphalitique, *Société de Neurologie de Paris*, meeting of May 5, 1921, *Rev Neurol (Paris)*, 1921, T. 37, n° 5 (May 1921), p. 462.

Babinski J. Intervention of 8 lines ["scopolamine"] (p. 706) à propos de Paulian et Bagdasar (travail du service du Pr Marinesco, de Bucarest) "A propos du traitement du parkinsonisme", *Réunion neurologique annuelle de la Société de Neurologie de Paris* (3-June 4, 1921), *Rev Neurol (Paris)*, 1921, T. 37, n° 6 (June 1921), pp. 703-706.

Babinski J. Intervention of 13 lines (p. 79) à propos de Jules Renault, Mme Athanassio-Bénisty et M.E. Hibert "Mouvements cloniques rythmés de l'hémiface droite, persistant pendant le sommeil et probablement consécutifs à une névraxite épidémique", *Société de Neurologie de Paris*, meeting of January 6, 1921, *Rev Neurol (Paris)*, 1921, T. 37, n° 1 (January 1921), pp. 77-80.

264. Babinski J, Jarkowski J, Plichet. Kinésie paradoxale. Mutisme parkinsonien, *Société de Neurologie de Paris*, meeting of April 7, 1921, *Rev Neurol (Paris)*, 1921, T. 37, n° 12 (December 1921), pp. 1266-1270.

267. Babinski J, Jumentié J. Hémisyndrome sympathique et médullaire à type irritatif, à évolution intermittente et rythmée, *Société de Neurologie de Paris*, meeting of December 1, 1921, *Rev Neurol (Paris)*, 1921, T. 37, n° 12 (December 1921), pp. 1251-1256.

Babinski J. Intervention of 15 lines (p. 74) à propos de Pierre Marie et Melle Gabrielle Lévy "Palilalie et syndrome parkinsonien par encéphalite épidémique", *Société de Neurologie de Paris* (January 12, 1922), *Rev Neurol (Paris)*, 1922, T. 38, n° 1 (January 1922), pp. 66-74. Résumé in *La Presse Médicale*, 1922, n° 7 (January 25), p. 75.

269. Babinski J, Jarkowski J. Hyperalgésie et réactions hyperalgésiques dans l'hémiplégie cérébrale, *Société de Neurologie de Paris*, meeting of February 2, 1922, *Rev Neurol (Paris)*, 1922, T. 38, n° 2 (February 1922), pp. 210-212 (Résumé in *La Presse Médicale*, February 15, 1922, n° 13, p. 140).

270. Babinski J, Charpentier. Automatisme et hyperalgésie dans l'hémiplégie cérébrale, *Société de Neurologie de Paris*, meeting of March 9, 1922, *Rev Neurol (Paris)*, 1922, T. 38, n° 3 (March 1922), pp. 300-302. (Résumé in *La Presse Médicale*, March 22, 1922, n° 23, p. 252).

272. Babinski J. Réflexes de défense, *Rev Neurol (Paris)*, August 1922, T. 38, n° 8, pp. 1049-1081. [Conférénce lone May 31, 1922, at the Royal Medical Society in London, [with cases presentation and projection of films].

273. Babinski J, Charpentier. Syndrome parkinsonien fruste post-encéphalitique. Troubles respiratoires, *Société de Neurologie de Paris*, meeting of November 9, 1922, *Rev Neurol (Paris)*, 1922, T. 38, n° 11 (November) pp. 1369-1377.

268. Babinski J, Jarkowski, Bethoux. Sarcome mélanique du cerveau à foyers multiples, consécutif à une néoplasie de la choroïde de même nature), *Société de neurologie de Paris*, meeting of March 9, 1922 (addendum to the meeting of January 12, 1922), *Rev Neurol (Paris)*, 1922, T. 38, n° 3 (March 1922), p. 331-336, (résumé in *La Presse Médicale*, 1922, n° 7 (January 25), p. 76).

271. Babinski J, Krebs, Plichet A. Torticolis spasmodique avec lésion du système nerveux central. Exostoses ostéogéniques multiples, *Société de Neurologie de Paris*, meeting of May 4, 1922 (addendum to the meeting of March 9, 1922), *Rev Neurol (Paris)*, 1922, T. 38, n° 5 (May 1922), pp. 587-593, (résumé in *La Presse Médicale*, March 23, 1922, n° 23, pp. 251-252).

270. Babinski J, Jarkowski J. Automatisme et hyperalgésie dans l'hémiplégie cérébrale, *Société de Neurologie*, meeting of March 9, 1922 (in *La Presse Médicale*, March 25, 1922, n° 24, p. 252).

Babinski J, Jarkowski J. Tumeur probable de la moelle, *Société de Neurologie de Paris*, meeting of March 9, 1922 [Pas de trace dans la *Revue Neurologique*]. Résumé in *La Presse Médicale*, March 22, 1922, n° 23, p. 252.

276. Babinski J, Jarkowski J. Sur le diagnostic des compressions spinales, *IVè Réunion Neurologique Internationale*, June 8-9, 1923, *Rev Neurol (Paris)*, 1923, T. 39, n° 6 (June), pp. 670-674.

274. Babinski J. Sur le traitement des tumeurs juxta-médullaires, *IVè Réunion Neurologique Internationale*, June 8-9, 1923, *Rev Neurol (Paris)*, 1923, T. 39, n° 6 (June), pp. 695-701.

Babinski J. A propos du procès-verbal. Sur l'anosognosie, *Société de Neurologie de Paris*, meeting of June 7, 1923, *Rev Neurol (Paris)*, 1923, T. 39, n° 6 (June), pp. 731-732.

277. Babinski J. A l'occasion du Procès-verbal. Sur l'épreuve du lipiodol comme moyen de diagnostic des compressions de la moelle, *Société de Neurologie de Paris*, meeting of February 7, *Rev Neurol (Paris)*, 1924, T. I, n° 2 (February), pp. 228-230.

278. Babinski J. De la section du spinal externe dans le torticolis spasmodique, *Société de Neurologie de Paris*, meeting of April 3, *Rev Neurol (Paris)*, 1924, T. I, n° 4 (April), pp. 452-457.

279. Babinski J. Sur la valeur du phénomène des orteils dans la sclérose en plaques, *Vè Réunion Neurologique Internationale 30-31 May*, *Rev Neurol (Paris)*, 1924, T. I, n° 6 (June), pp. 703-704.

Babinski J. Sur la démyélinisation dans la sclérose en plaques, *Vè Réunion Neurologique Internationale May 30-31*, *Rev Neurol (Paris)*, 1924, T. I, n° 6 (June), pp. 739-740.

Babinski J. Intervention of 25 lines (p. 250), on the paper by Souques et Blamoutier "Akinésie paradoxale glosso-labiée existant dans la station et disparaîssant dans le décubitus chez un parkinsonien," *Société de Neurologie de Paris*, meeting of February 7, *Rev Neurol (Paris)*, 1924, T. I, n° 2 (February), pp. 249-250.

Babinski J. Intervention of 6 lines (p. 813), on the paper by J. Poussepp (Dorpat) "La question de la localisation du signe du petit orteil par les cas de tumeurs du corps strié", *Société de Neurologie de Paris*, meeting of June 5, *Rev Neurol (Paris)*, 1924, T. I, n° 6 (June), pp. 812-813.

280. Babinski J, Jarkowski J. Quelques documents relatifs au diagnostic des compressions spinales, *Société de Neurologie de Paris*, meeting of March 6, 1924, *Rev Neurol (Paris)*, 1924, T. I, n° 3 (March), pp. 375-379. *[Discussions. To be published later in extenso]*

Babinski J. Intervention of 9 lines (p. 611), on the paper by Sicard, Haguenau, Coste "Vertèbre cancéreuse et para-cancéreuse. Aspects radiologiques : vertèbre blanche, noire, pommelée", *Société de Neurologie de Paris*, meeting of December 4, *Rev Neurol (Paris)*, 1924, T. II, n° 6 (December), pp. 608-611.

Babinski J, Jarkowski J. Addendum to the meetings of March 6, May 1 and July 3, 1924. Quelques documents relatifs aux compressions de la moelle, *Société de Neurologie de Paris*, meeting of December 4, *Rev Neurol (Paris)*, 1924, T. II, n° 6 (December), pp. 648-650.

Joltrain E, présenté par M. Babinski. Un nouveau cas d'anosognosie. *Société de Neurologie de Paris*, meeting of December 4, 1924, *Revue Neurologique (Paris)*, 1924, T. II, n° 6 (December), p. 638-640.

Babinski J. Allocution, meeting of January 11 (RéunionNeurologique de Strasbourg), *Rev Neurol (Paris)*, 1925, T. I, n° 2 (February), p. 242.

284. Babinski J. Eloge de J.-M. Charcot, Discours prononcé à la Sorbonne the May 26, 1925, in *Rev Neurol (Paris)*, June 1925, T.I, n° 6, pp. 746-756. Centenaire de Charcot et 25è anniversaire de la Société de Neurologie de Paris (p. 1120).

Babinski J. Intervention of 14 lines (p. 207), on the paper by Clovis Vincent "Foyer de ramollissement limité au noyau lenticulaire et à la tête du noyau caudé. Aucun symptôme strié", *Société de Neurologie de Paris*, meeting of February 5, *Rev Neurol (Paris)*, 1925, T. I, n° 2 (February), pp. 194-209.

Babinski J, de Martel Th. Tumeur de l'angle ponto-cérébelleux. Amélioration rapide après intervention chirurgicale, *Société de Neurologie de Paris*, meeting of February 5, *Rev Neurol (Paris)*, 1925, T. I, n° 2 (February), p. 209. [This communication will be published in the next issue].

281. Babinski J. Quelques considérations sur l'interrogatoire en clinique et les symptômes subjectifs, *Rev Neurol (Paris)*, 1925, T. I, n° 3 (March), pp. 297-310 (conférence faite le January 11, 1925 à la Réunion neurologique de Strasbourg).

Babinski J. Intervention of 3 lines (p. 246), on the paper by J.A. Barré "Tumeurs du cerveau et traumatismes crâniens", meeting of January 11 (Réunion neurologique de Strasbourg), *Rev Neurol (Paris)*, 1925, T. I, n° 2 (February), pp. 243-249.

Babinski J. Intervention of 11 lines (p. 354), on the paper by Lhermitte "Torticolis spasmodique", *Société de Neurologie de Paris*, meeting of March 5, *Rev Neurol (Paris)*, 1925, T. I, n° 3 (March), pp. 353-354.

282. Babinski J, de Martel. Th. Tumeur de l'angle ponto-cérébelleux. Amélioration rapide à la suite d'une extirpation intra-capsulaire par morcellement, *Société de Neurologie de Paris*, meeting of March 5, addenda to the meeting of February 5, *Rev Neurol (Paris)*, 1925, T. I, n° 3 (March), pp. 371-374.

Babinski J. Intervention of 16 lines (pp. 42-43), on the paper by Georges Guillain, Th. Alajouanine et M. Kalt "La forme myasthénique de l'encéphalite prolongée. - De quelques symptômes myasthéniques consécutifs à l'encéphalite épidémique", *Société de Neurologie de Paris*, meeting of January 7, *Rev Neurol (Paris)*, 1926, T. I, n° 1 (January), pp. 39-44.

Babinski J. Intervention of 24 lines (pp. 583-584), on the paper by J.A. Sicard et J. Haguenau "A propos de l'évolution d'une tumeur infundibulo-hypophysaire traitée par la radiothérapie", *Société de Neurologie de Paris*, meeting of April 15, *Rev Neurol (Paris)*, 1926, T. I, n° 5 (May), pp. 579-584.

Babinski J. Intervention of 15 lines (pp. 590-591), on the paper by Monier-Vinard et Pierre Puech "Syndrome de sclérose latérale amyotrophique post-traumatique", *Société de Neurologie de Paris*, meeting of April 15, *Rev Neurol (Paris)*, 1926, T. I, n° 5 (May), pp. 584-592.

Babinski J, Jarkowski. Intervention of 46 lines (pp. 619-620), on the paper by Serge Davidenk of (de Moscou) "Réflexes de défense, reproduisant le syndrome de la soi-disant "Surréflectivité hyperalgésique" dans un cas d'hémiplégie récente par thrombose artérielle", *Société de Neurologie de Paris*, meeting of April 15, *Rev Neurol (Paris)*, 1926, T. I, n° 5 (May), pp. 614-620.

285. Babinski J, Charpentier A, Jarkowski J. Paraplégie crurale par tumeur extra-dure-mérienne à la région dorsale. Opération. Guérison. (Sur l'épreuve du lipiodol), *Société de Neurologie de Paris*, meeting of December 2, *Rev Neurol (Paris)*, 1926, T. II, pp. 587-595.

Babinski J. Intervention of 11 lines (pp. 235-236), on the paper by Etienne Sorrel et Mme Sorrel-Dejerine "Paraplégie par tumeur juxta-médullaire prise pendant longtemps pour une paraplégie pottique. Ablation trop tardive de la tumeur. Persistance de la paraplégie", *Société de Neurologie de Paris*, meeting of February 3, *Rev Neurol (Paris)*, 1927, T. I, n° 2 (February), pp. 226-236.

Babinski J. Intervention of 13 lines (p. 498), on the paper by Clovis Vincent "La chirurgie des tumeurs intramédullaires en France en 1913. Sur un cas rapporté par Gendron, opéré avec succès par Th. De Martel", *Société de Neurologie de Paris*, meeting of April 7, *Rev Neurol (Paris)*, 1927, T. I, n° 4 (April), pp. 491-498.

Babinski J. Intervention of 22 lines (p. 501), on the paper by Albert Charpentier "A propos des communications de M. Bourguignon sur "l'innervation de quelques muscles de la face par les deux nerfs faciaux", *Société de Neurologie de Paris*, meeting of April 7, *Rev Neurol (Paris)*, 1927, T. I, n° 4 (April), pp. 498-502.

Babinski J. Intervention of 7 lines (p. 89), on the paper by Egas Moniz (de Lisbonne) "L'encéphalographie artérielle, son importance dans la localisation des tumeurs cérébrales", *Société de Neurologie de Paris*, meeting of July 7, *Rev Neurol (Paris)*, 1927, T. II, n° 1 (July), pp. 72-90.

Babinski J. Intervention of 37 lines (pp. 499-500), on the paper by L. Christophe (de Liège), présenté par M. Babinski "Sur la valeur diagnostique d'un arrêt du lipiodol intrarachidien", *Société de Neurologie de Paris*, meeting of November 3, *Rev Neurol (Paris)*, 1927, T. II, n° 5 (November), pp. 490-501.

Babinski J. Intervention of 26 lines (pp. 387-388), on the paper by A. Rouquier (de Lyon) "Syndrome moteur atypique, à forme hémiplégique, d'origine extrapyramidale, séquelle d'une névraxite", *Société de Neurologie de Paris*, meeting of March 1, *Rev Neurol (Paris)*, 1928, T. I, n° 3 (March), pp. 383-388.

287. Babinski J, Jarkowski J. Monoplégie crurale hypertonique, sans signes pyramidaux homolatéraux etavec anesthésie hiomolatérale. – Tumeur intramédullaire de la région lombosacrée, *Société de Neurologie de Paris*, May 2, 1929, *Rev Neurol (Paris)*, 1929, T. I, n° 5 (May), pp. 802-806.

288. Babinski J. Intervention of 66 lines (pp. 1171-1173), on the paper by A. Radovici "L'hystérie et les états hystéroïdes organiques", *Société de Neurologie de Paris*, meeting of June 5, *Rev Neurol (Paris)*, 1930, T. I, n° 6 (June), pp. 1164-1173.

Varia

1. Babinski J. Observations de rechutes pendant la convalescence de la fièvre typhoïde, *Journal des connaissances médicales*, 19 and 26 October 1882.

6. Babinski J. Epilepsie survenue chez un syphilitique et suivie de mort, reconnaissant pour cause une hémorragie méningée, *Revue de Médecine*, 1883.

7. Babinski J. Sur un cas de pseudo-pellagre, *Gazette Médicale de Paris*, 1884, p. 42.

9. Babinski J. Sur un cas de myélite chronique diffuse avec prédominance des lésions dans les cornes antérieures de la moelle, *Revue de Médecine*, 1884.

10. Babinski J, Dejerine. Note sur un cas de pneumonie tuberculeuse avec absence de bacille dans les crachats, *Revue de Médecine*, 1884.

8. Babinski J. Des modifications que présentent les muscles à la suite de la section des nerfs qui s'y rendent, *Comptes rendus de l'Académie des sciences*, January 7, 1884.

11. Babinski J. Sur les lésions des tubes nerveux de la moelle épinière dans la sclérose en plaques, *Comptes rendus de l'Académie des sciences*, June 8, 1884.

12. Babinski J. Recherches sur l'anatomie pathologique de la sclérose en plaques et étude comparative des diverses variétés de sclérose de la moelle, *Archives de Physiologie normale et pathologique*, February 15, 1885.

13. Babinski J. *Étude anatomique et clinique sur la sclérose en plaques*, Thèse, Paris, G. Masson, 1885.

16. Babinski J, Charrin. Sclérose médullaire systématique combinée, *Revue de Médecine*, 1886.

Babinski J. Recherches servant à établir que certaines manifestations hystériques peuvent être transférées d'un sujet à un autre sujet sous l'influence de l'aimant. Paris, A. Delahaye et E. Lecrosnier, 1886, 8 p. (Publications du "Progrès médical").

Babinski J. Recherches servant à établir que certaines manifestations hystériques peuvent être transmises d'un sujet à un autre sujet sous l'influence de l'aimant. *Le Progrès Médical*, 2ème série, 1886, T. IV, n° 47 (November 30), p. 1010-1011 (communication faite à la *Société de psychologie physiologique*, meeting of October 25, 1886). Résumé in *Annales Médico-Psychologiques*, 1891, T. I, pp. 144-145.

24. Babinski J. Faisceaux neuro-musculaires, *Archives de médecine expérimentale*, May 1, 1889.
26. Babinski J. Anatomie pathologique des névrites périphériques (Leçon faite à la Salpêtrière the May 30, 1890. *Gazette hebdomadaire de médecine et de chirurgie*, August 9, 1890.
29. Babinski J. Paraplégie flasque par compression de la moelle, *Archives de Médecine expérimentale et d'Anatomie pathologique*, March 1, 1891.
30. Babinski J. Hypnotisme et hystérie. Du rôle de l'hypnotisme en thérapeutique, Leçon faite à la Salpêtrière le June 23, 1891, *Gazette hebdomadaire*, July 25, 1891, n° 30, pp. 350-360. *Le Progrès Médical*, 1892, n° 47, p. 435 : "M. Babinski présente à la Société deux types de nouveaux marteaux percuteurs dus à M. Blocq."
32. Babinski J. *Notice sur les travaux scientifiques du Dr. J. Babinski*, January 1892, Paris, G. Masson, 1892, 26 pages.
39. Babinski J. *Des névrites*, in Charcot, Bouchard, Brissaud, "Traité de médecine", T.VI, Paris, G. Masson, 1894, pp. 649-834.
Babinski J. Des névrites périphériques, Congrès des aliénistes et neurologistes de France et des pays de langue Française, meeting of August 7, 1894, Analysis in *Rev Neurol (Paris)*, 1894, T. II, n° 16 (August 30), p. 483.
Babinski J. Coïncider le syndrome de Basedow et certains symptômes du myxoedème, Congrès des aliénistes et neurologistes de France et des pays de langue Française, meeting of August 2, 1895, Analysis in *Rev Neurol (Paris)*, 1895, T. III, n° 16 (August 30), p. 484.
Babinski J. communique le résultat de ses observations sur une modification du réflexe cutané plantaire dans certaines affections du système nerveux, *Le Progrès Médical*, 1896, N° 9, p. 137.
Babinski J. Intervention de 24 lines sur le réflexe cutané plantaire au *Congrès International de neurologie, psychiatrie, électricité médicale, hypnologie*, Bruxelles 1897, meeting of September 14, in *Le Progrès Médical*, 1897 (2è semestre), 3è série, T. VI, 25è année, n° 39 (September 25), p. 199.
Meeting of June 25, 1898, *Le Progrès Médical*, 1898, p. 7.
48. Babinski J. Du phénomène des orteils et de sa valeur sémiologique. *SeMayne Médicale*, 1898, 18, 321-322.
54. Babinski J, Charpentier. De l'abolition des réflexes pupillaires dans ses relations avec la syphilis, *Société de Dermatologie*, July 13, 1899.
59. Babinski J. Diagnostic différentiel entre l'hémiplégie organique et l'hémiplégie hystérique (Leçon faite à la Pitié), *Gazette des Hôpitaux*, n° 52, p. 521 (May 5, 1900) et n° 53, p. 533 (8 May 1900), analysis in *Rev Neurol (Paris)*, 1900, T. VIII, n° 16 (August 30), p. 809.
Babinski J. Sur les scléroses combinées, XIIIè Congrès International de Médecine, Paris, August 2-9, 1900, *Journal de Neurologie*, 1900, T. V, pp. 417-418.
87. Babinski J, Nageotte J. Lésions syphilitiques des centres nerveux. Foyers de ramollissement dans le bulbe. Hémiasynergie, latéropulsion et myosis bulbaires avec hémianesthésie et hémiplégie croisées. *Nouvelle iconographie de la Salpêtrière*, 1902, T. XV, n° 6 (November-December), pp. 492-512 [complement to the communication at the *Société de Neurologie de Paris* April 17, 1902, n° **80**].
105. Babinski J. Sur le traitement des affections de l'oreille et en particulier du vertige auriculaire par la rachicentèse, *Académie de médecine*, 28 December 1903. *Annales des maladies de l'oreille et du larynx*, T. XXX, February 2, 1904.
108. Babinski J. Introduction à la sémiologie des maladies du système nerveux. Des symptômes objectifs que la volonté est incapable de reproduire. De leur importance en médecine légale, Leçon faite à la Pitié, *Gazette des hôpitaux*, October 11, 1904.
112. Babinski J. Cyanose des rétines avec rétrécissement pulmonaire, sans cyanose généralisée, *Société d'Ophtalmologie*, December 6, 1904.
116. Babinski J, Melle Toufesco, De la cyanose des rétines dans le rétrécissement de l'artère pulmonaire, *Nouvelle Iconographie de la Salpêtrière*, n° 2, 1905.
Babinski J. *Des névrites*, in Bouchard, Brisseau, "Traité de Médecine", 2è édition, Paris, Masson et Cie, 1905, pp. 1-202.
125. Babinski J. Ma conception de l'hystérie et de l'hypnotisme (Pithiatisme), *Conférence faite à la Société de l'Internat des Hôpitaux de Paris (meeting of June 28, 1906)*, Chartres, Imprimerie Durand, 1906 (31 pages).
132. Babinski J, Chaillous. Du champ visuel et de la vision centrale dans l'atrophie tabétique des nerfs optiques, *Comptes-rendus de la Société d'Ophtalmologie de Paris*, February 7, 1907.
135. Babinski J. Some comments on the paper by M. Sollier entitled: "La définition et la nature de l'hystérie", *Archives générales de médecine*, March 1907.

134. Babinski J. Suggestion et hystérie. A propos de l'article de M. Bernheim intitulé: "Comment je comprends le mot hystérie", *Bulletin Médical*, March 30, 1907, 21:272-276.
137. Babinski J, Chaillous J. Résultats thérapeutiques de la ponction lombaire dans les névrites optiques d'origine intra-crânienne, *Société Française d'Ophtalmologie*, May 1907.
146. Babinski J. Some comments on the paper by M. Sollier entitled: "Définition de l'Hystérie en général et Hystérie infantile", *Presse Médicale*, December 21, 1907.
150. Babinski J. Traitement du vertige de Ménière par la ponction lombaire, Leçon faite à la Pitié, *Journal de Médecine et de Chirurgie pratiques*, June 10, 1908.
Babinski J. Some comments on the paper by M. Valobra entitled: "Contribution à l'étude des gangrènes cutanées spontanées chez les sujets hystériques", *Nouvelle Iconographie de la Salpêtrière*, November and December 1908.
155. Babinski J. Démembrement de l'hystérie traditionnelle. Pithiatisme. *Semaine médicale*, January 6, 1909, 29:3-8.
156. Babinski J. Some comments on the paper by M. Ettore Levi entitled: "Nouvelles recherches graphiques sur le phénomène de la trépidation du pied", *Encéphale*, January 1909.
161. Babinski J. Quelques documents relatifs à l'histoire des fonctions de l'appareil cérébelleux et de leurs perturbations, *Revue de Médecine interne et de thérapeutique*, May 1909, 1, pp. 114-129.
162. Babinski J. On the work of M. Ettore Levy entitled: "Quelques nouveaux faits relatifs à un cas d'Hystérie avec exagération des réflexes tendineux. Réponse aux critiques de M. Babinski", *Encéphale*, July 7, 1909.
165. Babinski J, Jarkowski. Sur la localisation des lésions comprimant la moelle. De la possibilité d'en déterminer le siège au moyen des réflexes de défense, *Académie de Médecine. Bulletin médical*, January 17, 1910.
167. Babinski J. Vertige voltaïque et lésions auriculaires, *Bulletins et Mémoires de la Société de Laryngologie, d'Otologie et de Rhinologie de Paris*, February 12, 1910.
Babinksi J. Crâniectomie dans un cas de tumeur cérébrale, *Journal de Médecine et de Chirurgie Pratiques*, 1909, 10 April, p. 252. Analysis in *Rev Neurol (Paris)*, 1909, T. XVIII, n° 14 (August 15), p. 987 and in *Le Progrès Médical*, 1909, n° 18, p. 234.
170. Babinski J. De la crâniectomie décompressive, *Académie de médecine. Bulletin médical*, April 20, 1910.
173. Babinski J. Utilité de la crâniectomie décompressive dans les tumeurs cérébrales, Leçon faite à la Pitié, *Journal de Médecine et de Chirurgie Pratiques*, June 10, 1910.
175. Babinski J. De l'hypnotisme en thérapeutique et en médecine légale, *Société médicale*, July 27, 1910.
Babinski J, Jarkowski J. Sur la localisation des lésions comprimant la moelle. De la possibilité d'en préciser le siège et d'en déterminer la limite inférieure au moyen des réflexes de défense, *Communication à l'Académie de médecine*, January 16, 1912.
190. Babinski J, Delherm L., Jarkowski J., Contribution à l'étude de la réaction de dégénérescence. Excitabilité faradique latente. Possibilité de la faire apparaître au moyen de la voltaïsation, *Société Française d'Electrothérapie*, March 1912.
191. Babinski J, Dagnan-Bouveret J. Emotion et hystérie, *Journal de Psychologie normale et pathologique*, March-April 1912, 9:97-146.
197. Babinski J. Réflexes tendineux et réflexes osseux, Leçons faites à l'hôpital de la Pitié recueillies par MM. Albert Charpentier et J. Jarkowski et revues par l'auteur, *Le Bulletin Médical*, 28è année, October 19, 1912, pp. 929-936; October 26, 1912, pp. 953-958; November 6, 1912, pp. 985-990; November 23, 1912, pp. 1053-1059. *Extrait du Bulletin Médical, October 19 and 26, November 6 and 23, 1912*. Paris, Imprimerie typographique R. Tancrède, 1912, 80 pages, Analysis in *Le Progrès Médical*, 1913, n° 17, p. 220.
198. Babinski J, Jarkowski J, Jumentié. Méningite cervicale hypertrophique, *Nouvelle Iconographie de la Salpêtrière*, January-February 1913, T. XXVI, pp. 10-19.
207. Babinski J, Tournay A. "Symptômes des maladies du cervelet", Premier rapport, XVIIè Congrès International de Médecine, Londres, August 6-12, 1913, Travaux de la section de Neuropathologie (section XI), Compte-rendu analytique par A. Barré, *Rev Neurol (Paris)*, 1913, T. XXVI, n° 18 (September 30), pp. 306-322.
208. Babinski J. *Exposé des travaux scientifiques*, Paris, Masson et Cie, 1913.
209. Babinski J. Désorientation et déséquilibration provoquées par le courant voltaïque, *Bulletin médical*, November 5, 1913.
211. Babinski J. Désorientation et déséquilibration spontanées et provoquées par le courant voltaïque, *Archives d'électricité médicale*, December 10, 1913.

Bulletin de l'Académie de médecine, 1914 (meeting of 21 July), 78è année, LXXII, 3è série, pp. 10–12.
224. Babinski J, Froment. Troubles physiopathiques d'ordre réflexe. Association avec l'hystérie, *Presse médicale*, July 9, 1915.
226. Babinski J, Froment. Les modifications des réflexes tendineux pendant le sommeil chloroformique et leur valeur en sémiologie, *Journal des Praticiens*, 1915, p. 686.
Babinski J, Froment. Les modifications des réflexes tendineux pendant le sommeil chloroformique et leur valeur en sémiologie, *Académie de Médecine*, October 15, 1915.
229. Babinski J, Froment. Paraplégie et Hypotonie réflexes avec surexcitabilité mécanique, galvanique et faradique, *Académie de Médecine*, January 11, 1916.
241. Babinski J, Froment, Heitz. Des troubles moteurs et thermiques dans les paralysies et la contracture d'ordre réflexe, *Annales de Médecine*, September–October 1916.
230. Babinski J, Froment. Contractures et paraplégies traumatiques d'ordre réflexe, *Presse médicale*, February 24, 1916.
245. Babinski J. A propos de la communication du Dr Bordier sur les réactions électriques d'hypothermie locale, *Bulletin de l'Académie de Médecine*, February 13, 1917.
252. Babinski J, Froment. Sur les troubles physiopathiques et réflexes, *Annales de la Faculté de médecine de Montevideo*, 1917.
248. Babinski J, Froment. Troubles physiopathiques d'ordre réflexe. Association avec l'hystérie. Evolution. Mesures médico-militaires, *Presse médicale*, July 9, 1917.
Babinski J, Dubois R. Tremblement du membre supérieur droit consécutif à une commotion par éclatement d'obus, *Journal du Praticien*, 1917, p. 330.
Babinski J, Froment J. *Hystérie–pithiatisme et troubles nerveux d'ordre réflexe en neurologie de guerre*, Paris, Masson et Cie, 1ère édition, 1917.
251. Babinski J, Froment J. *Hystérie-pithiatisme et troubles nerveux d'ordre réflexe en neurologie de guerre*, Paris, Masson et Cie, 2ème édition, 1918.
Babinski J, Froment J. *Hysteria or pithiatism and reflex nervous disorders in the neurology of war.* London, University of London Press, 1918.
256. Babinski J, Heitz. Les oblitérations artérielles traumatiques. Du rétablissement de la circulation après oblitération de l'artère principale d'un membre, *Archives des maladies du coeur, des vaisseaux et du sang*, n° 11, November 1918, p. 481.
258. Babinski J, Heitz. Les altérations artérielles traumatiques. Des troubles que détermine la lésion de l'artère dans les fonctions du membre blessé, *Archives des maladies du coeur, des vaisseaux et du sang*, December 1919.
Babinski J. Réflexes de défense [A lecture delivered at the Royal Society of medicine, London, with presentation of cases and cinematograph 9 films] *Brain*, 1922, Part 2, vol. 45, pp. 149–184. [Texte en français].
Babinski J, Chaillous J. Stase papillaire et craniectomie décompressive, *Congrès de la Société Française d'Ophtalmologie*, Paris, 8–11, May 1922 (in *La Presse Médicale*, May 11, 1922, n° 42, p. 460).
283. Babinski J. Syndrome cérébelleux, *Bulletin de l'Académie de Médecine*, April 23, 1925.

Olaf (pseudonym of Joseph Babinski) and Palau (1921)

Olaf et Palau, *Les détraquées*, In "Le Grand Guignol, le théâtre des peurs de la Belle Epoque", Foreword and notices by Agnès Pierron, Paris, Robert Laffont, 1995, pp. 808–839.

Œuvre scientifique (1934)

Babinski J. *Œuvre scientifique : recueil des principaux travaux*, publié par les soins de J.A. Barré, J. Chaillous, A. Charpentier, O. Crouzon, L. Delherm, J. Froment, Cl. Gautier, Ed. Hartmann, Ed. Krebs, R. Monier-Vinard, R. Moreau, A. Plichet, Aug. Tournay, Cl. Vincent, G.A. Weill, Paris, Masson et Cie, 1934.

His teacher's lessons

Two volumes of the *Leçons sur le système nerveux* by Charcot
Cornil V. Leçons professées pendant le premier semestre de l'année 1883-84 par M. Cornil, Professeur d'anatomie pathologique à la Faculté de médecine de Paris et recueillies par MM. Berlioz, Babinski, Gibier, Chantemesse, avec 25 figures intercalées dans le texte, Paris, Ancienne Librairie German Baillière et Cie, Félix Alcan éditeur, 1884.

Saturday clinical lectures

hématomyélie avec syndrome de Brown-Séquard (*Journal des Praticiens*, 1915, n° 4, p. 55 and *Journal des Praticiens*, 1914, p. 487),
hémisection traumatique de la moelle (Journal des Praticiens, 1915, n° 4, p. 55),
hémiplégie post-spasmodique (ou hémichorée post-hémiplégiqe) (*Journal des Praticiens*, 1915, p. 407),
paralysie faciale d'origine auriculaire (*Journal des Praticiens*, 1915, p. 8),
myopathies (*Journal des Praticiens*, 1915, p. 117),
hystérie (*Journal des Praticiens*, 1915, p. 134),
myasthénie (*Journal des Praticiens*, 1915, p. 215),
syndrome de Weber (*Journal des Praticiens*, 1915, p. 261),
parésie d'origine circulatoire (*Journal des Praticiens*, 1915, p. 390),
abcès cérébral latent (*Journal des Praticiens*, 1915, p. 517),
syndrome thalamique (*Journal des Praticiens*, 1916, p. 103),
diagnostic de maladie de Parkinson (*Journal des Praticiens 1916*, p. 165),
association hystéro-organique. Hémiplégie. Hémianopsie thermo-asymétrie (*Journal des Praticiens*, 1917, pCCCXXX)

Forewords

Charcot J-M. *Leçons du mardi à la Salpêtrière; Policliniques 1887-1888*. Notes de cours de MM. Blin, Charcot et Colin, Paris, Bureaux du Progrès Médical, Librairie A. Delahaye et Emile Lecrosnier, 1887. *Leçons du mardi à la Salpêtrière*; notes de cours de MM. Blin, Charcot [fils] et Colin; avant-propos de Jacques Sédat; préface de Joseph Babinski. – Paris: C. Tchou pour la Bibliothèque des introuvables, 2002, 2 vol. (XIX-748, p. 692) (*Collection Psychanalyse*) : Tome 1, Policliniques 1887-1888; Tome 2, Policliniques, 1888-1889.
Chiray M, Dagnan-Bouveret J. *La prothèse fonctionnelle des paralysies et des contractures*, Paris, A. Maloine et fils, 1919.
Fontecilla O, Sepulveda R M-A. *Le liquide céphalo-rachidien. Etudes cliniques*, Paris, A. Maloine et fils, 1921.
Bidou G. *Nouvelle méthode d'appareillage des impotents*, Paris, P.U.F., 1923, in-8°, 159 gravures.
Lavielle L et R. *Dax médical et thermal : études cliniques sur la station*, Paris, Maloine, 1930.
Moniz E. *Diagnostic des tumeurs cérébrales et épreuve de l'encéphalographie artérielle*, Paris, Masson et Cie, 1931.

Analyses published in the Revue Neurologique[5]

Analyse de Babinski J. "Du phénomène des orteils et de sa valeur sémiologique", *Semaine médicale*, 1898, n° 40, p. 321, in *Rev Neurol (Paris)*, 1899, T. VII, n° 2 (January 30), p. 63.

---

[5] These analysis figure in the Index of the *Revue Neurologique* under the name of Babinski.

Analyse de Babinski J. "Sur le réflexe du tendon d'Achille dans le tabes", *Gazette des Hôpitaux*, 1898, n° 128 (1 November 1898), p. 1182, in *Rev Neurol (Paris)*, 1899, T. VII, n° 6 (March 30), p. 63.

Analyse de Babinski J. Sur une forme de paraplégie spasmodique consécutive à une lésion organique et sans dégénération du système pyramidal, *Société Médicale des Hôpitaux de Paris*, meeting of March 24, 1899, *Bulletins et Mémoires de la Société Médicale des Hôpitaux de Paris*, 1899, T. XVI, 3è série, pp. 342–354, in *Rev Neurol (Paris)*, 1899, T. VII, n° 11 (June 15), pp. 425–426.

Work of Marinesco, reported by Babinski J., Sur deux cas de paraplégie flasque due à la compression du faisceau pyramidal sans dégénérescence de ce dernier, avec signe de Babinski et absence de réflexes tendineux et cutanés, *Société de Neurologie de Paris*, meeting of March 3, *Rev Neurol (Paris)*, 1904, T. XII, n° 6 (March 30), p. 332. [texte intégral in *Rev Neurol (Paris)*, 1904, T. XII, n° 5 (March 15), pp. 210–218.]

Analysis by Babinski J. "Sur le mécanisme du vertige voltaïque", *Société de Biologie*, March 14, 1903, Comptes-rendus p. 532, in *Rev Neurol (Paris)*, 1904, T. XII, n° 11 (June 15), p. 532.

Analysis by A. Léri on Babinski J. "Sur le traitement des affections de l'oreille et en particulier du vertige auriculaire par la rachicentèse", *Annales des maladies de l'oreille et du larynx*, February 1904, in *Rev Neurol (Paris)*, 1904, T. XII, n° 15 (August 15), p. 849.

Analysis by Babinski J. on "Sur les mouvements d'inclination et de rotation de la tête dans le vertige voltaïque", *Société de Biologie*, meeting of April 25, 1903, in *Rev Neurol (Paris)*, 1904, T. XII, n° 17 (September 15), pp. 947–948.

Analysis by A. Thomas on Babinski J. "Sur le traitement des affections de l'oreille et en particulier du vertige auriculaire par la rachicentèse", *Annales des maladies de l'oreille et du larynx*, February 1904, in *Rev Neurol (Paris)*, T. XII, n° 18 (September 30), p. 991.

Analysis by P. Sainton on Babinski J. "Méningite hémorragique fibrineuse. Paraplégie spasmodique. Ponctions lombaires. Traitement mercuriel. Guérison", *Bulletin de la Société médicale des Hôpitaux de Paris*, October 29, 1903, pp. 1083–1089, in *Rev Neurol (Paris)*, T. XII, n° 19 (October 15), pp. 1012–1013.

Analysis by P. Sainton on Babinski J. "Pemphigus hystérique", *Bulletins et Mémoires de la Société Médicale des Hôpitaux de Paris*, December 3, 1903, 6 lines de Babinski, in *Rev Neurol (Paris)*, 1904, T. XII, n° 19 (October 15), p. 1016.

Analysis by P. Sainton on Babinski J. "Sur l'albuminurie prétendue hystérique", *Bulletins et Mémoires de la Société Médicale des Hôpitaux de Paris*, December 3, 1903, p. 1334, in *Rev Neurol (Paris)*, 1904, T. XII, n° 19 (October 15), p. 1017.

Analysis by P. Sainton on Babinski J. "A propos de l'albuminurie prétendue hystérique", *Bulletins et Mémoires de la Société Médicale des Hôpitaux de Paris*, in *Rev Neurol (Paris)*, 1904, T. XII, n° 19 (October 15), p. 1017.

Analysis by A. Thomas on Babinski J. "Traité des maladies de l'enfance", 2è édition, publiée sous la direction de J. Gaucher et J. Comby, T. IV, *Maladies nerveuses*, par Comby, Babinski, Dupré, Méry et armand-Delille, Paris, Masson et Cie, 1905 [Babinski a rédigé l'article Méningites cérébro-spinale épidémique], in *Rev Neurol (Paris)*, 1905, T. XIII, n° 1 (January 15), p. 26.

Analysis by Thoma on Babinski J. "Introduction à la sémiologie des maladies du système nerveux", *Gazette des Hôpitaux*, October 11, 1904, n° 116, p. 1125, in *Rev Neurol (Paris)*, 1905, T. XIII, n° 11 (June 15), p. 583.

Analysis by Feindel on Babinski J, Melle Toufesco S. "De la cyanose des rétines dans le rétrécissement de l'artère pulmonaire", *Nouvelle Iconographie de la Salpêtrière*, an XVIII, fasc. 2, pp. 194–200, March–April 1905, in *Rev Neurol (Paris)*, 1906, T. XIV, n° 3 (February 15), p. 124.

Analysis by E. Feindel of the "Traité de médecine Bouchard-Brissaud, 2è édition, T. X, Maladies du système nerveux périphérique, Maladies nerveuses fonctionnelles ou de pathogénie indéterminée, Maladies mentales et syndromes mentaux", par J. Babinski, etc., Paris, Masson et Cie, 1904, in *Rev Neurol (Paris)*, 1906, T. XIV, n° 6 (March), pp. 257–258 [Babinski a rédigé le chapitre *Névrites*].

Analysis of Babinski J. "Hémispasme facial périphérique", par J. Babinski, *Nouvelle Iconographie de la Salpêtrière*, an XVIII, n° 4, pp. 419–424, July–August 1905, in *Rev Neurol (Paris)*, 1906, T. Xiv, n° 18 (September 30), pp. 858–859.

Analysis by Félix Patry on Babinski J, Nageotte J. "Note sur un cas de tabes à systématisation exceptionnelle", *Société de Biologie*, 1905, comptes-rendus p. 281, in *Rev Neurol (Paris)*, 1907, T. XV, n° 4 (February 28) p. 153.

Analysis by P. Londe on Babinski J. "Ma conception de l'hystérie et de l'hypnotisme", *Archives Générales de Médecine*, n° 35, August 28, 1906, in *Rev Neurol (Paris)*, 1907, T. XV, n° 4 (February 28), p. 159.

Analysis by Paul Sainton on Babinski J. "Contracture généralisée due à une compression de la moelle cervicale très améliorée à la suite de l'usage des Rayons X", *Bulletins et Mémoires de la Société Médicale des Hôpitaux de Paris*, December 6, 1906, pp. 1205-1210, in *Rev Neurol (Paris)*, 1907, T. XV, n° 9 (May 15), pp. 449-450.

Analysis by Feindel on Babinski J. "Suggestion et hystérie. A propos de l'article de M. Bernheim intitulé : "Comment je comprends le mot hystérie", *Bulletin Médocal*, an XXI, n° 24, March 30, 1907, pp. 273-277, in *Rev Neurol (Paris)*, 1907, T. XV, n° 13 (July 15), p. 672.

Analysis by Péchin on Babinski J. "Du champ visuel et de la vision centrale dans l'atrophie tabétique des nerfs optiques", *Société d'Ophtalmologie de Paris*, February 7, 1907, in *Rev Neurol (Paris)*, 1907, T. XV, n° 14 (July 31), pp. 716-717.

Analysis by P. Londe on Babinski J. "Quelques remarques sur l'article de M. Sollier intitulé : "La définition et la nature de l'hystérie", Archives Générales de Médecine, 1907, n° 3, p. 271, in *Rev Neurol (Paris)*, 1907, T. XV, n° 19 (October 15), p. 1055.

Analysis of Babinski J, Chaillous. "Résultats thérapeutiques de la ponction lombaire dans les névrites optiques d'origine intra-crânienne", Société Française d'Ophtalmologie, May 1907, *Rev Neurol (Paris)*, 1907, T. XV, n° 24 (December 30), pp. 1281-1282.

Analysis by Feindel on Babinski J. "Valeur sémiologique du signe d'Argyll-Robertson et de l'abolition du réflexe achilléen", La Clinique, p. 426, July 5, 1907, *Rev Neurol (Paris)*, 1908, T. XVI, n° 15 (August 15), p. 794.

Analysis by Paul Sainton on Babinski J. "Sur les prétendus troubles trophiques de la peau dans l'hystérie", *Bulletins et Mémoires de la Société Médicale des Hôpitaux de ParisParis*, December 12, 1907, pp. 1379-1383, *Rev Neurol (Paris)*, 1908, T. XVI, n° 15 (August 15), p. 816.

Analysis by Paul Sainton on Babinski J. "De la radiothérapie dans les paralysies spasmodiques spinales", *Bulletins et Mémoires de la Société Médicale des Hôpitaux de Paris*, n° 8, March 7, 1907, pp. 208-213, *Rev Neurol (Paris)*, 1908, T. XVI, n° 17 (September 15), pp. 925-926.

Analysis by Feindel on Babinski J. "Anesthésie généralisée et atrophie de la cuisse chez un accidenté du travail", *La Clinique*, n° 28, July 10, 1908, p. 441, *Rev Neurol (Paris)*, 1909, T. XVII/XVIII, n° 2 (January 30), p. 83.

Analysis par E. Feindel de Babinski J. "Importance diagnostique du phénomène des orteils", *Journal de Médecine et de Chirurgie Pratiques*, April 10, 1909, p. 250, *Rev Neurol (Paris)*, 1909, T. XVII, n° 13 (July 15), pp. 836-837.

Analysis by Feindel on Babinski J. "Hémiplégie hystérique avec mutisme datant de dix ans et suivie de guérison", *Journal de Médecine et de Chirurgie Pratiques*, April 10, 1909, p. 248, *Rev Neurol (Paris)*, 1909, T. XVII, n° 14 (July 30), p. 917.

Analysis by Feindel on Babinski J. "Crâniectomie dans un cas de tumeur cérébelleuse", *Journal de Médecine et de Chirurgie Pratiques*, April 10, 1909, p. 251, *Rev Neurol (Paris)*, 1909, T. XVIII, n° 14 (August 15), p. 987.

Analysis by E. Feindel on Babinski J. "Quelques remarques sur le mémoire de M. Ettore Levi intitulé: "Nouvelles recherches graphiques sur le phénomène de la trépidation du pied", *L'Encéphale*, An IV, n° 1, January 1909, pp. 40-44, *Rev Neurol (Paris)*, 1909, T. XVIII, n° 19 (October 15), p. 1226.

Analysis by E. Feindel on Babinski J. "Démembrement de l'hystérie traditionnelle. Pithiatisme", *La Semaine Médicale*, an XXIX, n° 1, January 6, 1909, pp. 3-8, *Rev Neurol (Paris)*, 1909, T. XVIII, n° 20 (October 30), pp. 1291-1293.

Analysis of Babinski J. "Quelques documents relatifs à l'histoire des fonctions de l'appareil cérébelleux et de leurs perturbations", *Revue mensuelle de médecine interne et de thérapeutique*, An I, n° 2, May 15, 1909, pp. 113-129, *Rev Neurol (Paris)*, 1909, T. XVIII, n° 23 (December 15), pp. 1474-1476.

Analysis of Babinski J. "propos du travail de M. Ettore Levi intitulé : "Quelques nouveaux faits relatifs à un cas d'hystérie avec forte exagération des réflexes tendineux", *L'Encéphale*, an IV, n° 7 (July 10, 1909), pp. 62-63, *Rev Neurol (Paris)*, 1910, T. XIX, n° 2 (January 30), p. 97.

Analysis of Babinski J. "Paralysie alterne (syndrome Millard-Gübler)", *Journal des Praticiens*, October 9, 1909, p. 645, *Rev Neurol (Paris)*, 1910, T. XX, n° 13 (July 15), p. 20 et n° 15 (August 15), p. 175.

Analysis by Feindel on Babinski J. "Quelques cas de tabes fruste", *Journal de Médecine et de Chirurgie Pratiques*, T. LXXXI, n° 11, June 10, 1910, p. 407, *Rev Neurol (Paris)*, 1911, T. XXI, n° 6 (March 30), p. 353-354.

Analysis by E. Feindel on Babinski J. "Utilité de la crâniectomie décompressive dans les tumeurs cérébrales", *Journal de Médecine et de Chirurgie Pratiques*, T. LXXXI, n° 11, June 10, 1910, p. 407, *Rev Neurol (Paris)*, 1911, T. XXI, n° 7 (April 15), p. 435.

Analysis by Babinski J. "De la crâniectomie décompressive", *Le Bulletin Médical*, an XXIV, n° 32, April 20, 1910, p. 371, *Rev Neurol (Paris)*, 1911, T. XXII, n° 13 (July 15), pp. 27-28.

Analyse by Feindel on Babinski J, Gendron A. "Leucocytose du liquide céphalo-rachidien au cours du ramollissement de l'écorce cérébrale", *Bulletin et Mémoires de la Société Médicale des Hôpitaux de Paris*, an XXVIII, March 28, 1912, pp. 370-374, *Rev Neurol (Paris)*, 1912, T. XXIV, n° 21 (November 15), pp. 498-499.

Analysis by E. Feindel on Babinski J, Jarkowski J. "Sur la localisation des lésions comprimant la moelle. Possibilité d'en préciser le siège et d'en déterminer la limite inférieure au moyen des réflexes de défense", *Le Bulletin Médical*, an XXVI, n° 5, January 17, 1912, p. 49, *Rev Neurol (Paris)*, 1912, T. XXIV, n° 13 (July 15), p. 20.

Analysis by Babinski J, Jumentié J. "Contribution à l'étude de l'hémorragie méningée", *Bulletins et Mémoires de la Société Médicale des Hôpitaux de Paris*, June 6, 1912, an XXVIII, p. 744, in *Rev Neurol (Paris)*, 1913, T. XXV, n° 1 (January 15), pp. 27-28.

Analysis of Babinski J. "Réflexes tendineux et réflexes osseux", *Bulletin Médical*, p. 929, 953, 985 et 1053, 19 et 26 October, 6 et November 23, 1912, in *Rev Neurol (Paris)*, 1913, T. XXV, n° 12 (June30), pp. 809-817.

Analysis par E. Feindel de Babinski J, Enriquez E, Durand (Gaston). "Pseudo-coxalgie et appendicite", *Bulletins et Mémoires de la Société Médicale des Hôpitaux de Paris*, July 18, 1913, an XXIX, n° 26, pp. 191-199, in *Rev Neurol (Paris)*, 1913, T. XXVI, n° 19 (October 15), pp. 413-414.

Analysis by E. Feindel on Babinski J, Jumentié J, Jarkowski J. "Méningite cervicale hypertrophique", *Nouvelle Iconographie de la Salpêtrière*, an XXVI, January February 1913, pp. 10-19, in *Rev Neurol (Paris)*, 1913, T. XXVI, n° 21 (November 15), p. 547.

Analysis by F. Allard on Babinski J. "Désorientation et déséquilbration produites par le courant voltaïque", *Archives d'électricité médicale*, December 10, 1913, pp. 10-19, in *Rev Neurol (Paris)*, 1914, T. XXVII, n° 6 (March 30), p. 409.

Analysis by E. Feindel on Babinski J, Dagnan-Bouveret J. "Emotion et hystérie", *Journal de Psychologie*, 1912, an IX, n° 2 (March-April), pp. 97-146, in *Rev Neurol (Paris)*, 1914, T. XXVII, n° 12 (June 30), pp. 819-821.

Analysis by F. Allard on Babinski J, Delherm, Jarkowski J. "Emploi simultané de deux courants en électrodiagnostic et en électrothérapie. La réaction faradique latente, la farado-galvanisation, la galvano-galvanisation", *Archives d'électricité médicale*, June 10, 1913, in *Rev Neurol (Paris)*, 1914, T. XXVII, n° 3 (February 15), p. 191.

Analysis of Babinski J, Weill GA. "Désorientation et déséquilibration spontanée et provoquée. La déviation angulaire", *Comptes-rendus de la Société de Biologie*, T. LXXIV, *n° 15 (April 26, 1913), p. 852*, *Rev Neurol (Paris)*, 2è semestre 1914-1915, T. XXVIII, n° 16 (April 1915), p. 254.

Analysis of Babinski J, Weill GA. "Mouvements réactionnels d'origine vestibulaire et mouvements contre-réactionnels", *Comptes-rendus de la Société de Biologie*, T. LXXV, *n° 27 (July 19, 1913), p. 98*, *Rev Neurol (Paris)*, 2è semestre 1914-1915, T. XXVIII, n° 16 (April 1915), p. 255.

Analysis of Babinski J, Froment J. "Les modifications des réflexes tendineux pendant le sommeil chloroformique et leur valeur en sémiologie", *Bulletins de l'Académie de Médecine*, T. LXXIV, October 19, 1915, p. 439, *Rev Neurol (Paris)*, 2è semestre 1914-1915, T. XXVIII, n° 23-24 (November-December 1915) "Neurologie de guerre", p. 986.

236. Analysis of Babinski J, Froment J. "Contractures et paralysies traumatiques d'ordre réflexe", *La Presse Médicale*, n° 11, p. 81, February 24, 1916, *Rev Neurol (Paris)*, 2è semestre 1914-1915, T. XXVIII, n° 4-5 (April-May 1916), pp. 687-688.

Analysis by E. Feindel. de Babinski J, Froment J. "Névrite irradiante ou contracture d'ordre réflexe", *Société Médicale des Hôpitaux de Paris*, meeting of May 18, 1916, *Bulletins et Mémoires de la Société Médicale des Hôpitaux de Paris*, 1916, XXXII, n° 15-16, p. 677, *Rev Neurol (Paris)*, 1916, T. XXIX, n° 11-12 (November-December 1916), pp. 425-426.

Analysis of Babinski J, Heitz J. "Oblitérations artérielles et troubles vaso-moteurs d'origine réflexe ou centrale. Leur diagnostic différentiel par l'oscillométrie et l'épreuve du bain chaud", *Société Médicale des Hôpitaux de Paris*, meeting of April 14, 1916, *Bulletins et Mémoires de la Société Médicale des Hôpitaux de Paris*, 1916, T. XL, 3è série, pp. 570–575, *Rev Neurol (Paris)*, 1916, T. XXIX, n° 11–12 (November–December 1916), p. 429.

Analysis by Mme A. Bénisty on Babinski J, Froment J. "Hystérie, pithiatisme et troubles nerveux d'ordre réflexe", 1 volume. *Rev Neurol (Paris)*, 1917 (1er semestre), n° 6 (June), pp. 322–324.

Analysis by E.F. on Babinski J. "A propos de la communication du docteur H. Bordier sur les réactions électriques d'hypothermie locale", *Bulletin de l'Académie de Médecine*, T. 77, n° 7 (February 13, 1917), p. 182. *Rev Neurol (Paris)*, 1917 (1er semestre), n° 6 (June), pp. 330–331.

Analysis by N.R. on Babinski J, Froment J, Heitz J. "Des troubles vaso-moteurs et thermiques dans les paralysies et les contractures d'ordre réflexe", *Annales de Médecine*, T. III, n° 5, September 1916. *Rev Neurol (Paris)*, 1917 (1er semestre), n° 6 (June), pp. 430–431.

Analysis by E. Feindel on Babinski J, Froment J. "Hystérie, pithiatisme et troubles nerveux d'ordre réflexe", 1 volume, 2ème édition (1918). *Rev Neurol (Paris)*, 1918 (1er semestre), T. 34, n° 5–6 (May–June), pp. 335–336.

Analysis of Babinski J. Froment J. "Les modifications des réflexes tendineux pendant le sommeil chloroformique et leur valeur en sémiologie",*Lyon Médical, November* 1915, *p. 347. Rev Neurol (Paris),* 1918 (2ndè semester), T. 34, n° 9–10 (September–October), p. 81.

Analysis by E. Feindel on Babinski J. Froment J. "Sur les troubles physiopathiques d'ordre réflexe", *Anales de la Facultad de Medicina de Montevideo*, T. II, fasc. 9–10 (October–November 1917), pp. 569–585. *Rev Neurol (Paris)*, 1918 (2è semestre), T. 34, n° 11–12 (November–December 1918), pp. 252–253.

Analysis of Babinski J, Heitz J. "Les oblitérations artérielles traumatiques; du rétablissement de la circulation après oblmitération de l'artère principale d'un membre", Archives des maladies du cœur, des vaisseaux et du sang, n° 11 (November 1918), p. 481, in *Rev Neurol (Paris)*, 1921, T. 37, n° 4 (April 1921), pp. 387–388.

Analysis by E. Feidendel on Babinski J. "Syndrome cérébelleux", *Bulletin de l'académie de Médecine*, T. 39, n° 16 (April 23, 1925), p. 422, in *Rev Neurol (Paris)*, 1925, T. II, n° 1 (July), p. 264.

Henri Babinski (alias Ali-Bab) papers

Ali-Bab. *Gastronomie Pratique. Études Culinaires suivies du Traitement de L'Obésité des Gourmands.* Paris, Ernest Fammarion, 1ère édition, 1907, 314 pages.

Ali-Bab. *Gastronomie Pratique. Études Culinaires suivies du Traitement de L'Obésité des Gourmands.* Paris, Fammarion, 7è édition, 1928.

Ali-Bab. *Encyclopedia of practical gastronomy* (translated by Elisabeth Benson), New York, McGraw-Hill Book Company, 1974.

Ali-Bab. *Gastronomie Pratique. Études Culinaires suivies du Traitement de L'Obésité des Gourmands.* Paris, Fammarion, 2001.

Babinski H. *Quelques mots sur les gisements aurifères de la Guyane française et en particulier sur les recherches des filons dans cette contrée. Suivis d'une notice sommaire sur les gisements appartenant à la Société de Saint-Elie.* Paris, Imprimerie Barthe et fils, 1888.

Babinski H. Obituary Bertrand Joseph Jean Marie Bruno Chaumond (1853–1888), *Bulletin de l'Association des anciens élèves de l'Ecole des Mines de Paris,* January–February 1888.

Babinski H. *Note sur une excursion dans le Canavese, présentée à la deuxième assemblée générale des actionnaires de la Société des placers aurifères du Piémont,* société anonyme à capital variable, Paris, Imprimerie Chaix, 1888.

Babinski H. *Note sur l'exploitation des alluvions aurifères du nord de l'Italie,* Paris, Imprimerie Chaix, 1889.

Babinski H. *Note sur les concessions réunies d'Adieu-Vat et de Bonne-Aventure, appartenant à la société des gisements d'or de Saint-Elie (Guyane française),* Paris, Imprimerie et Librairie centrales des chemins de fer, Imprimerie Chaix, 1890.

Babinski H. *Rapport sur une visite aux "Lauras diamantinas", gisements de diamant et de carbon de Lençoes, Palmeiras, San Antonio, Chique-Chique et Mar d'Hespanha, Etat de Bahia, (Brésil),* Paris, Imprimerie Chaix, 1897.

Babinski H. Obituary Léon Benoist (1855–1906) *Bulletin de l'Association des anciens élèves de l'Ecole des Mines de Paris,* 1907.

Babinski H. *Quelques conseils aux jeunes camarades qui désirent être chargés de missions*, Lille, Lefebvre-Ducrocq impr., 1914 (extrait du *Bulletin de l'Association amicale des Elèves de l'Ecole Nationale supérieure des Mines*, April 1914).
Babinski H. Obituary Joseph Obalski (1852–1915) *Bulletin de l'Association des anciens élèves de l'Ecole des Mines de Paris*, July–August 1915.
Babinski H. Obituary Leopold Michel (1846–1919) *Bulletin de l'Association amicale des anciens élèves de l'Ecole des Mines de Paris*, January–February–March 1920.
Babinski H. Preface to Pomiane E. de. *Bien manger pour bien vivre. Essai de gastronomie théorique*, Paris, Albin Michel, 1922.
Babinski H. Ceremony welcoming the Engineers of Cracow Mines School at the Association office in Paris. Translation from Polish of M. Babinski's speech. *Bulletin de l'Association des anciens élèves de l'Ecole des mines de Paris*, December 1923.

Dictionaries and encyclopaedias

French

Dictionnaire de Médecine Flammarion, Paris, Médecine-Sciences Flammarion, 1994.
Dictionnaire médical Masson, Paris, Masson, 1997.
Grand dictionnaire encyclopédique Larousse, 10 volumes, Paris, Librairie Larousse, 1982.
Grand Larousse en 5 volumes, Paris, Larousse éd., 1989.
WHO'S Who in France XXè siècle, Dictionnaire biographique des Français disparus ayant marqué le XXè siècle, Paris, Editions Jacques Lafitte, 2001 (1ère édition).
Ambrière M (sous la direction de). *Dictionnaire du XIXè siècle européen*, Paris, Puf, 1997.
Augé C. *Nouveau Larousse illustré, supplément* (s.d. circa 1906).
Colin A. *Dictionnaire des noms illustres en médecine, 1000 personnages célèbres de l'histoire médicale de l'antiquité classique au début du XX7 siècle*, Bruxelles, Prodim, 1994.
Galtier-Boissiere (sous la direction de). *Larousse médical illustré*, Paris, Librairie Larousse, circa 1932.
Hill GS. *Dictionary of medical and biological terms and medications*, Paris, Flammarion Médecine-sciences, 2005.
Julliard J, Winock M. (sous la direction de). *Dictionnaire des intellectuels français*, Paris, Seuil, nouvelle édition 2002.
Lépine P. *Dictionary of medical and biological terms*, Paris, Flammarion Médecine-Sciences, 1974.
Les noms en neurologie, Le Raincy, Congrès Relation, 2004.
Morel P. *Dictionnaire biographique de la psychiatrie*, Le Plessis-Robinson, Synthélabo, 1966.
Morel P. *Dictionnaire biographique de la psychiatrie*, Paris, Les empêcheurs de penser en rond, 1996.
Prévost M, Roman d'Amat (sous la direction de). *Dictionnaire de biographie française*, T. IV, Paris, Librairie Letouzay et Ané, 1948.
Rapin M (sous la direction de). *Le grand dictionnaire encyclopédique médical*, Paris, Flammarion, 1986.
Robert P (sous la direction de), rédaction générale : Alain Rey et Josette Rey-Debove. *Le grand Robert des noms propres. Dictionnaire universel alphabétique et analogique des noms propres*, Paris, Le Robert éd., 1980, 1989.
Vapereau G. *Dictionnaire universel des contemporains*, 5è édition, Paris, Librairie Hachette, 1980.
Vapereau G. *Dictionnaire universel des contemporains*, 6è éd., Paris, Librairie Hachette, 1893.

Polish

Slownik Jezyka Polskiego, Lwow, Worukarni Zakladu Ossolinskich, 1854 [*Polish Language Dictionary*, Lwow, Worukarni Zakladu Ossolinskich, 1854].
Wielka Encyklopedya Powszechna ilustrowana, Warszawa, Naklad Druk S. Sikorskiego, 40 tomes, 1891 [*Great Universal Illustrated Encyclopedia*, 40 vol., Warsaw, Naklad Druk S. Sikorskiego, 1891].

S. *Orgelbranda Encyklopedja Powszechna z ilustracjami i mapami*, Warszawa, S. Orgelbranda synow, 1898 [*S. Orgelbranda Illustrated (with maps) Encyclopaedia*, Warsaw, S. Orgelbranda ed., 1898].
Ilustrowana Encyklopedja Trzaski, Everta i Michalskiego, Opracowana pod redakcja Dra Stanislawa Lama, Warszawa, Nakladem Ksiegarni Trzaski, Everta i Michalskiego, 5 tomes, 1927 [*Traska Evert and Michalski Illustrated Encyclopaedia*, directed by stanislaw Lam, 5 volumes, Warsaw, Evert and Michalsk, 1927].
Slownik Jezyka Polskiego, Redaktor naczelny Witold Doroszewski, Warszawa, Panstwowe Wydawnictwo Wiedza Powszechna, 1958 [*Polish Language Dictionary*, Witold Doroszewski (ed. by), Warsaw, National Scientific Editions, 1958].
Encyklopedia Katolicka, Lublin, 1973 [*Catholic Encyclopaedia*, Lublin, 1973].
Wielka Encyklopedia Powszechna Pwn, Warszawa, Panstwowe Wydawnictwo Naukowe Pwn, 1978-1993 [*Great Universal Encyclopaedia PWN*, Warsaw, National Scientific Editions, 1978-1993].
Encyklopedia Powszechna Pwn, Wydanie Drugie, Warszawa, Pwn, 4 tomes, 1983 [*Universal Encyclopaedia PWN*, by Wydanie Drugie, Warsaw, 4 vol., PWN, 1983].
Zygmunt Gloger Encyklopedia staropolska ilustrowana, Warszawa, Wiedza Powszechna, 4 tomes, 1985 [*Cultured Illustrated Zygmunt Gloger Encyclopaedia*, 4 vol., Warsaw, Universal Editions, 1985].
Encyklopedia Staropolska, 2 tomes, Warszawa, Panstwowe Wydawnictwo Naukowe, 1990 [*Cultured Encyclopaedia*, 2 vol., Warsaw, National Scientific Edition, 1990].
Slownik Jezyka Polskiego, Redaktor naukowy : Pr Dr Mieczyslaw Szymczak, Warszawa, 3 tomes, Wydawnictwo Naukowe Pwn, 1993 [*Polish Language Dictionary*, Pr Dr Mieczyslaw szymczak (ed. by), 3 vol., Warsaw, National Scientific Editions, 1990].
Encylopedia Polski, Krakow, 1996 [*Polish Encyclopaedia*, Krakow, 1996].
Maly ilustrowany Leksykon Pwn, Warszawa, Wydawnictwo Naukowe Pwn, 1997 [*Brief Illustrated Lexicon*, PWN, Warsaw, National Scientific Editions PWN, 1997].
Mala Encyklopedia Powszechna Pwn, 1 tome, 1220 pages, Warszawa, Wydawnictwo Naukowe Pwn, 1997 [*Brief Universal Encyclopaedia PWN*, 1 vol., 1220 p., Warsaw, National Scientific Editions PWN, 1997].
Nowy Leksykon Pwn, 1 tome, 2030 pages, Warszawa, Wydawnictwo Naukowe Pwn, 1998 [*New Lexicon PWN*, 1 vol., 2030 p., Warsaw, National Scientific Editions PWN, 1998].
Wielka Encyklopedia Polski, Slowo wstene Jaroslaw Marek Rymkiewicz, 2 tomes, Krakow, Wydawnictwo Tyszard Kluszczynski, 2004 [*Great Polish Encyclopaedia*, Vol. 1, Krakow, Ryszard Kluczynski, 2004 (Foreword by Jaroslaw Rymkiewicz)].

Others

Chamber's Encyclopaedia. A dictionary of universal knowledge, London and Edinburgh, William & Robert Chambers, Limited, Philadelphia, JB Lippincott Company, 10 volumes, 1901.
Der Grosse Brodhaus. Handbuch des Missens in zwanzig bänden, Leipzig, JU Brodhaus, 20 tomes, 1929.
The Encyclopedia Americana, Editor in chief AH Mc Dannald, 30 volumes, New York, Chicago, Americana Corporation, 1946.
Dictionary of scientific biography, Editor in chief Gillispie CC, New York, Charles Scribner's sons, 1981 (8 volumes and supplements).
Encyclopaedia Britannica. A new survey of universal knowledge, Chicago, London, Toronto, Encyclopaedia Britannica, Ltd, 24 volumes, 1959.
Lietuviskoji Tarybine Enciklopedija, Vilnius, Leidykla "Mosklas", 9 tomes, 1976.

Medical journals archives

The following files have been systematically analysed:
Archives de Neurologie
Bulletins et Mémoires de la Société médicale des hôpitaux de Paris

Compte-rendus de la Société anatomique
Compte-rendus de la Société de Biologie
Le Progrès Médical
Revue Neurologique (Paris) from its foundation in 1893 to the death of Babinski in 1932.

Main printed sources

Adams RD, Victor M. *Principles of neurology* New York, McGraw-Hill 1977: 995–1001.
Addresses from various Neurological Societies, *Société Française de Neurologie*, meeting of June 2, 1958 (Centennial of J. Babinski's birth), *Rev Neurol (Paris)*, 1958(98):640–668.
    640: Germany (G. Schaltenbrand).
    643: Belgium (Van Gehuchten).
    648: Spain (Subirana).
    651: USA (Sir Percival Bailey).
    653: Hungary (T. Lehoczky).
    654: Italy (V. Néri).
    660: Portugal (Almeida Lima).
    663: Roumania (A. Kreindler).
    664: Switzerland (E Ott).
    664: Turkey (Ihsan Sükrü Aksel).
    666: Uruguay (V. Soriano).
Agulhon M. *La République*, Paris, Hachette, 1990.
Ajuriaguerra J. de, *L'œuvre scientifique du Dr André-Thomas*, in "Jubilé du Dr André-Thomas", Paris, Masson et Cie, 1955 (extrait de la *Rev Neurol (Paris)*,1955, 931, pp. 1–28).
Alajouanine Th. Leçon Inaugurale, November 21, 1947.
Alajouanine Th. Le centenaire de Babinski, *Sem Hôp Paris* 1958(34):1355–1364.
Album de l'Internat, Paris, G. Pascaud, 1921.
Andenaes S. Babinski reflex and the Cut reflex—a comparative study, *Acta Neurologica Scandinavica*, 1979, vol 60, pp. 260–263.
Anderson E, Haymaker W. Harvey Cushing (1869–1939) in Haymaker W, Schiller F, *The founders of neurology*, Sprinfield, Charles C Thomas, 2d ed,1970:543–54.
Andrezej P. Gasecki A, Kwiecinski H. On the legacy of Joseph Babinski, *Eur Neurol* 1995, 35: 127–130.
Annuaire statistique de la ville de Paris, XXIth year, 1900, Paris, Masson et Cie, 1902.
Anonymous. *Plans des hôpitaux et hospices civils de la ville de Paris. Levés par ordre du Conseil général d'Administration de ces établissements*. Paris, 1820.
Anonymous. Le choléra à Paris, *Le Concours médical*, 1884:642.
Anonymous. Hommage à Dr Georges-Hubert Esbach. *Le Progrès Médical*, 1890, T.XI, N° 9, 1st March.
Anonymous. Les médecins contemporains. M. le Dr Malassez, *Le Progrès Médical*, 1894(17):314.
Anonymous. Les médecins contemporains, Le Pr A. Chantemesse, *Le Progrès Médical*, 1897, T. V, n° 23 (5 June), pp. 361–363.
Anonymous. Inauguration d'un monument à la memories de J.-M. Charcot, *La Presse Médicale*, December 7, 1898, n° 100.
Anonymous. Inauguration d'un monument à la memories de J.-M. Charcot December 4, 1898, *Le Progrès Médical*, 1898, T. VIII, 3d series, N° 50 (10 December), p. 449.
Anonymous. *L'Assistance publique en 1900*, Administration générale de l'Assistance publique à Paris, Montévrain (Seine et Marne), Elèves de l'Ecole d'Alembert, 1900, p. 98.
Anonymous. Le groupe des médecins du Parlement, *Le Progrès Médical*, 1901, n° 15 (April 10), p. 253.
Anonymous. Variétés, *Annales Médico-Psychologiques*, 1903:346–347.
Anonymous. L'hôpital de la Pitié, *La France Médicale*, 1903:303–308.
Anonymous. La démolition de la Pitié, *Chron Méd*, 1903:387–390.
Anonymous. Le nouvel hôpital de la Salpêtrière, *Le Progrès Médical*, 1904(26):429.
Anonymous. Obituary. H. Parinaud 1844–1905, *Annales d'Oculistique*, 1905(133):321–337.
Anonymous. Nécrologie de Paul Poirier, *Le Progrès Médical*, 1907, T.XXIII, n° 19 :289–291.
Anonymous. Edouard Brissaud (1852–1909), *Rev Neurol (Paris)*, 1910, n° 1 (January 15), pp. 1–4.

Anonymous. *L'hôpital de la nouvelle Pitié (1905-1910)*, Montévrain, Ec. D'Alembert, 1910.
Anonymous. Le docteur Babinski, *Chanteclair*, 6th year, n° 89, October 1911(2).
Anonymous. *Inauguration du nouvel hôpital de la Pitié*, Montévrain, Ec. D'Alembert, 1913.
Anonymous. *Aux médecins morts pour la patrie (1914-18)*, Paris, Baillière/Doin/Masson, s.d.
Anonymous. Obituary. Professeur Chantemesse, *Le Progrès Médical* 1919(9):82.
Anonymous. Obituary of Dr Bucquoy, *Conseil de surveillance*, meeting of 1 July 1920, pp. 669-670.
Anonymous. Bucquoy (1829-1920), *La Presse médicale*, 1920, n° 48, pp. 892-893.
Anonymous. Le docteur Chaillous, *La Presse Médicale*, December 1924:2058.
Anonymous. Marie-Edmé-Jules Bucquoy, *Chron Méd* 1929, p. 203.
Anonymous. Allocution du Président à propos de la mort du Professeur Widal, *Rev Neurol (Paris)*, 1929, T. I, N° 2 (February), p. 205.
Anonymous. Death of Dr Babinski, *The British Medical Journal*, 1932, November 12, p. 892.
Anonymous. *Le Temps*, "Feuilleton du Temps of November 18, 1932": Psychologie et thérapeutique. Un neurologue de génie : Babinski.
Anonymous. Babinski, *The Lancet* 1932(19):1122.
Anonymous. Deaths, *Journal of American Medical Association* 1932(99):2045-2046.
Anonymous. Joseph FF. Babinski, 1857-1932, *The New England Journal of Medecine* 1932, 27, November 17, pp. 898-899.
Anonymous. Le docteur Babinski, *Chanteclair*, 28th year, n° 292, January-February 1933.
Anonymous. Pierre Marie (1853-1940). *Rev Neurol (Paris)*, 1939-1940(72):533-543.
Anonymous, Achille Souques (1860-1944), *Rev Neurol (Paris)*, 1945, T. 77, N° 1-2 (January-February 1945), p. 37.
Anonymous. *Cent ans d'Assistance publique à Paris (1849-1949)*, Administration Générale de l'Assistance publique à Paris, 1949.
Anonymous. JC L. Edouard Pozerski (April 20, 1875 - January 26, 1964), *Annales de l'Institut Pasteur*, June 1964(196):813-818.
Anonymous. Centenaire de Pierre Marie, *La Presse Médicale*, September 27, 1952, n° 60:1261-1263.
Anonymous. "About Henri Babinski", in Ali-Bab, *Encyclopedia of practical gastronomy* (translated by Elisabeth Benson), New York, McGraw-Hill Book Company, 1974, pp. 445-446.
Anonymous. Sir William Gowers (1845-1915), *Spine* 1996(721):1106-1110.
Anonymous. *Jozef Feliks Franciszek Babinski (1857-1932)*, Oficyna Wyd. Politechniki Opolskiej. Opole 2000.
Anonymous. Joseph Babinski (1857-1932), *Revista peruana de Neurologia*, 2002(8):31-40.
Anonymous. A short history of the reflex hammer, *Practical Neurology*, 2003 Dec(3):366-371.
Anonymous. Ecole polonaise des Batignolles, l'âme ardente de la Pologne, *Parisdixsept, Journal d'information de la Mairie du dix-septième arrondissement*, 2005 april(39):16-17.
Antle M. *Cultures du surréalisme : Les Représentations de l'autre*, éds Acoria, coll. Les Mots en partage, 2001, 194 p. http://www.cavi.univ-parisParis3.fr/Rech_sur/cult_surr.htm.
Anton G. Über die Selbstwahrnehmung der Herderkrankungen des Gehirns durch den Kranken bei Rindenblindheit und Rindentaubheit [On the selfperception of focal brain lesions in patients with cortical blindness or cortical deafness], *Archiv für Psychiatrie und Nervenkrankheiten (Berlin)*, 1899, 32:86-127.
Armand-Delille P. Voyages et conférences médicales dans les Républiques Baltes, *La Presse Médicale*, May 2, 1934, n° 35, pp. 715-717.
Association des anciens élèves de l'école polonaise. Procès-Verbal 1865-1897 (N° 1-62. Manquent les N° 11, 16, 20, 22-23, 26, 29, 31, 40 à 44, 47 à 49, 51, 60-61). *Bulletin littéraire et scientifique*.
Aubry G. *Le syndrome de coagulation massive du liquide céphalorachidien*, Paris, Steinheil, 1909.
Auckler E. *Le professeur J. Dejerine (1849-1917)*, Paris, Masson, 1922.
Audureau J. *A propos de quelques tumeurs encéphaliques opérées*, Angers, Germain et G. Grassain, 1898.
Auvray M. *Les tumeurs cérébrales*, Paris, Henri Jouve, 1896.
Babinski L. Sylwetka Jozefa Babinskiego na tle jego zycia codziennego, *Neurol Neurochir Pol* 1969(III):543-546.
Babonneix L. J.-A. Sicard (1872-1929), Meeting of the *Société de Neurologie* February 7, 1929, *Rev Neurol (Paris)*, 1929(I):161-164.
Bailey P. Joseph Babinski (1857-1932). The man and his works, *World Neurology*, 1961(2):134-140.
Bailey P. *Pierre Marie*, in Haymaker W, Schiller F. "The founders of neurology", 2d ed., Springfield, Charles C Thomas, 1970, p. 476.
Bailey H, Bishop WJ. *Notable names in medicine and surgery*, London, HK Lewis & Co, 1944.

Ballet G. *Recherches anatomiques et cliniques sur le faisceau sensitif et les troubles de la sensibilité dans les lésions du cerveau*. Thése, Paris, Goupy et Jourdan Impr. and Progrès Médical, A. Delahaye et E. Lecrosnier, 1881.
Ballet G. *Traité de pathologie mentale*, Paris, Dom, 1903.
Barbara JG. Les étranglements annulaires de Louis Ranvier (1871), Société des Neurosciences, *La lettre N°28, Histoire des Neurosciences*, 2005, p. 3.
Bariety M, Coury C. *Histoire de la médecine*, Paris, Fayard, 1963.
Barraquer-Bordas L. Sobre el diagnostico clinico de las formas espinales monotipicas de esclerosis multiple. El valor del signo del abanico en el adulto, *Revista de Neurologia (Spain)*, 2001, 33 (11, Dec 1-15), pp. 1046-1048.
Barraquer-Bordas L. Sobre la probable dualidad del signo del abanico. Hipotesis clinicofisiopatologicas, *Neurologia (Spain)*, Jun-Jul 2001, 16(6) pp. 272-274.
Barraquer-Ferre L. Contribution à l'étude du réflexe plantaire pathologique, *Neurol (Rev Neurol (Paris)*, 1930, T. I (1st semester), n° 2 (February), pp. 174-182.
Baruk H. Babinski (1857-1932), *Revue philosophique de la France et de l'étranger*, Paris, Presses Universitaires de France, 1959, pp. 459-465.
Baruk H. *Des hommes comme nous*, Paris, Robert Laffont, 1976, pp. 28-32.
Beauvoir S de. *Tous les hommes sont mortels*, Paris, Gallimard, 1946.
Bélanger C. What do you know about Joseph Babinski? *Le Journal Canadien des Sciences Neurologiques*, 1989, 16(1): 4-7.
Benedikt M. Tremblement avec paralysie croisée du moteur oculaire commun. *Bull Méd (Paris)*, 1889, 3: 547-548.
Bénézit E. *Dictionnaire des peintres, sculpteurs, dessinateurs et graveurs*, Paris, Gründ, nouvelle édition, 1999.
Benson E. *About Henri Babinski*, in Ali-Bab, "Encyclopedia of practical gastronomy" (translated by Elisabeth Benson), New York, McGraw-Hill Book Company, 1974, pp. 445-446.
Bercherie P. *Les fondements de la clinique. Histoire et structure du savoir psychiatrique*, Paris, Navarin éd., 1980, pp. 180-185.
Bernard D, Gunthert A. *L'instant rêvé, Albert Londe*, Nîmes, Editions Jacqueline Chambon, 1993.
Bernheim H. *Hypnotisme, suggestion, psychothérapie*. Paris, Doin 1891 (3ème ed.).
Bezançon F. Hommage au professeur Cornil, *La Presse Médicale*, 1904, annexe, n° 21, pp. 161-166.
Bianchon H. [pseudonym of Maurice de Fleury]. *Nos grands médecins d'aujourd'hui*, Paris, Société d'éditions scientifiques, 1891.
Bidou G. *La scoliose et son traitement*, Paris, Maloine, 1913.
Bidou G. *Nouvelle méthode d'appareillage des impotents*, Paris, P.U.F., 1923.
Bidou G. *Principes scientifiques de récupération fonctionnelle des paralytiques*, Paris, Le livre pour tous, 1927.
Bidou G. *La thérapie mécanique*, Paris, Vuibert, 1929.
Billy A. *Paris vieux et neuf, La rive gauche*, Paris, Eugène Rey, 1909.
Binet JL. *Edouard Vuillard et Henri Vaquez*, Communication at the *Académie des beaux-arts*, meeting of December 15, 2004, pp. 69-75.
Birch CA. *Names we remember. 56 eponymous medical biographies*, Beckenham, Ravenswood pub., 1979, pp. 9-10.
Blanchard (Docteur), Le syndrome du baptême, *Le Progrès Médical*, 1898(VIII):504-505.
Blondel C. *Eusapia Palladino : la méthode expérimentale et la "diva des savants"*, in Bensaude-Vincent B, Blondel C. "Des savants face à l'occulte, 1870-1940", pp. 143-171.
Bodin J. *Contre Freud. Critique de toute psychologie de l'inconscient*, Paris, Masson, 1927, analysis in Rev Neurol (Paris), 1927(I):264.
Bogousslavsky J. Marcel Proust's Lifelong Tour of the Parisian Neurological Intelligentsia: From Brissaud and Dejerine to Sollier and Babinski, *Eur Neurol* 2007(57):129-136.
Boisseau J. *Traitement local des gommes syphilitiques par les injections d'iodure de potassium*, Paris, G. Steinheil, 1906.
Boisseau J. Hystérie et simulation. L'accident pithiatique n'est autre chose qu'un accident simulé, *Annales médico-psychologiques*, 1949, T. II, N° 2 (July), pp. 121-167 and N° 3 (October), pp. 249-286. Cf. chapitre 15.
Bolzinger A. *Freud et les Parisiens*, Paris, Campagne Première/Recherche, 2002.
Bonduelle M. In memoriam: W. Jakimowicz (1904-1972), *Rev Neurol (Paris)*, 1973(129):290.
Bonduelle M. Notice biographique de Georges Guillain (1876-1961), *Rev Neurol (Paris)*, 1977(133):661-666.
Bonduelle M. Charcot et les Daudet, *La Presse Médicale* 1993(22):1641-1648.

Bonduelle M. De la Revue neurologique à la Société de Neurologie : 1893-1899, *Rev Neurol (Paris)*, 1995(151):307-310.
Bonduelle M. Histoire de la Société Française de Neurologie: 1899-1974, *Rev Neurol (Paris)*, 1999(155):785-801.
Bonduelle M, Gelfand T, Goetz CG. *Charcot : un grand médecin dans son siècle.* Paris, Michalon, 1996.
Bonnet M. *La rencontre d'André Breton avec la folie, Saint-Dizier, August—November 1916.* http://entretenir.free.fr/breton3.html.
Bourdillon Ch. *De la crâniectomie décompressive dans les syndromes d'hypertension intracrânienne. Résultats éloignés.* Thése de doctorat en médecine, Paris, Vigné, 1925.
Bourgeois H. Le vertige voltaïque dans les affections de l'oreille interne. Epreuve de Babinski. *Le Progrès Médical* 1917(34):279.
Bourguignon G. Les conditions périphériques du réflexe plantaire normal et du signe de Babinski. Etude de la chronaxie motrice et sensitive. *Rev Neurol (Paris)*, 1927(I):1081.
Bourneville, Le concours d'agrégation en médecine, *Le Progrès Médical* 1892(XV):223.
Bourneville D. Le concours d'agrégation en médecine, *Le Progrès Médical* 1892(XV):239-240.
Bourneville. Les concours d'agrégation : une série de citations, *Le Progrès Médical*, 1892(XV):421-422.
Bourniol L. *Contribution à l'étude du syndrome de Babinski-Froment*, Thése de doctorat en médecine, Faculté de Médecine de Montpellier, Montpellier, Imprimerie Emmanuel Montane, 1928.
Boveri P. Sur la présence ou disparition du phénomène de Babinski suivant la position du malade, *Rev Neurol (Paris)*, 1916(7):143-144.
Bratkowski S. Inzynierowie Babinscy, *Kwartalnik Historii Nauki I Techniki* 1975(XX):295-311.
Breatnach CS. Sir Gordon Homes, *Medical History* 1975(18):194-200.
Bredin J.-D. *L'Affaire*, Paris, Julliard, 1983.
Breton A. *Manifeste du surréalisme*, Paris, Aux éditions du sagittaire, 1924.
Breton A. *Nadja*, Paris, Gallimard, 1928, pp. 47-62.
Breton A (sous la direction de). *Le Surréalisme même*, N° 1, October 1956, Paris, Pauvert, incluant les 2 encarts ("Les détraqués" et "Le royaume de la terre", scénario inédit de Abel Gance et N. Kaplan).
Breuer J, Freud S. Le mécanisme psychique des phénomènes hystériques. Communication préliminaire. 1892. In Freud S, Breuer J "Études sur l'hystérie". Paris, Puf, 1956, pp. 1-13.
Briquet P. *Traité clinique et thérapeutique de l'hystérie.* Paris, Plon, 1859.
Brissaud E. *Anatomie du cerveau de l'homme; morphologie des hémisphères cérébraux, ou cerveau proprement dit.* Paris, Masson, 1893.
Broca P. Diagnostic d'un abcès situé au niveau de la région du langage; trépanation de cet abcès. *Rev Anthropol*, 1876, 5:244-248.
Broca A, Maubrac P. *Traité de chirurgie cérébrale*, Paris, Masson et Cie 1896, reviewed in *Le Progrès Médical* 1896,TIII,n° 24,381.
Broche F. *Léon Daudet, le dernier imprécateur.* Paris, Robert Laffont, 1992.
Brouilhet AR. *Les héros sans gloire*, Paris, Charles Lavauzelle, 1927, p. 233.
Brueyre M. *Conseil supérieur de l'assistance publique*, T.IX, fascicule 68, 1898-1899, p. 55.
Bruns J., Tooth M.H. Le traitement des tumeurs du cerveau, *Rev Neurol (Paris)*, 1913, T.XXVI, pp. 343-347.
Brunschweiler (Lausanne). A propos du réflexe de Babinski dans la sclérose latérale amyotrophique, *Revue Neurologique (Paris)*, 1925, T. I, n° 6 (June), pp. 848-851.
Bulletin de l'Association des anciens élèves de l'Ecole des Mines de Paris, January-February 1888.
Bulletin de l'Association des anciens élèves de l'Ecole des Mines de Paris, 1907.
Bulletin de l'Association des anciens élèves de l'Ecole des Mines de Paris, July-August 1915.
Bulletin de l'Association amicale des anciens élèves de l'Ecole des Mines de Paris, January-February-March 1920.
Bulletin Polonais, littéraire, scientifique et artistique, N° 114 (January 15, 1898), p. 31.
Cahen G. Le nouvel hôpital de la Pitié, *La revue Philanthropique*, 1911-1912, T. I, pp. 648-650.
Carrie PA. Ed. Enriquez, *La Presse Médicale*, 1928, n° 55, pp. 876-877.
Cesbron H. *Histoire critique de l'hystérie.* Paris, Asselin et Houzeau 1909.
Cestan, Dupuy-Dutemps. Sur le signe pupillaire d'Argyll-Robertson, XIIè Congrès des médecins aliénistes et neurologistes de France et des pays de langue française, Grenoble, August 1-7, 1902, abstract in *Le Progrès Médical*, 1902, 31st year, 3nd série, T. XVI, n° 33 (August 16, 1902), p. 106.
Charbonnel A. *Liaisons et discrimination cérébello-vestibulaires*, Société Française de Neurologie, XXIIè RéunionNeurologique Internationale (Paris, 2 June 4, 1958), Rapports, Le cervelet, Paris, Masson et Cie, 1958.pp. 77-128.

Charcot JM. Foreword, In *Leçons sur les fonctions motrices du cerveau*, by François François-Franck, Paris, 1887.
Charcot JM. *Leçons du mardi à la Salpêtrière*; notes de cours de MM. Blin, Charcot [fils] et Colin; avant-propos de Jacques Sédat; préface de Joseph Babinski. - Paris : C. Tchou pour la Bibliothèque des introuvables, 2002, 2 vol. (XIX-748, 692 p.) (*Collection Psychanalyse*).
Charcot JM. De la contracture hystérique. Œuvres complètes. *Leçons sur les malaldies du système nerveux*. Tome I:347-66. Paris, Progrès médical, Bataille 1892.
Charcot JM. *Leçons sur les localisations cérébrales*. Paris, Alcan 1893.
Charcot JM. Leçon du mardi January 17, 1888. *Leçons du mardi 1887-1888*. Paris, Bureaux du Progrès médical 1888.
Charcot JM. Leçon du mardi January 24, 1888. *Leçons du mardi 1887-1888*. Paris, Bureaux du Progrès médical 1888.
Charcot JM. De l'hémianesthésie hystérique. *Leçons sur les maladies du système nerveux*. Paris, Progrès médical, 1892: 300-346.
Charcot JM. De l'hystéro-épilepsie. *Leçons sur les maladies du système nerveux*. Paris, Progrès médical 1892:367-85.
Charcot JM. La foi qui guérit. *Revue hebdomadaire*. Paris: Plon, 1892.
Charcot JM, Bouchard C. Nouvelles recherches sur la pathogénie de l'hémorragie cérébrale, *Archives de Physiologie Normale et Pathologique*, 110-127, 643-665, 725-734.
Charcot JM, Bouchard C, Brissaud E. *Traité de médecine*, Paris, G. Masson, 1891-1893.
Charpentier A. *Un grand médecin. J. Babinski (1857-1932)*, Paris, La Typographie François Bernouard Dr, 1934.
Charpentier A. *Babinski (Joseph)(1857-1932)*, in Dr M. Genty, "Les biographies médicales", T.VI, Paris, Librairie J.B. Baillière et fils, 1937-1939, pp. 17-32.
Charpentier A. *Relations entre les troubles des réflexes pupillaires et la syphilis*, Thèse de médecine, Paris, 1899.
Charpentier A. Babinski, *Le Figaro*, dimanche October 30, 1932, p. 2.
Charpentier A. "Relations entre les troubles des réflexes pupillaires et la syphilis", thése, Paris, 1899.
Chenivesse P. Grand Guignol et aliénisme, 6è *Congrès de l'Association Européenne pour l'Histoire de la Psychiatrie*, Paris, Hôpital Sainte-Anne, 22-24 September 2005.
Chipault A. *Chirurgie opératoire du système nerveux*, 2 vols, Paris, Rueff et Cie, 1894-1895.
Chipault A. Etudes de chirurgies médullaires, Historique, Chirurgie opératoire, Traitement. Paris, F. Alcan, 1894.
Chipault A. Rapport de l'origine des nerfs rachidiens avec les apophyses épineuses, *Archives de Neurologie*, 1895, TXXIX, n° 102 :150-151.
Chipault A. Manuel opératoire de la ponction vertébrale lombo-sacrée, *Archives de Neurologie*, 1895, TXXIX, 472.
Chipault A. *Travaux de neurologie chirurgicale*, Paris, L. Bataille et Cie, 1896.
Chipault A. Rachicocainisation, *Société de Biologie*, meeting of June 29, 1901, analysed in Le Progrès Médical 1901,3[d] series,T.XIII, n° 23 :375-376.
Chipault A. *Etat actuel de la chirurgie nerveuse*, 3 vol, Paris, J. Rueff, 1903.
Chiray M, Dagnan-Bouveret J. *La prothèse fonctionnelle des paralysies et des contractures*, Paris, A. Maloine et fils, 1919.
Chorobski J. Speech of M. Jerzy Chorobski (Varsovie), *Société Française de Neurologie*, meeting of June 2, 1958 (Centenaire de la naissance de J. Babinski), *Rev Neurol (Paris)*, 1958, T. 98, n° 6, pp. 637-639.
Clarac F, Lechevalier B. Albert Gombault (1844-1904), a pioneer in neurosciences, *Rev Neurol (Paris)*, 2006, 162, n° 2, pp. 253-263.
Claude H. L'hypertension intracrânienne, *Le Journal Médical Français*, May 1915, n° 5.
Claude H, Bourguignon G, Baruk. Signe de Babinski transitoire dans un cas de démence précoce, *Rev Neurol (Paris)*, 1927, T. I, n° 6 (June), p. 1078.
Claude H., Lévy-Valensi M. *Maladies du cervelet et de l'isthme de l'encéphale*. Paris, Librairie J.B. Baillière, 1922, in Brouardel et Thoinot, Gilbert et Thoinot, "Nouveau Traité de Médecine", fascicule XXXII.
Collier JS. An investigation upon the Plantar Reflex, with reference to the significance of its variations under pathological conditions, including an inquiry into the aetiology of acquired pes cavus, *Brain*, 1899, 23: 71-99.

Collins J. Syphilis and the nervous system, *The Journal of the American Medical Association*, 1913, vol LXI, n° 11 (September 13), pp. 860–866.
Cone TE Jr, Khoshbin S. Botticelli demonstrates the Babinski reflex more than 400 years before Babinski; pediatrics in art. *American Journal of Diseases of Children*, 1978 Feb, 132(2): 188.
Cornil V. *Titres et travaux scientifiques*, Paris, Imprimerie E. Martinet, 1872.
Cornil V. *Notice sur les titres et travaux*, Paris, Parent, 1882.
Cornil V. Leçons données pendant le premier semestere de l'année 1883–84 by M. Cornil, Professor of Pathological Anatomy at the Paris Medical School and collected by MM. Berlioz, Babinski, Gibier, Chantemesse, avec 25 figures inserées das le texte, Paris, Ancienne Libriairie German Baillière et Cie, Félix Alcan éditeur, 1884.
Cornil V, Babes V. *Les bactéries et leur rôle dans l'anatomie et l'histologie pathologiques des maladies infectieuses*, 1 volume et Atlas. Paris, F. Alcan, 1885.
Cornil V., Ranvier L. *Manuel d'histologie pathologique*. Paris, F. Alcan, 1869.
Cornil V, Suchard E. Note sur le siège des parasites de la lèpre, Société médicale des hôpitaux de Paris, meeting of June 10, 1881, *Mémoires de la Société Médicale des Hôpitaux de Paris*, 1881, T. XVIII (2nd series), pp. 151–154.
Cossa P. Jules Boisseau, *La Presse Médicale*, March 18, 1961.
Cossa P. Babinski, précurseur des méthodes de choc électrique, *Annales Médico-Psychologiques*, 108è année, T. I,March 1950, pp. 325–330.
Crimslik HL, Ron M. Conversion hysteria : history, diagnostic issues and clinical practice. *Cognitive neuropsychiatry* 1999; 4 :165–80.
Crosby EC. Jean Nageotte (1866–1948), *in* Haymaker W, Schiller F. In "The founders of neurology", Springfield, Charles C Thomas, 2d ed., 1970, pp. 133–136.
Crouzon O. *Des scléroses combinées de la moelle*, Paris, G. Steinheil, 1904.
Crouzon O. Allocution de M. Crouzon, Président, Société de Neurologie de Paris, meeting of January 10, 1924, *Rev Neurol (Paris)*, 1924, N° 1 (January), pp. 81–82.
Crouzon O. Jean Jarkowski (1880–1929), *La Presse médicale*, 1930, n° 14, p. 246.
Crouzon O. *Discours d'ouverture de la Chaire d'Assistance Médico-Sociale*, given on 22 November, 1937 à la Faculté de Médecine de Paris.
Cuba JM. Influencia de la medicina francesa en la medicina peruana, *Revista peruana de Neurologia*, 2002, 8(1): 31–40.
Dagognet F. "Le grand déchiffreur : J. Babinski" in Dagognet F. *Savoir et pouvoir en médecine*, Le Plessis Robinson, Institut Synthélabo, Collection les Empêcheurs de penser en rond, 1998, pp. 99–103.
Dalkowska A, Pecold K. Professor Witold J. Orlowski. Obituary for the 10th anniversary of his death [article in Polish] *Kin Oczna*. 1999, 101(1): 59–62.
Dandy WE. *The Brain*, Hagerstown, Maryland, WF Prior Company, 1966.
Darier J. Anatomie pathologique du tabès, *Gazette hebdomadaire de médecine et de chirurgie*, January 30, 1892, 2è série, T. XXXIX, n° 5, p. 1.
Darmon P. Des suppliciés de la Grande Guerre: les pithiatiques. *Histoire, Économie et Société*, 2001; 20:49–64.
Dartigues L. *Faisceau Scriptural*, vol.3, Paris, G.Dom, 1932.
Daudet L. *Les morticoles*, Paris, Bibliothèque Charpentier, Charpentier et Fasquelle, 1894.
Daudet L. *Devant la douleur*, Paris, Nouvelle Librairie Nationale, 1922.
Daudet L. *Les oeuvres dans les hommes*, Paris, Nouvelle Librairie Nationale, 1922, pp. 197–243.
Daudet L. "Babinsky" (sic), *Action française*, October 30, 1932.
Daudet L. *Souvenirs littéraires*, Paris, Bernard Grasset, Le Livre de Poche, 1968, pp. 133–134.
Daudet L, *Souvenirs et polémiques*, Paris, Robert Laffont, 1992, p. 166.
Davis FB. Three letters from Sigmund Freud to André Breton, *J Am Psychoanal Assoc*, 1973, 21(1): 127–194.
De Bélina. *Les polonais et la Commune de Paris*, Paris, Librairie générale, 1871 (138 p.).
De Bélina. *Les polonais et la Commune de Paris*, Paris, Librairie générale, 1871 (138 p.). Annexe: "Mémoire justificatif du Comité de l'émigration polonaise", Paris, July 5, 1871, Prince L. Czartoryski et al.
De Caro GM, Brunori A, Giuffre R. Neurosurgery in Rome, *Ann Ital Chir*, 1998,69:249–284.
D'Echerac A (G. Dargenty). *L'Assistance publique. Ce qu'elle fut; ce qu'elle est*, Paris, G. Steinheil, 1909, pp. 355–356.

Déchy A. *Le signe d'Argyll-Robertson et la cytologie du liquide céphalo-rachidien*, Thése de doctorat en médecine, Paris, Tome X, n° 109, 1902-1903.
Dejerine J. Sur l'abolition du réflexe cutané plantaire dans certains cas de paralysies fonctionnelles accompagnées d'anesthésie (hystéro-traumatisme), *Société de Neurologie de Paris*, meeting of February 4, 1915, *Rev Neurol (Paris)*, 1914-1915, T. XXVIII, n° 19 (July 1915), pp. 521-529.
Dejerine J. *Sémiologie des affections du système nerveux*, in Ch.Bouchard "Traité de pathologie générale," T. V, Paris, Masson, 1901, pp. 359-1168.
Dejerine J. Clinique des Maladies du Système Nerveux, Leçon inaugurale. *La Presse médicale*, n° 26, April 1, 1911.
Dejerine J. *Sémiologie des affections du système nerveux*, Paris, Masson, 1914.
Dejerine J, Thomas A. L'atrophie-olivo-ponto-cérébelleuse, *Nouvelle Iconographie de la Salpêtrière*, 1900, 13 : 330-370.
Dejerine J, Thomas A. *Traité des maladies de la moelle épinière*, Paris, J. B. Baillière, 1902.
Dejerine J. with the collaboration of Mrs Dejerine-Klümpke, *Anatomie des centres nerveux*, 2 vol. Paris, Rueff, 1890-1901.
Delage R. *Emmanuel Chabrier*, Paris, Fayard, 1999.
Delaporte S. *Les médecins dans la Grande Guerre 1914-1918*, Paris, Bayard, 2003.
Delbet P. A propos de la trépanation décompressive, *Société de Chirurgie*, March 22, 1911. Analysis in *Rev Neurol (Paris)*, 1911, T. Xxii, n° 13 (July 15), pp. 26-27.
Delherm L. *Le traitement par l'électricité de la constipation habituelle et de la colite muco-membraneuse*, Paris, Henri Jouve, 1903.
Delorme. Tumeurs cérébrales et trépanation décompressive, *Société de Chirurgie*, March 29, 1911. Analysis in *Rev Neurol (Paris)*, 1911, T. XXII, n° 13 (July 15), p. 25.
Devoize JL. "The other" Babinski's sign: paradoxical raising of the eyebrow in hemifacial spasm. *Journal of Neurology, Neurosurgery and Psychiatry*, April 2001, 70(4) p. 516.
Dieulafoy G., *Manuel de pathologie interne*. Paris, G. Masson Editeur, 1895, T. II, Chapitre IV - Maladies du cervelet, pp. 100-101.
Divers auteurs *Ce que la France a apporté depuis le début du XXè siècle*, Paris, Flammarion, 1946, pp. 256-264.
Domanski CW. Julian Ochorowicz (1850-1917) et son apport dans le développement de la psychologie du XIXè siecle. *Psychologie et Histoire*, 2003, vol. 4, 101-114.
Dore G. *Le nouveau Paris*. Emile de Labédollière, Barcelona, Sacelp, 1986.
Dohrmann GJ, Nowack WJ. The upgoing great toe optimal method of elicitation. *Lancet* 1973, 17: 339-341.
Dreze C. Charcot 1825-1893, *Louvain Médical*, 2001, 120, pp. 33-66.
Drèze C. André Breton, de la médecine et la psychiatrie à la surréalité, *Louvain Médical*, 2003, 122: 367-374.
Dubarry JJ. Note sur la communication princeps de Babinski concernant le réflexe cutané plantaire, *Hist Sc Méd*, 1989, n° 2, pp. 145-146.
Dubas F. Bibliothèque idéale. Histoire de la controverse sur les anévrysmes miliaires de Charcot et Bouchard, *Rev Neurol (Paris)*, 2006, T. 162, n° 3, pp. 400-405.
Duckett S. Etude de la fonction cérébelleuse par François Pourfour du Petit (1710), *L'Encéphale*, 1964, n° 2, pp. 291-298.
Dufour H. Relations existant entre les troubles pupillaires, la syphilis, le tabes et la paralysie générale. *Société Médicale des Hôpitaux de Paris*, June 13, 1902, abstract in *Le Progrès Médical*, 1902, T. XV, n° 25 (21 June), p. 411.
Dumas G. *Le surnaturel et les Dieux d'après les maladies mentales (essai de théogénie pathologique)*, Paris, Puf, 1946.
Dumesnil R. *Histoire illustrée de la Médecine*, Ed. Histoire et Art, Plon, 1935 et 1950; Huguet F. Les professeurs de la faculté de médecine de Paris. Dictionnaire biographique 1794-1939, Paris, Cnrs, mpr, 1991.
Durand I. *Les médecins-ministres dans les gouvernements français de 1871 à 1858*, Thése de Médecine, Faculté Necker-Enfants-malades, Paris, 1985; Les médecins ministres, *Le Progrès Médical*, 1905, 34è année, 3è série, n° 4 (28 January), p. 60.
Durand G, Carrie PA. Ed. Enriquez, *La Presse Médicale*, 1928, n° 55, pp. 876-877.
Duret H. *Tumeurs de l'encéphale : Rapport au congrès de chirurgie*, 1903, F.Alcan edit, 393-407.
Duret H. *Les tumeurs de l'encéphale : manifestations et chirurgie*, Paris, F. Alcan, 1905.
Edelman N. *Les métamorphoses de l'hystérique. Du début du XIX e siècle à la Grande Guerre*. Paris, Éditions de la découverte 2003.

Edelman N. *Histoire de la voyance et du paranormal, du XVIIIè siècle à nos jours*, Paris, Editions du Seuil, 2006.
Ellis JD. *The physician-legislators in France, Medicine and politics in the early Third Republic, 1870-1914*, Cambridge, Cambridge University Press, 1990.
Enriquez E, president. Allocution, *Rev Neurol (Paris)*, 1918, T. I, N° 1-2 (January-February), pp. 69-71.
Enriquez E, Laffitte, Bergé, Lamy. *Traité de médecine*, Paris, Octave Doin et fils, 1909.
Escourolle R, Gray F, Hauw JJ. Les atrophies cérébelleuses, *Rev Neurol (Paris)*, 1982, 138 (12) : 953-955.
Esmonet C. La gastronomie pratique, *Le Progrès Médical*, 1912, T. 17, p. 216.
Fauconnet E. *Joseph Babinski, et la naissance de la neurochirurgie française*, Thése de Médecine, Faculté de Rennes, 1985.
Faure JL. Charles Périer (1836-1914), *La Presse Médicale*, 1914, n° 81 (December 24), p. 743.
Faure M. *Histoire des cours de l'Institut Pasteur*, fascicule dactylographié, 14 pages, Paris, Institut Pasteur, 1987.
Ferrier D. Annual meeting: section of Neurology, *Br Med J*, 1898, 2, 964-970.
Fierro A. *Histoire et mémoire du nom des rues de Paris*, Paris, Parigramme, 1999.
Fine EJ, Ionita CC, Lohr L. The history of the development of the cerebellar examination. *Seminars in Neurology*, December 2002, vol. 22, n° 4, pp. 375-384.
Finelli PF. Reflex hammer with built-in pin, *Neurology*, March 1991, vol. 41, p. 344.
Flatau E. De la radiothérapie des tumeurs du cerveau et de la moelle, *Rev Neurol (Paris)*, 1924, T. I, N° 1 (January), pp. 23-40 et N° 2 (February), pp. 176-191.
Flatau E, Sawicki B. Kyste hémorragique intradural du sac spinal, *Rev Neurol (Paris)*, 1924, T. II, N° 6 (December), pp. 589-596.
Flatau E. De la valeur diagnostique du signe de l'érection dans la méningite tuberculeuse, *Rev Neurol (Paris)*, 1925, T. I, N° 5 (May), pp. 590-591; Flatau E. Recherches expérimentales sur la perméabilité de la barrière nerveuse centrale, *Rev Neurol (Paris)*, 1926, T. II, N° 6 (December), pp. 521-540.
Fleury M. de. *Le médecin*, Paris, Hachette, 1927.
Fontecilla O, Sepulveda R M-A. *Le liquide céphalo-rachidien. Etudes cliniques*, Paris, A. Maloine et fils, 1921.
Fosseyeux M. *Catalogue des manuscrits des archives de l'Assistance publique*, Paris, Berger-Levrault, 1913.
Fournier A. *De l'ataxie locomotrice d'origine syphilitique*, Paris, G. Masson, 1876.
Fournier A. *Traitement de la syphilis*, Paris, Rueff, 1893, quoted by Tilles G, Wallach D. Le traitement de la syphilis par le mercure. Une histoire thérapeutique exemplaire, *Histoire des Sciences Médicales*, 1996, T. XXX, n° 4, pp. 501-510.
Fraenkel T. *Carnets de guerre 1916-1918*, Paris, Éditions des Cendres, 1990, (http://entretenir.free.fr/breton69.html).
Freeman W. *Charles Foix (1882-1927)*, in Haymaker W, Schiller F. "The founders of neurology", Springfield, Charles C Thomas, 2d ed., 1970, pp. 116-120.
Freeman W. *Alfred Vulpian*, in Haymaker W, Schiller F. "The founders of neurology", Springfield, Charles C Thomas, 2d ed., 1970.
Freeman W. *Edouard Brissaud (1852-1909)*, in Haymaker W, Schiller F. "The founders of neurology", Springfield, Charles C Thomas, 2d ed., 1970, pp. 417-420.
Freitas GR de, Moll J, Araujo AQ, The Babinski-Nageotte syndrome. *Neurology*, June 12, 2001, 56(11) p. 1604.
Freitas GR de, Andre C. Absence of the Babinski sign in brain death. A prospective study of 144 cases. *Journal of Neurology*, 2005, 252, pp. 106-107.
Freud S. Quelques considérations pour une étude comparative des paralysies motrices organiques et hystériques. *Archives de Neurologie* 1893, 26: 29-43.
Freud S. L'hérédité et l'étiologie des névroses (1896) In *Névroses, psychoses et perversions*. Paris, Puf 1978 pp. 47-59.
Freud S. *Abriss der Psychanalysis*, Gesamte Werke XVII, 1938, 134.
Freud S. L'étiologie de l'hystérie. In *Névorses, psychoses et perversions*. Paris Puf 1978 pp. 83-112.
Freud S. Charcot. Wiener Medizine Wochenschrift 1893. Traduction française in *Résultats, idées et problèmes*. Paris, Puf 1984, pp. 61-73.
Freud S. *Correspondance 1873-1939*, traduction A. Berman, Paris, Gallimard, 1966.
Fröhlich A. *Ein Fall von Tumor der Hypophysis cerebri ohne Akromegalie*, Wiener klinische Rundschau, 1901, 15: 833-836; 906-908.

Froin G., Inflammations méningées avec réactions chromatique, fibrineuse et leucocytique du liquide céphalo-rachidien, *Gazette des Hôpitaux*, September 3, 1903.
Froment J (travail du service du docteur Babinski). La paralysie de l'adducteur du pouce et le signe de la préhension, *Société de Neurologie de Paris*, meeting of October 7, 1915, *Rev Neurol (Paris)*, 2è semestre 1914–1915, T. XXVIII, n° 23–24 (November–December 1915) "Neurologie de guerre", pp. 1236–1240.
Froment J, Bonnet P, Colrat A. Hérédodégénérations rétinienne et spino-cérébelleuse; variantes ophtalmoscopiques et neurologiques présentées par trois générations successives, *J Med Lyon*, 1937: 153–163.
Fulton J. Joseph François Félix Babinski 1857–1932, *Archives of Neurology and Psychiatry*, January 1933, 29:168–174.
Fulton J.F. Science in the clinic as exemplified by the life and work of Joseph Babinski, *The Journal of Nervous and Mental diseases*, 1933, (77):121–133.
Galinowski A. *L'enseignement à la faculté de médecine de Paris au début de la 3ème République et le décret du June 20, 1878*, Thèse de médecine, Créteil, University Paris-XII, 1979.
Garcin R. L'œuvre de Babinski, *Société Française de Neurologie*, meeting of June 2, 1958 (Centenaire de la naissance de J. Babinski), *Rev Neurol (Paris)*, 1958, T. 98, N° 6, pp. 619–631.
Gasecki A. Jozef Babinski wspoltworca wspolcaesnej neurologii i neurochirurgii. *Neurologia i Neurochirurgia Polska*, 1997, 31(3):641–656.
Gasecki A, Hachinski V. On the names of Babinski. *Canadian Journal of Neurological Sciences*, 1996;23:76–79.
Gasecki A, Kwiecinski H. On the legacy of Joseph Babinski, *Eur Neurol*, 1995, 35, pp. 127–130.
Gastinel P. La ponction lombaire thérapeutique, *Le Progrès Médical*, 1914, n° 2, p. 19 and n° 24, p. 283.
Gauchet M, Swain G. *Le vrai Charcot*. Paris, Calman-Lévy, 1997.
Gelfand T, (annotation, translation, and commentary). "Mon cher Docteur Freud": Charcot's unpublished correspondence to Freud, 1888–1893, *Bulletin of History of Medicine*, 1988, 62: 563–588.
Gelfand T, Kerr J. Freud and the history of psychoanalysis, Hillsdale NJ, London, Tne Analytic Press, 1992.
Gendron A. *Etude clinique des tumeurs de la moelle et des méninges spinales.Contribution à l'étude des localisations médullaires en hauteur.* Medical thesis, Paris, Maloine, 1913.
Geny C. Signe de Babinski : on nous aurait trompé ? *Jim on-line*, November 3, 2005.
Ghosh D, Pradhan S. "Extensor toe sign" by various methods in spastic children with cerebral palsy, *Journal of Child Neurology*, 1998, vol 13, n° 5 (may), pp. 216–220. Comment in *Journal of Child Neurology*, 1999, may, 14(5), pp. 337–340.
Gieysztor A et al. *Histoire de la Pologne*, Warszawa, Pwn éditions scientifiques de Pologne, 1971.
Gilles de la Tourette G. *Traité clinique et thérapeutique de l'hystérie d'après l'enseignement de la Salpêtrière*. Tome I: Hystérie normale ou interparoxystique, Paris, Plon, 1891.
Giroire H. *Clovis Vincent 1879–1947, pionnier de la neurochirurgie française*, Paris, Olivier Perrin, 1972.
Glowacki J. Prace naukowe Josefa Babinskiego zwiazane z zagadnieniami neurochirurgii, *Archivum Historii Meycynyd (Warsz)*, 1969(XXXII):437–441.
Goetz CG. *Charcot, The Clinician, The Tuesday Lessons*, New York, Raven Press, 1987.
Goetz CG. Charcot and the aging brain. *Archives of neurology* 2002(59):1821–1824.
Goetz CG, Bonduelle M, Gelfand T. *Charcot, Constructing neurology*, New York, Oxford University Press, 1995.
Goetz CG, Pappert EJ. Early American professorships in neurology, *Annals of Neurology*, 1996, Aug, 40 (2), p. 258–263.
Goldflam S. Sur la valeur clinique du signe de Gordon, Réflexe paradoxal des fléchisseurs, Phénomène paradoxal des orteils et du mollet, *Rev Neurol (Paris)*, 1925(I):590–591.
Goldflam S (de Varsovie). Zur Lehre von den Hautreflexen an den Unterextremitäten (insbesondere des Babinskischen Reflexes [Contribution à l'étude des réflexes cutanés du membre inférieur (en particulier du réflexe de Babinski)], Neurologisches Centralblatt, 1903, n° 23 (December 1), p. 1119 et n° 24 (December 15), p. 1137; analysis in *Rev Neurol (Paris)*, 1905(XIII):971–972.
Gomez-Fernandez L, Calzada-Sierra DJ. Pseudobabinski, *Rev Neurol (Spain)* 2001(32):799.
Gordon A. Le phénomène des doigts, *Rev Neurol (Paris)*, 1912, n° 20 (October 30), pp. 421–424.
Gracon G. *Les catholiques polonais en France (1919-1949)*, Thésis de médecine, Lille III – Charles de Gaulle, April 7, 2003 [http://www.univ-lille3.fr/theses/garcon-gabriel/html/these_front.html].

Grant R. The neurological assault on the great toe (1893–1911), *Scot Med J* 1987, 32, pp. 057–059.
Grasset J. *Traité pratique des maladies du système nerveux*, Montpellier, Coulet, P., Delahaye & Lecrosnier, 1881.
Greenblatt S, Dagi TF, Epstein MH. A history of neurosurgery in its scientific and professional contexts. The American Association of Neurological surgeons, Park Ridge, Illinois, 1997.
Greenblatt SH, Smith DC. *The emergence of Cushing's leadership: 1901 to 1920*. In Greeenblatt SH, Dagi TF, Epstein MH. "A history of neurosurgery In its scientific and professional contexts", Parke Ridge Illinois, The American Association of Neurological Surgeons, 1997.
Grmek MD. *Histoire de la pensée médicale en Occident, 3. Du romantisme à la science moderne*, Paris, Editions du Seuil, 1999.
Guillain G. *Chaire de clinique des maladies du système nerveux, Leçon d'Ouverture du Professeur Georges Guillain (December 20, 1923)*, La Presse Médicale of the 26 January 1924.
Guillain G. Discours du Professeur G. Guillain, Président de la Société *Rev Neurol (Paris)*, 1925,T1, n° 6 (June), p. 1155–1158.
Guillain G. Préface à Bidou G. *Principes scientifiques de récupération fonctionnelle des paralytiques*, Paris, "Le livre pour tous", 1927.
Guillain G. J. Babinski (1857–1932), *La Presse Médicale*, 1932 (12 November), 91:1705–1707.
Guillain G. Allocution par Georges Guillain sur la mort de M. Jean Darier, *Société Médicale des Hôpitaux de Paris*, meeting June 10, 1938, pp. 1018–1020.
Guillain G. *J.-M. Charcot, 1825–1893, Sa vie, Son œuvre*, Paris, Masson et Cie, 1955, p. 62.
Guillain G. *Gustave Roussy (1874–1948)*, in Haymaker W, Schiller F. "The founders of neurology", Springfield, Charles C Thomas, 2d ed., 1970, pp. 510–513.
Guillain G, Barré JA. *Travaux neurologiques de guerre*, Paris, Masson, 1920.
Guillain G, Bertrand I. *Anatomie topographique du système nerveux central*, Paris, Masson, 1926.
Guillain G, Bidou. Sur la récupération fonctionnelle des grandes paralysies, *Académie de médecine*, n° 18, May 4, 1926.
Guillain G, Mathieu P. *La Salpêtrière*, Paris, Masson, 1925.
Guilly P. *Duchenne de Boulogne*, Paris, Librairie J.B. Baillière & Fils, 1936, p. 95, 145, 148.
Guilly P. Vie en survol de Gilles de la Tourette ou les caprices de la postérité, *La Presse Médicale*, March 9, 1985, 14 (10) : 569–570.
Guillaumat L, Maurax PV, Offret G. *Neuro-Ophtalmologie*, Paris, Masson et Cie Editeurs, 2 vol., 1959.
Guiot G. Clovis Vincent 1879–1947, *Surgical Neurology*, 1973, 1 : 189–190.
Gunderson CH. *Essentials of clinical neurology*, New York, Raven Press, 1990.
Gusmao S. Broca et les débuts de la neurochirurgie moderne, *Histoire des Sciences médicales*, 2002, T.36, n° 4, pp. 423–427.
Guyon F, Bazy P. *Atlas des maladies des voies urinaires. Maladies de l'urètre et de la prostate*, Paris, Doin, 1886, 380 p. et 50 planches.
Haberberg G. *De Charcot à Babinski : étude du rôle de l'hystérie dans la naissance de la neurologie moderne*, Thesis de doctorat en médecine, Faculté de médecine de Créteil, 1979.
Hallion M. Allocution de M. Hallion, président, à l'occasion du décès de M. Clunet, membre de la Société, *Rev Neurol (Paris)*, 1917, T. I, N° 4–5 (April–May), pp. 244–246.
Hamonet C. Note Historique, La prescription médicale par Babinski, *Journal de Réadaptation médicale*, 1999, 19, N°1, p. 29.
Hartenberg P. Les nouvelles idées sur l'hystérie. *Presse médicale* 1907; 15:469.
Hautant A. Rapport sur l'étude clinique de l'examen fonctionnel de l'appareil vestibulaire, 8è Réunion Neurologique Internationale (1–2 June 1927), *Rev Neurol (Paris)*, 1927, T. I, n° 6 (June), pp. 908–976.
Haymaker W, Schiller F. *The founders of neurology*, Springfield, Charles C Thomas, 2d ed., 1970.
Hayem G. Professor Vulpian, *Revue Internationale de l'Enseignement*, December 15, 1887, Paris, Armand Colin et Cie, 1887.
Haustgen T, Bourgeois ML. Dr Jules Séglas (1856–1939), president of the *Société Médico-Psychologique*, sa vie et son œuvre, *Annales médico-psychologiques*, 2002, vol 160, n° 10 (December), pp. 701–712.
Heltman V. *Emigracja polska od 1831 do 1863*. Krotki rys historyczny, Lipsk, 1865.
Herman E. *Jozef F. Babinski, Jego zycie i dziela*, Panstwowy Zaklad Wydawnictw Lekarskich, 1965.
Hillairey J. *Dictionnaire historique des rues de Paris*, Paris, Les éditions de Minuit, 1963.
Holmes G. On certain tremors in organic cerebral lesions. *Brain*, 1904, 27: 325–337.
Holmes G. *A form of familial degeneration of the cerebellum*. Brain, Oxford, 1907(30):466–489.

Holmes G. The symptoms of acute cerebellar injuries due to gunshot injuries, *Brain*, 1918(40):461-535.
Horsley V. Remarks on ten consecutive cases of operations upon the brain and cranial cavity to illustrate the details and safety of the method employed, *Br Med J*, 1887(1):863-865.
Horsley V. Surgical versus the expectant treatment of intracranial tumour, *Br Med J*, 1910:1833-1835.
Huard P. Présentation, il y a 100 ans par Constantin Paul de son stéthoscope bi-auriculaire autostatique á l'Academie de Médecine, *Bull Acad Natl Med*, 1981(165):1117-1121.
Huard C, Billy A. (dessins de Charles Huard, texte d'André Billy). *Paris vieux et neuf. La rive gauche*, Paris, Eugène rey, 1909.
Huet. Discours de M. Huet, Président, á l'occasion de la mort du Professeur Gilbert Ballet, *Rev Neurol (Paris)*, 1916, n° 6 (June), pp. 896-898.
Huguet F. *Les professeurs de la faculté de médecine de Paris. Dictionnaire biographique 1794-1939*, Paris, Cnrs, Inrp, 1991, pp. 568-569.
Hulmann M. Inauguration d'un service de neuro-chirurgie à l'hôpital de la Pitié, *La Presse Médicale*, June 21, 1933, p. 1008.
Hulmann M. Inauguration á l'Hopital Cochin d'un monument á la memoire du Professeur Widal, *La Presse Médicale*, July 19, 1933, n° 57, pp. 1159-1160.
Hulmann M. Jubilé des vingt-cinq années de services hospitaliers du Dr. Delherm, *La Presse Médicale*, October 18, 1933, n° 83, p. 1624.
Hurst AF. Dr. Babinski, *The British Medical Journal*, 1932, November 26, p. 988.
Ignatius J. "Babinski positiivinen" Joseph François Félix Babinski 1857-1932 [article en finlandais], *Duodecim*, 1993, 109, pp. 254-256.
Iragui V. The Charcot-Bouchard controversy, *Archives of Neurology* 1986(43):290-295.
Jaboulay M. La trépanation décompressive (La mobilisation de la voûte du crâne), *Lyon Médical* 1896(LXXXIII):73-75.
Jakimowicz W. Josef Babinski (w stulecie urodzin) [article in Polish], *Zjazs Neurologow I Neurochirurgow W R*, 1959, N° 3, pp. 411-415.
Janet P. Quelques définitions de l'hystérie. *Archives de Neurologie* 1893; 25:417-38, and 26:1-29.
Janet P. *Contribution à l'étude des accidents mentaux chez les hystériques*. Thèse de médecine. Paris, 1893.
Janet P. La psycho-analyse, Rapport au XVIIè Congrès International de Médecine de Londres (6-13 August 1913), in *Rev Neurol (Paris)*, 1913, T.XXVI, n° 18 (30 September), pp. 371-372.
Jarkowski J. Essai d'application thérapeutique de l'osmium, en particulier dans la sclérose en plaques (Note préliminaire), *Rev Neurol (Paris)*, 1929, T. I, n° 4 (April), pp. 631-633.
Jayle F. L'hôpital de la Pitié, *La Presse Médicale*, 1912, n° 53, pp. 557-564.
Joffroy A. Speech prononced by Professor Joffroy, Société de Neurologie de Paris, meeting of July 6, 1899, *Rev Neurol (Paris)*, 1899, T. VII, pp. 506-509.
Jolly J. Louis Ranvier (1835-1922). Notice biographique, *Archives d'Anatomie microscopique*, 1922(XIX):1-72.
Julliard J, Winock M. (edited by). *Dictionnaire des intellectuels français*, Paris, Seuil, new edition 2002.
Jumentié, DE Martel Th. Deux cas de tumeurs sous-corticales diagnostiquées et localisées par la clinique travail du service du professeur Dejerine), *Rev Neurol (Paris)*, 1910, T.XIX, n° 8 du 30 April, pp. 529-532.
Keen WW. Three successful cases of cerebral surgery including the removal of a large intra cranial fibroma, resection of damaged brain tissue and resection of the cerebral cortex for the left hand. With remarks on the general technique for such operations, *Trans Am Surg Assoc*, 1888,6:293-347 (cited in *Le Progrès Médical*, 1890, n° 14(5 April), p. 278.
Kenez J. Joseph Babinski (1857-1932) a francia klinilai neurologia egyk uttöreje, *Orvosi Hetilap*, 1984, vol. 125, n° 4, pp. 222-228.
Khalil R. *Vie et œuvre de Babinski*, in Conférences lyonnaises d'Histoire de la Neurologie et de la Psychiatrie, Lyon, Documentation médicale Oberval, 1982, pp. 255-280.
Kiple KF (edited by). *The Cambridge world history of human disease*, Cambridge, Cambridge University Press, 1993.
Kieniewicz S. *Historia Polski 1795-1918*, Warszawa, Widawnictwo Naukowe Pwn, 1998.
Klippel M. Homage to Professor Joffroy, *Rev Neurol (Paris)* 1908(XVI):1326-1327.
Koehler PJ, Okun MS. Important observations prior to the description of the Hoover sign, *Neurology* 2004(63):1693-1697.
Kother J. Le Petit Journal du Passé-28/08/2005 Le Guide des Connaisseurs http://www.leguidedesconnaisseurs.be/article1126.html

Koupernik C. In memoriam: Auguste Tournay, 1878–1969. *Revue de Neuropsychiatrie Infantile* 1969(17):331–332.

Krasnianski M, Neudecker S, Schluter A, Zierz S. Babinski-Nageotte's syndrome and Hemimedullary (Reinhold's) syndrome are clinically and morphologically distinct conditions. *Journal of Neurology* 2003(250):938–942.

Krause F (de Berlin). *Chirurgie du cerveau et de la moelle épinière*, traduit par le docteur Julien Bourguet, Préface du professeur M. Jeannel (de Toulouse), 2 vol, 1912, Société d'editions scientifiques, Paris, Analysis in *Rev Neurol (Paris)*, 1912(XXIV):640.

Krebs E. Du diagnostic et des indications opératoires dans les complications récentes et tardives des traumatismes cérébraux fermés, *Rev Neurol (Paris)*, 1939(71):369–388.

Krebs E. Nécrologie J. Babinski 1857–1932, *L'Encéphale* 1863(XXVIII):72–80.

Kyle R, Shampo M. Jozef Brudzinski, *Jama*, 1979 April, 241(15), p. 1620.

Kyle R, Shampo M. Jean-Baptiste-Etienne-Charcot, *Jama*, 1984; 252(2), p. 257.

L'Assistance publique en 1900, Administration générale de l'Assistance publique à Paris, Montévrain (Seine et Marne), Elèves de l'Ecole d'Alembert, 1900.

La Presse Médicale, 1915, supplément au n° 5, 4 February), "Have you looked at the last Forain?".

Labédollière E de. *Le nouveau Paris, Histoire de ses vingt arrondissements en 1860*, Paris, Gustave Barba libraire-éditeur, 1860.

Laignel-Lavastine M. Hommage à Joseph Jumentié, *Société de Neurologie de Paris*, meeting of june 7, 1928, *Rev Neurol (Paris)*, 1928, T. II, N° 1 (July), pp. 146–147.

Laignel-Lavastine M. *Recherches sur le plexus solaire*, Paris, Georges Steinheil, 1903.

Laignel-Lavastine M. Allocution, Société de Neurologie de Paris, meeting of January 12, 1928, *Rev Neurol (Paris)*, 1928, T. I, N° 1 (January), pp. 94–95.

Laignel-Lavastine M. Leçon Inaugurale de la Chaire d 'Histoire de la médecine et de la chirurgerie, November 20, 1931, Paris, Faculté de Médecine, p. 9.

Laignel-Lavastine M. (edited by). *Histoire générale de la médecine, de la pharmacie, de l'art dentaire et de l'art vétérinaire*. Paris, A. Michel, 1936/1949.

Lang JL. *Georges Heuyer, fondateur de la pédopsychiatrie. Un humaniste du XXè siècle*, Paris, Expansion Scientifique Publications, 1997.

Lannois, Durand. Deux cas de tumeurs de l'angle ponto-cérébelleux (tumeurs de l'acoustique opérées chirurgicalement), *Rev Neurol (Paris)*, 1909, T.XVII, n° 10 (30 May), p. 674.

Lanska DJ, Dietrichs E. Reflekshammerens historie, *Tidsskr Nor Loegeforen* 1998, 118 (n° 30), pp. 4666–4668.

Lanteri-Laura G. "L'hystérie, matrice de la sémiologie neurologique", in Poirier J et Poirier JL, (sous la direction de), *Médecine et philosophie à la fin du XIXè siècle*, Cahier de l'Institut de Recherche Universitaire d'Histoire de la connaissance, des idées et des mentalités n° 2, Créteil, Université Paris-Xii, 1978, pp. 141–148.

Lanzino G, Di Pierro CG, Laws ER Jr. One century after the description of the "sign": Joseph Babinski and his contribution to neurosurgery. *Neurosurgery*, apr 1997, 40(4) : 822–828.

Laplane D, Bonduelle M. Le débat sur l'hystérie, *Rev Neurol (Paris)*, 1999, 155 (10): 815–821.

Lareng L. Auguste Tournay. *Anesthésie Analgésie (Paris)*. 1969 Jan–Feb; 26(1):5–10.

Laveran, Obituary of Dr Bucquoy, *Bulletin de l'Académie de Médecine*, 1920, 27, pp. 4–5.

Lavielle L et R. *Dax médical et thermal : études cliniques sur la station*, Paris, Maloine, 1930.

Laws ER. "Schools" of neurosurgery: their development and evolution. In Greeenblatt SH, Dagi TF, Epstein MH. "A history of neurosurgery In its scientific and professional contexts", Parke Ridge Illinois, The American Association of Neurological Surgeons, 1997.

Ledoux MP et G. *Un homme, une oeuvre. Ferdinand-Jean Darier (1856–1938)*, Longpont-sur-Orge, Société historique, 1987; http://www.whonamedit.com/doctor.cfm/514.html.

Lees AJ. Georges Gilles de la Tourette. The man and his times, *Rev Neurol (Paris)*, 1986, 142 (11), pp. 808–816.

Le Gendre P. *Charles Bouchard, son œuvre et son temps (1837–1915)*, Paris, Masson et Cie, 1924.

Legrand du Saulle, *Les Hystériques - Etat physique et état mental - Actes insolites, délictueux et criminels*, Paris, Librairie J.-B. Baillière, 1891, cited in *Le Progrès médical*, 1886, T.III, n° 22 (29 May), pp. 400–401.

Le Grand Guignol, le théâtre des peurs de la Belle Epoque, Préface et notices par Agnès Pierron, Paris, Robert Laffont, 1995.

Lejars F. *Traité de chirurgie d'urgence*, Paris, Masson, 1901.

Lejars F. *Exploration clinique et diagnostic chirurgical*, Paris, Masson, 1923.
Lejonne P, Lhermitte J. Atrophie olivo-rubro-cérébelleuse, *Nouvelle Iconographie de la Salpêtrière*, 1909, 22 : 605-619.
Lemonnier P (Président de l'Association). Biographie de Ceslas Waliszewski (1852-1897), avec notes de notre condisciple Babinski, *Bulletin de l'Association amicale des anciens élèves de l'Ecole des Mines*, June 1898.
Leon-Sarmiento FE, Prada LJ, Torres-Hillera M. The first sign of Babinski. *Neurology*, Oct (1 of 2) 2002, 59 (7), p. 1067.
Leon-S FE, Prada LJ, The true Sign of Babinski. *Arch Pathol Lab Med* (United States), Jun 2001, 125(6), p. 723.
Léonard J. "Le corps médical au début de la IIIè République", in Poirier J et Poirier JL, (sous la direction de), *Médecine et philosophie à la fin du XIXè siècle*, Cahier de l'Institut de Recherche Universitaire d'Histoire de la connaissance, des idées et des mentalités n° 2, Créteil, Université Paris-XII, 1978, pp. 9-21.
Léonard J. *La médecine entre les pouvoirs et les savoirs*, Paris, Aubier Montaigne, 1981.
Leri A. *Cécité et tabès (étude clinique)*, Paris, J. Rueff, 1904.
Le Sourd L. Le docteur Joseph-François-Félix Babinski (1857-1932), *Gazette des hôpitaux*, 105th year, n° 92, November 16, 1932, p. 1681.
Les grands travaux hospitaliers, 1911. Un nouvel hôpital. La Pitié. Paris, Berger-Levrault, 1913.
Les maîtres de la médecine et de la chirurgie en France et à l'étranger, s.l.n.d. Album de photos, Babinski p .49.
Letulle M. Rapport sur la candidature de M. Babinski comme membre associé par M. Letulle, *Société Anatomique de Paris* meeting of May 25, 1884, *Bulletins de la Société Anatomique de Paris*, 1884, LVIII year, 4th series, T. VIII, pp. 265-267.
Letulle M. Victor Cornil (1837-1908), *La Presse Médicale*, 1908, annexe, n° 32, pp. 273-275.
Letulle M. Malassez (1843-1909), *La Presse Médicale*, 1909, n° 104 (29 December), pp. 1017-1022.
Letulle M. Bucquoy (1829-1920), *La Presse Médicale*, 1920, 48, pp. 892-893.
Lhermitte F. *Le syndrome cérébelleux. Etude anatomo-clinique chez l'adulte*, Société Française de Neurologie, XXIIè Réunion Neurologique Internationale (Paris, June 2-4, 1958), Rapports, Le cervelet, Paris, Masson et Cie, 1958.pp. 7-49.
Lhermitte J. Les petits signes de l'hémiplégie organique et leur valeur sémiologique, *NeurolParis-Rev Neurol (Paris)*, 1911, T. 22, n° 19 (October 15, 1911), pp. 407-417. Analysis in *Le Progrès Médical*, 1911, n° 48, p. 590.
Lhermitte J. Babinski (1857-1932), Hommage prononcé á l'Académie nationale de médecine to the meeting of December 10, 1957, *Bulletin de l'Académie nationale de médecine*, December 10, 1957, 32-33:727-740.
Lichterman BL. Roots and routes of Russian neurosurgery (from surgical neurology towards neurological surgery), *Journal of History of Neurosciences*, 1998,7(2):125-135.
Liévre JA. L'œuvre d'André Léri, *Semaine des Hôpitaux*, 1971, May 26;47(25), pp. 1630-1637.
Lisowski W. Professor Josef Babinski (1857-1932) - pioneer of contemporary classical neurology, *Materia Medica Polona*, 1986, fasc 3 (59), pp. 179-182.
Liste générale des anciens élèves de l'Ecole Polonaise, Paris, Imprimerie polyglotte A. Rueff-Heymann, 1908 (courtesy of Dr Pierre Konopka).
Loeper M. Nécrologie GM Debove, *Le Progrès Médical*, 1920, n° 48, p. 517.
Loeper M. Babinski, *Le Progrès médical*, November 5, 1932, n° 45, p. 1885.
Loeper M. Nécrologie. A.Chauffard, *Le Progrès Médical*, November 12, 1932, n° 46, p. 1947.
Loeper M. Nécrologie. Pierre Marie, *Le Progrès médical*, April 1940, n° 17-18, p. 348.
Logre (Dr.) Un Maître Français : Babinski, *La Revue du Médecin*, February 1930.
Lucas-Championnière J. La décompression cérébrale par l'ouverture du crâne et ses indications, *Journal de Médecine et de Chirurgie Pratiques*, T. LXXXI, n° 19, October 10, 1910, p. 721, Analysis *in Rev Neurol (Paris)*, 1911, T. XXI, n° 7 (15 April), p. 435.
Lyons AE. *The crucible years 1800 to 1900: Macewen to Cushing*. In Greeenblatt SH, Dagi TF, Epstein MH. "A history of neurosurgery in its scientific and professional contexts", Parke Ridge Illinois, The American Association of Neurological Surgeons, 1997.
Lyons JB. Sir Victor Horsley, *Medical History*, 1967, T II, n° 4:361-373.
Lyons JB. Josef Babinski 1857-1932, *Nursing Mirror, Midwives Journal*, 1975, vol. 141, n° 18 (30 October), p. 53.
Mabin D. Proust ou la parole d'un insomniaque, *La Presse médicale*, 1993, Tome 22, n° 32, pp. 1663-1665.

Mac Arthur LL. Accès chirurgical aseptique au corps pituitaire et à sa région. *The Journal of the American Medical Association*, 1912, T. LVIII, n° 26 (29 June), p. 2009. Analysis in *Rev Neurol (Paris)*, 1913, T. XXV, n° 4 (28 February), p. 212.

Mac Ewen W. Intracranial lesions: tumour of the dura mater. *Lancet*, 1881, 2, 541–543.

Magnan. Nécrologie de Ch. Périer, Président, *Bulletin de l'Académie de Médecine*, 1914 (meeting of December 22), 78th year LXXII, 3d series, p. 418.

Maynot R. "Babinski", *La Vie Médicale*, n° 22, November 10, 1932, p. 977.

Malassez. Décès et obsèques de Monsieur Cornil, discours de Malassez. *Bulletins de l'Académie de Médecine*, 1908, n° 16, pp. 480–483.

Malle BF. The social cognition of intentional action. In Halligan PW, Bass C, Oakley DA: *Malingering and illness deception*. Oxford, Oxford University Press 2003 : 83–92.

Marie P. Sur l'hérédo-ataxie cérébelleuse, *Semaine Médicale*, 1893, 13:444–447.

Marie P (ed. by). *La pratique neurologique*, Paris, Masson, 1911.

Marie P. Eloge de J.-M. Charcot, éloge prononcé à l'Académie de médecine the May 26, 1925, in *Rev Neurol (Paris)*, June 1925, T.I, n° 6, pp. 731–745, Centenaire de Charcot et 25è anniversaire de la Société de Neurologie de Paris.

Marie P, Crouzon O. Le phénomène du jambier antérieur (phénomène de Strümpell), *Société de Neurologie de Paris*, meeting of July 2, 1903, *Rev Neurol (Paris)* 1903, T. XI, n° 14 (July 30), pp. 729–731.

Marie P, DE Martel TH, Chatelin. Dix huit mois de chirurgie nerveuse dans le service du Professeur P. Marie à la Salpêtrière, Société de Neurologie de Paris, meeting of July 10, 1913. *Rev Neurol (Paris)*, 1913, T XXVI:132–134.

Marie P, Foix Ch, Alajouanine Th. De l'atrophie cérébelleuse tardive à prédominance corticale. *Rev Neurol (Paris)*, 1922, T. 38, n° 7, pp. 849–885 et n° 8, pp. 1082–1111.

Marinesco G. Sur quelques résultats obtenus avec le "606" dans le traitement des maladies nerveuses, *La Presse Médicale*, n° 8, January 28, 1911.

Marinesco G, Minea J. L'emploi des injections de sérum salvarnisé "in vitro" et "in vivo" sous l'arachnoïde spinale et cérébrale dans les tabes et la paralysie générale, *Rev Neurol (Paris)*, 1914, T. XXVII, n° 5 (March 15), pp. 336–347.

Martel de Th. Technique de la trépanation du crâne. *Journal de Chirurgie*, 1910, n° 4 (April 15), pp. 357–367, Analysis in *Rev Neurol (Paris)*, 1911, T.XXII, n° 13 (July 15), p. 28.

Martel de Th. Opération d'une tumeur de la moelle. *Société de Neurologie de Paris*, meeting of July 10, 1913. *Rev Neurol (Paris)*, 1913, T.XXVI, p. 117.

Martel de Th, Chatelin C. Tumeur du lobe frontal droit. Opération en deux temps, ablation de la tumeur. *Rev Neurol (Paris)* 1913, TXXV, n° 2, January 30: pp. 139–142.

Martel De Th, Chatelin C. *Les blessures du crâne et du cerveau*, Paris, Masson ed, 1917.

Martin, *Le Progrès Médical*, 30 août 1930.

Martin du Gard R, Tardieu J. *Lettres croisées (1923–1958)*, Paris, Nrf Gallimard, 2003, p. 240.

Massey EW, Sanders L. Babinski's sign in Medieval, Renaissance, and Baroque art. *Arch Neurol*, 1989, 46 : 85–88. Comment in: *Archives of Neurology*, oct 1989, 46(10): 1046; *Archives of Neurology* oct 1989, 46(10): 1047; *Archives of Neurology*, mar 1990, 47(3), p. 253.

Massey EW. Babinski's sign in Medieval, Renaissance, and Baroque art. *Archives of Neurology*, 1990, 47, p. 253.

Massie R. Charcot et Babinski : au-delà de la simple relation professeur-élève, *The Canadian Journal of Neurological Sciences* 2004(31):422–426.

Mathot (Dr). Causerie médicale. Nouveau Palmarès. A M. Babinski, ingénieur, *Journal des Praticiens*, 1914, p. Clxi.

Mauran L. Troubles nerveux et pithiatisme chez les soldats français, pendant la Grande Guerre, *Histoire des Sciences Médicales*, 1995(XXIX):63–69.

McHenry LC. *Garrison's History of Neurology*, Springfield Illinois, Charles C Thomas Publisher, 1969.

Mellergard P, Ljunggren B. Akademikerna gjorde tummen ner för Babinski *[Les universitaires rejetèrent Babinski]*, *Läkartidningen*, 1989, vol 86, n° 3, pp. 149–151.

Ménégaux G. In memoriam Thierry de Martel, 1875–1940, *Mém Acad Chir (Paris)*, 1953, 79 (1–3), pp. 87–99.

M.G, V.D. Joseph Chaillous, *La Presse Médicale*, n° 35, May 2, 1934, p. 717.

Michaux L. Georges Heuyer (1884–1977), *Nouv Presse Med*. 1978 Feb 4;7(5):383–384.

Mijolla A de. Les lettres de Jean-Martin Charcot à Sigmund Freud (1886–1893). Le crépuscule d'un dieu, *Revue Française de Psychanalyse* 1988:702–25.

Milian G. *Le Progrès Médical* 1907(XXIII):884.
Milian G. Le Professeur V. Cornil 1837–1908, *Le Progrès Médical*, 1908:199.
Mollaret P. Obituary. Georges Guillain (1876–1961), *La Presse Médicale* 1961(69):1696–1706.
Mondor H. Les 150 ans de l'Internat, Discours prononcé à la Sorbonne en 1951 à l'occasion des festivités des 150 ans de l'Internat, http://www.aaihp. fr/150ans.html#top
Monier-Vinard R. *Neurologie*, Paris, Masson, 1935.
Monier-Vinard R. Speech of M. Monier-Vinard, President, *Rev Neurol (Paris)*, 1939(71):54–56.
Monier-Vinard R. *Neurologie*, 2ème édition entièrement révisée, Paris, Masson, 1943.
Monin E. Les huitres, *Journal de la Santé* 1889(VII):260.
Moniz E. Dr Joseph Babinski, *Lisboa Médica* 1932(IX):1065.
Moniz E. L'encéphalographie artérielle, son importance dans la localisation des tumeurs cérébrales. *Rev Neurol (Paris)*, 1927(II):72–90.
Moniz E. Injections intracarotidiennes et substances injectables opaques aux rayons X. *Presse médicale*, Paris, 1927, 35: 969–971.
Moniz E. *Diagnostic des tumeurs cérébrales et épreuve de l'encéphalographie artérielle*, Paris, Masson, 1931.
Moniz E. *L'angiographie cérébrale*, Paris, Masson, 1934.
Moniz E. *La leucotomie préfrontale. Traitement chirurgical de certaines psychoses*, Torino, 1937.
Moreau R. Maxime Laignel-Lavastine, *Société Française de Neurologie*, meeting of November 5, 1953, *Rev Neurol (Paris)*, 1953(89):274–276.
Moreau R. Hommage à la mémoire de Joseph Babinski à l'occasion du 100è anniversaire de sa naissance, *Bull Mém Soc Méd Hôp Paris* 1958(74):449–457.
Mouquin M. Obituary of Charles Laubry (1872–1960), *La Presse Médicale* 1961(69):703–704.
Nageotte J. *Tabès et paralysie générale*, Paris, G. Steinheil, 1893.
Nageotte J. Note sur un nouveau microtome à cerveau, *Société de Biologie*, meeting of March 11, 1899, *Comptes-rendus hebdomadaires des Séances et Mémoires de la Société de Biologie*, 1899:202–203.
Nageotte J. Présentation d'un microtome du cerveau, XIIIth International Congress of Medicine, meeting of August 3, Comptes-Rendus Section de Neurologie, pp. 145–146, Paris, Masson et Cie éditeurs, 1900.
Nageotte J. Névrite radiculaire subaiguë. Dégénérescences consécutives dans la moelle (racines postérieures) et dans les nerfs périphériques (racines antérieures), *Rev Neurol (Paris)*, 1903, T. XI, n° 1 (January 15), p. 1.
Nageotte J. Note sur les fibres endogènes grosses et fines des cordons postérieurs et sur la nature endogène des zones de Lissauer, *Société de Biologie*, meeting of December 19, 1903, *Comptes rendus hebdomadaires des Séances et Mémoires de la Société de Biologie*, 1904, p. 1651.
Nageotte J. Sur la nature et la pathogénie des lésions radiculaires de la moelle qui accompagnent les tumeurs cérébrales, *Rev Neurol (Paris)*, 1904, n° 1 (January 15), p. 1.
Nageotte J. *La structure fine du système nerveux*. Paris, Maloine, 1905.
Nageotte J. *Notice sur les travaux de M. J. Nageotte*, Paris, Imprimerie de la Cour d'Appel, 1911.
Nayrac P. In memoriam Auguste Tournay (1878–1969), *Rev Neurol (Paris)*, 1969 Mar (120):196–7.
Nicati, Rietsch. *in* Archives de physiologie normale et pathologique, Paris, 1885: 6: 72.
Nicolas S. *L'hypnose: Charcot face à Bernheim*. Paris, L'Harmattan 2004.
Noir J. Nécrologie. Emile Duclaux, Membre de l'Institut et de l'Académie de Médecine, *Le Progrès Médical*, 1904, 33è année, 3è série, T. XIX, n° 19 (May 7), pp. 316–317.
Noir J. Souvenirs évoqués par la mort de deux maîtres : Chauffard et Babinski, *Concours Médical* 1932(52):3733–3734.
Nomenclature officielle des voies de Paris. http://www.v1.paris.fr/Carto/Nomenclature/2819.nom.html.
Nos docteurs, répertoire photo-biographique et annuaire du corps médical, Paris, Hirschlern, 1902.
Notes pour servir à l'histoire du spiritisme scientifique. La vie trépidante d'Eusapia Palladino. Eusapia Palladino et le Palladinisme. http://www.sdv.fr/pages/adamantine/eusapiapalladino.htm.
Nothnagel H. *Traité clinique du diagnostic des maladies de l'encéphale basé sur l'étude des localisations*, Translation by Dr P. Kéraval, Foreword by Professeur Charcot, Paris, Adrien Delahaye & Emile Lecrosnier, 1885.
Oakley DA. Hypnosis, and suggestion in the treatment of hysteria. *In* Halligan PW, Bass C, Marchall JC eds. *Contemporary approaches to the study of hysteria. Clinical and theoretical perspectives*. Oxford, Oxford University Press 2001, pp. 312–329.
Oakley DA, Ward NS, Halligan PW, Frackowiak Rsj. Differential brain activations for malingered and subjectively "real" paralysis, *In* Halligan PW, Bass C, Oakley DA, eds. *Malingering and illness deception*. Oxford, Oxford University Press, 2003, pp. 67–84.

Onanoff J. *Sur un cas d'épithélioma (étude histologique)*, Thése, Faculté de médecine de Paris, Paris, Ollier-Henry, 1892.
Opara J. W sprawie artykulu: A. Gasecki: Jozef Babinski wspoltworca wspolcaesnej neurologii i neurochirurgii [Jozef Babinskin co-founder of contemporary neurology and neurosurgery], *Neur Neurochir Pol*, 1997, 3: 641. [Letter concerning the paper of A. Gasecki : Josef Babinski co-founder of contemporary neurology and neurosurgery (N. Nch. Pol., 1997, 3, p. 641), *Neurologia i Neurochirurgia Pol*ska, 1997(6):1272-1273.
Oppenheim H. in discussion, p. 612, de Koenig W. Ueber die bei Reizung der Fussohle zu beobachtenden Reflexerscheinungen mit besonderer Berücksichtigung der Zehenreflexe bei den verschiedenen Formen der cerebralen Kinderlähmung, *Neurologisches Centralblatt*, 1899(18):610-613.
Oppenheim H. Zur Pathologie des Hautreflexe an der unteren Extremitäten, *Monatsschr Psychiatri Neurol*, 1902, 12, pp. 421-423. (cited by Goetz CG. History of the extensor plantar response: Babinski and Chaddock signs, *Seminars in Neurology* 2002(22):391-398).
Orden AO. Que Babinsky ? Babinski, *Medicina (Buenos-Aires)*,1999(59):119.
Orzechowski K. Josef Babinski w dziejach ubieglego okresu neurologii. *Lekarz Wojskowy*, 1933(1):1-10.
Orzechowski C, Mitkus W. De la forme parkinsonienne des tumeurs de la région infundibulo-hypophysaire, *Rev Neurol (Paris)*, 1925(II):1-17.
Pallardy G, Pallardy MJ, Wackenheim A. *Histoire illustrée de la radiologie*, Paris, Roger Dacosta, 1989.
Parizel PM, Makkat S, Jorens G et al. Brain stem haemorrhage in descending transtentorial herniation (Duret hemorrhage), *Intensive Care Medicine* 2002(28):85-88.
Passouant P. Personality: Dr. Auguste Tournay. *International Journal of Neurology*, 1965;5(2):217-21.
Pasteur Vallery-Radot. Otfrid Foerster (1873-1941), *Rev Neurol (Paris)*, 1942(74)72-74.
Paul C. Stéthoscope flexible, *Le Progrès médical* 1881(IX):375.
Pearce JMS. Babinski and his sign, *Journal of Neurology, Neurosurgery and Psychiatry* 1988(51):1163.
Pearce JMS. *Fragments of Neurological History*, London, Imperial College Press, 2003.
Pearce JMS. Hermann Oppenheim (1858-1919), *Journal of Neurology, Neurosurgery and Psychiatry* 2003(74):569.
Pearce JMS. The Argyll Robertson pupil, *Journal of Neurology, Neurosurgery and Psychiatry* 2004(75):1345.
Pearce JMS. Sir Gordon Holmes (1876-1965), *Journal of Neurology, Neurosurgery and Psychiatry* 2004(75):1502-1503.
Pearce JMS. Parinaud's syndrome. *J Neurol Neurosurg Psychiatry* 2005(76):99.
Pecker J. Thierry de Martel 1875-1940, *Surgical Neurology* 1980(13):401-403.
Pérec G. *Quel petit vélo chromé au fond de la cour?* Paris, Denoel, 1966.
Philippon J. The development of neurological surgery at the Salpêtrière Hospital, *Neurosurgery*, May 1996, 38(5):1016-1022.
Philippon J. L' œuvre de Babinski, *Bull Acad Natle Méd* 2007, 191, n° 7, p. 1319-1327.
Pieron H. Obituary of M. J. Babinski, *Compte-rendus de la Société de Biologie*, meeting of November 5, 1932:494-495.
Pinto F. A short history of the reflex hammer, *Practical Neurology*, 2003, (3):366-371.
Plichet A. *Babinski (1857-1932)*, in Dumesnil R. and Bonnet-Roy F. (edited by), "Les médecins célèbres", Genève, Editions d'Art L. Mazenod, 1947, pp. 250-251.
Plichet A. Le syndrome subjectif des blessés du crâne. *La Presse Médicale*, 1955, n° 32, p. 473.
Poirier J. Joseph Babinski, une personnalité complexe, *Bull Acad Natle Méd* 2007, 191, n° 7, p. 1343-1354.
Poirier J, Babinski histologist and anatomo-pathologist, *Romanian Journal of Morphology and Embryology*, 2008, 49(2), 262-269.
Poirier J. L'autre Babinski, *Neurologies*, Avril 2008, vol. 11, n° 107, p. 219-225
Poirier J, Chértien F. Désiré Bourneville (1840-1909), *Journal of Neurology*, 2000, 247 (6): 481.
Poirier J, Chértien F. Gustave Roussy (1874-1948), *Journal of Neurology*, 2000, 247 (11): 888-889.
Poirier J, Chértien F. Pierre Marie (1853-1940), *Journal of Neurology*, 2000, 247 (12): 983-984.
Poirier J, Derouesné C. La neurologie à l'Assistance publique et en particulier à la Salpêtrière avant Charcot, *Rev Neurol (Paris)*, 2000, 156(6-7), pp. 607-615.
Poirier J, Signoret JL (ed. by). *De Bourneville à la sclérose tubéreuse. Un homme. Une époque. Une maladie.* Paris, Médecine-Sciences Flammarion, 1991.
Poirier P. *Topographie crânio-encéphalique.Trépanation*, Paris, Lecrosnier et Babe,1891. (Review in the *Progrès Médical* 1891, TXIII, n° 6:114-116).

Pomiane E de. *Bien manger pour bien vivre. Essai de gastronomie théorique*, Paris, Albin Michel, 1922, [prizewinner of the Académie Française].
Pomiane E de. *Cooking With Pomiane*, North Point Press, 1976.
Postel J, Allen DF. *L'oeuvre historique de Gilbert Ballet (1853-1916)* : http://www.bium.univ-paris5.fr/sfhm/histoire3.htm.
Pozerski E. *L'Ecole polonaise ou l'esprit de 1830*, edited by the Association des Anciens Elèves de l'école polonaise, 15 rue Lamandé, Paris, 78 pages.
Pozerski de Pomiane E. *Souvenirs d'un demi-siècle à l'Institut Pasteur*, type-written brochure, 73 pages, s.l.n.d.
Prigratano GP, Schacter DJ. *Awareness of deficit after brain injury. Clinical and theoretical issues*. New York, Oxford University Press, 1991.
Pruzinski A. Profesor Dr Hab. nauk med. Eufemiusz Herman – Nestor Polskiej Neurologii, *Neurologia i Neurochirugia Polska* 1982(5–6):306–328.
Quercy P, Quercy D. Pierre Janet. L'hypnotisme, la suggestion, l'hystérie. La définition de l'hystérie. La rencontre de Freud, *Annales médico-psychologiques* 1949(II):287–314.
Ramsay-Hunt J. Dyssynergia cerebellaris myoclonica primary atrophy of the dentate system. A contribution to the pathology and symptomatology of the cerebellum. *Brain* 1921(44): 490–538.
Ranvier L. *Leçons sur l'histologie du système nerveux*, recueillies par M. Ed. Weber, 2 vol., Paris, Libraire F. Savy, Paris, 1878.
Ranvier L. *Leçons d'anatomie générale sur le système musculaire*, recueillies par M. J. Renaut. Paris, Bureaux du Progrès médical, 1880.
Ravaut P. Intervention (pp. 707–709), concerning the report of J.A. Sicard (with discussions) "Syphilis nerveuse et son traitement", *Réunion neurologique annuelle de la Société de Neurologie de Paris* consacrée à "Formes cliniques de la syphilis nerveuse et leur traitement" (9–10 July 1920), *Rev Neurol (Paris)*, 1920(XXXVI):609–748).
Ravina A. Plichet André (1888–1965), *La Presse médicale* 1965(17):993–995.
Raymond F. *L'étude des maladies du système nerveux en Russie. Rapport adressé à M. le ministre de l'Instruction publique par F. Raymond*, Paris, G. Doin éditeur, 1889.
Raymond F. *Etiologie du tabes dorsal*, Paris, Aux bureaux du Progrès Médical, Veuve Babé et Cie, 1892.
Recondo J de *Sémiologie du système nerveux. Du symptôme au diagnostic*, 2nd ed, Paris, Médecine-Sciences Flammarion, 2004.
Reddaway WF, Penson JH, Halecki O, Dyboski R. *The Cambridge History of Poland. From Augustus II to Pilsudski (1697–1935)*, Cambridge University Press, 1941.
Rey A. (Ecole des Mines de Paris, classe de 1876), Nécrologie de Henri Babinski, in *Bulletin de l'Association des Anciens élèves de l'Ecole des mines de Paris*, 1931. http://www.annales.org/archives/x/babinsky.html.
Richet Ch. *Traité de métapsychique*, Paris, Félix Alcan, 1922 (new edition in 1923).
Richter DH. *Emigracja polska do Ludow Europy*, Wroclaw, 1848.
Ricou P, Leroux-Hugon V, Poirier J. *La bibliothèque Charcot à la Salpêtrière*, Paris, éditions Pradel, 1993.
Rist E. *25 portraits de médecins français, 1900–1950*, Paris, Masson, 1955, pp. 57–63.
Rivet L. Joseph Babinski (1857–1932), *Bull Mém Soc Méd Hôp Paris*, 1932(34):1722–1733.
Robertson A. On an interesting series of eye symptoms in a case of spinal disease, with remarks on the action of belladonna on the iris, *Edinburgh Medical Journal* 1869(14):696–708.
Robertson A. Four cases of spinal spinal myosis: with remarks on the action of light on the pupil, iris, *Edinburgh Medical Journal*, 1869, vol. 15, pp. 487–193, cité par Pearce Jms, The Argyll Robertson pupil, *Journal of Neurology, Neurosurgery and Psychiatry* 2004(75):1345.
Roger H. Bouchard (1837–1915), *La Presse Médicale*, 1915, supplement for N°53 (November 4), pp. 402–406.
Rosenblum S. *Du développement du système nerveux au cours de la première enfance. Contribution à l'étude des syncinésies, des réflexes tendineux et cutanés et des réflexes de défense*, Paris, Le François, 1915.
Rothmann M (de Berlin). "Les symptômes des maladies du cervelet et leur signification", Deuxième rapport, XVIIè Congrès International de Médecine, London, August 6–12, 1913, Travaux de la section de Neuropathologie (section XI).
Roudinesco E. *La bataille de cent ans. Histoire de la psychanalyse en France, vol. I (1885–1939)*, Paris, Ramsay éd., 1982.

Roussy G. *La couche optique (étude anatomique, physiologique & clinique). Le syndrome thalamique.* Paris, G. Steinheil, 1907.
Roussy G. Charles Foix (1882-1927), *Rev Neurol (Paris),* 1927, T. I, N° 4 (April), pp. 441-446.
Roussy G. Centenaire de Vulpian, *Rev Neurol (Paris),* 1927, T. I, N° 6 (June), pp. 1159-1160.
Roussy G. Eulogy of Mrs Dejerine-Klumpke (1859-1927), *Rev Neurol (Paris),* 1927, T. II, N° 6 (December), pp. 635-642.
Roussy G. Notice nécrologique sur M. Jean Darier (1856-1938), *Comptes Rendues de l'Académie de Médecine,* meeting of June 28, 1938, pp. 737-742.
Sabin TD. Should we bother to look for the Babinski sign? *Journal Watch Neurology,* 2006 January 26, 2006(126):1-1.
Sahadevan MG. A hundred years of the Babinski reflex, *Journal of the Royal College of Physicians of London,* 1996, Vol. 30, n° 1 (January/February), p. 83.
Salwa W, Bautsch A, Lados A, Szura H, Chlipalska J, Chlipalski J, Lone R, Grabowska K. Dorobek naukowy Panstwowego Szpitala dla Nerwowo I Psychicznie Chorych im. J. Babinskiego w Krakowie-Kobierzynie w okresie piecdziesiecioletniego istnienia (1917-1967), *Przegl Lek.* 1967;23(9), pp. 660-665.
Sartre JP. *Les mots,* Paris, Gallimard, Collection Folio, 1964, p. 214.
Satran R. Joseph Babinski in the competitive examination (Agrégation) of 1892, *Bull N Y Acad Med.* 1974(50):626-635.
Satran R. Fulgence Raymond, the successor of Charcot, *Bull N Y Acad Med* 1974(50):931-942.
Satran R. Chekhov and Rossolimo. Careers in medicine and neurology in Russia 100 years ago, *Neurology* 2005(64):121-127.
Schaefer, Ueber einen antagonistischen reflex, *Neurologisches Centralblatt* 1899(22):1016-1018.
Schiller F. The reflex hammer. In memoriam Robert Wartenberg (1887-1956), *Medical History* 1967(11):75-85.
Schmahmann JD. Disorders of the cerebellum: ataxia, dysmetria of thought, and the cerebellar cognitive affective syndrome, *J Neuropsychiatry Clin Neurosci* 2004(16):367-378.
Science and Learning in France: The Society for American Fellowships in French Universities, 1 vol, 454 pages, 1917.
Sézary A. Raymond Monier-Vinard (1878-1944), *La Presse Médicale* 1944(17):274-275.
Sicard A. *Les injections sous-arachnoïdiennes et le liquide céphalo-rachidien. Recherches expérimentales et cliniques,* Paris, Georges Carré and C. Naud, 1900.
Sicard A. Etude des différents réflexes sous le contrôle de la bande d'Esmarch, *Société de Neurologie de Paris,* meeting of December 4, 1919, *Rev Neurol (Paris),* 1919, n° 12 (December), pp. 948-950.
Sicard A, Forestier J, *Rev Neurol (Paris),* 1921,28:1264-1266.
Sicard JA, Forestier J. Méthode générale d'exploration radiologique par l'huile iodée (Lipiodol). *Bull Mém Soc Méd Hôp Paris,* 1922, pp. 460-463.
Sicard JA, Forestier J, Laplane L. Radiodiagnostic lipiodolé au cours des compressions rachidiennes. *Rev Neurol (Paris),* 1923,6:276.
Signoret JL. Une leçon clinique à la Salpêtrière (1887) par André Brouillet, *Rev Neurol (Paris),* 1983, 12, pp. 693-694.
Singer C, Ashworth Underwood E. *A Short History of Medicine,* Oxford University Press, New York & Oxford, 1962, p. 735.
Souques A. *Etapes de la neurologie dans l'Antiquité grecque (d'Homère à Galien),* Paris, Masson et Cie, 1936.
Sournia JC. *Histoire de la médecine et des médecins,* Paris, Larousse, 1991.
Spillane JD. *The doctrine of the nerves. Chapters in the history of neurology,* Oxford, Oxford University Press, 1981.
Stakenburg M. A reflex hammer for accurate measurement of reflex latency, *Electroencephalography and Clinical Neurophysiology,* 1979, 46 : 613-614.
Starr MA, *Brain surgery,* New York, William Wood & Co, 1893.
Stewart TG, Holmes G. Symptomatology of cerebellar tumours; a study of forty cases, *Brain* 1904(27):522-549.
Strachey J. *Bibliography and Author Index. The Standard Edition of the Complete Psychological Works of Sigmund Freud,* vol. 1 (1886-1899), London, Hogarth, Toronto, Irwin, 1966.
Strümpell AV. Ueber das Verhalten der Haut- und Sehnenreflexe bel Nervenkranken, *Neurologishes Centralblatt* 1899(18):617-619.
Suchard E. Note sur les lésions histologiques de l'ongle incarné ou onyxis latéral, *Société Anatomique,* meeting of December 19, 1884, *Progrès médical* 1885(II):202.

Suchard E. *Technique générale et somMayre des autopsies cliniques*, in "Clinique médicale de la Charité, leçons et mémoires" by Professor Potain and collaborators, Paris, Masson, 1894, pp. 1011–1056.
Swift H, Ellis A. Le traitement direct de la syphilis du système nerveux central, New York Neurological Society, April 1, 1913, *Journal of Nervous and Mental Disease* 1913:467–470.
Tada M, Tada M, Ishiguro H, Hironta K. Babinski-Nageotte syndrome with ipsilateral hemiparesis. *Archives of Neurology* 2005(62):676–677.
Tan TC, Black PMcL. The contributions of Otfrid Foerster (1873–1941) to neurology and neurosurgery, *Neurosurgery* 2001(49):1231–1236.
Tarlau M. The extensor toe reflex, *Archives of Neurology* 1989(46):1047.
Tashiro K. Kisaku Yoshimura and the Chaddock reflex, *Archives of Neurology* 1986(43):1179–1180.
Tasmira J. (Pod redakcja) *Zarys Historii Polski*, 861 pages, Warszawa, Panstwowy Instytut Wydawniczy, 1979.
Tatu L, Moulin T, Monnier G. The discovery of encephalic arteries. From Johann Jacob Wepfer to Charles Foix. *Cerebrovasc Dis*, 2005; 20: 427–432.
Terrier F, Péraire M. *L'opération du trépan*, Paris, Alcan edit, 1895.
Thewlis MW. 1932 – The death of Babinski, *Medical Times*, 1972 sept, 100 (9): 40–44.
Thiebaut F. Obituaries. JA Barré (1880–1967), *Journal of the Neurological Sciences*, Amsterdam, 1968, 6: 381–382.
Thomas A. *Le cervelet, étude anatomique, clinique et physiologique*, Paris, G. Steinheil éd., 1897.
Thomas A. *La fonction cérébelleuse*, un volume de l'*Encyclopédie scientifique*, Paris, Doin éditeur, 326 pages, 1911, analysis in *Le Progrès Médical*, 1911, T. XXXI, n° 25 (June 24, 1911), p. 311.
Thomas A. Durupt A. *Localisations cérébelleuses*, Paris, Vigot, 1914.
Thomas A. *Pathologie du Cerveau et du Cervelet. Pathologie du Cervelet*, In G.H. Roger GH, Widal F, Teissier PJ., "Nouveau Traité de Médecine", Fascicule XIX, Paris, Masson, 1925.
Thomas A. *Équilibre et Équilibration*. Paris, Masson, 1940.
Thuilleaux M. Le roman psychiatrique d'André Breton, January 16, 2004, http://www.psydesir.com/ced/imprimer.php?id_article=6
Thuillier J. *Monsieur Charcot de la Salpêtrière*. Paris, Robert Laffont, 1993.
Tilles G, Wallach D. Le traitement de la syphilis par le mercure. Une histoire thérapeutique exemplaire, *Histoire des Sciences Médicales*, 1996(XXX):501–510.
Ting Chang, The limits of the gift. Alfred Chauchard's donation to the Louvre, *Journal of the History of Collections*, 2005, 17(2), pp. 213–221.
Tollemer L.-A, *Maladies du cervelet*, in Charcot JM, Bouchard C, Brissaud E, "Traité de médecine", Paris, G. Masson,1894. T. VI, pp. 245 – 272.
Toupet R. Chirurgie de l'hypophyse, *Revue de Chirurgie*, 1912, an XXXII, n° 6 (10 June), pp. 899–945. Analysis in *Rev Neurol (Paris)*, 1913, T. XXV, n° 4 (28 February), pp. 212.
Tournay A. *L'homme endormi. Essai d'une introduction historique et critique à la séméiologie du sommeil naturel*. Thése. Paris, G. Steinheil éditeur, 1909.
Tournay A. *Neurologie*, Paris, Gaston Doin (Les consultations journalières), 1926.
Tournay A. *Sémiologie du sommeil. Essai de neurologie expliquée*, Paris, Doin, 1934.
Tournay A. Allocution à propos du décès de M. Thierry de Martel, *Rev Neurol (Paris)*, 1939–1940, 72 (2è semestre), N° 7, pp. 705–710.
Tournay A. Discours du Président, sortant, Société de Neurologie de Paris, meeting of January 9, 1941, *Rev Neurol (Paris)*, 1941, T. 73, N° 1-2 (January–February), pp. 24–26.
Tournay A. Nécrologie de M. Pierre Marie, *Rev Neurol (Paris)*, 1941, T. 73, n° 11–12 (November–December): 618–621.
Tournay A. Joseph Babinski (1857–1932), *Médecine de France*, 1953, n° 43, pp. 3–10.
Tournay A. Babinski dans la vie, *La Presse Médicale*, 1958, 66:1485–1489.
Tournay A. Les régulations organiques de l'affectivité, *Bulletin de psychologie, édité par le Groupe d'Etudes de Psychologie de l'Université de Paris*, Opening lecture, January 12, 1966, pp. 1–51.
Tournay A. *La vie de Joseph Babinski*, Amsterdam, Elsevier, 1967.
Tournay A. Chauchard P, Sorre M. "Conditions et régles de vie", Livre VI, in Piéron H. (sous la direction de), *Traité de psychologie appliquée*, Paris, Puf, 1958.
Trepsat Ch. Traitement d'un tiqueur par la psychanalyse, *Le Progrès Médical*, 1922, N° 16 (22 April), pp. 182–184.
Trillat E. *Histoire de l'hystérie*, Paris, "Médecine et histoire" Seghers, 1986.

Trocmé F. *De la thérapeutique palliative dans les tumeurs de l'encéphale. Méthodes décompressives (ponction lombaire et trépanation palliative)*, Thése, Paris, Henri Jouve éditeur, 1909.
Trouillas P. *Le syndrome cérébelleux*, http://spiral.univ-lyon1.fr/polycops/NeuroInterFac/NeuroInterFac-3.5.html
Trouillet R, Gely-Nargeot MC, Derouesné C. Unawareness of deficits in Alzheimer's disease: a multidimensional approach, *Psychologie et NeuroPsychiatrie du Vieillissement* 2003(1):99–110.
Vaintray (Dr). Le Docteur Babinski, *Le Correspondant Médical*, October 31, 1907.
Vallery-Radot P. *Deux siècles d'histoire hospitalière, de Henri IV à Louis-Philippe (1602–1836)*, Londres, Paris, New York, Editions Paul Dupont, 1947, p. 79.
Vallery-Radot P. L'ancien hôpital d'Aubervilliers, *La Presse Médicale*, November 12, 1949, n° 72, pp. 1062–1063.
Van Bogaert L. Nécrologie. Joseph Babinski, *Journal de Neurologie et de Psychiatrie*, 1932, T.XXXII, n° 11, p. 890–891.
Van Bogaert L. Auguste Tournay (1878–1969), *Journal of Neurological Sciences*, 1970 Feb;10(2):197–198.
Van Gehuchten A. Le phénomène des orteils, *Journal de Neurologie*, 1898, T.III, n° 8, pp. 153–155.
Van Gehuchten A. A propos du phénomène des orteils, *Journal de Neurologie*, 1898, T.III, n° 14, pp. 284–286.
Vaquez H. Les troubles pupillaires dans les lésions aortiques. *Société Médicale des Hôpitaux de Paris*, meeting of February 7, 1902, in *Le Progrès Médical*, 1902, 3è série, T. XV, n° 7 (February 15), p. 103.
Vaquez H. *Précis de thérapeutique*, Paris, Librairie J.-B. Baillière et fils, 1907.
Vaquez H. Joseph Babinski (1857–1932), *Bulletin de l'Académie de Médecine* 1932(35)1264–1273.
Vasse P. Babinski et la transmission de pensée, *Revue Métapsychique*, Nouvelle série N°11 (July–August–September 1950), pp. 148–151.
Veith I. Four thousand years of hysteria. In Horowitz MJ. *Hysterical personality*, New York, Aronson, 1977 : 7–94.
Villaret M. Great steps in hydro-climatology, Inaugural Lesson of the Chair of Hydrology and of therapeutic climatology, *La Presse Médicale*, 1928, n° 95 (28 November), pp. 1513–1518.
Villey R. *Histoire du diagnostic médical*, Paris, Masson, 1976, pp. 166–168.
Vincent C. J. De quelques causes d'erreur dans le diagnostic des syndromes d'hypertension intracranienne et dans celui de la localisation des tumeurs cérébrales, *Société de Neurologie de Paris*, meeting of November 10, 1910, *Rev Neurol (Paris)*, 1911(XXI):209–217.
Vincent C. J. Babinski (1857–1932), *Rev Neurol (Paris)*, 1932(2):441–446.
Vincent C. Leçon inaugurale, *Presse Médicale*, 1939, 1, n° 40 :761–766.
Vires, Calmettes (communiqué par M. Souques), Recherches sur le phénomène des orteils (signe de Babinski), *Société de Neurologie de Paris*, meeting of June 7, 1900, *Rev Neurol (Paris)*, 1900(VIII):535–536.
Vitu Auguste. *Paris*. Paris, P. Quantin, 1890 (450 dessins inédits d'après nature).
Voldmann D. Guérir du cancer et mourir de vieillesse : histoire de l'hospice Paul-Brousse de 1905 à 1975, *Asclepio*, 1983(35):317–326.
Voorhers IW. Chirurgie de l'hypophyse avec considérations particulières sur la méthode endonasale de Hirsch, *Medical Record*, 1912(2180):282. Analysis in *Rev Neurol (Paris)*, 1913(XXV):212.
Vuilleumier P. Hysterical conversion and brain function. *Progress in Brain Research* 2005; 150: 309–329.
Vuillemier P, Chichero C, Assal F, Schwartz S, Slosman D, Landis T. Functional neuroanatomical correlates of hysterical sensorimotor loss. *Brain* 2001(124):1077–1090.
Vuilleumier P. Anosognosia: the neurology of beliefs and uncertainties, *Cortex* 2004(40):9–17.
Walshe F. Sir. The Babinski plantar response, its forms and its physiological and pathological significance, *Brain* 1956(LXXIX):529–556.
Walshe F. What place for Babinski in modern neurology, *Société Française de Neurologie*, session of June 2, 1958 (Centennial of the birth of J. Babinski), *Rev Neurol (Paris)*, 1958(98):632–636.
Wartenberg R. Babinski reflex and Marie–Foix flexor withdrawal reflex. Historical note, *A.M.A. Archives of Neurology and Psychiatry* 1951(65):713–716.
Wartenberg R. *Joseph François Félix Babinski, In* Haymaker W, Schiller F. "The founders of neurology", 2d ed., Springfield, Charles C Thomas, 1970, pp. 397–399.
Weil A. *Hermann Oppenheim (1858–1919), in* Haymaker W, Schiller F. "The founders of neurology", 2d ed., Springfield, Charles C Thomas, 1970, pp. 492–495.

Weil MP. Sur un cas de méningite syphilitique incurable par le mercure et guérie par le dioxydiamidoarsenobenzol, *Société de thérapeutique*, meeting of December 10, 1913, analysis in *Rev Neurol (Paris)*, 1914(XXVII):762.
Weinstein EA, Kahn RL. *Denial of illness: symbolic and physiological aspects*, Springfield, Ch Thomas, 1955.
Wertheimer P., David M. Naissance et croissance de la neurochirurgie, *Neurochirurgie* 1979(25):249-363.
Weschler IS. *Charles Elsberg (1871-1948)*, in Haymaker W, Schiller F. "The founders of neurology" 2d ed, Springfield, Charles C Thomas, 1970:552-554.
Widal F, Sicard A. In Bouchard C, "Traité de pathologie générale", Paris, Masson, 1900, T. VI, p. 621.
Widal F, Sicard A, Ravaut P. *Bull Soc Méd hôp Paris*, January 18, 1901.
Widlöcher D. L'hystérie, cent ans après. *Rev Neurol (Paris)* 1982;138:1053-60.
Wieviorka A. (edited by). *Justin Godart, Un homme dans son siècle (1871-1956)*, 2nd ed., Paris, Cnrs Editions, 2005.
Wilkins RH, Brody IA. Babinski's sign, *Arch Neurol* 1967(17):441-446.
Wilkins RH. *Treatment of craniocerebral infection and other common neurosurgical operations at the time of Lister and Macewen*, In Greeenblatt SH, Dagi TF, Epstein MH. "A history of neurosurgery In its scientific and professional contexts", Parke Ridge Illinois, The American Association of Neurological Surgeons, 1997.
Willms J. *Paris, Capital of Europe, From the Revolution to the Belle Époque*, New-York, Holmes & Meier Publishers, Inc, 1997, p 309.
Willoughby EW, Eason R. The crossed upgoing toe sign: a clinical study, *Annals of Neurology* 1983(14):480-482.
Wirotius JM. Histoire de la rééducation, *Encycl Med Chir (Elsevier, Paris), Kinésithérapie-Médecine physique-Réadaptation*, 26-005-1-A-10, 1999, 25 p.
Wolinetz E. *Neurochirurgie du praticien* (foreword by A. Tournay), Paris, Masson, 1953.
Yoshimura K. On Babinski's phenomenon, *Igaku Chuo Zasshi*, 1906(4):533-549, 824-841, 939-955 (cited by Tashiro K. Kisaku Yoshimura and the Chaddock reflex, *Archives of Neurology* 1986(43):1179-1180).
Yoshimura K. Ueber das Babinski'sche phænomen, Aus der medicinischen Facultät der Kaiserlich Japanischen Universität zu Tokio, Bd. Viii, Heft 2, 1908, S. 220.
Zabriskie EG. *Joseph Jules Dejerine*, in Haymaker W, Schiller F. "The founders of neurology", 2d ed., Springfield, Charles C Thomas, 1970, p. 426.
Zamoyski A. *The Polish way. A thousand-year history of the Poles and their culture*, London, John Murray, 1987.
Zeldin T. *Histoire des passions françaises, I, Ambition et Amour*, Paris, Seuil, 2002.

Index

Académie de médecine, 16, 28, *29*, 37, 56, 70, 87, 89, 90, 92, 93, 95, 107n.18, 114, 116, 121, 124, 140, 142, 143, 182, 187, 195, 271, 326, 328, 331, 334, 347, 357
Académie des sciences, 16, 37, 59, 89, 90, 91, 93, 95, 110, 122, 124, 139, 142, 144, 195, 328, 335
Achard, Charles (1860–1944), 110, 112, 193, 236
  Manuel de Médecine (1896), 236
Achilles reflex, 197–198, 224, 237–238, 241, *242*
Acromegaly (Pierre Marie disease), 202, *203*, 223, 326
Adiadochokinesia, 253, 255, 258, 261, 262, 263–264
Adie, William John (1886–1935), 202
Adiposo-genital syndrome, *203*, *204*
Aggregation/Agrégation
  (associate professorship),
   viii, 10, 12n.12, 97, 98, 114, 144
  1892 Competition for, 105–113
    Babinski's failure in candidacy for, viii, 10, 27, 167, 187, 217, 335, 345–346, 347, 362
    de la Tourette's failure in candidacy for, 12n.12

Ajuriaguerra, J. de (1911–1993), 333
Alajouanine, Théophile (1890–1980), 328, 330, 332, 351, 360
Alfonso XIII, King of Spain, (1886–1941), 47, 164
Alfort school, 325
Ali-Bab (Joseph's brother Henri), viii, 37, 48, 57, 68–73, 82–83, 357, 362 *See also* Babinski, Henri (1855–1931) (brother)
Alienist, 94, 119, 321
Allegri, Antonio (Correggio) (1494–1534), 222
Allen-Checkley sign, 232, 233
Allips, Miss, *156*, 157
Alzheimer, Alois (1864–1915), 342
Ambroise Paré Hospital, 180
American Neurological Association, 16
American Neurological Society, 343
Amyotrophic lateral sclerosis, 7, 133
Anatomical Society, 133, 330–139, 140–141 *See also* Société anatomique de Paris
Anatomopathology, 90, 137, 140, 141, 143, 145–149
Anatomy, 93, 99, 100, 105, 122, 127, 144, 145, 267, 272, 276, 326, 328, 332, 333, 341

Anatomy (*Cont.*)
  Nageotte's research on connective tissue and of the nervous system, 144
  Poirier's book on cranioencephalic topography, 267
Aneurysms, 202, 208, 211, 336
Annales de Médecine, 195
Annales Médico-psychologiques, 176
Anosodiaphoria, 27, 205, 206
Anosognosia, 27, 189, 196, 205–206, 211
Anton, Gabriel (1858–1933), 205
Anton syndrome, 205
Anton-Babinski syndrome, 206, 347
Aortic aneurysm of the aorta, 202, 211
Aphasia, 176, 189, 194, 268, 326, 332
Aragon, Louis (1897–1982), 46
Archiv fur Psychiatrie und Nervenkrankheiten, 236
Archives de Médecine, 250
Archives de Neurologie, 128, 188, 315
Archives de Physiologie Normale et Pathologique (1868), 7
Argyll-Robertson sign, 188, 199–201, 215, 287
Art, 7–8, 19–21, 40, 46, 49, 178
  Belle Epoque, the, 14–15
Arthropathies, 191, 197
Articular pathology, 307
Assistance Publique, Paris, 97, *153*, 154–155
Association d'enseignement médical des hôpitaux de Paris (Association for medical education of the Hôpitaux de Paris), 162
Asynergy, 249, 253, 256–257, 258, 262, 263–264
Athetosic movements, 207–208
Aubervilliers Hospital, 112
Aubry, Georges, 287
Autosuggestion, 301, 305–306, 311, 312, 316, 317, 319
Auvray, Maurice (1868–1945), 268
  medical thesis on first results of cranial surgery, 268

Babès, Victor (1854–1926), 140
Babesiosis, 140

Babinski, Aleksander (1823–1899) (father), viii, 3–6, 61–65
Babinski, Antoni (1812–1847) (uncle), 80–81
Babinski, Henri (1855–1931) (brother), viii, 3, 8, 10, 25, 36, 37, 55, 57, 59, 65–77, 82–83, 183, 288, 328
  Gastronomie Pratique, 48, 83
  Bien manger pour bien vivre, 82
  See also Ali-Bab (Joseph's brother Henri)
Babinski, Jan Josef (1873–1921), 81
Babinski, Joseph (1857–1932), vii, 3
  competitions for:
  1892 agrégation
    Bureau Central, *104*
  love of native Poland, 54–61
  relationship with brother Henri, 74–77, 360
  youthful impressions, 3–6
  See other entries under Babinski
Babinski, Jozef *See* Babinski, Joseph; entries under Babinski
Babinski, Léon (1891–1973), 40, 43, 44, 47–49, 57, 62n.42, 86, 183
Babinski, Stanislas A., 82
Babinski, Waclaw (1887–1957), 81–82
Babinski hammer, 30, 237, 238, *239*, 240, 252
Babinski platysma sign, 235
Babinski reflex, 223, 231
Babinski sign, vii, viii, ix, 70, 188, 196, 217–233, 345, 346, 352, 355, 357
  and spinal automatism reflexes, 245
  techniques used in searching for, 247–248
Babinski syndromes, 202–205, 347
Babinski the teacher, 167–179
  foreign students and, 183–185
  nonresident students' devotion to, 179–182
  Saturday lessons, 160–161
  students and close friends to, 169–179
  training foreign physicians, 183–185
Babinski the therapist, 159–160, 283–295
Babinski vault (Montmorency cemetery), 80

Babinski's career, 8–12, 15–16, 126–127, 151–152
  candidacy for Nobel Prize, 345–346
  as *médecin des hôpitaux* at La Pitié, 152–158
  private practice, 162–165
  and Société anatomique, 133–149
  and teachers, 12–25
  voluntary military service, 9, 54
  See also hysteria; pithiatism
Babinski's circle of friends/associates, 85–93
  intimate friends, 86–94
  students who became friends, 95–96
Babinski's death, 20–21, 51, 80
Babinski's education, 4, 8–15, 115–131
Babinski's eminent patients, 163–164
Babinski's eminent students, 168–169
Babinski's interest in therapy, 283–294
  development of neurosurgery, 290
  rehabilitation of handicapped, 290–292
Babinski's neologisms, 27–28
Babinski's papers and publications, 169, 187–189, 189–194, 206–208
  anatomopathology and histology, 145–149
  Compendium, 102
  contributions to:
    cerebellar symptomatology, 251–257
    vestibular symptomatology, 258–260
  medical thesis, 9–10
  Notice sur les travaux scientifiques (1892), 34
  Oeuvre scientifique, 209–216
  toe phenomenon and hysteria, 10–11
  See also Babinski syndromes; big toe extension; toe phenomenon
Babinski's personality, 23–34, 39–46, 156
  absence of political or religious commitment, 36–38
  appreciation of the arts/theatre, 39–40, 43–46
  attachment to his native country, 54–61
  fascination with paranormal phenomena, 34–35
  Léon Babinski's vignette of, 47–51
  work ethic, 24–28, 214–216
Babinski's professional relationships

Charcot's school:
  agreement with, 317, 319
  differing with, 302, 305–307
  Freud, 314–317
  Pierre Janet, 313
Babinski's public image, 345–363
  affiliations with scientific associations, 10, 189–194
  attitude to "name syndrome," 346–347
  limited place in publications, 354–358
  posthumous reputation, 348–351
  street names, 358–360
  See also Société de Neurologie de Paris
Babinski's research and studies, 145–148, 193, 208–209
  debate on hysteria with Janet, 313–314
  hypnotism, 11–12
  hysteria and pithiatism, 302–313, 317–318
  main tasks, 15–16
  nervous diseases, 143–144, 189, 196–202
  neurology, 321–343
  study of semiology, 195–196
  study of syphilis, 197–201
  technique of cerebral angiography, 362
  toe phenomenon, 10–11, 36, 229
  See also hysteria; pithiatism
Babinski's semiology, 195–196
Babinskiego, Josefa, 360
Babinski-Fröhlich syndrome, 202, 247
Babinski-Froment syndrome, 202, 204, 347
Babinski-Nageotte syndrome, 347
Babinski-Rabiner hammer, 240 *See also* Babinski hammer
Babinskis, extended family, 80–82
Babinski-Vaquez syndrome, 202, 215, 347
Babinski-Weill test, 259–260
Bacteriology, 90, 92, 140, 336
Bailey, Sir Percival (1892–1973), vii, 353
Bainville, Jacques (1879–1936), 86
Balbiani, Edouard-Gérard (1823–1899), 142
  Archives d'anatomie microscopique (1897), 142
Ball, Benjamin (1834–1893), 333

Ballet, Gilbert (1853–1916), 128, 130n.28, 205, 334
   thesis on anatomoclinical research, 334
   Traité de pathologie mentale (1903), 334
Baranyi, A. (1876–1936), 185
Bariety, Maurice (1897–1971), 354
   L'histoire de la médecine, 354
Barré, Jean Alexandre (1880–1967), 28, 36, 96, 168, 169, 194, 195, 198, 258, 328, 337
   inversion of the ulnar reflex, 243
Barré sign (in pyramidal syndrome), 175
Barré-Liéou syndrome, 175
Barré-Masson syndrome, 175
Baruk, Henri (1897–1999), 31, 32, 352, 356
Basedow disease, 207, 284, 326
Basic sciences, 6, 7, 16–18
Batignolles School *See* Polish School (Paris)
Baudelaire, Charles (1821–1867), 8
Bazy, Pierre (1853–1934), 36, 85, 89, 90, 162
   Atlas des maladies des voies urinaires, 89
Beaujon Hospital, 89, 336
Beavor, Charles E. (1854–1908), 341
Bechtrew sign, 232
Béclère, Antoine (1856–1939), 162, 358
Bekhterev, Vladimir (1857–1927), 266, 343
Benjoin colloidal reaction, 160
Bennet, Hughes (1848–1901), 265
Benoist, Léon (1855–1906), 73–74
Berbez, Paul, 130n.28, 333
Bergman, Ernst Von (1836–1907), 266
   technology of antisepsis after Lister, 266
Bergouignan, Michel (1907–1970), 208
   "Influence of the aneurysms of the aorta on lung diseases," 208
Bergson, Henri (1859–1941), 14, 36
   Essai sur les données immédiates de la conscience (Time and free will: an essay on the immediate data of consciousness), 14
Bernard, Claude (1813–1878), 6, 12, 142, 152, 189, 354
   Introduction to the Study of Experimental Medicine, 6
Bernays, Martha (Freud's fiancée), 314

Bernheim, Hippolyte (1840–1919), 14, 16, 300, 305–306, 317, 337
   De la suggestion et de ses applications à la thérapeutique (Suggestive therapeutics: a treatise on the nature and uses of hypnotism), 14
   Nancy school, 305
Besnier, Ernest Henri (1831–1909), 87
Bicêtre Hospice/Hospital, 86, 89, 94, 116–120, 143, 144, 177, 321, 325, 326, 330, 331, 332, 360
Bidou, Gabriel (1878–1959), 291, 292
Big toe extension, 221–222, 236, 239–240, 245, 247–248 *See also* Babinski sign; toe phenomenon
Billy, André (1882–1971), 154
Bing sign (in pyramidal lesions), 229
Bizet, Georges (1838–1875), 8
   Carmen (1875), 8
Blin, Emmery (1863–?), 128, 193n.28
   Leçons du mardi, 128
Blindness/total blindness, 177, 205
Blocq, M. Paul (1860–1896), 130, 238
Blum, Léon (1872–1950), 93
Boguslawski, Alojzy (1812–1847), 80–81
Boisseau, Jules (1877–1961), 168, 175
Bonduelle, Michel, ix, 113
   Charcot: Constructing Neurology, ix
Bordet, Jules (1870–1961), 197
Botticelli, Sandro (1445–1510), 222
Bouchard, Charles (1833–1899), 7, 24, 92, 105, *106*, 107, 110, 113, 128, 182, 236, 334, 335, 336
   lightning pain observed in tabes dorsalis, 7
Boulevard Haussmann, 11, 40, 47, 48, 85, 163, *165*
Boulevard du Montparnasse, 3, 4n.1, 63, 79, 85
Boulloche, Pierre (1864–1923), 193, 236
Bourdillon, Charles (1891–1963), 168
   decompressive craniotomy, 168
Bourgeois, Henri, 259
Bourgeois, Léon (1851–1925), 110, 111
Bourneville, Désiré-Magloire (1840–1909), 7, 36, 38, 98, 105, 128, 321, 325, 358

recommended anonymous
examinations, 98
Boyce, Sir Rupert (1863–1911), 266
Boznanska, Olga (1865–1940), 48, 163
Brain, 39, 157, 189, 208, 270, 271, 273, 274,
275, 276, 282, 297, 319, 332, 334,
337356, 362
changes in hysteria, 300
cortical function, 341
pathological study of, 158
See also brain tumors
Brain compression, 211
Brain lesions, 39, 268
Brain microtome, 143
Brain tumors, 168, 183, 205, 210, 277, 266,
268, 273, 276, 280, 296, 337, 362 See
also cerebral tumors
Bramwell, Byron (1847–1931), 341
work on diseases of the spinal cord, 341
Braque, Georges (1882–1963), 19
Bredin, Jean-Denis, 36
L'Affaire, 36
Breton, André (1896–1966), 20, 43–46
concept of surrealism, 20
Le Surréalisme, meme (review), 44
Nadja (journal), 45
Brissaud, Edouard (1852–1909), 12, 36,
128, 130n.28, 164, 189, 192, 193,
236, 325, 326, 328, 331, 336–337
Leçons sur les maladies nerveuses, 337
Revue Neurologique (co-founder), 337
Traité de Médecine, 337
British Journal of Psychology, 16
British Medical Association, 266
The British Medical Journal, 110
Broca, Pierre Paul (1824–1880), 6, 87, 141,
267, 268, 297, 326, 355
Brocq, Louis-Anne-Jean (1856–1928), 87
Brouardel, Paul (1837–1936), 130, 354
Brown, Sanger (1852–1928), 251
Brown-Séquard, Charles (1817–1894), 7,
12, 110, 189, 244
Brown-Séquard syndrome, 162, 190,
213, 246
Brudzinski, Josef (1874–1917), 357n.55
Bruns, L. (1858–1916), 253, 255, 276
adiadochokinesia, 253
Buck hammer, 240

Bucquoy, Jules (1829–1920), 9, 101,
121–124
Brudzinski, Josef (1874–1917), 357n.55
eponymic sign in meningitis, 357n.55
Bulbar disorder, 212
Bulletin de l'Association des anciens élèves
de l'Ecole des Mines de Paris, 59
Bulletin de la Société Médicale des
Hôpitaux de Paris, 197
Bulletin Médical, 195, 237
Bulletin polonais littéraire, scientifique
et artistique, 65
Bulletins de la Société Anatomique de
Paris, 188
Bulletins et Mémoires de la Société
Médicale des Hôpitaux de
Paris, 188
Bureau central, 10, 97, 101–102, 104,
143n.36, 151, 154
Bureau des recherches géologiques
et minières, 67
Bychowski, Zygmunt, 1860–1935), 235n.88
Bychowski sign, 230n.88

Calmette, A. (1863–1933), 33, 355
The Cambridge World History of Human
Disease, 355
Cardiac diseases, 157
Cardiac edema, 90
Caruso, Enrico (1873–1921), 40
Central nervous system, 189, 199,
210, 215, 218, 231, 300–301,
326, 328 See also nervous system;
peripheral nervous system/
peripheral nerves
Cerebellar asynergy, 27, 211, 264
Cerebellar ataxia, 252–253, 261, 262, 275
Cerebellar catalepsy, 27, 249, 253, 257–258,
261, 263
Cerebellar disorders, 212
Cerebellar lesions, 158, 250–251, 255,
256, 258
Cerebellar symptomatology, 15, 27, 196,
234, 246, 249–250, 261–264
Babinski's contribution to, 251–260
Cerebellar syndrome, 56, 212, 257,
263–264, 332
Cerebellopontine angle tumors, 158, 274

Cerebellum, 16, 121, 188, 249, 256, 260–262, 263
Cerebral tumors, 273–277 *See also* brain tumors
Cerebrospinal fluid, 90, 144, 160, 168, 287–288, 331, 334
  cytodiagnosis of, 201, 208
  Wassermann reaction, 197
Cerebrospinal meningitis, 219, 287
Cestan, Raymond (1872–1934), 168, 176, 337
  thesis on Little syndrome (1899), 176
Cestan-Chenais brain stem syndrome, 176
Cézanne, Paul (1839–1906), 14, 19
Chabrier, Emmanuel (1841–1894), 164
Chacornac, 49, 50, 86
Chaddock, Charles Gilbert (1861–1936), 228
  translated into English of Babinski's papers, 185
Chaddock reflex *See* lateral malleolus sign
Chaillous, Joseph (1872–1934), 96, 157, 169, 198
Champeaux Cemetery (Montmorency), 21, 57, 80, *81*
Chanteclair (satirical review), 347
Chantemesse, André (1851–1919), 139–140, 358
  Eberth bacillus, 140
  thesis on tuberculosis meningitis, 139
Charbonnel, Maurice (1884–1946), 258
Charcot, Jean-Baptiste) (1867–1936), 130n.28, 75
Charcot, Jean-Martin (1825–1893), viii–ix, 7, 10, 11–12, 14–15, 23–24, 43, 46, 60, 70, 75, 94, 112–113, 124–127, 136–137, 154, 158, 162, 192–193, 236, 244, 267, 269, 346, 350, 354, 355–357, 358
  concept of hereditary degeneration, 319
  concepts on hysteria, 298–300, 302
    role of emotion in, 301, 311–312, 313
  "contemplative method,"
    of examination, 250–251
  Dreyfus affair, 13, 36
  Freud's visit to Salpêtrière, 314–318
  interest in therapeutics, 282, 283
  Leçons du mardi, 128, 314

Leçons sur les maladies du système nerveux (Lessons on Diseases of the Nervous System), 7
  and pupils, 128–130, 334–336
  relationship with Babinski, 101, 105–110, 129–132, 188–189, 194–195, 297
  and Société anatomique, 140–141
Charcot-Bouchard aneurysms, 336
Charcot-Marie-Tooth disease, 326
Charité Hospital, 93, 94, 107, 116, 185, 330, 336
Charles Foix Hospital (Ivry), 360
Charpentier, Albert (1872–?), 24, 35, 36, 43, 61, 86n.3, 95, 131, 157, *163*, 165, 168, *169*, 179, *181*, 195, 199, 310, 315, 330, 351, 363
Charrin, Albert (1856–1907), 86, 92, 191
Chaslin, Philippe (1857–1923), 59
Chauchard Collection, 40, 49
Chauffard, Emile (1855–1932), 348, 349, 363
Chaumond, Joseph Jean Marie Bruno (1853–1888), 73
Chef de clinique (chief resident) *See* chief residents (*chefs de clinique*)
Cheyne-Stokes respiration, 225
Chicago Neurological Society, 230
Chief residents (*chefs de clinique*), v, 10, 11, 12n.12, 31–32, 98, 101, 157, 294, *299*, 331, 333
  Babinski, 130n.28, 167, 188
  Charcot, 124–131, 133, 137, 326, 334
  Maxime Laignel-Lavastine, 182
  Raymond Cestan, 176
Chipault, Antony (1866–1920), 267, 268, 269, 282
  "Chipault laws," 268
Chiray, Maurice (1877–?), 180, 291, 294–295
  La prothèse fonctionnelle des paralysies et des contractures (Functional prosthesis in paralyses and contractures), 180
Chirurgien des Hôpitaux de Paris, 97, 272
Cholera epidemics (1884, 1885 and 1892), 9, 13, 133n.2, 137, 152

INDEX   *435*

Chopin, Frédéric (1810–1849),
    40, 49, 53, 59
Chorobski, Jerzy (1902–1986), 183, 353
Cirrhosis, 157
Claude Bernard Hospital, 6, 12, 142, 152,
    201, 354
Claude, Henri (1869–1946), 31, 86n.4, 182,
    195, 189, 262, 334
    Histoire de la médecine
        (History of medicine), 182
    Nouveau traité de médecine
        (A new treatise on medicine), 262
Clemenceau, Georges (1841–1929),
    88, 93, 111
Clinic for the Study of Diseases of the
    nervous system, 326
Clinic of Cutaneous and Syphilitic
    Diseases (at Saint-Louis
    Hospital), 199
Clinicians, viii, ix, 79, 94, 133, 136, 140,
    158, 175, 188, 251, 279, 331, 335,
    350, 355, 361, 363
Clinique des Maladies Nerveuses
    (in Kazan), 358
Clinique Geoffroy Saint-Hilaire, 154
Clonus *See* spinal epilepsy
Clovis, Vincent (1879–1947), 18, 36, 55, 75,
    86n.4, 95, 145, 157, 168, 180, 195,
    269, 271, 274, *275*, *281*, 293, 282,
    332, 351, 362
    assistance to Babinski in diagnosis
        of pithiatism, 310
    first professor of neurosurgery in
        France, 282
    hostility to technique of radiology, 279
Clunet, Jean (1878–1917), 177n.13
Cochin Hospital, 90, 94, 124
Collège de France, 6, 12, 25n.7, 87, 92, 93,
    135, 136, 141–145, 178
College of Physicians and Surgeons
    of New York, 342
Colin, 128
    Leçons du mardi, 128
Compagnie Universelle de Panama, 13
Competitive examination, viii, 97–112,
    113–114
Complete clonus *See* spinal epilepsy
*Comptes-rendus de l'Académie des
    Sciences,* 195
*Comptes-rendus Hebdomadaires des
    Séances et Mémoires de la Société
    de Biologie,* 188
Comte, Auguste (1798–1857), 14
Congrès des aliénistes et neurologists
    (Bordeaux, August 1895), 207
Connective tissues, 142, 144
Consciousness, 14, 206, 313, 316, 319, 330
Conseil d'Etat, 111, 112
Conseil de Surveillance de l'Assistance
    Publique, 346, 348
Conseil national de la Résistance, 145
Cornell sign, 231
Cornil, Victor (1837–1908), 9, 24, 37, 38,
    90, 93, 101, 103, 110, 130, 135,
    136–139, 142, 143
    and chair of pathological anatomy,
        136–137
    Charcot's comment on, 24n.7
    and karyokinesis and
        anatomopathological
        processes, 137
    Manuel d'histologie pathologique
        [Handbook on pathological
        histology], 136
    and pathological anatomy of leprosy, 93
    political activities, 138–139
    and residency of Babinski, 121–124, 133,
        145, 321
    and Société anatomique, 140–141
    Traité d'histologie pathologique
        (co-editor), 330
Corrège *See* Allegri, Antonio (Correggio)
Cortical blindness, 205, 206
Courbet, Gustave (1819–1877), 5, 7–8
    realism movement in painting, 7–8
Coury, Charles (1916–1973), 354
    L'histoire de la médecine, 354
Cracow, 53, 55, 61, 74, 79
Cranial surgery, 268, 277
Crookes, William (1832–1919), 35
Crouzon, Octave (1874–1938), 36, 95, *163*,
    168, 169, 177, 195, 235n.88
    study of cranial and facial
        malformations, 177
Crouzon's disease (hereditary craniofacial
    dysostosis), 177

Crural nerve palsy, 237
Crural paraplegia, 191, 213, 218
Cruveilhier, Léon-Jean-Baptiste
    (1791–1874), 122, 136, 141, 363
Curie, Marie (1867–1934), 12, 18, 36,
    56, 74
Curie, Pierre (1859–1906), 12, 18, 36, 74
Cushing, Harvey (1869–1939), 18, 270,
    271, 273, 281, 342
CUT (crossed upgoing toe) sign, 231
Cytology, 90, 144, 168
Czartoryski, Ladislau Prince (1828–1894),
    64, 77
    "Mémoire justificatif du Comité de
        l'émigration polonaise," 64

D'Ache, Caran (1858–1909), 29n.29
    Psst (anti-Semitic journal), 29n.29
D'Arsonval, Jacques-Arsène (1851–1940),
    92, 110, 291
    works on bacteriology and microbial
        diseases, 92
Da Vinci, Leonardo (1503–1507), 222
Dagnan-Bouveret, Jean (?–1918), 95, 180,
    291, 294–295
    *La prothèse fonctionnelle des paralysies
        et des contractures* (Functional
        prosthesis in paralyses and
        contractures), 180
Dagnan-Bouveret, Pascal (1852–1929), 180
Dagognet, François (1957–2001), 355
Dandy, Walter (1886–1946), 271
    technique of injecting air into brain
        ventricles, 271
Darier, Jean–Ferdinand (1856–1938), 9, 62,
    85, 86n.4, 87–88, 90, 162
    Nouvelle pratique dermatologique
        (editor in chief of), 88
Darier sign (in urticaria pigmentosa), 87
Darier-Ferrand, dermatofibrosarcoma
    protuberans of, 87
Darier-Roussy's hypodermic sarcoids, 87
Darier-White syndrome, 87
Darwin, Charles (1809–1882), 6
    Origin of Species (1865), 6
Daudet, Alphonse (1840–1897), 94
    Morticoles (satire of university and
        hospital circles), 94

Daudet, Léon (1867–1942), 19, 23, 36, 37,
    69, 86, 128n.21, 328, 335
Dax médical et thermal (book, 1930), 293
De Abreu Freire, Antonio Caetano, 183
De la Tourette, Georges Gilles
    (1857–1904), 12, 15, 102, 103, 105,
    112, 128, 130n.28, 300, 321, 325,
    355, 358, 360
    *L'Hypnotisme et les états analogues
        au point de vue médico-légal*
        (Hypnotism and analogous
        conditions in forensic
        medicine), 15
    *La nouvelle iconographie de la
        Salpêtrière*, 12
De Martel, Thierry (1876–1940), 75, 86n.4,
    272, 274, 275, *276*, 277, *278*, 280,
    281, 282
De Mirabeau, Sibylle Gabrielle Riquetti
    (1849–1932), comtesse de Martel,
    75, 275
De Pomiane, Edouard Pozerski
    (1875–1964), 57, 82–83, 90, 79n.111
De Pressensé, Francis, 37
De Swiecinski, Georges Clément
    (1878–1958), 61
Debove, Georges-Maurice (1845–1920),
    106, 128, 130n.28, 143, 236, 336
    Manuel de Médecine (1896), 236
Debussy, Claude (1862–1918), 19, 20
    Après-midi d'un faune, 20
    Pelleas et Mélisande, 19
Déchy, Albert, 168, 201
Decompressive craniectomy, 211
Decompressive craniotomy, 168, 276
Decompressive techniques, 211, 290
Defense reflexes, 196, 211, 213,
    245–248, 271
Dejerine, Jules (1849–1917), 16, 24, 32–33,
    38, 55, 74, 113, 122, 158, 164, 189,
    193, 195, 223, 240, 250, 261, 273,
    325, *327*, 330, 332, 342, 355–356,
    357, 358, 359
    and Charcot, 311
    confrontation with Pierre Marie, 1
        89, 326
    head of Bicêtre's department
        of neurology, 330

membership of the *Commission du fonds*, 164
Semiologie des affections du système nerveux (Semiology of diseases of the nervous system), 238
working with Babinski, 341–342
Dejerine-Klumpke, Augusta (1859–1927), 74, *327*
Dejerine-Roussy syndrome, 326, 333, 356
Dejerine-Sottas neuropathy (1893), 201, 326
Dejerine-Thomas olivopontocerebellar atrophy (1900), 249
Delherm, Louis (1876–1953), 26, 96, 157, 158, 168
  thesis on electrical treatment of common constipation, 157
Delorme, Ed (1847–1929), 274
Denial, 206
Descartes, René (1596–1650), 14
Diabetes, 101, 157, 201
Diadococinesia, *27*
Diaghilev, Sergei (1872–1929), 20
  Ballets Russes, 20
Diagnosis, vii, 95, 101n.6, 157, 160, 176, 188, 195, 196, 199, 211, 213, 269, 274, 310, 360, 362
  Babinski's meticulousness in, 201, 224, 252, 264, 271, 272, 279, 282, 354, 355
  of hysteria, 303, 307, 311, 317–318
  pupil irregularity and syphilis, 200
  X-rays in, 266
Dictionnaire des intellectuels français, 354
Dictionnaire des polonais ayant participé à la Commune de Paris, 63
Dieulafoy, Georges (1839–1911), 143, 176, 251, 363
Digestive tract diseases/digestive tract pathology, 124, 336
Diphtheria, 18, 103, 148, 152
Disseminated epidemic encephalomyelitis (Flatau-Redlich disease), 60
The Doctrine of the Nerves: Chapters in the History of Neurology, 355
Dombrowski, Jaroslav (1836–1871), 5
Dorland's Medical Dictionary, 234–235
Doumer, Paul (1857–1932), 91

Dreyfus affair (1894–1899), 13, 18–19, 25, 29–31, 36–39, 48–49
Du Bellay, J. (1522–1560), 73, 83
Du Saulle, Legrand (1830–1886), 116–119, *120*
Dubois, Paul-Charles (1848–1918), 326
  "Les manifestations fonctionnelles des psychonévroses", 326
Duchenne, Guillaume (1806–1875), 6–7, 250, 355, 356
  electrotherapy and neurology, 7
  De l'électrisation localisée, 7
Duclaux, Émile (1840–1904), 37, 354
Dufour, M., 189, 200
Duguet, 151
Dumas, Georges (1866–1946), 182, 185, 294
Dupré, Ernest (1862–1921), 189, 193, 224, 334, 352
Dupuytren, Guillaume (1777–1835), 355
Durand Restaurant, 130
Durante, Francesco (1844–1934), 266
  resection of olfactory groove meningioma, 266
Duret, Henri (1849–1921), 270, 337
Duval, Mathias (1844–1907), 105, 127, 135
Dysmetry, 253, 255, 261, 262–264
  See also hypermetry

Eberth bacillus, 140
Ecole des hautes études en sciences socials, 38, 178
École des mines de Paris, 8, 59, 62, 65, 66, 73, 77
École normale supérieure, 91, 144
École pratique des hautes études, 59, 93
École préparatoire (École supérieure polonaise), 62
École supérieure polonaise (École préparatoire), 62
Edinger, Ludwig (1855–1918), 341
  founder of modern comparative anatomy of nervous system, 341
Ehrlich, Paul (1854–1915), 18, 286
606/salvarsan/Ehrlich salt/neo-salvarsan, 286
Eiffel Tower, 13

8th International Neurological Meeting (1927), 259
Einstein, Albert (1879–1955), 18, 91
  treatise o n special relativity, 18
Electric shock treatment (sismotherapy), 288 *See also* electrotherapy
Electrodiagnostics, 158, 260
Electrotherapy, 7, 128, 158, 166, 288–289
Elsberg, Charles A. (1871–1948), 34, 270, 271, 272, 342
Encéphale (journal), 195
Enfants-Malades Hospital, 124, 125
Enriquez, Edouard (1865–1928), 86, 92, 95, 192
Epilepsy, 6, 214, 219, 268, 293, 300, 304
  See also spinal epilepsy
Epithelioma, 141, 202
Erb, Wilhelm Heinrich (1840–1921), 185, 236, 341
  patellar tendon reflex, 236
Erb-Goldflam disease, 60, 359
  See also myasthenia
Erick, Pierre, 124 *See also* Parinaud, Henri (1844–1905)
Errera, Antoine, 64
  "La Garde nationale sous la Commune de Paris, 1871", 64
Esbach, Georges Hubert (1843–1890), 94
  inventor of the albuminometer, 94
Esbach's tube, 94
Esmarch bandage, 34, 211, 225
Eugénie, Empress (1826–1920), 107n.18
Evangélique Hospital (Warsaw), 183
Exposé des travaux scientifiques du Dr Babinski (1913), 209–210, 225n.29, 228n.48
Externat des Hôpitaux de Paris (part-time nonresident student) See *externat* examinations
Externat examinations, 97, 98–99, 100, 114
Externs/externes, 8, 59, 97–98, 116, 170–174

Facial hemispasm, 213, 235
Facial neuralgia, 214, 331
Facial palsy, 30, 157, 162
Facio-scapulo-humeral muscular dystrophy (Landouzy-Dejerine syndrome, 1885), 326
Faculté de médecine de Paris, 8, 98
Faisans, 154n.5
Falguière, Alexandre (1831–1900), 130
Fallot, 355
Fauconnet, Evelyne, 222
Favre, Jules (1809–1880), 139
Feindel, Eugene (1862–1930), 193n.28
Ferdinand, Franz (Austrian archduke) (1863–1914), 19
Fernand Widal Hospital, 90
Féré, Charles (1852–1907), 25, 86, 94, 130n.28
  thesis on functional disorders of sight, 94
  Alienist at Bicêtre, 86
Fernand Widal Hospital, 90
Ferrier, Sir David (1843–1928), 341
Fierro, A., 358
Filipowicz, Wladyslaw, 183
Flammarion, Camille (1842–1925), 35
Flatau, Edward (1868–1932), 60
Flatau's law, 60
Flatau-Redlich disease (disseminated epidemic encephalomyelitis), 60
Flaubert, Gustave (1821–1880), 8
  Madame Bovary, 8
Flourens, Marie-Jean-Pierre (1794–1867), 7, 12, 250
Foch, Field Marshal Ferdinand (1851–1929), 89, 90–91
Foerster, Otfrid (1873–1941), 185
Foix, Charles (1882–1927), 185, 245, 250, 272, 332, 360, 363
Follin, Eugène (1823–1867), 141
Forain, Jean-Louis (1852–1931), 29, 36
  Psst (anti-Semitic journal), 29n.29
Forensic medicine, 119
Forestier, Jacques (1890–1978), 272
Fournier, Alfred (1832–1914), 87, 199
Fraenkel, Théodore (1896–1964), 44
France, 3–5, 26, 46, 55, 57–58, 61–62, 71, 74, 78–79, 81, 92, 158, 159, 160n.33, 193, 240, 273, 338, 349, 352, 359, 361, 363
  child psychiatry in, 182

INDEX 439

importance of hysteria in, 297–298
neurosurgical developments in, 267–271, 274, 275, 281–282, 283, 290, 321, 342
Paris Commune, 63–65, 78
physicians elected to public life, 37–39
Polish emigration, 53–54
political climate, 18–19
political situation in, 12–13
radiotherapy in, 289
syphilis problem in, 196–197
France, Anatole (1844–1924), 36, 40
Franco-Prussian War (1870), 4–5
Frazier, Charles Harrison (1870–1936), 270, 342
    retrogasserian neurotomy and spinal cordotomy, 270
Free Faculty of Lille, 337
Freeman, Walter (1895–1972), 184
French Army Health Service, 310
French neurosurgery *See* neurosurgery
French Revolution, 4
French Guyana, 13n.14, 67–68
Freud, Sigmund (1856–1939), 11, 16, 45, 206, 342
    and Charcot, 298, 301
    Breton's fascination for, 46
    Everyday Life (1904), 16
    The Interpretation of Dreams (1900), 16
    Salpêtrière visit, 128–129, 314–318
Froin Georges (1874–1932), syndrome, 287
Frölich, Alfred (1871–1953), 202
Froment, Jules (1878–1946), 55, 96, 169, 204n.74, 277, 307, *308*
Froment sign, 204n.74
Fulton, John F. (1899–1960), 86, 95, 224, 226

Galezowski, Jean, 79n.111, 124
Galezowski, Xavier (1833–1907), 79n.111, 124, 125
Gallois, Paul, 101
"galvanic vertigo," *See* voltaic vertigo
Galvez, Pedro, 62
Gambetta, Léon (1838–1882), 139
Garcin, Raymond (1897–1971), 352
Gasne, 130n.28

Gastronomie pratique (1928), 48, 83, 68–73, 83, 362
Gaucher, Ernest (1854–1919), 114, 175, 286
Gaucher's disease, 114
Gauckler, E., 326
    Nouveau Traité de Médecine (1911), 326
Gaussel, Amans, 1871–1937), 235n.88
Gautier, Claude (1884–1955), 96, 169
Gazecki, A., 44, 56
Gazeta Narodowa (Polish newspaper), 64, 70
Gazette Hebdomadaire de Médecine et de Chirurgie, 110, 195
Gellé, 130n.28
Gendron, André (1880–1932), 168, 272
    thesis on spinal tumors, 168
General anesthesia, 241, 307
General paralysis, 199–200, 201
Gengou, Octave (1875–1957), 197
George Washington University, 184
Germany, 7, 19, 59, 184, 266, 282, 338, 341, 342, 353
Gley, Eugène (1857–1930), 24, 25n.7
Godlee, Sir Rickman John (1849–1925), 265
Goldflam, Samuel (1852–1932), 60, 162, 223
Goldstein, 356
Golgi, Camillo (1843–1926), 7, 148
Gombault, Albert (1844–1904), 30, 128, 130n.28, 144, 193, 321, 330–331
Goncourt, Edmond (1822–1896), 75
Goncourt, Jules (1830–1870), 75
Gonda, Victor (1889–1959), 230
Gonda sign, 230
Gonda-Allen sign, 230, 233
Gordon, Alfred (1874–1953), 228n.49, 231, 233
Gordon sign, 228, 233
Gosset, Antonin (1872–1944), 274, 358
Gowers, Sir William Richard (1848–1915), 185, 229, 236, 265, 341
    Clinical Lectures on Diseases of the Nervous System, 341
Gowers's knee jerk, 236
Grancher, Joseph (1843–1907), 38, 140, 143

Grande Encyclopédie de Pologne (2004), 356, 357
Grasset, Joseph (1849–1918), 33, 158, 235n.88, 250, 337
Grasset sign, 235n.88
Grasset-Bychowski sign, 235n.88
Grasset-Gausse sign, 235n.88
Grasset-Gaussel-Hoover sign, 235n.88
Gréard, 130
Great Britain, 7, 19, 272, 338, 349
Greenblatt, S., 282
Grévy, Jules (1807–1891), 139
Grimm, Jacob (1785–1863), 75
Grimm, Wilhelm (1786–1859), 75
Guibout, Eugène (1820–1895), 121–124
Guignard, Léon (1852–1928), 9, 86, 95
Guillain, Georges (1876–1961), 86, 95, 113, 128, 160, *163*, 169, 194n.35, 291, 328, 330, 337, 346, 356
 Revue d'Oto-neuro-ophtalmologie (founder), 175
Guillain-Barré syndrome, 175, 328
Guillain-Barré-Strohl syndrome, 175
Guinon, Georges (1889–1891), 128, 130nn.28, 31, 193n.28

Habich, Edward Jan (1835–1909), 61n.40
Hachinski, V., 44, 56, 231
Halsted, William Stewart (1852–1922), 270
Hammond, William A. (1828–1900), 342
Hanot, Victor Charles (1844–1896), 106
Hartmann, Edward, 96, 169
Haussmann, Georges Eugène (1809–1891), 8, 13, 86
Hayem, Georges (1841–1933), 122, 363
Head faradization, 158
Head, Sir Henry (1861–1940), 341
Health Service (1804), 97
Heart disease, 87, 93, 116, 305
Hecaen, Henri (1912–1983), 333, 28
Heitz, J., 208, 310
 vasomotor disturbances of reflex, 208
Hematology, 142
Hematoma, 277, 289
Hematomyelia, 162
Hemiasynergy, 204, 212, 253

Hemiplegias, 144, 157, 162, 164, 191, 204, 205, 206, 211, 212, 218, 227, 235, *243*, 304
Henneguy, Louis-Félix (1850–1928), 142
Henryk *See* Babinski, Henri
Hereditary craniofacial dysostosis (Crouzon's disease), 177
Hereditary cerebellar ataxy, 326
Hereditary cleidocranial dysostosis, 326
Hereditary hypertrophic neuropathies, 201
Heredity, 6, 204, 301, 312, 313, 316, 319
Herman, E., 50, 202n.70
Hertz, Cornelius, 13n.13
Hess, Walter Rudolph (1881–1973), 184
 work on diencephalon, 184
Heuyer, Georges (1884–1977), 168, 182
Hindfelt, B., 231
Hirtz, Edward (1869–1936), 162
Histoire du diagnostic médical (History of medical diagnosis), 355
Histophysiology, 142
Hoffmann, Paul (1868–1959), 196
 discovery of *Treponema pallidum* (1905), 196
Hoffmann sign, 230
Holmes, Sir Gordon Morgan (1876–1965), 251, 253, 262, 263, 264, 341
Holmes familial olivocerebellar atrophy (1907), 249
Hoover sign, 235n.88
Hoover, Charles Franklin (1865–1927), 235n.88
Horsley, Sir Victor Alexander (1857–1916), 185, 185, 265, 266, 267, 270, 272, 273, 274, 275, 337, 341, 353
 Horsley's trepanation technique, 266
Hospice des Incurables, 325
Hospice for Abandoned Children, 152
Hospital system in France, 92, 97, 109, 152, 328, 330
Hôtel-Dieu Hospital, 124
Huchard, H. (1842–1910), 208
 "Influence of the aneurysms of the aorta on lung diseases," 208
Hugo, Jeanne (1869–1941), 94
Hugo, Victor (1802–1885), 8, 40, 94
 Hernani (play), 40

Alienist at Bicêtre, 86
Huppert, Karl-Hugo (1832–1904), 255
Hurst, A. F., 159
Hydatid cyst, 102, 290
Hydrotherapy, 116
Hypermetry (unrestrained movements), 27, 249, 253, 254–255, 261, 263, 276
See also *dysmetry*
Hypoglossal nerve, 207
Hypotonia, 253, 262, 307
Hypotony, 262–264
Hypertrophic pulmonary osteoarthropathy, 326
Hysteria, viii, 10, 12–16, 30–31, 157, 159, 162, 187, 188, 192, 213, 238, 282, 302–304, 297–319, 333, 336, 337, 356
   Babinski's development of thought on, 302, 131, 135, 306–313, 317
   Charcots' conceptions of, 298–300, 301, 303–304, 316
   etiology of, 301
   hypnosis and suggestion in, 11, 14–15, 305–306
   present theories of, 318–319
   psychic analysis of, 301, 315–317
   See also pithiatism
Hysteric hemiplegias, 222, 223
Hysteric migraine, 191
Hysterical paralysis, 313–314

Iena University, 251
Impartiality, 111, 141, 292
Infectious diseases, 12, 152, 154, 294
Ingres J.A. (1780–1867), 40
   "La Source", 40
Insanity, 7, 92, 154, 285
Institut de Myologie, 360
Institut du Cancer (built 1934–35), 333
Institut général psychologique, 36
Internal medicine, 90, 105, 116, 153, 156, 167, 325, 334, 341
Internat des Hôpitaux de Paris (full-time resident) See *internat* examinations
Internat examinations, 97, 99–100, 114
   competition for the residency Gold Medal, 100–101

Interne provisoire (provisional resident), 128
Internes, 8, 97, 170–175
Intraspinal tumors, 332, 362
   See also spinal cord tumors; spinal tumors

Jaboulay, Mathieu (1860–1913), 267, 268, 274
   pioneer in experimental kidney transplantation, 268
Jackson, Hughlings (1835–1911), 6, 185, 355, 356
   coordination and cerebral cortex, 6
Jacksonian convulsions, 267
Janet, Pierre (1859–1947), 12, 14–15, 16–17, 59, 127, 176, 193n.28, 299, 301, 312, 317, 319
   concept of dissociation of psychic processes, 319
   concept of hereditary degeneration, 319
   Journal de Psychologie Normale et Pathologique, 312
   own conception of hysteria, 313–314, 316
Janville, Comtesse de Martel (1850–1932), 275
Jarkovski, Jean (1880–1929), 20, 50, 57–58, *156*, 157, 165, 183, 243
   Babinski's volunteer assistant and friend, 183
   thesis on Parkinsonian paradoxical kinesis, 58
Jassy Hospital (Romania), 176
Jaurès, Jean (1859–1914), 178
Jendrassik, E. (1858–1921), 241
Jendrassik's maneuver, 241
Jewish Hospital, 160
Joffroy, Alix (1844–1909), 25, 101, 128, 130nn.28, 31, 193, 330, 334
   first president of the Société de neurologie de Paris, 334
Johnston, S.C., 232, 234
Jolly, Justin-Marie (1870–1953), 142
Journal des Débats, 111
Journal Officiel, 111
Jumentié, Joseph (1881–1928), 86n.4, 134, 158, 198, 252, 274

Jumentié, Joseph (*Cont.*)
  thesis on pathological anatomy and
    cerebellopontine angle tumors, 158
Juster, E., 230

Keen, William Williams (1837–1932), 266
  first removal of a brain tumor in United
    States, 299
Khalil, R., 42, 44n.91
Kidney, 90, 157, 268
King's College Hospital (Edinburgh), 185
Kinnier-Wilson, Samuel A. (1878–1937),
    185, 341
Kinnier Wilson disease, 185
Klippel, Maurice (1858–1942), 25, 193
Knee reflex, 197–198, 237, 241, *245*, 243
Koch, Robert (1843–1910), 12, 137, 140,
    160, 270
  origin of tuberculosis (the tubercle
    bacillus), 12
  study of karyokinesis, 137
Kocher, Emil Theodor (1841–1917), 270
Kojevnikoff, Alexis J. (1836–1902), 343
Korsakoff, Sergei (1854–1900), 60, 343
Kozhevnikoff, Alexis (1836–1902), 60
  *Atlas of the Human Brain and
    Description of the Course of the
    Nerve Fibers*, 60
Krause, Fedor (1856–1937), 266, 270, 276
Krauss, William Christopher
    (1863–1909), 240
Krawczyk, Mieczysalw, 231
Krebs, Edouard (1883–1971),
    96, 177, 195, 351
  recipient of Babinski Fund, 195

L'Action Française (right-wing daily
    newspaper), 19, 37
L'Aurore (large circulation newspaper), 13
  published Émile Zola's "J'Accuse"
    (1898), 13
L'Echo de Paris (large circulation
    newspaper), 110
L'oeuvre scientifique (Babinski's major
    research papers), 169, 187, 206,
    209–213
La Gazette des Hôpitaux, 110
La Justice (newspaper), 111

La Pitié Hospital, 10, 46, 58, 57, 185, 222,
    281, 332
  Babinski as head of department (1895),
    112, 151–161, 268, 271–272,
    290–292, 325, 330
  Babinski's study of neurological
    diseases, 162, 321
  beginning of Babinski's career, 10
  training periods of Babinski's
    residency, 121
  wartime activity in, 277, 310
La Presse Médicale, 58, 178, 195
*La prothèse fonctionnelle des paralysies
    et des contractures* (Functional
    prosthesis in paralyses and
    contractures), 180
La Rochefoucauld Hospital, 87
La Semaine Médicale, 102n.10
Labbé, Marcel (1870–1939), 168, 177, 185
Labor unions, 12, 19, 29n.29
Labyrinthic disorders, 210, 212, 259,
    260, 263
Laënnec, René. (1781–1826), 79, 156, 351
Lagrange, Count de, 67
Laignel-Lavastine, Maxime (1875–1953),
    24, 86n.4, 168, 182, 334, 346, 354
  Histoire de la medicine, 354
Lama, Stanislawa, 357n.55
  Ilustrowana Encyklopedja Trzaski;
    357n.55
  Mala Encyklopedia Powszechna,
    357n.55
Lamalou-les-Bains, 283n.3
Lamy, Henri (1865–1909), 130n.28
Lancet, 362
Landau, W., 233
Landouzy, Joseph (1845–1917), 182,
    326, 335
Landouzy-Dejerine syndrome
    (facio-scapulo-humeral
    muscular dystrophy, 1885), 326
Landowski, 130n.28, 193n.28
Lannois, Maurice (1856–1942), 274
  direct approach to cerebellopontine
    angle tumors, 274
Lapicque, Louis, 59
Lariboisière Hospital, 116, 143, 325
Laroche, Guy, 160

Lasègue, Ernest Charles (1816–1883), 336
Lateral malleolus reflex of Balduzzi, 229
Lateral malleolus sign, 228–229
Laubry, Charles (1872–1960), 36, 86, 93
   development of sphygmomanometer, 93
   study of congenital heart diseases and coronaropathies, 93
Lavielle, Louis, 292
   Dax médical et thermal (1930), 293
Lavielle, René, 292
   Dax médical et thermal (1930), 293
Le Figaro (large circulation newspaper), 81, 347, 349
Le Gendre, P., 105
Le Journal des Praticiens, 70, 160, 195, 335
Le Matin (large circulation newspaper), 109, 110, 283
Le Petit Parisien (newspaper), 348
Le Progrès Médical (journal), 7, 25n.7, 70, 94n.32, 98, 105, 109, 111, 135n.5, 162, 188, 195, 237, 267
   news about neurosurgical developments, 267
   praise of Babinski, 162–163
   praise of Cornil's lectures, 136–137
Le Surréalisme, même, 44
Le Temps (newspaper), 164, 361
Lead poisoning, 101, 157
Lecène, Paul (1878–1929), 272
   French general surgeon, 272
Léchelle, 160, 327
Leçons du mardi, 128, 314
Lejars, Félix (1863–1932), 86, 92, 274
   Traité de chirurgie d'urgence, 92
Lejonne and Lhermitte olivorubrocerebellar atrophy (1909), 249
Lenin, Vladimir (1870–1924), 178
Léonard, Jacques, 355
   La médecine entre les pouvoirs et les savoirs, 355
Leredde, Emile (1866–1926), 33
Léri, André (1875–1930), 86n.4, 168, 177
Léri's disease (melorheostosis), 177
Les polonais et la Commune de Paris (book), 63
Lesueur, Eustache (1616–1655), 40

Letulle, Maurice (1853–1929), 55, 136, 141, 333
Lévy-Valensi, Joseph (1879–1943), 262, 334
   Nouveau traité de médecine, 262
Leygues, M. (minister of education) (1857–1933), 131
Lhermitte, François (1921–1998), 263
Lhermitte, Jean (1877–1959), 86n.4, 353, 356
Lhermitte–Trelles syndrome (lymphoblastic infiltration of the peripheral nervous system), 356n.49
Ligue des droits de l'homme, 37–38
Lima (Peru), 47, 61, 62, 75
Limoges Hospital, 125
Lister, Joseph (1827–1912), 6, 265, 266
Literature, 7–8, 19–21, 52, 178, 294–295
   Babinski's liking for, 40
   Belle Epoque, the, 14–15
   Vulpian's liking for, 122
Littré dictionary, 76
Locomotor ataxia, 157, 250, 262
Loeper, Maurice (1875–1961), 55, 335
Londe, Albert (1858–1917), 12, 130nn.28, 31
   La nouvelle iconographie de la Salpêtrière, 12
Longet, François-Achille (1811–1871), 250
Lopez, Miguel Jimenez, 185
Lucas-Championnière, Paul (1843–1913), 162, 267
Luciana, Luigi (1840–1919), 250
]Lumbar punctures, 213, 214, 269, 273, 296, 287–288
Lumbroso, Cesare (1836–1909), 35
Lumière, Auguste (1862–1954), 20, 75, 359
Lumière, Louis (1864–1948), 20, 75, 359
Lung pathologies, 157
Lungs, 124, 136
Lutenbacher, 206
Luys, Jules Bernard (1828–1897), 128, 330
Lycée Descartes, 4
Lycée Impérial Louis-le-Grand, 4
Lymphoblastic infiltration of the peripheral nervous system (Lhermitte–Trelles syndrome), 56n.49
Lymphocytosis, 201

Macewen, Sir William (1848–1924), 265, 270
Madonick, J., 233
Magnet, influence of, 34, 35n.54, 192, 302
Mairet, Albert (1852–1935), 106
Maison des élèves de la Patrie, 152 *See also* La Pitié Hospital
Maison Dubois, 90
Maison Mathieu, 239n.104
Malassez, Charles (1842–1909), 142, 143, 144
   Malassezia furfur, 143
Malassez cell (instrument for counting of blood cells), 143
Malassezia furfur (cause of pityriasis versicolor), 143
Mandal Bechtrew sign, 231
Manuel d'histologie pathologique, 142
Manuel de Médecine (1896), 236
Maranon, Grégorie, 184
Marfan, Antoine (1858–1942), 114
Marie cerebellar hereditary ataxia (1893), 249
Marie de Médicis (1573–1642), 152
Marie, Pierre (1853–1940), viii, 24, 30, 33, 36, 38, 86, 86n.4, 102, 103, 113, 128, 130nn.28, 31, 143, 176, 183, 206, 223, 229, 235n.88, 245, 250, 277, 282, 321, 325, 326, 328, *329*, 330–333, 349, 352, 354, 356, 357, 358, 360, 363
   and Babinski, 30
   chair of pathological anatomy, Paris Medical School (1908 to 1917), 136
   co-founded the *Revue Neurologique*, 192, 193, 194n.32, 337
   described acromegaly, 326
   dispute on aphasia with Dejerine, 189
   experimental work on cerebellum, 249, 250, 251
   and Freud, 299
   guidance to colleagues, 177, 185, 269
   inversion of the ulnar reflex, 243
   thesis on Basedow disease, 326
Marie-Foix-Alajouanine syndrome (ataxia of the cerebellum in the elderly), 249
Marinesco, Georges (1864–1938), 350

   collaborator of *Revue Neurologique*, 193n.28
Marion, Georges (1869–1960), 267
Martin Du Gard, Roger (1881–1958), 185
Mathieu, M., 238, 328
Maubrac, P., 268
Maupassant, Guy de (1850–1893), 14
McBurney, Charles (1845–1913), 266
Medea, Eugenio (1873–1967), 350
Médecin des hôpitaux, ix, 12, 19n.111, 87, 90, 92, 93, 136, 140, 325, 331
   Babinski's position, 16, 103, 151–153, 192, 330
   competitive examinations for, 101–102
   salary of, 162
Médecin-aliéniste, 92, 143, 155
Médecine Moderne, 107, 109
Médicat des Hôpitaux de Paris, 97, 101–104, 124
Medicine, vii, 6–8, 45, 96, 113, 115n.2, 128, 283–284, 330, 334, 346, 354–356, 363
   Babinski's love for, 49, 50, 321, 354–356
   competitive examinations for, 97, 101–104, 111, 113–114
   Cornil's dual career, 136
   Pierre Janet's views on psychology, 317
   progress in, 12, 16–18
   social aspects of, 270
   Wallon's dual training, 144
Meige, Henry (1866–1940), 128, 193, 194n.32, 229, 240, 333
   modified and standardized Skoda's reflex hammer, 240
Melorheostosis (Léri's disease), 177
Mendel, Gregor (1822–1884), 6
Ménière, Prosper (1899–1962), 355
Ménière's disease, 114
Ménétrier, Pierre (1859–1935), 114
Meningitis, 208, 213, 219, 271, 286, 287, 289, 357n.55
Mercury treatment (of syphilis), 33, 198, 213, 226, 285–286, 287
Metchnikoff, Ilya (1845–1916), 18
   phagocytic theory of immunity, 18
Meyerson, Ignace (1888–1983), 59
   comparative historical psychology, 59

Meynert, Theodor Hermann (1833–1892), 205
Michel, Leopold (1846–1919), 74
Microorganisms, 6, 18, 286
Miller, T. M., 234
Mills, Charles K. (1845–1931), 342
Mine Engineering School of Cracow, 74
Mingazzini, Giovanni (1859–1919), 343
Mirabeau, Comte de (1749–1791), 275
Mirbeau, Octave (1848–1917), 283
Mistinguett (Jeanne Bourgeois) (1875–1956), 40, 61
Mitchell, Silas Weir (1829–1934), 342
Mitkus, W., 60
Mlochowski, de Belina, 63–64
  Les polonais et la Commune de Paris, 63
Moebius, Paul Julius (1853–1907), 313
Mondor, Henri, 358, 363
Monet, Claude (1840–1926), 8, 93
Monier-Vinard, Raymond (1878–1944), 96, 168, 169, 179, 180, 351
Moniz, Egas (1874–1955), 20n.22, 38, 72, 73, 76, 96, 168, 195, 183–184, 229, 278, 350
  Confidences d'un chercheur scientifique, 73
  creation of psychosurgery, 184
  first Portuguese scientist to win a Nobel Prize, 183
  inventor of cerebral angiography, 279, 362
Montmorency cemetery, *21*, 39, 51, 57, 79, 80, *81*
Montreal Neurological Society, 358
Morax, Victor (1866–1935), 157
Moreau, René (1886–1973), 86, 92, 96, 168, 169, 360
Morphine, 191, 284–286
Motz, Boleslaw (1865–1935), 50, 57
Mouninou, Henri (Babinski's patient), 158, 251, *252*
Mouquin, M. (1891–1964), 93
Mugnier-Vogt, Cécile (1875–1962), 75
Multiple sclerosis, 7, 10, 30, 101, *138*, 142, 201, 212, 244
Munich school of neuropathology, 342
Muscular disorders/muscular dystrophies, 162, 213, 326

Musée de l'Assistance publique, Paris ("Babinski's microtome"), 143
Musée Dupuytren, 140
Myasthenia, 60, 162
Myopathies, 191, 213, 227
Myxedema, 207

Na Czystem Hospital (Warsaw), 202n.70
Nadja (journal), 45
Nageotte, Jean (1866–1948), 59, 134, 141, 143, 144, 158, 168, 198, 325, 356
  research on microscopic anatomy of the connective tissue, 144
Nancy Hospital, 106, 176, 337
Nancy school, 305
Napoléon III (1808–1873), 4, 97
National Guard (French), 5, 62, 75, 64
National Hospital (Great Britain), 338
National Hospital for Nervous Diseases (Queens Square), 185, 338, 341
National Hospital for the Paralyzed and the Epileptic (London), 265
Nationalism/nationalist insurrection, 5, 19, 37n.59, 65
Navy sanatorium, 124
Neelon, F. A., 221
Nepotism, 98, 110, 111
Néri, Vincenzo (1882–?), 31, 184
Nervous diseases, 44, 122, 136, 155, 193, 200, 325, 336, 342, 372
Nervous system, ix, 9, 6, 11–12, 101, 121, 124, 136, 210, 215, 218, 219, 223, 268, 269, 274–275, 305
  acquiring new dimensions in, 270–271, 282
  Babinski's study of, 143–144, 189, 237, 244–245, 277
  chair for, 321–330
  and hysterical diathesis, 301
  pathology, 121, 124, 236
  and syphilis, 196–202
    mercury treatment of, 285–286
  and vasomotor nerves and sympathetic nerves, 6
  and voltaic vertigo, 259
  See also central nervous system; peripheral nervous system/ peripheral nerves

Netter, Just-Arnold (1855–1936), 103
Neuralgias, 157, 288, 290
Neurasthenia, 157, 214, 290, 331
Neurochirurgie du praticien, 179
Neuroimagery, vii, 232
Neurological centers, 45, 158, 176, 291, 294, 295, 321, 332
Neurological community, 206, 223
Neurological diagnosis, vii, 189, 195–196, 282 See also neurological semiology
Neurological Institute, New York, 342
Neurological pathologies, 157, 162, 224
Neurological semiology, viii, 180, 208, 222, 249, 353, 354, 368, 360
Neurological Society of Paris, 205, 280
Neurology, 6–7, 113, 321–324, 335–343
  in Babinski's times, 321–324, 335–336
  in combat conditions, 16, 309–310, 312, 331
  in provinces of France, 115
  Salpêtrière chair for the study of diseases of the nervous system, 325–332
  Ste. Anne Hospital clinical chair for mind and brain diseases, 333–334
  world, 337–343
  See also neurology
Neurology (journal), 233
Neuromuscular fascicles, 139, 148
Neuromuscular spindles, 139, 142, 148, 191
Neuronal anatomy, 60
Neuropsychological mechanisms, 206
Neurosurgery, 168, 183, 184–185, 246, 265–266, 270, 290, 337–343, 360
  Babinski's role in, 290
  defense reflexes, 245–246
  in France, 15, 18, 267–282
  See also neurology
New England Journal of Medicine, 349
New York Neurological Institute, 270
New York Neurological Society, 343
Nicati, 140
Nissl, Franz (1860–1919), 342
Noïca, D., 33, 184
Nonpyramidal diseases, 212, 257, 263–264, 332

Nonresident student (*externe*), 45, 59, 94, 113, 143n.36
  Babinski's career as, 8–11, 98–112, 116, 157
  Babinski's pupils, 45, 59, 87, 94, 95–96, 159, 167, 168, 179–183
  tests for selection of, 114
Nos grands médecins d'aujourd'hui, 355
Nothnagel, Hermann, 251
Nouveau Traité de Médecine (1911), 262, 326
Nouvelle pratique dermatologique, 88
Nystagmus, 258, 259, 263, 264

Obalski, Joseph (1852–1915), 59, 74
Oberlé, Gérard, 69
Ochorowicz, Julian (1850–1917), 35
  "hypnoscope," 35n.54
Oeuvre des prisonniers militaires (charitable organization for prisoners of war), 124
Offenbach, Jacques (1819–1880), 8
  La belle Hélène (operatta, 1864), 8
  La vie parisienne (operatta, 1866).8
Official residency (*interne titulaire*), 121–123
Olaf, 43–46
  Les détraquées (The mad ones), 43–46
Onanoff, J. (1859–?), 202
Opéra Comique, 8
Oppenheim, Hermann (1858–1919), 30, 227, 228n.48, 233, 266, 341
  Lehrbuch der Nervenkrankheiten, 341
Oppenheim sign, 227, 228n.48, 233
Optic neuritis, 125, 226, 287
Organic disorders, 300–304, 307, 317
Organic hemiplegia, 191, 211, 217, 222, 227, 235
Organic lesions, 201, 224, 218, 219
Orsini, Felice (1819–1858), 4
Orthopedic Institute, Berck, 291
Orzechowski, C., 60, 183
Oulmont, N. (1815–1864), 130n.28
Outpatients, 16, 152, 154–155, 158, 159, 165, 176, 315, 333, 348

Pachymeningitis, 271, 289
Palais Garnier, 8

Palau, Pierre (1885-1966), 43, 44
Palladino (Paladino), Eusapia
    (1854-1918), 35
Palsy/experimental palsy, 148-149
Panama scandals (1892), 13
Paradoxical knee reflex of Benedikt, 243
Paranormal phenomena, 14, 34-36
Paraplegia, 157, 211, 212, 213, 218, 219,
    287, 289
Parinaud, Henri (1844-1905), 42, 124, 157
Paris, 3-4, 10, 13, 18-21, 47-50, 56, 57, 58,
    61-65, 68-74, 77-79, 159, 163, 285,
    325, 346, 349, 361, 362
  Babinski's preference for, 26-27, 75-76
  "Bloody Week" in, 5-6
  center of medical science, 354-355
  French Congress of Surgery held in, 266
  Haussmann's transformation of, 86n.4
  home to scientific associations/publica-
    tions, 178, 179, 189-190, 197, 250,
    289, 337-338, 348, 350
  hospital districts of, 154-155, 332, 363
  Right Bank society of, 86
  scientific publication/papers from, 7-8,
    192-193, 195, 250
  streets named for physicians, 358-360
Paris Commune, viii, 5, 12, 38, 47, 61-65
Paris hospital system/Parisian hospital
    system, 10, 85, 92n.21, 93, 97, 113,
    375 See also hospital system
Paris Medical School, 136-140, 159
Paris Opéra, vi, 8, 20n.19, 39, 40, 48, 49
Parkinson's disease, 11, 20, 27, 50, 65,
    285, 331
Parmentier, 130n.28
Partial clonus See spinal epilepsy
"Partially disabled", 293-294
The Pasteur Institute, 12, 18, 37, 38, 57
Pasteur, Louis (1822-1895), 6, 12, 18, 37
  microorganisms and process
    of fermentation, 6
Pathological anatomy, 7, 87, 93-94, 158,
    176, 189, 272, 321, 326, 333
  Babinski's involvement in, 10-11,
    121, 133-149, 187, 188, 190, 200,
    325, 361
  chair of pathological anatomy at Paris
    Medical School, 136-140

Cornil's contribution to study of,
    136-137
Patient treatment, viii, 283
Paul, Constantin (1833-1896), 116, *120*
  invented the flexible stethoscope, 116
Paul-Brousse regional hospital, 332
Pavlov, Ivan P. (1849-1936), 18, 343
  conditioned reflexes, 18
Pechkranc, Stanislaw (1865-1921),
    202n.70
Pechkranc-Babinski-Frölich syndrome,
    202n.70
Pérec, Georges (1936-1982), 352
Père-Lachaise cemetery, 80
Periaxial diffuse encephalitis
    (Shilder disease), 60
Periaxile nevritis, 30
Périer, Charles (1836-1914), 121-124, 359
Peripheral facial palsy, 235
Peripheral motor neuron dysfunction, 234
Peripheral nervous system/peripheral
    nerves, 210, 236, 280-282, 290
Peripheral neuritis, 107, 191
Peripheral neuropathies, 227
Perron, Charles (1862-1934), 61n.40
Peruvian Geographical Society, 62n.40
Pétain, Philippe (1856-1951), 47, 164
Peter Bent Brigham Hospital, 342
Petri, Julius Richard (1852-1921), 140
Philippe, Claude (1865-1903), 330, 331
Physical Therapy Institute, Grenoble, 291
Physiopathic disorders, 28, 188, 214,
    307-308, 310
Picard, Émile (1856-1941), 16, 36, 85, 91
  Traité d'analyse, 91
Picasso, Pablo (1881-1973), 19
Pick, Arnold (1851-1924), 342
Pierre Marie disease See acromegaly
    (Pierre Marie disease)
Pierret, 130n.28
Pinel, Philippe (1845-1926), 358
Piotrowsk phenomenon, 229
Pithiatism, ix, 16, 27, 176, 188, 210, 213,
    297-319, 330
  Joseph's departure from Charcot's
    conceptions, 306-314
  present theories of hysteria, 318-320
  See also hysteria

Pitres, Albert (1848–1928), 127, 128, 130n.28, 194, 311, 337
Pityriasis versicolor, 142
Plan Langevin-Wallon, 145
Plateau, Marius (1886–1923), 36
   L'Action Française, 36
Pleurésies, 119, 157
Plichet, André (1888–1965), 96, 169, 177, 178, 195, 363
   joint recipient of Babinski Foundation Prize, 177, 195
   Tryptique (journal), 178
Pneumonias, 103, 157
Podkolinski, Félix, 183
Poirier, Paul (1857–1907), 267
   book on cranioencephalic topography (1891), 267
Poland, 3–4, 28, 39, 47, 62, 53–54, 59, 60, 62, 65, 68, 78–79, 82, 124, 346, 349
   Babinski's attachment to, 55, 80, 357, 361, 363
   street signs in, 358–360
Polish School (Paris), 4, 77–78
Porte d'Aubervilliers Hospital, 10, 152
Potain, Carl Edouard (1825–1901), 87, 93–94, 106, 107
Pott's disease, 289
Pozerski, Edouard, 57, 78, See also de Pomiane
Presse Médicale (journal), 128n.21, 178, 195
Private practice, 25, 86, 97–98, 113–114, 162–165, 279
Proust, Marcel (1871–1922), 20, 164
   À la recherche du temps perdu (Remembrance of things past), 20
Provisional resident (*interne provisoire*), 116–119, 167
Pseudo-sciatica, 234
Pseudo-tabes, 198, 212
Psst (anti-Semitic journal), 29n.29
Psychiatry, 16, 92n.21, 168, 228, 236, 294, 337, 341–342
   André Breton's relationship with, 45
   Legrand du Saulle's publications on, 119
   Raymond Cestan, 176
   Georges Heuyer and child psychiatry, 182
   impact of war, 309
   hysterical symptoms, 312–313, 317–318
   Freud's work, 317
Psychological Bulletin, 16
Psychological mechanisms, 206, 316
Psychophysiology, 94
Pupillary reflex/pupillary light reflex, 168, 211, 214
Pupillary semiology, 196
Purves Stewart, Sir James (1869–1949), 272
Pussep, Ludwig Martynovich (1875–1942), 266
Putman, James G. (1846–1918), 342
Pycocyanic infection, 191
Pyramidal tract, 221, 225, 228, 230, 235

Queen's Square hammer, 240
Quincke, Heinrich Irenaeus (1842–1922), 268
Quinquaud, Charles-Eugène (1841–1894), 106
Quinze-Vingts Hospital, 157

Rabiner, Abraham (1892–1986), 30, 240
   Babinski-Rabiner hammer, 240
Radiologues des hôpitaux, 158
Radiology, 105, 158
Radiotherapy, 158, 214, 289–290
Raffaello, Sanzio (Raphael) (1483–1520), 222
Ramsay Hunt, James (1874–1937), 342
   dentorubroatrophy (1921), 249
Ranvier, Louis (1835–1922), 87, 93, 101, 133, 135, 136, 141–144, 356
   Archives d'anatomie microscopique (co-founder), (1897), 142
   Traité d'histologie pathologique (co-editor), 330
   Manuel d'histologie pathologique (co-author), 142
Rationalism, 14, 19
Ravaut, Paul (1872–1934), 201, 286
Rayer, Pierre (1793–1867), 189
Raymond, Fulgence (1844–1910), 12
Raymond-Cestan syndrome (tumor of the peduncles), 176
Raynaud, Maurice (1834–1881), 355
Réaction de Bordet-Wassermann (BW), 197

Reflex hammer, 30, 237, 238–240
Reflexes, ix, 217–234
  defense reflexes, 245–248
  tendon and bone, 236–244
  See also Babinski reflex; Babinski sign; big toe extension; toe phenomenon
Rehabilitation of handicapped, 290–292
Renan, Ernest (1823–1892), 40
Renaut, Louis (1844–1917), 143
Renoir, Auguste (1841–1919), 14
Residency Gold medal competitive examination, 100–101
Réunion Neurologique Internationale (1924), 30
Revista de neuropsiquiatria (journal), 356
Revue d'Oto-neuro-ophtalmologie, 176
Revue de Médecine (journal), 195
Revue Neurologique (journal), 12, 16, 24, 188, 197
Rhizomelic spondylosis, 326
Ribot, Théodule (1839–1916), 313
Riboulet, Pierre (1928–2003), 360
Richardière, Henri, 101, 110
Richer, Paul (1849–1933), 12, 122, 127, 128, 130nn.28, 30, 193, 194
  La nouvelle iconographie de la Salpêtrière, 12
Richet, Charles (1850–1935), 18, 35n.54, 47n.54, 363
  Traité de métapsychique, 35n.54
  work on anaphylaxis, 35
Riddoch, Georges (1888–1947), 272
Rietsch, Maximilien, 140
Rimbaud, Arthur (1854–1991), 5
Rist, Edouard (1871–1956), 168
Rivet, Lucien (1878–1968), 113, 167
Rivoire, André (1872–1930), 87
Robin, Charles (1821–1885), 24, 37, 38, 128, 135, 141, 142, 154n.5, 358
Robineau, Maurice (1870–1950), 272
  pioneer for trigeminal retrogasserian neurotomy, 273
Roch, Maurice (1878–1967), 230
Rochon-Duvigneaud, André (1863–1952), 193n.28
Roentgen, Wilhelm (1845–1923), 12, 266
  discovery of X-rays, 12

Roger, G.H. (1860–1946), 90, 182n.38, 226, 346
Romberg, Moritz Heinrich (1795–1873), 7
  tabes dorsalis lesions on dorsal columns of spinal cord, 7
Rosenblum, Sophie, 59, 168
Rossolimo sign, 228
Rossolimo, Grigorii Ivanovich (1860–1928), 216–217
  anal reflex, 217
Rothmann, Max. (1868–1915), 254
Roussy, Gustave (1874–1948), 24, 86n.4, 136, 332
Roux, Émile (1853–1933), 18
Royal Society of Medicine (London), 16, 350
Rubens, Peter Paul (1577–1640), 222
Ruault, Albert (1850–1928), 193n.28
Russell, J. S. R. (1863–1939), 250
Russian Military Medical Academy, 266

Sabouraud, Raimond (1864–1938), 87
Saint-Antoine Hospital, 92, 116, 121, 124
Saint-Louis Hospital, 87, 101, 121, 175, 199
Salary, 114, 128, 162–163
Salpêtrière Hospital, viii, ix, 7, 11, 59, 92, 110, 119, 143, 144, 152, 177, 185, *275, 276,* 331, 332, 360, *361*
  Babinski's tenure in, 188, 302, 321
  Chair for the Study of Diseases of the Nervous System at, 11–12
  Charcot as head of department in, 122, 124–132, 153–154, 325–326
  clinics devoted to functional recovery, 291
  Freud's visit to, 314–318
  quarrel on hysteria, 16
  second neurological department, 330
  specialized in neurology, 86
Salpêtrière school, viii, 110, 188, 256, 302, 305, 317
Sarcoidosis, 201
Scarlet fever, 103, 164
Schaefer, Georges (1882–?), 227
Schaefer sign, 227
Schaudinn, Fritz (1871–1906), 196
  discovery of *Treponema pallidum* (1905), 196

School of Fine Arts, 127
School of Pharmacy, Paris
Sciatica, 128, 197, 214, 234, 289, 302, 290
Sciences, 6–7, 115
Scientific journals, 7, 55, 187, 209, 355, 356
Scientific Society of Warsaw, 60
Scopolamine, 225, 284–285
Second Empire (of Napoléon III), 4
Sée, Germain (1818–1896), 106, 107, 109
   Médecine Moderne, 107, 109
Séglas, Jules (1856–1939), 86, 92
Seguin, Edward C. (1843–1898), 342
Semaine médicale, 102n.10, 195
Semiologie des affections du système nerveux, 237
Sémiologie du sommeil [Sleep semiology] (1934), 179n.26
Semiology, 133, 135, 159, 188–189, 195–196, 199, 210–211, 223, 236–237, 361–362
Semi-simulator, 308, 319
Sensory deficits, 205–206
Sergent, Emile (1867–1943), 162
Serodiagnosic technique, 90
Seventeenth International Congress (London), 16
Shaltenbrand, Georges (1897–1979), 31, 227
Sherrington, Sir Charles (1857–1952), 18, 353
Shilder disease (periaxial diffuse encephalitis), 60
Sicard, Jean-Athanase (1872–1929), 29, 183, 201, 272, 284, 331
Sicard-Forestier technique (spinal cord compression), 362
Sieur, Celestin (1860–1955), 274
Simon, Jules (1814–1896), 139
Simulation, 195, 306–307, 308–311, 319
Sismotherapy (electric shock treatment), 288 *See also* electrotherapy
Skoda, Josef (1805–1881), 240
Skoda hammer, 238
Société anatomique de Paris, 10, 133–135, 140–149 *See also* Anatomical Society
Société de biologie, 10, 94, 148, 188, 189, 190, 218, 281

Société de médecine légale, 119
Société de Neurologie de Paris, 11, 16, 30, 31, 32, 58, 60, 95, 155, *163*, 177–178, 179, 182, 197, 275–276, 335n.35, 337–338, 346, 350–351
   Babinski Foundation Prize from, 177
   Babinski's bequest to, 195
   Babinski's presidential address at, 182
   commemoration of Vulpian centennial by, 194
   and military psychiatry, 309
   presentation of papers and discussion at, 197–199, 207, 271–272, 289, 311
   Revue Neurologique (official journal from 1899), 193, 326–327
Société de neurologie de Buenos-Aires, 350
Société de pédiatrie, 144
Société française d'ophtalmologie, 177
Société française de cardiologie, 93
Société française de neurologie, 263, 337, 352
Société internationale de cardiologie, 93
Société Mathématique de France, 62n.40
Société Médicale des Hôpitaux de Paris, 32, 188, 192, 197, 199, 238, 241, 293
Société médico-psychologique, 92, 119
Society for Polish Workers in France, 58n.30
Södebergh (Goteborg), 350
Sodium salicylate, 284–285, 289
Sorbonne university, 37, 59, 86n.4, 91, 131, 294
Souques, Achille (1860–1944), 127, 162, 189, 330
Sournia, Jean-Charles, 354
   L'histoire de la medicine et des médecins, 354
Spasmodic paralysis, 33
Spasmodic paraplegia, 157, 212, 213, 287
Spasmodic torticollis, 207, 212, 280, 290
Spiller, William J. (1863–1940), 342
Spillmann, Louis François (1975–1940), 106
Spinal cord compressions, 188, 213, 222, 272, 279, 362

Spinal cord tumors, 168, 196, 271, 273 See also intraspinal tumors; spinal tumors
Spinal epilepsy, 244–245
Spinal tumors, 271–273, 290 See also intraspinal tumors; spinal cord tumors
Spondylotic pseudo-tabes, 27
St. Joseph Hospital, 333
St. Petersburg Hospital, Russia, 124
Starr, Moses Allen (1854–1932), 266, 342
Stewart-Holmes maneuver (1904), 253
Stookey hammer, 240
Stransky sign, 232
Strasburg University, 58
Stravinsky, Igor (1882–1971), 20
  Sacre du Printemps, 20
Striate muscles, 192
Strikes, 4, 19
Strowski, F., 86
Strümpell, Adolph (1853–1925), 218
Strümpell phenomenon, 235n.88
Strümpell sign, 227
Strümpell-Lorrain disease, 218n.6
Strychnine poisoning, 219, 225
Suchard, Eugène (1852–1915), 86, 93
  pathological anatomy of leprosy, 93
Surrealism, 20, 46
Sydenham chorea, 285
Syphilis, 7, 18, 103, 164, 196–202, 331
  Babinski's papers on, 189
  Boisseau's thesis on, 175
  mercury treatment of, 285–286
  relationship with pupillary reflex, 168
  test for, 160
Syphilitic myelitis, 157
Szapiro method, 231

Tabes, 134, 157, 177, 191, 197, 198–200, 212, 236, 249, 241, 255, 285, 293
Tabes arthropathies, 169
Tabes dorsalis/tabes dorsalis lesions, 7
Taylor, Madison (1855–1931), 240
  "tomahawk reflex hammer", 240
Teissier, Pierre-Joseph (1851–1932), 90, 262
  Nouveau traité de médecine, 262
Tendon and bone reflexes, 236–243
Tenon Hospital, 89, 152, 360

Tenth International Medical Congress (Berlin, 1890), 266
Terrier, Félix (1837–1908), 267
Tetanus, 191, 284
Therapeutics, vii, 107n.18, 116, 151, 189, 210, 214, 283
Thermal asymmetry, 27
Thévenard diseases, 201
Thibierge, Georges (1856–1926), 154n.5, 193n.28
Thiers, Adolphe (1797–1877), 6
Thomas, André, 32, 86n.4, 158
Throckmorton sign, 231
Tinel, Jules (1879–1952), 31
Toe abduction, 224
Toe phenomenon, 10–11, 36, 188, 218–222
  See also Babinski sign; big toe extension
Tooth, Howard Henry (1856–1925), 276
Toulouse Lautrec, Henri de (1864–1901), 14
Tournay, Auguste (1878–1969), 28, 43, 50, 95, 112, 113, 157, 168, 169, 178, 179, 180, *181*, 195, 226, 238, 254, 330, 351
Toxins, 18, 207
Traité de chirurgie d'urgence (Treatise on surgical emergencies), 92
Traumatic hysteria, 301, 316
Travaux de Neurologie Chirurgicale (journal), 268
Treaty of Versailles, 54, 183
Trelles, Oscar (1904–1990), 355, 356n.49
  Revista de neuro-psiquiatria (founder), 365n.49
Trémolières, Fernand (1875–1958), 168
Tremor, 103, 157, 208, 262, 263
Treponema pallidum, 18, 196
Tribune Médicale, 110
Tripier, Raymond (1838–1916), 106
Trocmé, Francis, 168
Troemner, Ernest L. O., 240
Trophic disorders, 204, 306, 307, 311, 318
Trousseau, Armand (1856–1910), 116
Tryptique (journal), 178
Tuberculosis (the tubercle bacillus), 12, 136, 140, 157, 172, 196
  cholera vibrio, 12

Tuberculosis meningitis, 139
Turner, William Aldren (1864–1945), 250
22nd International Neurological Meeting (Paris, 1958), 263
XVIIth International Congress of Medicine (London, 1913), 317
Typhoid fever/typhoid, 25, 102

United States, vii, 7, 16, 35, 184, 202n.70, 229, 240, 266, 270, 272, 281, 338, 342, 349, 353
Universités populaires, 38
University of Paris, ix, 37, 93, 116, *117*, 124, 285
University of Warsaw, 16

Val-de-Grâce Hospital, 46
Van Bogaert, Ludo (1897–1989), 185, 343
Van Gehuchten, Arthur (1861–1914), 30, 223, 343, 353
Van Gijn, A., 226
Van Gogh, Vincent (1853–1890), 14
Vaquez, Henri (1860–1936), 9n.7, 16, 20, 23, 25, 26, 36, 49, 55n.8, 72, 80, 85, 86, 87, *88*, 92, 93, 112, 164, 165, 178, 203, 285, 358, 363
   Archives des Maladies du Coeur, des Vaisseaux et du Sang, 87
   polycythemia vera (later known as polyglobuly or Vaquez disease), 87
   Precis de therapeutique, 72, 285
Varicose veins., 157, 331
Variot, Gaston (1855–1930), 162
Vasomotor disorders/vasomotor disturbances, 204, 208, 220, 306, 307, 311, 318
Vasomotor nerves, 6
Vecqueret, Karol, 50
Verleugnung (*denial*), 206
Verneuil, Stanislas (1823–1895), 128, 141
Vernon hammer, 240
Versailles, 4, 54, 183
Vertebral reflexes, 243
Vertigo, 204, 214, 251, 258, 287, 347
   See also voltaic vertigo
Vestibular semiology, ix, 211, 258–261
Villaret, Maurice (1877–1946), 168, 182
Villey, R., 355

Histoire du diagnostic médical, 355
Vincent, Clovis (1879–1947), 18, 36, 55, 75, 95, 133, 157, 168, 180, 195, 258, 265, 269, 271, 274, *275*, 276, 278, 279, *281*, 282, 310, 332, 351, 362, 363
Virchow, Rudolph (1821–1902), 6, 140, 142
   Cellular Pathology, 6
Vires, 33
Visual anosognosia, 205
Vogt, Oskar (1870–1959), 74
Volitional equilibration, 27
Voltaic vertigo, 32, 158, 191, 249, 258–259, 261, 288 *See also* vertigo
Von Monakow, Constantin (1853–1930), 356
Vuillard, Edouard (1868–1940), 87
Vulpian, Alfred (1826–1887), 7, 9, 12, 24, 101, 113, 121–122, *123*, 133, 135, 136, 141, 158, 194, 244, 250, 282, 307, 330, 358
   chair of pathological anatomy, 136
   discovery of adrenaline (1856), 7
   experimental work in animals, 250
   studies on normal and pathological histology, 145

Wages, 12, 167 *See also* salary
Waliszewski, Ceslas (1852–1897), 74
Wallon, Henri (1879–1962), 144–145
   thesis on boisterous child, *l'enfant turbulent*, 144
Walshe, Sir Francis (1885–1973), 188n.4, 219, 224, 226, 352
Walther, 274
War pathology, 307, 328, 331
War surgery, 277
Warsaw, 47, 50, 53, 56, 68n.14, 59, 60, 61, 73, 81, 82, 353
Warsaw Neurological Society, 16
Warsaw School of Medicine, 16
Warsaw University, 55, 58, 61n.40
Wartenberg, Robert (1887–1956), 184, 222, 232
Wassermann test, 198
Wassermann, August Paul von (1866–1925), 197
   development of Wassermann

test/reaction 1906), 197, 198
Watts, James Winston (1904–1994), 184
Weill, G. A., 96
Weren, Henryeta (1819–1897) (mother), 3–6, 61, 65
Weren-Babinksa, Henryeta *See* Weren, Henryeta (1819–1897) (mother)
Wernicke, Karl (1848–1905), 205, 297, 326, 341
Westphal, Carl Friedrich Otto (1833–1890), 60, 160, 236, 341, 356
Westphal sign, 197, 198n.46, 236, 241
Widal, Fernand (1862–1929), 29, 85–86, 90, *91*, 92, 114, 168n.3, 201, 262, 331, 358, 363
  Nouveau traité de medicine, 262
  serodiagnosic technique, 90
Wilson's disease, 341
Wolinetz, E., 179

Wood, Horatio C. (1841–1920), 342
World Fair (1889), 13
World War I, 16, 20, 38, 53, 60, 124, 158, 176, 177, 183, 208, 229, 270, 277–280, 280
Wright, Orville (1871–1948), 75
Wright, Wilbur (1867–1912), 75
Wurtz, Robert, 110, 112

Yersin, Alexandre (1863–1943), 18
  discovery of plague bacillus, 18
Yoshimura, Kisaku (1879–1945), 229

Zacchariadès, 142
Zamoyski, Count Maurice, 58–59
Zola, Émile (1840–1902), 13, 37
Zurich Society of Psychiatry and Neurology, 358